INTEGRATED PHYSIOLOGY and PATHOPHYSIOLOGY

INTEGRATED PHYSIOLOGY and PATHOPHYSIOLOGY

Julian L. Seifter, MD

James G. Haidas Distinguished Chair in Medicine, Brigham
and Women's Hospital
Master Clinician Educator, Brigham and Women's Hospital
Associate Professor of Medicine
Harvard Medical School
Boston, MA, USA

Elisa C. Walsh, MD.

Instructor in Anesthesia
Department of Anesthesia, Critical Care and Pain Medicine
Massachusetts General Hospital
Boston, MA, USA

David E. Sloane, MD, EdM

Instructor in Medicine
Division of Allergy and Immunology
Brigham and Women's Hospital
Dana Farber Cancer Institute
West Roxbury VA Medical Center
Harvard Medical School
Boston, MA, USA

Artist, illustrator, or editorial assistant
(if to appear on the title page):

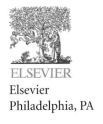

ELSEVIER
Elsevier
Philadelphia, PA

Elsevier
1600 John F. Kennedy Blvd.
Ste 1800
Philadelphia, PA 19103-2899

INTEGRATED PHYSIOLOGY AND PATHOPHYSIOLOGY,
Copyright © 2022 by Elsevier, Inc. All rights reserved.

ISBN: 978-0-323-59732-6

Notice

Library of Congress Control Number: 2021932143

Content Strategist: Elyse O'Grady
Content Development Specialist: Meghan B. Andress
Publishing Services Manager: Deepthi Unni
Project Manager: Radjan Lourde Selvanadin
Design Direction: Bridget Hoette

Printed in India

Last digit is the print number: 9   8   7   6   5   4   3   2   1

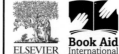

Working together
to grow libraries in
developing countries

www.elsevier.com • www.bookaid.org

To Betsy, Andrew, Ellie, and Lori,
and in Memory of Charles

Julian Seifter

With love and gratitude to
Marcia
Richard
Susan
Barry and Sandi
Tsila
Nesya, Avi, Moshe, Shalva, and Talya

And in loving memory of
Joe
Irv and Fay

לַכֹּל זְמָן וְעֵת לְכָל־חֵפֶץ תַּחַת הַשָּׁמָיִם:

A time for all, and a season for everything under the heavens.
(Ecclesiastes 3:1)

David Sloane

PREFACE

You probably suspect that knowing the basic concepts and selected details of human physiology is critically important. Not just for understanding the clinical manifestations of diseases, but for designing and monitoring rational treatment. By asking the question "What processes are at work to cause this patient's symptoms and signs?" you are already on the way to asking and answering the subsequent and related questions "What can we do to help this patient?" and "How can we know—what can we observe and what can we measure to determine—if treatment is working?"

But even more than this, a solid knowledge of physiology may help increase your powers of observation of patients. When you know physiology, you have a sense of what to look, listen, feel, and even smell for. Mastering physiology and thinking about it actively when you encounter a patient augments your consciousness and sharpens your perception. It makes you sensitive to important details and helps you distinguish between what to prioritize in the flow of data. It helps you think mechanistically and creatively, dynamically, and carefully.

This book can help you build that mastery of physiology. It cannot do everything for you—you will have to work at it and on yourself—because it is not an encyclopedia of physiology with every detail. Instead it has expanded bullet points with clear explanations describing medically relevant physiologic processes in health and disease.

Here are a few of the salient features of this text that are the result of pedagogic considerations.

Structure and Function: Most chapters start off reviewing the basic human body structures (from gross anatomy down to molecules) germane to the physiology. Structure and function are inextricably intertwined and reinforce each other. You need to know the basic composition and arrangement of the systems to understand dynamic processes, and learning those processes will help to organize and recall the structures because you know what they do.

Case studies: Case studies are narratives that help organize information in conceptual and realistic ways. They may not be studies of large populations in randomized controlled trials, but they are critical evidence that complement such studies. Cases can demonstrate the variety of disease phenotype among individuals.

Boxes: Often, the history of the understanding of a disease starts with observation of its character, then moves to treatment (sometimes discovered serendipitously), and only thereafter to investigating the basic mechanisms, as science fills in the gap between observation and treatment. The smallpox vaccine, for example, was developed well before the cellular and molecular mechanisms of immunology that reveal how that vaccine works were discovered. But for pedagogic purposes, we often present information in an order different from the historical record of observation, treatment, and molecular insight. Typically, there is a discussion of the genetic basis of a disease in a Genetics Box, then a description of how the disease arises in a Development

Box, and thereafter a consideration of the treatment of that disease in a Pharmacology Box. The focus of the text is always on the science and mechanisms of disease, not pathology or clinical pharmacology.

Clinical Correlation boxes focus on clinically relevant applications of physiology, while Fast Fact boxes highlight the selected facts that are useful to store in long-term memory so that when you are thinking analytically, you have them at the ready.

Themes: Several principles apply broadly to physiology and thus cross numerous organ systems. These are principles of nature that you must be able to see clearly in different contexts.

One of these themes is *dynamism*: physiology always suggests motion as critical to life. For anything to happen in the body, there must be forces at work. All physiologic phenomena, from moving blood to moving ions, depend on gradients of pressure or concentration, gravitational force, and electrical force. Part of mastering physiology means looking for a driving force, seeking a reason for things to move. Why and how (mechanistically) do things happen in the body? Ohm's law, for example, is one of many important force-flow relationships. We are talking about energy, and how pressure gradients drive fluid flow and how voltage gradients drive current.

A second theme is *homeostasis*: there are several forms of this, and they work on different levels of resolution from the molecular up to the whole human organism. Negative feedback systems maintain physiologic variables like pH, body temperature, and the extracellular concentration of potassium within a range of utility. Positive feedback mechanisms result in explosive phenomena, such as operate in malignancies. Other systems are "feed forward" or anticipatory.

None of these systems is dichotomous—rather, physiologic processes work on a continuum by gradations. We often tell students "Most of the time, you are better off answering a question with a range rather than a number." There are two such ranges. One is the range of values found in a population of healthy individuals. The second is the range of values that a variable can take in a given individual based on perturbations from a homeostatic set point and physiologic compensatory mechanisms.

For example, there is no single normal value for the serum sodium, but there is a range of, for example, 136 to 143 mEq/L in a given laboratory, and within a given person, the variability is generally tighter, such as less than 5%. Physiologic ranges are determined by measuring the given variable in a large number of healthy volunteers, determining the mean and the standard deviation, and then defining the lower limit of the range as the mean minus two standard deviations and the upper limit of the range as the mean plus two standard deviations.

Just because something is found to be statistically significant does not indicate its physiologic importance. Only experience can tell us that. For example, if the thyroid stimulating hormone (TSH) is slightly elevated or the platelet count is mildly low, that does not mean that the patient necessarily has a disease.

But the inverse is true as well—just because a lab value is within the range does not mean that there is not a significant pathologic process at work. For example, a patient in respiratory distress from a severe asthma attack may have a partial pressure of carbon dioxide within the normal physiologic range when measured on an arterial blood gas, but given the context of the asthma exacerbation, this normal value is actually an ominous sign that the patient is starting to tire and may die. Because there are multiple influences on many physiologic variables, you have to think about the context in which a given finding is present to determine its meaning.

Two key parts of thinking globally about homeostasis are considering: (1) flows into and out of the body, and (2) multiple overlapping regulatory systems. Examples of the former include the daily intake and output of sodium and water. An example of the latter is the sometimes additive and sometimes antagonistic activities of various mediators, metabolites, hormones, and neurotransmitters in the control of vascular tone.

Vasoconstrictors and vasodilators may be at work simultaneously to provide fine control. In addition, a given mediator or substance, such as adenosine or oxygen, can have counterintuitive effects, such as vasoconstriction or vasodilation, depending on the location and the context in which it operates. This can be caused by different receptors for a given mediator or the effects of other influences such as medications. A patient with anaphylaxis who takes a beta adrenergic blocker (which works through cyclic adenosine monophosphate [cAMP]) may not respond to the adrenergic receptor agonist epinephrine, but can be treated with glucagon, which generates cAMP via a distinct glucagon receptor. This text does not cover pathophysiology exhaustively, but emphasizes the mechanisms of disease states as they are are grounded in the basic physiology.

We hope that this text will be a helpful contribution to your growth in thinking critically about physiology.

JS
EW
DS

ACKNOWLEDGEMENTS

We had critical assistance and invaluable expertise from many at Elsevier.

Elyse O'Grady, content strategist par excellence, oversaw the project with grace, kindness, and patient persistence. While she maintained a broad view of the project, that did not prevent her from working on specific details, especially regarding clear figures. We want to acknowledge the contributions of authors of other textbooks published by Elsevier.

Megan Andress and Kathleen Nahm were content development specialists who did the critical work of gently reminding us of deadlines and coordinating with other staff at Elsevier once drafts were submitted.

Radjan Lourde Selvanadin was the project manager who ferried drafts to proofs and tirelessly inquired into and corrected details.

Most importantly, we are indebted to the too numerous to count medical and dental students who asked questions and motivated us to think broadly and deeply about physiology, explain it lucidly, and link it meaningfully to clinically relevant pathophysiology.

CONTRIBUTORS

The precursor to this text was co-authored and co-edited with Austin Ratner, MD, and his positive influence on the organization, writing, and thinking behind the present book endures. An earlier version of the revised manuscript benefited from important contributions from four students at Harvard Medical School who deserve special thanks. Jasmine Thumb edited the neurology material, clarifying and adding new sections. Caleb Yeung edited the skeletal muscle chapter. Helen Xu edited the renal section. Dmitriy Timerman reviewed multiple chapters including those in the cardiac and pulmonary sections. While the text underwent major changes since their contributions, their hard work catalyzed that transformation, for which we are grateful.

CONTENTS

Foundations

General Principles of Physiology

FOUNDATIONS OF HOMEOSTASIS

Life functions (e.g., growth and development, reproduction, breathing, cognition, movement, self-defense, and responses to environmental stress) require either the input of energy into the body or the transformation of energy from one form to a more useful form by the body. For anything to happen in an organism, there must be a force, an energy, or work in the form of some gradient—chemical, mechanical, or electrical. The human body is not at equilibrium with the environment, although conditions may be fairly constant, in which the body is in or near a steady state.

The important physiologic force-flow relationships relate "intensive" and "extensive" properties of state. These are called conjugate properties.

- Intensive properties have to do with each part of a system at large and are not additive. Chemical potential, electrical potential, temperature, and pressure are intensive properties of a system.
- Extensive properties, such as mass, moles, volume, charge, and entropy are additive.

For example, all the moles (extensive) of a part of a solution add up to the total moles of substance, whereas the concentration (intensive) in each part of a solution is not additive. The concentration of salt in the harbor is the same at high and low tide, but the volume and the moles of (sodium) Na^+ are different: There is a greater volume of solution and greater mass of Na^+ at high tide. But the stable concentration, the ratio of moles to volume, exemplifies that the quotient of two extensive properties (solution volume and Na^+ mass in this example) is the conjugate intensive property (concentration).

The difference of an intensive property at two points of a system is the "driving force" for the conjugate extensive property:

- Electrical gradients (intensive) drive flow of charge (extensive).
- Pressure gradients (intensive) drive flow of volume (extensive).
- Chemical gradients (intensive) drive flow of moles (extensive).

This chapter provides an overview of homeostasis, the tendency of the body's physiologic systems to maintain a relatively stable state and internal milieu despite changing external and internal environments by keeping physiologic variables within acceptable ranges. Some background information and appendices available on the companion website for this text provide detail on general properties of cell membranes, mechanisms by which solutes and water traverse membranes, membrane transport, mechanisms by which cells receive and respond to signals, and how cells in the body communicate with each other, all of which are means by which homeostasis occurs.

TRANSPORT PROCESSES IN LIFE

Dynamic processes govern the movement of fluids and gases within the body do not necessarily occur across cell membranes. The transport of fluids, such as blood and water like solutes, requires a driving force, such as a pressure gradient. The consequent movement depends on the nature of any barrier and the magnitude and direction of the pressure gradient.

- The heart is a pump that generates a pressure, driving blood through the circulation system, where the force is the hydrostatic, (or in a moving fluid hydraulic) pressure gradient and the flow is blood flow.
- The flow of gases in the respiratory tree follows the same pressure gradient rules, but unlike liquids, gases are compressible fluids.

Fluids (liquids and gases) not only flow through tubes and across cell membranes, but they can leave the circulation by crossing capillary basement membranes into the extravascular space surrounding cells, joining the interstitial fluid.

CELL MEMBRANE STRUCTURE AND TRANSPORT FUNCTIONS

The contents of cells are sealed off from the extracellular environment by a lipid barrier called the plasma membrane that protects the cell's interior from the changing conditions of the extracellular environment and helps maintain the specific chemical milieu supporting intracellular metabolic processes. Additional background information about the structure and function of the plasma membrane can be found in the online appendix to this chapter.

TYPES OF MEMBRANE TRANSPORT

Because the plasma membrane is made up predominantly of hydrophobic (lipophilic) molecules, other hydrophobic molecules are able to enter or exit cells by dissolving into or through the membrane. Hydrophilic (lipophobic) molecules, however, must cross the plasma membrane through water-filled channels or via specific carrier proteins.

Transport Across the Plasma Membrane

Transport across the plasma membrane occurs by several mechanisms, including:

- Diffusion
- Osmosis
- Endocytosis
- Exocytosis
- Protein-mediated transport

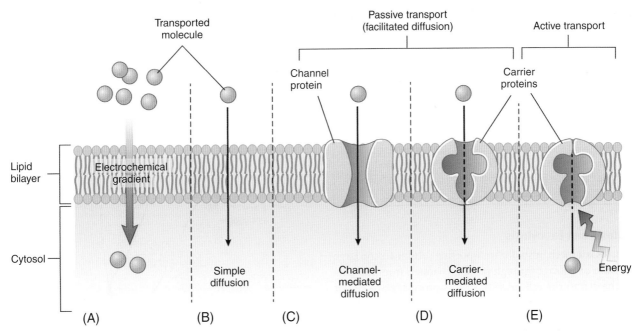

Fig. 1.1 The transport of solutes across the plasma membrane. A. An electrochemical gradient favors the movement of a solute from the extracellular to the intracellular space. B. If the solute is small and lipid-soluble, it may pass through the membrane via simple diffusion. C. The solute may require a channel protein to facilitate passive diffusion across the membrane. D. The facilitated diffusion may require a carrier protein to passively carry the solute down its gradient. E. In active transport, the carrier protein requires metabolic energy to fulfill its transport function because transport of the solute against its electrochemical gradient costs energy.

(Fig. 1.1). We would like to post appendices on the website for this text.

Diffusion and Osmosis

The diffusion of molecules across the plasma membrane is not carrier-mediated and does not require the expenditure of chemical energy directly produced by cells, but it depends on electrochemical gradients at adjacent points. Some solutes are permeable through plasma membranes or between cells and may therefore diffuse across the barrier. One such form of diffusion is nonionic diffusion, in which a small electroneutral molecule crosses the cell membrane.

The magnitude and direction of solute diffusion across cell membranes are described quantitatively by Fick's law of diffusion:

$$J = P \times A \times (C_1 - C_2)$$

where:
- J represents the net rate of diffusion of a solute from compartment 1 into compartment 2. As there may simultaneously be transport from compartment 2 to compartment 1, the meaning of net transport is that the sign of the next transports is determined by which direction (C_1 to C_2 or C_2 to C_1) dominates. When they are equal, this is called "steady state." As it describes the movement of material across a membrane per unit time, it has units such as $\frac{moles}{seconds}$;
- P is the permeability coefficient of the barrier separating the two compartments and is proportional (inversely) to molecular size and (directly) to mobility of the solute molecule in the medium (diffusivity) and inversely related to the thickness of the membrane and the viscosity of the medium. It has units such as $\frac{micrometers}{seconds}$ and so resembles a velocity;
- A denotes the surface area for diffusion in units, such as m²; and
- C_1 and C_2 represent the respective concentrations of the molecule across the permeability barrier in typical concentration units of mass per unit volume, such as $\frac{moles}{m^3}$.

Thus small, uncharged molecules diffuse easily across a large surface area with a steep concentration gradient (i.e., P, A, and ($C_1 - C_2$) are all large), whereas large or highly charged molecules will not diffuse easily and will require protein-mediated transport to cross the membrane. A small surface area (A) or small concentration gradient ($C_1 - C_2$) will likewise limit the rate of diffusion. When solutes are charged, the determination of gradients is more complicated because one must account for charge differences, or voltage, across the membrane.

Osmosis is the diffusion of water across a semipermeable membrane from a solution of low solute concentration (which thus can be thought of as a solution of high water concentration) to one of higher solute concentration (and thus lower water concentration). The concentration of "free" water molecules is greater in a solution with a lower solute concentration because less water is occupied in charge interactions with the solute. The increased amount of free water molecules on one side of a membrane drives the diffusion of water from low solute concentration to high. Like diffusion, osmosis does not require energy expenditure by cells (see Clinical Correlation Box 1.1).

Endocytosis and Exocytosis

Endocytosis is a mechanism for transporting substances too large for diffusion or passage through protein channels from the outside of the cell to the cell interior. In this process, extracellular material is brought into the cell without actually passing through the lipid bilayer (Fig. 1.2), as the material is surrounded by the plasma membrane and enclosed within a small sphere of bilayer that pinches off the cell membrane. This envelope derived from the membrane is called a vesicle. Vesicles can move within the cytoplasm, and their contents are still extracellular, topologically speaking. Endocytosis, an energy-dependent process, has other names depending on the material taken up.

- It is called phagocytosis when particulate matter enters the cell.
- It is called pinocytosis when soluble small molecules in a volume of fluid enter.
- It is called receptor-mediated endocytosis when specific extracellular molecules are bound to integral proteins before being endocytosed.

Exocytosis is the opposite process, whereby intracellular material in a vesicle is expelled from the cell when the vesicle fuses with the plasma membrane. Like endocytosis, exocytosis requires energy. Endocytosis and exocytosis also allow the shuttling of receptors or transporters from the plasma membrane to an intracellular compartment, not for catabolism as in Figure 1.2, but to regulate the insertion or removal of the receptor, channel, or transporter in the plasma membrane in the appropriate circumstances.

An example of reversible vesicle movement is the addition and removal of aquaporins, water channels, to the plasma membrane of renal collecting duct cells under the control of antidiuretic hormone (ADH, also called vasopressin). When ADH concentrations increase, this hormone stimulates the fusion of collecting duct intracellular vesicles with embedded transmembrane aquaporins with the cell membrane, thus adding the water channels and increasing the resorption of free water from the urine into the blood. When ADH concentrations decrease, the opposite occurs: The plasma membrane vesicles pinch off and move into the cytoplasm, removing the aquaporins. See the renal section, Chapter 18, for additional information.

Facilitated Diffusion and Active Transport

An unequal distribution of a charged substance on the two sides of the cell membrane will cause a chemical gradient and an electrical gradient to coexist as an electrochemical gradient.

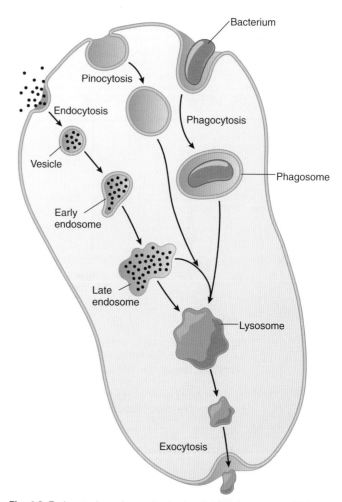

Fig. 1.2 Endocytosis and exocytosis. A cell can take up material by enclosing it in an envelope of lipid bilayer that pinches off of the plasma membrane. When the engulfed material is solid, the process is called phagocytosis. When the enveloped material is mostly liquid, the process is called pinocytosis. Because the substances remain inside membrane-enclosed spheres called vesicles, they are topologically still "outside" the cell. After being metabolized, the cell can extrude waste materials by fusing the vesicle back to the plasma membrane. This process of exocytosis is the reverse of endocytosis. It is used by the cell to export important products made intracellularly into the extracellular environment.

Sometimes cells need to take up ions or molecules from the extracellular space into the cytoplasm or move intracellular substances out of the cell against forces that oppose such transport. This occurs:

1. When a molecule is too large or too hydrophilic to diffuse freely through the plasma membrane, even if a concentration gradient favors the movement; and
2. When the cell needs to transport a substance "up" a chemical, electrical, or electrochemical gradient.

By "up" a gradient we mean a process that leads to a decrease in entropy and a corresponding positive change in Gibbs free energy, while by "down" a gradient we mean a process that leads to an increase in entropy and a corresponding negative change in Gibbs free energy. The latter reactions may proceed spontaneously, but the former do not and always require an input of energy. When the Gibbs free energy is 0, that state is equilibrium.

This is the same idea as chemical reactions: those that require energy to proceed "up" a gradient or against forces are termed endergonic, while those that proceed "down" a gradient or with forces are exergonic. Most exergonic reactions in biological systems are exothermic, such as the cleavage of ATP by ATPases in muscle mitochondria. Movement against opposing forces occurs by specific protein transporters (carriers or channels) embedded in the cell membrane. These proteins are carriers for facilitated diffusion (situation 1) or active transporters (situation 2), depending on whether they move molecules down or up an electrochemical gradient, respectively.

Facilitated diffusion is the movement of a substance that cannot freely cross the membrane down an electrochemical gradient. Such a process does not require metabolic energy because it works "downhill," much like simple diffusion, except that the net flux of molecules is much greater because of facilitation by the protein carrier or channel (Fig. 1.3):

- The insulin-dependent glucose transporter allows plasma glucose to enter cells via facilitated diffusion.
- Various ion-specific channels for Na^+, potassium (K^+), chloride (Cl^-), and other species participate in facilitated diffusion because they allow ion entry into cells only in the presence of a favorable "downhill" electrochemical gradient. Many ion channels are gated, meaning that they alternate between an open and a closed conformation, depending on the presence of an "opening" stimulus (Fig. 1.4).
  - Ion channels that open in response to an extracellular hormone are termed ligand-gated ion channels. For example, the nicotinic acetylcholine receptor, nAChR, is a ligand-gated Na^+ channel triggered by acetylcholine at the synaptic cleft.
  - Some ion channels open when the resting membrane electrical potential of the plasma membrane reverses, a process known as depolarization. Such channels are called voltage-gated ion channels.

- A mechanical-gated channel opens under the influence of hydrostatic or osmotic pressure (see Fig. 1.4).

Active transport requires energy and is either primary or secondary, depending on the source of the energy used.
- Primary active transporters use adenosine triphosphate (ATP) directly to carry specific ions against an electrochemical gradient.
  - The ubiquitous Na^+,K^+-ATPase, is a protein pump that transports both Na^+ and K^+ against their respective electrochemical gradients (Fig. 1.5). By simultaneously transporting three Na^+ ions out of the cell and two K^+ ions in, the Na^+,K^+-ATPase (also called "the Na^+,K^+ pump") maintains high extracellular and low intracellular Na^+ concentrations and high intracellular and low extracellular K^+ concentrations. The activity of this pump is increased by intracellular Na^+ and by extracellular K^+. Each transport cycle of the Na^+,K^+ pump results in the net loss of a cation from the intracellular compartment. The establishment and maintenance of such ion gradients are responsible for the resting membrane electrical potential discussed in Chapter 2.
  - Other active transporters are the Ca^{2+}-ATPases in the sarcoplasmic reticulum, renal tubules, intestine, and cardiac muscle. They sequester cytosolic Ca^{2+} within the sarcoplasmic reticulum or transport Ca^{2+} against an electrochemical gradient out of the cell.
  - The H^+/K^+-ATPase, located on the lumenal surface of gastric parietal cells, pumps hydrogen (H^+) against an unfavorable electrochemical gradient into the lumen of the stomach, acidifying gastric contents.

Secondary active transport involves a pump like the Na^+,K^+-ATPase and a cotransporter. First, the pump establishes a Na^+ gradient. Then, the Na^+ diffuses down its concentration gradient across the cotransporter into the cell. The cotransporter couples this movement of Na^+ to the movement of another

Fig. 1.3 Facilitated diffusion. A. Solute S has an electrochemical gradient favoring movement into the cell, but it is unable to cross the plasma membrane via simple diffusion either because S is too large or too hydrophilic to cross the membrane. It enters via facilitated diffusion with the help of a carrier protein in an energy-free manner. B. Solute S enters by facilitated diffusion with the help of a carrier protein without additional energy expenditure. In the model shown, the carrier can exist in two conformational states: state 1, in which solute S binds to the protein on the outside, and state 2, in which the solute diffuses into the cell. This arrangement is known as a "ping-pong" mechanism. The initial rate of transport rate occurs when the concentration of S inside the cell is zero and the solute is only present extracellularly. In this situation, transports can only occur in one direction (into the cell). Once enough solute S crosses into the intracellular compartment, the electrochemical gradient decreases and the same transporter may facilitate the movement of S out of the cell. This is known as bidirectional transport. Depending on which direction dominates determines the net transport. When the inward and outward movements of S are equal the system reaches steady state.

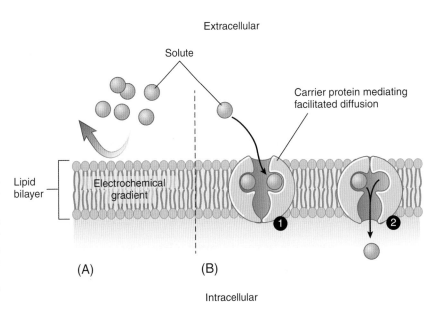

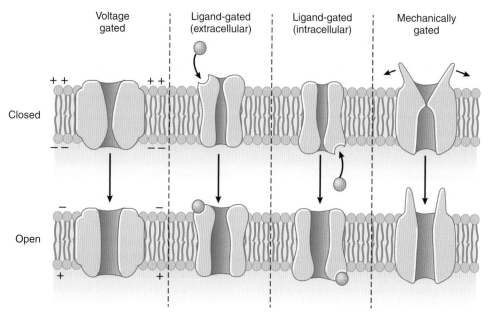

Fig. 1.4 Gated membrane protein channels. A gated channel is one that alternates between a closed state, which does not allow solutes to go down their electrochemical gradient, and an open state, which does. Such channels may be opened in response to changes in the membrane electrical potential (voltage-gated), the presence of an extracellular or intracellular ligand-gated, or the application of a mechanical force such as stretch or pressure (mechanically-gated).

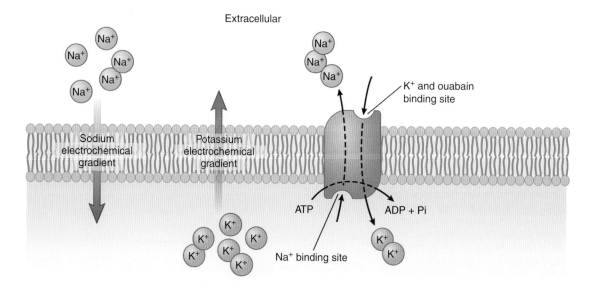

Fig. 1.5 The Na^+,K^+-ATPase active transporter. Na^+ has an electrochemical gradient favoring movement into the cell, whereas K^+ has a gradient favoring movement out of the cell. The Na^+,K^+-ATPase creates and maintains these gradients by moving Na^+ out of the cell and K^+ into the cell, against their respective gradients. Each iteration of the transporters moves three Na^+ out and two K^+ in and uses one molecule of ATP as the energy source. Each iteration contributes to the resting membrane potential because more positive charges move out of the cell than in, so the cell interior is relatively negative compared with the extracellular space. Such a transporter is electrogenic. Since ATP production is much greater with aerobic respiration in mitochondria, these organelles often accumulate near the plasma membrane and the function of the Na^+,K^+-ATPase is sensitive to the need for oxygen. *ATPase*, Adenosine triphosphatase; *K^+*, potassium; *Na^+*, sodium.

solute into the cell. ATP is used indirectly, in that transmembrane gradients created by primary active transporters (e.g., the Na^+,K^+-ATPase) are used to drive the transport of other solutes against unfavorable concentration or electrochemical gradients.

- When a secondary active transporter moves two solutes in the same direction, it is called a symporter (Fig. 1.6). Examples of symporters are:
  - The Na^+-K^+-$2Cl^-$ cotransporter found in the ascending limb of the renal tubule.
  - Sodium-glucose transport protein (SGLT)-2 is a facilitated diffusion transporter in proximal tubule cells of the nephron that links the resorption of filtered glucose to the resorption of Na^+. Inhibitors of this symporter constitute an important class of drugs to treat diabetes mellitus.
  - The Na^+-glucose cotransporter in the intestinal mucosa.
  - The Na^+-amino acid cotransporter in the proximal renal tubule.
- An antiporter transports two solutes in opposite directions across the cell membrane (see Fig. 1.6).
  - The Ca^{2+}/Na^+ antiporter found in cardiac muscle uses the Na^+ gradient created by the Na^+,K^+-ATPase to drive intracellular Ca^{2+} out of cells against its electrochemical gradient. Note that calcium has $2+$ charges and sodium just $1+$. Unless two Na^+ ions were transported, the transporter would carry a net $1+$ charge and would be "electrogenic".
  - The electroneutral Cl^-/bicarbonate (HCO_3^-) antiporter prevents the cytosol from becoming too basic during

intracellular accumulations of HCO_3^- by extruding intracellular HCO_3^- and taking up Cl^- in exchange.

A carrier that transports Na^+ coupled to a neutral solute, such as D-glucose, enables glucose to be transported in a 1:1 ratio with Na^+. Because cells almost always have a large and inwardly-directed Na^+ gradient (i.e., Na^+ in extracellular fluid is high and is kept low in the cell by the Na^+,K^+ pump) there is potential energy in the Na^+-gradient that is almost high enough to remove the full amount of glucose from the urinary or intestinal lumen where these transporters exist (SGLT 2) because the Na^+ concentration in the lumen is much greater than the glucose concentration.

Some coupled transporters have a stoichiometry different from 1:1. Consider the cotransport of Na^+ and HCO_3^- out of a cell. Because of the action of the electrogenic Na^+,K^+-ATPase that generates a relative negative charge in the interior of the cells, for Na^+, an electrochemical gradient opposes the movement of this ion out of the cell. For HCO_3^-, the chemical gradient opposes the movement of this ion out of the cell, but the electrical gradient favors it. The coupling of $1\ Na^+$ to $1\ HCO_3^-$ in a Na^+/HCO_3^- cotransporter would thus lack sufficient energy to extrude HCO_3^-. If, however, the transporter had the stoichiometry of coupling $1\ Na^+$:$3\ HCO_3^-$, then it would be electrogenic, carrying a net negative charge. Because the inside of the cell is negative, there can be an outwardly directed HCO_3^- gradient only if the magnitude of the electrical gradient exceeds the electrochemical gradient for Na^+ and the chemical gradient for HCO_3^-. Increasing the stoichiometry to $3HCO_3^-$:1

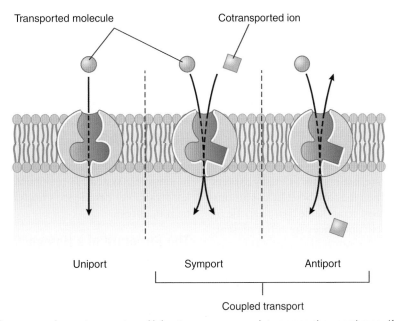

Uniport   Symport   Antiport

Coupled transport

Fig. 1.6 Plasma membrane transporters. Uniporters carry one solute across the membrane. If this movement is down the electrochemical gradient, it requires no added energy, but if it is against the gradient, energy must be spent. Cotransporters move more than one solute. Symporters carry two solutes in the same direction, while antiporters transfer them in opposite directions. If both solutes are moving down their respective gradients, no energy is needed. If one of the solutes is going down its gradient, it may supply enough energy to move the other against its gradient. If both solutes are transported against their gradients, energy is required.

Na^+ raises the driving force for extrusion of HCO_3^- to the third power, providing ample energy for such a transporter to extrude HCO_3^- and defend against cell alkalinization.

SIGNAL TRANSDUCTION

To harmonize and coordinate physiologic functions, organ systems, organs, tissues, and cells must communicate with each other. These integrated communication systems work on different scales or level of resolution. Among those on the smallest scale, as the cell membrane is a barrier not only to matter but to information, messages have to traverse it. Various signal transduction networks carry information from outside the cell to various receptors embedded in the cell membrane or present in the cytosol, by means of signaling molecules called ligands, and biochemical alterations in the cell occur in response to contact between receptors and their ligands. The complex biochemical chain reactions culminate in changes in cell function and gene expression.

CELL-CELL COMMUNICATION

On lager scales of resolution, cell-to-cell communication occurs when one or more cells send a signal to alter the function of a target cell.
- When the target cell is the same as the signaling cell, such communication is called autocrine.
- When the target cell is adjacent to the signaling cell, such communication is called juxtacrine.
- When the target cell is not adjacent but a relatively short distance away (a few cell radii) from the signaling cell, such communication is called paracrine.
- When the target cell is a relatively great distance away from the signaling cell, such communication is called endocrine and the signaling molecules are called hormones. The endocrine system is the network of hormone secreting tissues commonly referred to as "glands." See the endocrine section (see Chs. 28–36).

HOMEOSTASIS

"A fairly constant or steady state, maintained in many aspects of the bodily economy even when they are beset by conditions tending to disturb them, is a most remarkable characteristic of the living organism. Because circumstances are often present, which, if not controlled, would profoundly modify the constancy of the state, we must assume that controlling factors are at hand ready to act whenever the constancy is imperiled" (Walter B. Cannon, 1926).

Walter B. Cannon, the eminent American physiologist, first proposed the term homeostasis for the efforts of the body to maintain the values of physiologic variables within a given range. The term is an elision of the Greek homeo- meaning "same" and Latin -stasis meaning "standing." Homeostatic processes defend the body against the perturbing forces of the environment. If water is scarce, homeostasis conserves water to keep the amount of fluid in our bodies constant. If the environment is hot, homeostasis purges heat to maintain a constant body temperature.

When homeostatic processes are working properly, the body achieves a steady state, a condition in which the inputs of matter and energy to a system equal the outputs. Homeostasis maintains such a state over the long term but not necessarily from instant to instant. For example, ingestion of a large amount of water will temporarily expand the total body water. Within minutes to hours, however, homeostatic mechanisms will remove excess water through urination, restoring the steady state level of body water volume.

Although inputs of matter and energy equal outputs in a steady state, this does not mean the internal system is similar in content to the external environment, in which case there would be equilibrium. On the contrary, in a steady state the system maintains its differences from the environment. For example, in a healthy steady state, the dietary intake of potassium must equal the elimination of potassium to maintain a body fluid potassium concentration within strictly regulated limits. Similarly, the system is not internally uniform in a steady state. For example, most of the body's potassium is concentrated inside cells, while most of the body's sodium is concentrated outside cells. In a steady state, there are concentration gradients and there is flow through the system. Homeostasis not only controls matter and energy exchange with the outside environment, but it also preserves the concentration gradients and other polarities of the internal environment. In contrast to a steady state, equilibrium exists when there is no net flow. When conditions are globally uniform, there are no concentration or electrochemical gradients at all, and there is no net flow through the entire system; the condition we colloquially call death.

Explaining how the body's homeostatic mechanisms maintain a steady state is the aim of physiology. Pathophysiology is the study of how and why the body's homeostatic mechanisms fail, and what happens when they do.

AN ELECTROMECHANICAL EXAMPLE OF HOMEOSTASIS

Cruise control in an automobile is a nonbiologic example of a homeostatic system. It maintains a constant speed (the regulated variable) despite variations in the road (the environmental influences).

The Structure of a Homeostatic System

A simple homeostatic system consists of four components (Fig. 1.7):
- Sensor: This is the speedometer, which determines the speed of the car and relays the information to a computer elsewhere in the car.
- Control center: This is the car's onboard computer, which compares the input from the sensor (the speedometer) with the speed programmed for the cruise control (65 miles per hour [mph], for example). The computer then determines whether the car should speed up, slow down, or continue at its present speed.

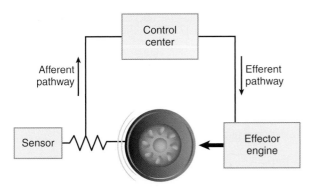

Fig. 1.7 The basic components of a homeostatic system. This simple model of a cruise control system has a sensor that detects the current speed of the car. The sensor sends this information via the afferent transmission pathway to the computer control center, where a comparison of the current speed is made with the set point. The control center makes a decision to increase, decrease, or maintain the speed. It sends a signal via the efferent transmission pathway to the effector engine to adjust the work it does to affect the speed appropriately.

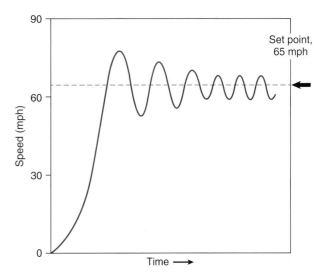

Fig. 1.8 Fluctuations of a variable around a set point. A homeostatic system, such as cruise control, increases the variable when it is under the set point and decreases it when it is above the set point. Depending on the gain of the system, the variable "floats" around the set point. Other stimuli may perturb the variable, necessitating further work by the homeostatic system to correct the perturbation.

- Effector: This is the engine, which translates the commands of the computer into action to alter the car's speed back toward the set point.
- Transmission pathways: This is the wiring in the car's electrical system. The speedometer sends information to the computer along an incoming or afferent pathway, and the computer sends information to the engine along an outgoing or efferent pathway.

These four basic components are found in biologic as well as nonbiologic control systems.

The Function of a Homeostatic System

Despite varying topography, a car's cruise control system constantly maintains the set speed. However, the car's speed is not always precisely 65 mph, for example; the cruise control system is always reacting to, rather than anticipating, outside conditions. Only a "perceived" decrease in speed by the speedometer can trigger the computer to rev up the engine. Therefore the car must already be climbing a hill, for example, and slowing down to a speed less than 65 mph before the car's computer "realizes" it should signal the engine to work harder. The more sensitive the system is to deviations from the set point, the higher the system's "gain." The higher your cruise control's gain, the less will be the variation from the set point speed of 65 mph.

Likewise, if the car starts down a hill and surpasses the set point speed, this information is relayed to the computer, causing the engine to perform less work and allowing the car to slow down back toward the set point of 65 mph. The result is that the speed of the car fluctuates around 65 mph. The amplitude and frequency of the fluctuations depend on both changing outside conditions and the system's gain (Fig. 1.8).

Feedback Systems

Fluctuations around a preset value are characteristic of homeostatic systems. A feedback system is one in which the system adjusts its activity by monitoring its own output. Feedback can be either negative or positive. Three types of systems—negative-feedback, positive-feedback, and feed-forward—contribute to human body homeostasis.

- A negative-feedback system responds to an altered output by restoring the variable toward a predetermined set point (Fig. 1.9). In the case of cruise control, an increase in speed slows down the engine, either by decreasing the flow of gas to the engine or by applying the brakes (or both). A decrease in speed prompts the computer to increase speed back toward the set point (65 mph) by augmenting effective engine activity, either by increasing the flow of gas to the engine or by decreasing the braking force (or both). Because negative-feedback systems check themselves, they are very stable and are crucial to the maintenance of homeostasis in the body, contributing to the control of various physiologic variables, such as blood pressure and the concentration of blood glucose. Some processes of feedback regulation are considered compensations. Examples of compensatory mechanisms include:
- Changes in respiratory or renal functions in response to a challenge in acid-base balance (see chapter 22 on Acid Base Balance).
- Thickening of the muscle of the left ventricle in response to hypertension to enable a greater force of contraction.
- Long-term adaptations in structure and function of cells and organs help maintain the normal steady state. In adaptation to the low inspired oxygen of high altitude, there is an increase in number of oxygen-carrying red blood cells in the circulation.
- A positive-feedback system responds to a disturbance in steady-state conditions by moving the variable farther away from the initial set point (Fig. 1.10):
- Population "explosion" exemplifies positive feedback. As the birth rate increases, there will be a larger population

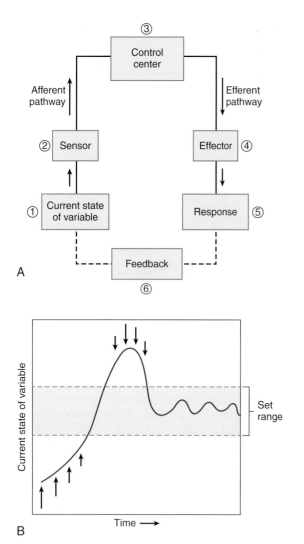

Fig. 1.9 A negative-feedback system. A. A model of the system. B. The system's function and the changes in the variable. The curve represents the value of the variable, and the *arrows* represent the work done by the homeostatic system to return the variable to the set range. The length of the arrow is proportional to the effort exerted or the work performed by the system.

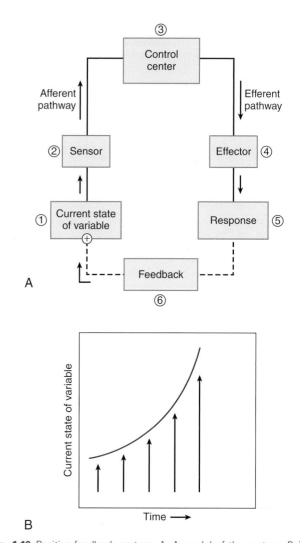

Fig. 1.10 Positive-feedback system. A. A model of the system. B. The system's function and the changes in the variable. In a positive feedback system, the response moves the variable farther away from the starting point.

and subsequently a greater birth rate—exactly the opposite behavior a negative-feedback system would exhibit.

- In economics, an example of positive-feedback systems would be increased prices leading to an increased cost of living, which would in turn promote increased wages, increased cost of production, and ultimately even higher prices.

The explosive behavior of positive-feedback systems makes them inherently unstable. While they are less common than negative-feedback systems in maintaining the steady state in the body, positive-feedback systems do play a role in human physiology.

- The opening of some voltage-gated cell membrane ion channels, leading to the initiation of an action potential in neurons, depends on a positive-feedback system. As the membrane potential increases from the resting potential, the channels open, allowing more positively charged ions to

enter the cell. This further increases the membrane potential, thereby triggering more channels to open (see Ch. 2).
- Such systems either possess an intrinsic mechanism or depend on a companion antagonistic system that limits or decreases the activity of the system and resets the physiologic variable to its original set point.
- Unlike feedback systems, a feed-forward system is proactive; it has a sensor that anticipates environmental changes and prompts the system to act before the alterations begin to affect it (Fig. 1.11). Consider a cruise control system linked to a global positioning system showing the topography of the road. Anticipating an uphill climb, for example, the computer would know to tell the engine to work harder before the topography changes. Thus the system could maintain its set point speed even before changing conditions perturb it. As an example of a physiologic feed-forward system, imagine yourself about to participate in the traditional Running of the Bulls event in Pamplona, Spain. As you anticipate the necessary exertion, your autonomic nervous system

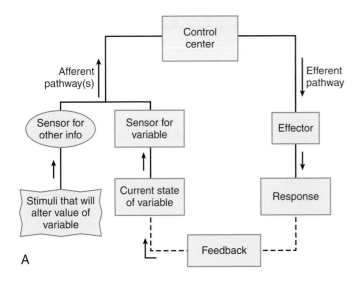

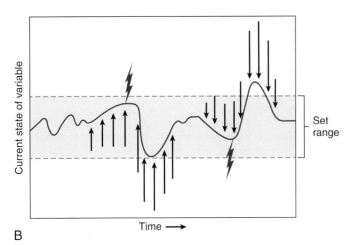

Fig. 1.11 A feed-forward system. A. The control center uses information beyond the current state of the variable and anticipates that the variable is going to be "pushed" from the set range by some stimulus. It therefore activates the compensatory mechanism(s) preemptively, so that the time and degree of perturbation of the variable may be limited. B. The curve shows that the system begins to adjust the variable before the stimuli (lightning bolts) affect the variable.

increases the strength and rate of contraction of your heart, providing increased cardiac output even before your leg muscles demand more oxygen-laden blood to fuel your dash to safety. The production of saliva in anticipation of a good meal (the so called "cephalic phase of digestion") is another example of a physiologic feed-forward system.

Fueling Homeostasis

In the presence of oxygen, the body typically converts chemical energy in ingested food into other forms of chemical energy, most importantly ATP. As long as it has an adequate stock of ATP, the body can convert this chemical energy into whatever form it needs to maintain homeostasis. For example, when body temperature drops, ATP in skeletal muscles fuels contraction, causing shivering, and the thermal energy released in the

process increases body temperature. The chemical energy of the body can be converted to mechanical, thermal, and electrical energies that support all biologic processes. Almost a quarter of the body's energy expenditure is devoted to keeping potassium inside cells and sodium outside cells.

Components of a Homeostatic System in the Body

In the body, receptors are the body's sensors that detect chemical, electrical, or mechanical changes. The body's transmission pathways include neural and vascular "highways," as well as the chemical transmitters or signaling molecules (neurotransmitters, hormones, metabolites) that carry information along the pathways. The body's control centers are the nervous system and endocrine system, which determine the body's responses to changes in its environments (external and internal). Its effectors are muscles, secretory tissues, and other end organs that ultimately produce the body's response to a given stimulus.

A major difference between many physiologic homeostatic systems and the electromechanical homeostatic systems exemplified by cruise control is that physiologic homeostatic systems often have a set range instead of a set point. This means that many physiologic variables do not have a single normal value but a normal range of values. For example, the normal range of serum potassium is 3.5 to 5.0 mmol/L.

Understanding each homeostatic mechanism in the body requires knowing the specific components of the particular system. What is the receptor, and to what is it responding? How is information transmitted from the receptor to the control center and from there to the effector? What is the effector, and how does it modulate one or more physiologic variable(s)? What is the body's response to its own modified function? Analyzing homeostatic mechanisms in a systematic way provides insight into the normal function of cells, tissues, organs, and organ systems in the body and into the causes and results of diseases.

PATHOPHYSIOLOGY

Physiologic homeostatic systems can fail to serve homeostasis in one or more of three ways: intrinsic defects, extrinsic defects, and deleterious long-term effects of acute compensatory changes.

With intrinsic defects, the system itself malfunctions. An intrinsic defect is an inherited or acquired dysfunction in any component of the system—sensor, transmission pathway, control center, or effector. This is the case in type I diabetes mellitus, in which the immune system destroys insulin-producing beta islet cells in the pancreas, leading to hyperglycemia (i.e., high blood glucose levels). This beta cell deficiency constitutes sensor, control center, and transmission pathways defects because pancreatic beta cells sense the plasma glucose concentration and respond by secreting insulin when the concentration is above the normal set range (see the Endocrine section). Patients with type 1 diabetes no longer have enough beta cells to produce an adequate supply of insulin to maintain glucose homeostasis. In type 2 diabetes mellitus, there is a peripheral tissue resistance to insulin action. Insulin may be secreted at increased amounts owing to hyperglycemia, but the end-organ effector sites cannot respond normally to the insulin (dysfunction in the effector tissues of the system).

With extrinsic defects, a homeostatic system responds in a normal manner but is responding to an abnormal stimulus, and in trying to "do its job" propagates a disease state. For example, a patient in congestive heart failure may have a cardiac left ventricle that can no longer pump blood effectively. This pump failure leads to a backup of blood in the lungs and a deficiency in perfusion (i.e., supply of blood) to peripheral tissues, including the kidneys. In response, the kidneys react as they do whenever they are inadequately perfused—they secrete the hormone renin, setting off a hormonal cascade (the renin-angiotensin-aldosterone axis) that ultimately causes increased salt (and water) reabsorption by the nephrons. The body thus holds on to more fluid. This response is expected from a normal, though underperfused, kidney. However, in this situation, the problem is not a deficiency in total body volume as might be seen in dehydration or hemorrhage. Rather, there is a loss of "effective circulating volume," leading the kidneys to respond as if there were insufficient total body volume. In conserving salt and water, the kidneys unwittingly worsen the problem, further overloading the heart, and the lungs are liable to "drown" from retention of even more fluid that cannot be pumped forward fast enough by the failing heart (see the Cardiovascular section). Here the kidney's homeostatic mechanisms are working properly, but their function exacerbates the situation for the damaged heart. There is an intrinsic defect of the heart and an extrinsic abnormality involving the kidney.

Deleterious long-term effects of acute compensatory changes result when the body's attempts to maintain homeostasis are initially helpful but ultimately counterproductive. This is the cost of running for a long time (chronically) a homeostatic mechanism intended for short-term (acute) use. Consider, again, a case of congestive heart failure because of left ventricular dysfunction. There is inadequate blood pressure to sufficiently perfuse peripheral tissues. The decrease in systemic blood pressure is sensed by the arterial baroceptors (See Clinical Correlation Box 1.2: Autonomic Control of Arterial Blood Pressure and the Cardiovascular section). These baroceptors, sensing decreased perfusion pressure, trigger more sympathetic and less parasympathetic outflow, leading to peripheral vasoconstriction. Although leading to a higher blood pressure through an increased vascular resistance in the short term, this response forces the failing heart to pump against even higher resistance, which further compounds the heart failure over the long term.

Using medication, surgery, radiation, and other modalities, therapeutic interventions aim to reverse or correct pathophysiologic functioning of homeostatic mechanisms. Managing congestive heart failure may include augmenting the heart's ability to pump blood, changing the hemodynamics of blood flow through the arteries, or interfering with the kidney's efforts to activate the renin-angiotensin-aldosterone axis. The clinician's job is to know how control systems like those at work in congestive heart failure ought to function, how and why they sometimes do not, and what to do in such situations.

Clinical Correlation Box 1.2
Autonomic Control of Arterial Blood Pressure

Many neurohormonal systems act in concert to maintain blood pressure (see the cardiovascular and renal chapters). Arterial blood pressure is a function of cardiac output (how frequently and how intensely the heart muscle contracts) and blood vessel resistance. Suppose there is a drop in blood pressure. How does the body respond? First, pressure-sensitive receptors (baroceptors) in the carotid sinuses and aortic arch detect the pressure drop. The receptors actually are stretch receptors that detect a pressure change across the vessel wall. In response to this blood pressure drop, the carotid-sinus receptors decrease their rate of stimulation of cranial nerves IX and X. These cranial nerves ultimately synapse on neurons in the medulla of the brain stem, which respond to the decreased rate of stimulation by increasing sympathetic nervous system activity and decreasing parasympathetic activity (see Ch. 4). This alteration in autonomic outflow mediates three changes: increased heart rate, increased contractility of the cardiac ventricles, and vasoconstriction of systemic arteries and veins (increasing blood vessel resistance); all of which help increase blood pressure. This increase is sensed by the baroceptors, which subsequently increase their rate of firing, causing a compensatory readjustment of sympathetic and parasympathetic outflow (Fig. 1.12). Conversely, an increase in blood pressure sensed by the baroceptors triggers a decrease in heart rate, ventricular contractility, and blood vessel resistance; changes that all lead to a decrease in blood pressure. In either case, blood pressure is restored toward the previous level. The components of this homeostatic mechanism are:

Sensors: Baroceptors in the carotid sinus.

Afferent transmission pathway: Cranial nerves IX and X.

Control center: Neurons in the medulla oblongata.

Efferent transmission pathway: Sympathetic and parasympathetic nerves.

Effectors: Cardiac myocytes and vascular smooth muscle.

This system is a classic negative-feedback system.

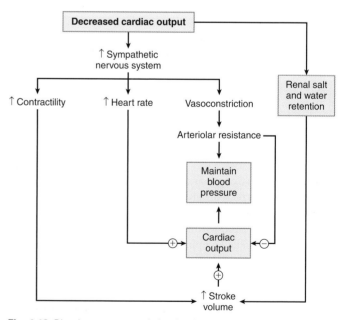

Fig. 1.12 Blood pressure regulation by the autonomic nervous system (ANS). A decrease in cardiac output leads to a decrease in blood pressure below the set range is detected by the system and leads to changes in heart contraction and blood vessel resistance that increase the pressure. An increase in blood pressure above the set range is detected by the system and results in the opposite changes in the heart and blood vessels that lower the pressure.

Introduction to Diagnosis

"To explain the phenomena in the world of our experience, to answer the question 'why?' rather than only the question 'what?,' is one of the foremost objectives of empirical science."
Carl G. Hempel (1948)

Diagnosis is the medical term for scientific explanation or hypothesis. An explanation takes a set of facts and seeks a general law of the universe from which those facts might be logically deduced.

For example, why does the apple fall downward from the limb of the tree? We note that both the apple and earth have mass, and recall the law of gravity—two bodies with mass will attract each another.

To use another example, a patient arrives in your clinic with a fever, runny nose, and a cough—why? We may apply three known laws of physiology:

1. A law of microbiology: People commonly acquire bacterial and viral infections in the upper respiratory tract.
2. A law of immune response: Infections will activate macrophages.
3. A law of immune system behavior: Macrophages will secrete interleukins, which alter the hypothalamic set point for temperature regulation and lead to fever, whereas inflammatory cells activated at the mucus membranes lead to vasodilation, leakage of fluid from the vascular space, and increased mucus production.

Thus this patient's presenting symptoms adhere to known medicobiological laws, making an upper respiratory infection as a plausible explanation. However, we could also consider a rival explanation—could this all be caused by allergies, for example?

A list of more than one possible explanation for clinical observations is called a differential diagnosis. The only way to distinguish between two equally plausible explanations is to gather more data and to reconsider the two explanations in light of the new data. For example, we could ask the patient about his exposures to other sick people and to possible allergens, such as dust, pets, or pollen. We could draw the patient's blood and measure the concentrations of various kinds of immune cells.

Say the patient denies any contact with allergens and any history of allergies. Then, as he considers his recent past, he suddenly remembers that his cousin who came to dinner had a terrible cold. Finally, a complete blood count (CBC) shows high numbers of neutrophils, which we know to be elevated in the response to some infections but not in response to allergies. Now, we can more confidently say that an upper respiratory infection better explains all the data than allergies.

Thus we test clinical hypotheses to select one diagnosis from a pool of differential diagnoses. Our hypothesis testing falls into two broad categories:

1. Asking questions about the history of the present illness and other medical history;
2. Obtaining objective information from the physical examination, blood tests, imaging studies, and so on (see Fast Fact Box 1.1.1).

Fast Fact 1.1.1

Subjective complaints predicting the presence of an underlying illness are termed symptoms, whereas objective findings predicting presence of an underlying illness are called signs. For example, the report of frequent coughing is a symptom, whereas a temperature of 102° F is a sign. But note that if you the caregiver observe the patient coughing, then cough is also a sign.

After gathering subjective and objective data, we work in two directions sequentially. First, we have to combine the observations we have made so far with previous experience, material learned previously, and imagination to construct a reasonably broad differential diagnosis. Second, we try to narrow our differential diagnosis and plan a course of action. The plan may include further testing to acquire more data, which can be used to further pare down our list of differential diagnoses. The plan may also include treatments to reduce or control symptoms. Often, a treatment tried empirically, is also useful as a "bioassay" to test one or more of the hypotheses in the differential diagnosis list. If a treatment for a given disease process does not help the patient, that decreases the likelihood that that particular diagnosis is correct in this case. But if the treatment is very helpful, it provides circumstantial evidence in support of that diagnosis. The benefit of such an approach is that it starts to address the patient's desire to feel better (especially if the treatment works), but its utility may be limited by many treatments having multiple effects that might improve symptoms that are consistent with more than one of the diagnoses on the differential. For example, a nasal steroid inhaler might help the patient's runny nose and cough whether they are caused by a viral infection or allergies.

Once a likely explanation is found, the plan will include a treatment aimed at relieving the underlying illness(es) (see Clinical Correlation Box 1.1.1).

Clinical Correlation Box 1.1.1

The mnemonic "SOAP" summarizes the format of clinical reasoning used in many medical presentations and notes in the patient's chart.

Subjective
  How is the patient feeling?

Objective
  Vital signs, fluid input/output, physical examination, and testing results.

Assessment
  What do you think may be going on, and why? What is keeping the patient in the hospital?)

Plan
  What will you do to treat or test?

Knowledge of physiology is critically important to making diagnoses thoughtfully and using active thinking to reason and not simply pattern recognition. Illnesses and their treatments may act at the cellular and molecular level, but illnesses are generally known to their sufferers by dysfunction or reaction at the organ level. To trace a path from an illness to its manifestations, we must know:

1. The role of each organ system in normal physiology;
2. How one system affects one or more other system(s);
3. The consequences that occur when an organ system under- or overperforms.

As you go through the case studies, try not to concern yourself too much with mastering the details of the featured illnesses and their treatment protocols. Rather, take the opportunity to familiarize yourself with the process of diagnosis, by which physiologic principles are used to infer an explanation from among several possibilities. Follow the course of the illness and try to appreciate how its progression can be predicted (and hence better treated) from a knowledge of the physiologic laws of the body.

Neurophysiology

An Overview of Nerve Cell Physiology and Electrophysiology

INTRODUCTION

The nervous system actively participates in, regulates, and integrates all the other body systems. The nervous system is broadly divided into:
- The central nervous system (CNS) (see Ch. 3).
  - Composed of brain and spinal cord.
- The peripheral nervous system (PNS) (see Ch. 4).
  - Composed of the autonomic nervous system (ANS) and somatic nervous system.

This chapter focuses on the structure and cellular physiology of the functional unit of the nervous system, neurons (nerve cells).

NERVE CELL STRUCTURE AND FUNCTION

The neuron is the basic cellular unit of the nervous system. The human brain contains approximately 10^{11} neurons, with each making roughly 1000 synapses with other neurons. Thus there are about 10^{14} synaptic connections in the human brain, forming a "neural network" allowing the highly interconnected nerve cells to communicate with one another.

Nerve Cell Morphology

Although neurons share many characteristics similar to other cells, they also possess specialized structures that enable information to be processed in an organized manner. Although the precise structure of neurons is dependent on their function, all share several basic features (Fig. 2.1 and Table 2.1):
- Dendrites: Short, highly branched cytoplasmic extensions.
  - Function: Receive afferent signals from the environment.
  - Located near the cell body (soma).
- Cell body (soma).
  - Function: Contains nucleus and molecular machinery necessary for gene expression, protein production, and cell metabolism.
- Axon: Long, cytoplasmic extension.
  - Function: Transmits signals from soma to end organs or other neurons.
  - Proteins and other substances are ferried along microtubule "highways" in the axon by specific transport proteins.
    Kinesins (anterograde transport).
    Dyneins (retrograde transport) (see Clinical Correlation Box 2.1 and (Fast Fact Box 2.1).

Clinical Correlation Box 2.1

Certain pathogens exploit retrograde transport to invade the nervous system. Upon exposure to distal axon terminals, they are able to "hitch-hike" back to the cell soma. Known examples include tetanus toxin, herpes simplex virus, rabies virus, and poliovirus. Thus onset of symptoms will be delayed according to the length of time required for retrograde transport.

Fast Fact Box 2.1

Anterograde: Substances move away from the soma.
Retrograde: Substances return to the soma.

- Myelin: Phospholipid-rich sheath surrounding axons.
  - Function: Insulates neurons and facilitates nerve transmission over long distances.
  - Composed of the plasma membrane of specialized glial support cells (Fig. 2.1 and Table 2.2).
    - In the CNS, support cells are called oligodendrocytes and support many neurons.
      - In the PNS, support cells are called Schwann cells and support one neuron.
  - Phospholipid fat in the myelin sheath gives axons a white appearance.
    White matter = myelinated axons.
    Grey matter = unmyelinated cell bodies.
- Terminal boutons: Specialized endings of axon.
  - Function: Allows communication to target tissues or other neurons via synapse.
- Synaptic cleft.
  - Function: Maintains association of presynaptic and postsynaptic elements.
  - Extensive cytoskeletal elements allow maintenance of structure.
  - Site of enzymatic degradation of excess neurotransmitter.

The presynaptic axon terminal, synaptic cleft, and postsynaptic dendrite comprise the synapse (Fig. 2.2). Fundamentally, there are two different types of synapses:
- Chemical: Convert an electrical signal into a chemical signal, which is then received by chemical receptor. More highly regulated.
- Electrical: Allow ions to flow directly between neurons from the presynaptic to postsynaptic membranes without loss of signal strength.

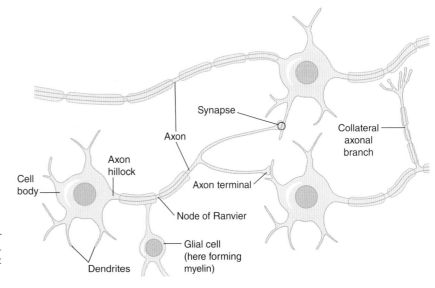

Fig. 2.1 General neural structure common to central and peripheral neurons. (Modified from Nolte J. *Elsevier's Integrated Neuroscience*. Philadelphia, PA: Elsevier. 2007. Fig. 1.1.)

TABLE 2.1	**Neuron Classifications Based on Number of Dendrites and Axons**
Classification	**Description**
Unipolar	One dendrite or one axon (i.e., sensory neurons)
Pseudo-unipolar	One process that branches into a dendrite and an axon
Bipolar	One dendrite and one axon
Multipolar	Multiple dendrites and axons

TABLE 2.2	**Different Types of Support Cells of the Neuron, Known as Neuroglia**	
Neuroglia	**Description**	**Function**
Astrocytes	Stain positive for glial fibrillary acidic protein (GFAP)	Repair neurons, provide nutritional support, maintain the blood-brain barrier, regulate CSF composition
Ependymal cells	Single cell layer, lines the ventricles	Produce CSF in the choroid plexus, circulate CSF
Microglia	Irregular nuclei, little cytoplasm	Become phagocytic in response to tissue damage
Oligodendroglia (oligodendrocytes)	Found in the CNS	Myelinate up to 30 neurons each
Schwann cells	Found in the PNS. Gaps between cells are called nodes of Ranvier	Myelinate only one axon each. Secrete growth factors and create a pathway for axonal regeneration

CNS, Central nervous system; *CSF,* cerebrospinal fluid; *PNS,* peripheral nervous system.

Nerve Cell Membrane

As in other cells, the cell membrane is a lipid bilayer with embedded proteins. In neurons, the plasma membrane serves three crucial roles:

- Maintains the integrity of the intracellular environment.
- Allows reception of signals.
- Regulates changes in electrochemical state of the nerve cell.

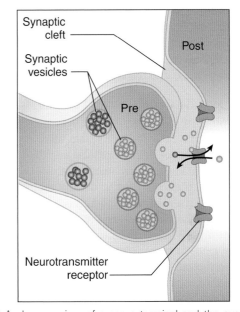

Fig. 2.2 A close-up view of a nerve terminal and the synapse. The terminal bouton on the left contains a number of membrane bound vesicles, small subcellular compartments holding chemical neurotransmitters. The synaptic cleft between the terminal bouton and the target cell has enzymes that can cleave neurotransmitter molecules once they are released from the nerve terminal. The cell membrane of the presynaptic neuron has embedded ion channels and the N^+-K^+-ATPase transporter, while the plasma membrane of the postsynaptic target cell has embedded neurotransmitter receptors. When a neurotransmitter molecule binds to the post synaptic receptor ligand gated channel, the channel assumes an open conformation allowing Na^+ (blue sphere) and K^+ (red sphere) to flow down their respective electrochemical gradients (Na^+ into the post synaptic cell and K^+ out of the post synaptic cell). Note how the neurotransmitter-containing vesicles and the neurotransmitter receptors cluster at the synapse, where a nerve terminus is juxtaposed with the target cell membrane. (Modified from Nolte J. *Elsevier's Integrated Neuroscience*. Philadelphia, PA: Elsevier. 2007. Fig. 3.3.)

Two classes of membrane proteins essential to nerve cell function are ion channels and neurotransmitter receptors:

- Ion channels are found in specialized regions of the axon cell membrane and regulate the passage of ions, such as Na^+, K^+, Cl^-, and Ca^{2+} into or out of the cell.
  - Ungated channels are constituitively open to their specific ion.
  - Gated channels
    Exist in three possible states (Fig. 2.3):
      Closed = specific ion cannot cross the cell membrane.
      Open = specific ion is permitted to cross the cell membrane.
      Locked = specific ion cannot cross the cell membrane and the receptor cannot open.
    - Two subclasses are essential to neuronal function:
      Voltage-gated ion channel is more likely to be open when there is a change in the electrical potential of the nerve cell membrane.
      Ligand-gated ion channel is more likely to be open when a specific neurotransmitter binds to it.
- Neurotransmitter receptors are present on the dendrites and on the plasma membrane of nonneuronal target cells. These receptors bind their respective neurotransmitter ligands that have been released into the synaptic cleft (see Fig. 2.2).

Nerve Cell Ions, Resting Membrane Potential, and Electrochemical Gradients

The plasma membrane is semipermeable, allowing some substances to pass between the intracellular and the extracellular spaces while restricting the movement of others.

Two types of gradients exist in driving the movement of substances across the plasma membrane:

- Chemical gradients occur when the concentration of a solute differs on one side of the membrane from the other.
  - Solute tends to move from the area of higher concentration to that of lower concentration until equilibrium is established.
- Electrical gradients occur when the solute possesses an electrical charge.
  - Na^+, K^+, Ca^{2+}, Cl^-, and HCO_3^- are electrically charged solutes whose intracellular and extracellular concentrations are tightly controlled.
  - Transmembrane movements are the basis of electrochemical signaling in neurons and muscle cells.

At baseline, the intracellular space is electrically negative compared with the extracellular space. Three factors play into this.

1. The interior of a cell contains negatively charged solutes, such as proteins and nucleic acid macromolecules such as DNA and RNA that cannot traverse the cell membrane.
2. The Na^+,K^+-ATPase enzyme in the plasma membrane transports three Na^+ out of the cell and two K^+ into the cell, meaning a net loss of one positive charge from the cytoplasm.
3. Leakage of K^+ out of the cell down its chemical gradient through membrane channels removes more positive charges from the cell.

The baseline electrical polarization of the cell membrane is called the resting membrane potential (Em). Mathematically, Em is conventionally defined as the difference in electrical potential between the inside and the outside of the cell: $E_m = E_{in} - E_{out}$. A typical human neuron has an E_m of -60 to -70 mV.

A combined electrochemical gradient acting on each of the major ions thus regulates its movement (Fig. 2.4). The sum of the chemical and electrical potential of ion X is called the electrochemical potential (μ) and is defined by the equation:

$$\mu = \mu_0 + RTln[X] + zFE \qquad \textbf{(Eq. 2.1)}$$

μ_0 is the reference state electrochemical potential in mV; R = 8.3145 J/(°K)(mol) is the universal gas constant; T is the absolute temperature in degrees Kelvin, approximately 310° K at body temperature; ln[X] is the natural logarithm of the concentration of the ion X; z is the electrical charge on ion X (+1 for K^+ and Na^+, +2 for Ca^{2+} and Mg^{2+}, and −1 for Cl^- and HCO_3^-); F = 9.6485×10^4 Coulombs/mol is the Faraday constant; and E is the electrical potential in mV.

The difference in electrochemical potential across a cell membrane is defined as $\Delta\mu = \mu_{in} - \mu_{out}$. Because μ_0 is constant, substituting Equation 2.1 and combining like terms yields:

$$\Delta\mu = RTln([X]_{in}/[X]_{out}) + zFE_{in} \qquad \textbf{(Eq. 2.2)}$$

$\Delta\mu$ is called the electrochemical potential difference. It quantifies the electrochemical gradient, the combined chemical and electrical forces acting on an ion X. As Equation 2.2 depicts, the electrochemical gradient acting on a particular ion with respect to a particular cell depends on:

1. The ratio of the intracellular and extracellular concentrations of the ion.
2. The ion's charge.
3. The E_m of the particular cell (see Fig. 2.4).

When the ion is in chemical and electrical equilibrium (i.e., no net flow in either direction), there is no net charge generated and thus $\Delta\mu$ must equal 0. Given this, we can rearrange Equation 2.2 to yield the following equation:

$$E_m = RTln([X]_{in}/[X]_{out}) - zF \qquad \textbf{(Eq. 2.3)}$$

Converting from natural logarithm to log10 and substituting in the known values of R, T, and F results in the Nernst equation.

$$E_m = (-61.54 \text{ mV}/z)log_{10}([X]_{in}/[X]_{out}) \qquad \textbf{(Eq. 2.4)}$$

This is the Nernst potential, or equilibrium potential that results from an ion being in equilibrium at the measured intracellular and extracellular concentrations. The Nernst potential depends on the particular ion's charge and its distribution across the cell membrane (Table 2.3). The Nernst equilibrium potential is a simplification of a more complex equation describing the steady state potentials for every ion gradient in the cellular and extracellular space. This equation, known as the Goldman equation, is as follows: Em = (-61.54 mV)log[($P^{K*}[K^+]^{in}/P^{K*}[K^+]^{out}$) + ($P^{Na*}[Na^+]^{in}/P^{Na*}[Na^+]^{out}$) + ($P^{Cl-*}[Cl^-]^{out}/P^{Cl-*}[Cl^-]^{in}$) + ...)]. The contribution of each ion is determined by the magnitude of the electrochemical gradient and the permeability or conductance of the membrane to that ion. In the resting potential state, where the membrane permeability to K^+ is much greater ($P^{K+} >>> P$ for other ions) than that of other ions because the K^+ channels are open while those for other ions are closed, the resting membrane potential is very near the Nernst potential for K^+, as the Goldman equation simplifies to something close to the

Na$^+$ channel

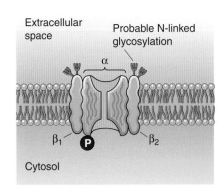

Ca^{2+} channel

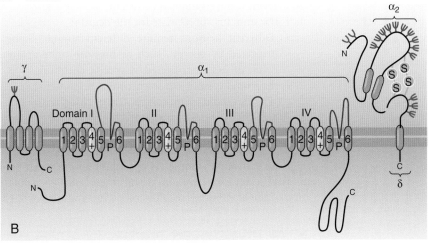

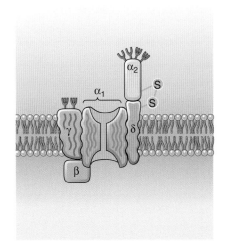

K$^+$ channel

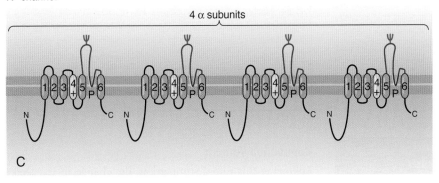

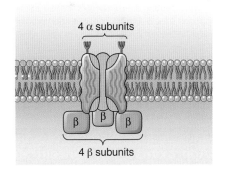

Inactivation of K$_V$-type channels

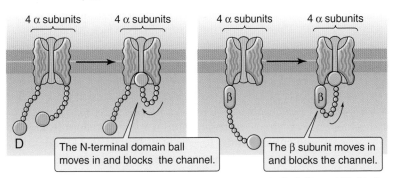

Fig. 2.3 Ion channels selective for (A) Na$^+$, (B) Ca^{2+}, and (C) K$^+$. Gated channels, such as the K$_V$ type channel can be in one of three states: closed, open, or locked ("blocked"). (From Moczydlowski EG. Electrical excitability and action potentials. In: Boron WF, Boulpaep EL, eds. *Medical Physiology*, Third Edition. Philadelphia, PA: Elsevier. 2017. Figs. 7.12 and 7.18.)

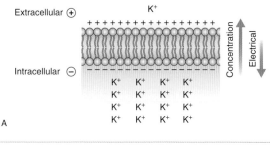

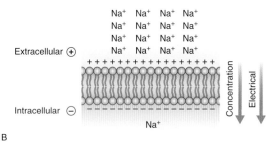

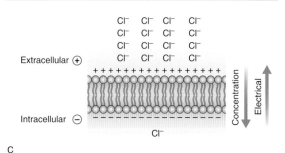

Fig. 2.4 Electrochemical gradients of K⁺, Na⁺, and Cl⁻. A. A large concentration gradient favors the movement of K⁺ out of the cell, but the negative resting membrane potential, $E_m = -60$ to -70 mV, partially opposes this. B. Both a concentration gradient and an electrical gradient favor the movement of Na⁺ into the cell. Only the relative impermeability of the cell membrane and the action of the Na⁺,K⁺-ATPase maintain this high Na⁺ electrochemical gradient. C. Cl⁻ has a concentration gradient similar to Na⁺, but because its charge is -1 the negative resting membrane potential opposes the movement of Cl⁻ into the cell.

TABLE 2.3	**Nernst Potentials and Approximate Ion Concentrations for Various Ions**			
X	z	[X]$_{in}$	[X]$_{out}$	E$_X$
K⁺	+1	120 mM	4 mM	−91 mV
Na⁺	+1	10 mM	140 mM	+70 mV
Cl⁻	−1	9 mM	105 mM	−65.6 mV

K⁺ Nernst equation. The Goldman equation describes a steady state situation, while the Nernst equation is a simplified, special case of that state that describes an equilibrium situation.

Nerve Cell Function

Neurons receive and transmit information in the form of electrochemical impulses. This is a binary process—the neurons are either "on" or "off."

Activation Thresholds

To turn "on," a neuron requires the following components:
1. Stimulus
2. One or more receptors for that stimulus
3. An intact plasma membrane
4. Ion channels
5. Ion gradients (see Fast Fact Box 2.2)

Fast Fact Box 2.2

An activating stimulus will depolarize the membrane, or make it less negative with respect to extracellular space. An inhibitory stimulus will hyperpolarize the membrane, or make it more negative.

To determine if a stimulus is sufficient, we may ask:
1. Is the stimulus appropriate for the neuron?
   - Different neurons require different stimuli. Some are triggered by energy (such as pressure or temperature) while others are triggered by specific chemicals.
2. Is the stimulus sufficient for neuronal response? (Fig. 2.5)
   - The threshold membrane potential (usually around −55 to −50 mV) must be attained.
   - A subthreshold stimulus will depolarize the membrane slightly, but not to threshold.

If an activating stimulus is appropriate for a given neuron and sufficient for activation, it will trigger further depolarization of the membrane (see Physiology Integration Box 2.1).

Physiology Integration Box 2.1

A subthreshold stimulus causes a few gated Na⁺ channels in the specific area of the membrane where the stimulus was received to open, increasing the local membrane conductance (g$_{Na}$⁺) and membrane permeability (P$_{Na}$⁺) to Na⁺ and allowing positive charges to flow into the neuron. This shifts resting membrane potential (E$_m$) away from its resting value, depolarizing the membrane segment toward the Nernst potential for Na⁺ of +70 mV. However, the magnitude of membrane depolarization is insufficient to reach threshold, and E$_m$ decays back down to its resting value.

Conduction Velocity

Following this initial stimulation, the change in E$_m$ decreases exponentially because of resistance of the cytoplasm. This change depends on two essential variables:
- Distance from the site of membrane stimulation (Fig. 2.6).
- Time from the initial stimulus (see Figs. 2.5 and 2.6).

Voltage (V) decreases with distance traveled down the axon (x) and a length constant, λ, according to:

$$V = V_o e^{-(x/\lambda)} \tag{Eq. 2.5}$$

where λ is the distance for which a change in membrane potential declines to 37% of its initial value (V$_o$). It is dependent on membrane resistance (rm) and cytoplasm resistance (ri):

$$\lambda = \sqrt{(r_m / r_i)} \tag{Eq. 2.6}$$

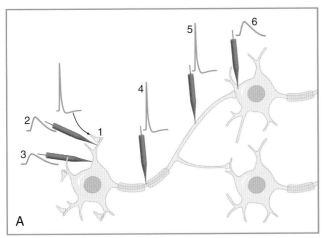

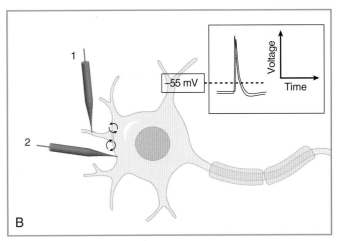

Fig. 2.5 A. Chemical and electrical signaling by neurons. Chemical signals (neurotransmitters) released from presynaptic terminals (1) cause local production of graded potentials in postsynaptic sites (2); these become smaller and slower (3) as they spread from their site of production. Action potentials are used to convey large, constant-amplitude signals (4, 5) over long distances; these in turn invade axon terminals and cause transmitter release, resulting in graded potentials in other neurons (6). B, Passive, decremental spread of current (and voltage) from one neuron (1) to another (2) through an electrical synapse. There is little delay, and the direction of the voltage swing is unchanged. (A, From Nolte J. *Elsevier's Integrated Neuroscience*. Philadelphia, PA: Elsevier. 2007. Fig. 2.1. B, From Nolte J. *Elsevier's Integrated Neuroscience*. Philadelphia, PA: Elsevier. 2007. Fig. 3.1.)

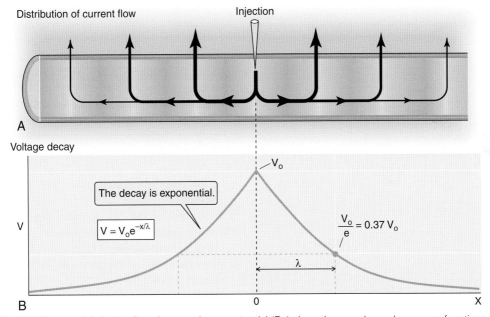

Fig. 2.6 Exponential decay of resting membrane potential (E_m) along the neural membrane as a function of distance from stimulus. (From Moczydlowski EG. Electrical excitability and action potentials. In: Boron WF, Boulpaep EL. *Medical Physiology*, Third Edition. Philadelphia, PA: Elsevier. 2017. Fig. 7.22B and C.)

Similarly, the conduction velocity (v) depends on distance traveled, as well as a time constant, τ:

$$v = x / \tau \qquad \text{(Eq. 2.7)}$$

where τ is the time it takes for the membrane to charge to 63% of the final membrane potential. It is dependent on the neuron's membrane resistance (R_m) and capacitance (c_m):

$$\tau = R_m c_m \qquad \text{(Eq. 2.8)}$$

These principles explain how myelination affects electrical propagation.

- Myelin $\rightarrow \uparrow r_m \rightarrow \uparrow \lambda \rightarrow \uparrow$ propagation distance.
- Myelin $\rightarrow \uparrow$ membrane thickness $\rightarrow \downarrow c_m \rightarrow \uparrow$ conduction velocity (see Fast Fact Box 2.3).

This allows the rapid conduction of electrical signals down some of the longest axons (up to 1 m long) in our bodies.

Action Potential Generation and Voltage-Gated Ion Channels

When a stimulus depolarizes the membrane to the threshold
value, it triggers a self-propagating membrane depolarization
cascade called an action potential (AP)—the "on" state of the
nerve cell (see Fig. 2.4). An AP is either full-sized or not elicited,
also known as the all or nothing response.

The basis of the AP is the sequential opening and subsequent
locking of voltage-gated ion channels (Fig. 2.7).
- Voltage-gated Na$^+$ channels are sensitive to changes in Em.
- Depolarization to threshold triggers conformational shift in
  voltage-gated Na$^+$ channels → increased opening.
- ↑ conductance of Na$^+$ → ↑ influx of Na$^+$ → further depolarization of E_m toward ENa$^+$.

This positive feedback loop is responsible for the explosive
depolarization phase of the AP (Fig. 2.8).

Like most positive feedback loops, the depolarization phase
of the AP (see Fig. 2.8) eventually has to be limited and reversed

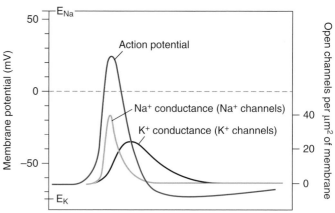

Fig. 2.8 Changes in membrane permeability and ion conductances with
an action potential (AP). When a stimulus causes membrane depolarization sufficient to drive resting membrane potential (E_m) to the threshold
potential, there is an explosive increase in the membrane's permeability
to Na$^+$ (PNa$^+$) and therefore in Na$^+$ conductance (gNa$^+$) as voltage-gated
Na$^+$ channels open and allow Na$^+$ to enter the cell. This depolarizes the
membrane, explaining why the rapid depolarization phase of the AP is
concurrent with the increase in PNa$^+$ and gNa$^+$. At the peak of the AP,
PNa$^+$ and gNa$^+$ decrease rapidly as the voltage-gated Na$^+$ channels lock.
The voltage-gated K$^+$ channels open more slowly than the Na$^+$ channels,
and the peak in PK$^+$ and gK$^+$ coincides with membrane repolarization.
Because the K$^+$ channels close slowly, unlike the Na$^+$ channels that
quickly lock, the efflux of K$^+$ drives E_m beyond the resting value toward
EK$^+$, briefly hyperpolarizing the membrane.

for the neuron to return to its resting state. This, again, occurs
because of conformational shifts in the voltage-gated Na$^+$
channels.
- Membrane depolarization eventually leads to transition to
  the locked state (see Fig. 2.7).
    - ↓ Na$^+$ influx.
    - Inability to respond to depolarizing stimulus (refractory
      state).
- ↑ Na$^+$ outflow via ungated ion channels and Na$^+$,K$^+$-
  ATPase.

The reversal of the AP, or membrane repolarization, is also
driven by voltage-gated K$^+$ channels:
- Depolarization causes voltage-gated K$^+$ channels to shift from
  the closed state to the open state → ↑ K$^+$ efflux (Fig. 2.9) (see
  Fast Fact Box 2.4).

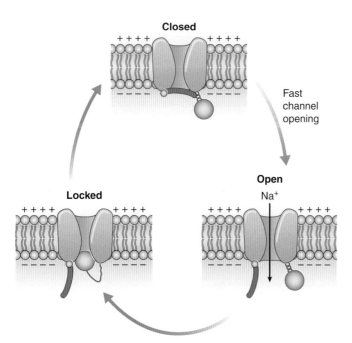

Fig. 2.7 Voltage-gated ion channels shift sequentially among three
states. At rest, the voltage-gated Na$^+$ channel is closed. When membrane depolarization occurs, it increases the probability that the channel
will open, allowing Na$^+$ to enter the cell. After some time in the open
state, membrane depolarization causes the channel to enter the locked
state. Only membrane repolarization can reset the channel to the
closed state. During the time that most of the Na$^+$ channels are locked,
the neuron is unable to respond to additional stimuli and is in the refractory state.

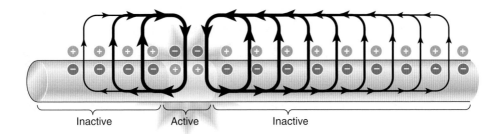

Fig. 2.9 Propagation and amplification of an action potential in an unmyelinated axon. (From Moczydlowski EG. Electrical excitability and action potentials. In: Boron WF, Boulpaep EL. *Medical Physiology*, Third Edition. Philadelphia, PA: Elsevier. 2017. Fig. 7.21A).

- K^+ exits the cell down its electrochemical gradient (which is made steeper because E_m was driven so far from EK^+ by the AP).
- Positive charge is removed from the interior of the cell and restores the charge distribution of the resting state.

The voltage-gated K^+ channels differ in two important ways from the voltage-gated Na^+ channels:

1. The K^+ channels open more slowly in response to membrane depolarization than the Na^+ channels. Repolarizing efflux of K^+ starts as the Na^+ channels begin to lock.
2. Some K^+ channels do not lock in response to prolonged depolarization. At the end of the AP, when the Na^+ channels are locked or closed and the K^+ channels have not yet reverted to the closed state, the continued flow of K^+ out of the cell causes a transient hyperpolarization—that is, E_m becomes more negative than the resting value, approaching EK^+ more closely (see Fig. 2.8). Thereafter, the K^+ voltage-gated channels close, and E_m returns again to its resting value.

Myelin, Nodes of Ranvier, and Saltatory Conduction

APs must be continually reinforced as they propagate down the axon. This occurs via electrotonic conduction, or local current flows. The following process is repeated continuously along the axon starting with the site of initial stimulus (Fig. 2.10):

- Greater inward flow of Na^+.
- Depolarization of adjacent membrane segments.
- Increased conductance to Na^+ in adjacent membrane segments.
- Triggering of "new" APs (depolarizing currents). This is a case of a positive feedback process (see chapter 1).

In this fashion, the APs are regenerated with the same size and shape as they travel down the axon. Furthermore, because the voltage-gated Na^+ channels in the region behind the AP are in their locked refractory state, the AP must propagate unidirectionally (see Fig. 2.10).

Recall that the propagation speed of the AP down the axon depends on membrane resistance. Although increasing the cross-sectional area of the axon can reduce this resistance, this solution is inherently limited. Instead, the myelin sheath becomes essential in ensuring rapid AP propagation in addition to preventing the loss of the conducting signal.

To further improve the conduction of the AP, the myelin sheath restricts AP regeneration to specific "gaps" that occur in the sheath every 1 to 2 mm called the nodes of Ranvier. In these

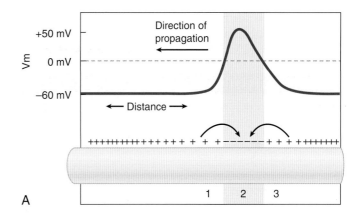

A

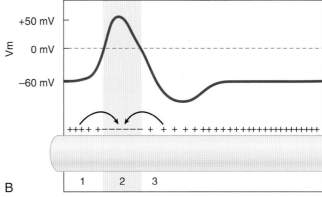

B

Fig. 2.10 Triggering and propagation of an action potential (AP). A. An AP occurs when a region of the neuron membrane is depolarized to the threshold value. The positive charges that flow into the cell quickly diffuse, creating local currents. This passive electrotonic conduction depolarizes adjacent segments of the membrane. B. The action potential (2) moves unidirectionally because local currents can initiate an action potential in an area of the membrane that has not been stimulated past the refractory period (1) but cannot do so in an area of the membrane that is recovering from an AP and is in the refractory state (3).

regions, there are higher densities of voltage-gated Na^+ and K^+ channels at the nodes than at those portions of the cell membrane covered by myelin. There are two main advantages to this adaptation:

1. By strategically locating the ion channels at the nodes rather than expressing them homogeneously on the axon membrane, the total number of proteins the neuron has to synthesize decreases.

2. By increasing the efficiency, the rate, and the range of electrotonic conduction (through the mechanisms discussed in the prior section), fewer Na$^+$ ions are needed to enter the cell, which saves work for the Na$^+$,K$^+$-ATPase.

The axon membrane is thus divided into two qualitatively distinct regions:

- The regions covered by myelin allow the AP to be rapidly propagated but do not regenerate it.
- The nodes of Ranvier regenerate the AP, but this occurs more slowly than local transmission by electrotonic conductance.

Thus the AP appears to start, move rapidly down the axon, slow down at a node of Ranvier to regenerate, and then continue down the axon quickly until it reaches the next node. Such a pattern is the basis for saltatory conduction from the Latin word *saltare* meaning "to jump" (Fig. 2.11) (see Clinical Correlation Box 2.2).

Clinical Correlation Box 2.2

Loss of the myelin sheath, as occurs in demyelinating diseases, such as multiple sclerosis, can cause profound neurologic dysfunction because saltatory conduction fails and action potentials are propagated slowly or even decay completely before reaching their end-target (Fig. 2.11).

Transmission Across the Synapse

Once the AP finally reaches the axon terminals, it is unable to cross the synaptic cleft to reach the next neuron or target cell. Thus the AP must be transformed from a membrane voltage into a transmissible, chemical signal.

The language that allows the AP to cross the synaptic cleft is that of the neurotransmitters. A variety of important neurotransmitters (Table 2.4) can carry out different effects depending on the receptor they bind to:

- At rest, these chemical substances are stored in membrane-bound vesicles clustered at the axon terminals.
- When an AP depolarizes the terminal membrane, specialized voltage-gated Ca^{2+} channels open.
- Like Na$^+$, Ca^{2+} has a large electrochemical gradient favoring its influx into the cell; thus this causes a nonnegligible increase in [Ca^{2+}]$_{in}$ (Fig. 2.12A).
- ↑ [Ca^{2+}]$_{in}$ causes neurotransmitter vesicles to fuse with the cell membrane of the axon terminals and release neurotransmitters into the synaptic cleft (Fig. 2.12B).

Once released, neurotransmitters diffuse across the synaptic cleft and bind to receptors on the surface of a target cell.

- These neurotransmitter receptors are ligand-gated ion channels that open in response to the binding of their ligands (Fig. 2.12C).

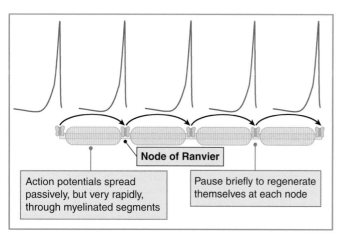

Node of Ranvier

Action potentials spread passively, but very rapidly, through myelinated segments

Pause briefly to regenerate themselves at each node

Fig. 2.11 Saltatory conduction of an action potential (AP) down a myelinated axon. An AP is generated when the membrane at a node of Ranvier is depolarized to threshold. Local currents carry the depolarization down the axon and an intact myelin sheath prevents leakage of current across the membrane, increasing the rate and the distance over which electrotonic conduction can occur. When the depolarization reaches the next node of Ranvier, it slows down and regenerates the action potential. The alternating velocity at which the AP propagates is called saltatory conduction. If the myelin sheath is damaged or lost, as occurs in diseases, such as multiple sclerosis, charges leak out of the membrane, causing the AP to slow down or even dissipate completely before it reaches the next node of Ranvier. (From Nolte J. *Elsevier's Integrated Neuroscience.* Philadelphia, PA: Elsevier. 2007. Fig. 2.20.)

TABLE 2.4 Different Types of Neurotransmitters in the Central Nervous System and Their Functions		
Neurotransmitter	**Description**	**Clinical Implications**
Acetylcholine	• In the PNS and CNS • Muscarinic and nicotinic receptors	• Decreased levels: Alzheimer dementia
Dopamine	• Synthesized from tyrosine • Precursor to norepinephrine	• Increased levels: psychosis, mania, and schizophrenia • Decreased levels: Parkinson's disease
γ-Aminobutyric acid (GABA)	• Main inhibitory NT in the CNS	• Decreased levels: anxiety, epilepsy
Glutamate	• Main excitatory NT in the CNS	• Increased levels: epilepsy, schizophrenia, Alzheimer's disease
Glycine	• Inhibitory NT • Controls glutamate activity in the brain	• Indirect clinical effects through modulation of glutamate
Histamine	• Role in sleep modulation and satiety	• Decreased levels: sedation, increased appetite (weight gain)
Norepinephrine (NE)	• Precursor to epinephrine	• Increased levels: major depressive disorder • Decreased levels: anxiety
Serotonin	• Monamine NT • Synthesized from tryptophan • Regulates body temperature, sleep, mood, sexuality	• Increased levels: schizophrenia • Decreased levels: major depressive disorder, bipolar disorder, anxiety disorder

CNS, Central nervous system; *NT,* neurotransmitter; *PNS,* peripheral nervous system.

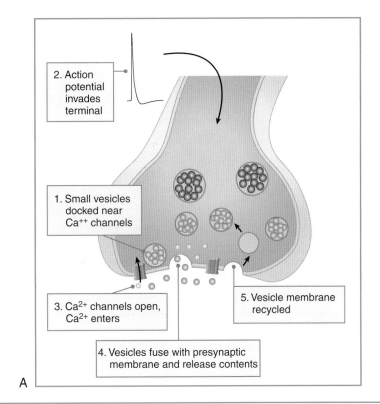

2. Action potential invades terminal

1. Small vesicles docked near Ca++ channels

3. Ca2+ channels open, Ca2+ enters

5. Vesicle membrane recycled

4. Vesicles fuse with presynaptic membrane and release contents

A

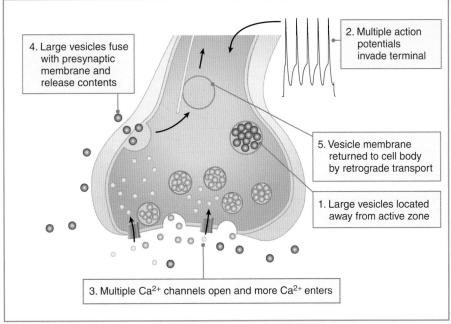

4. Large vesicles fuse with presynaptic membrane and release contents

2. Multiple action potentials invade terminal

5. Vesicle membrane returned to cell body by retrograde transport

1. Large vesicles located away from active zone

3. Multiple Ca2+ channels open and more Ca2+ enters

B

Fig. 2.12 Trans-synaptic transmission. A. An action potential reaches the axon terminals and the depolarization of the terminal membrane opens voltage-gated Ca^{2+} channels. B. The influx of Ca^{2+} causes neurotransmitter vesicles to fuse with the plasma membrane and release neurotransmitter molecules into the synaptic cleft.
Continued

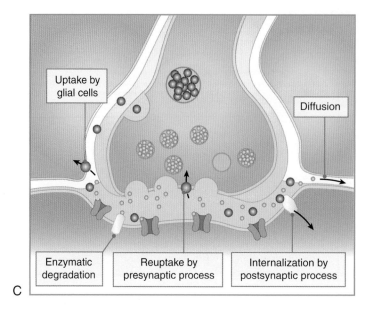

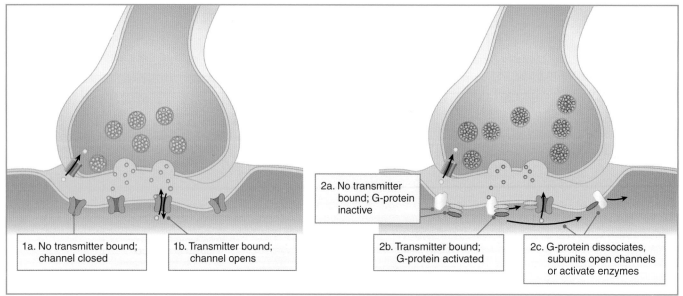

Fig. 2.12, cont'd C. The neurotransmitter diffuses across the synapse and binds to ligand-gated ion channels on the dendrites of the postsynaptic neuron, depolarizing the membrane. D. If sufficient activating stimuli reach the postsynaptic neuron, an action potential will be generated and conducted. Meanwhile, enzymes in the synaptic cleft metabolize the neurotransmitter so that signaling is limited. (From Nolte J. *Elsevier's Integrated Neuroscience*. Philadelphia, PA: Elsevier. 2007. Figs. 3.6, 3.7, 3.8, and 3.9.)

- If the neurotransmitter receptor is a ligand-gated Na^+ channel, sufficient signal leads to depolarization of the postsynaptic cell membrane and a new AP is generated (Fig. 2.12D).
- If the neurotransmitter receptor is a ligand-gated K^+ channel, the membrane of the postsynaptic cells is hyperpolarized, decreasing the likelihood that the target cell will be activated.

To limit the effect of neurotransmitters, these molecules are either broken down by specialized enzymes resident in the synaptic cleft or taken up and recycled by the axon terminals of the presynaptic neuron. For example, one neurotransmitter, acetylcholine (ACh), is broken down by acetylcholinesterase (see Clinical Correlation Box 2.3).

Clinical Correlation Box 2.3

In myasthenia gravis (MG), a neuromuscular junction (NMJ) autoimmune disease, circulating antibodies block acetylcholine (ACh) receptors on the postsynaptic membrane of the NMJ and thus inhibit the excitatory effect of ACh. Acetylcholinesterase inhibitors (such as neostigmine and pyridostigmine) can be administered to slow the enzymatic degradation and recycling of ACh in the synaptic cleft, allowing ACh to stay in the cleft longer to stimulate the receptors that are still functional.

PATHOPHYSIOLOGY OF NEURONS, GLIA, AND ELECTRICAL CONDUCTION

When the neural tissue operates properly, it integrates and transmits signals rapidly to and from the brain. When neural tissue does not function normally because of causes, such as demyelination, tumor, or disturbances of the basic molecular machinery, signal transmission both to and from the brain may be compromised.

Demyelinating Diseases

Recall that the myelin sheath made by oligodendrocytes (in the CNS) or Schwann cells (in the PNS) decreases the time constant, τ, of a neuron allowing for faster conduction of signals transmitted through the nerve cell. Furthermore, the myelin sheath decreases capacitive losses through the neural cell membrane, increasing the length constant, λ.

The pathophysiology of demyelinating disease revolves around impaired signal conduction:
- Loss of myelin $\rightarrow \uparrow \tau, \downarrow \lambda \rightarrow \downarrow$ conduction velocity and $\downarrow$ propagation distance
- Impaired conduction may affect both afferent (sensory) and efferent (motor) functions, as well as more complex processes, such as cognition.
  - Symptoms depend on the type of nerve involved.

Demyelinating disease may be classified in two broad categories (Table 2.5):
- Myelinoclastic: Normal myelin is destroyed by toxic, chemical, or autoimmune substances.
- Leukodystrophic: Abnormal myelin degenerates.

If possible, treatment centers around slowing the rate of demyelination. In the case of multiple sclerosis, for example, intravenous corticosteroids and several immunomodulatory agents, such as interferons, natalizumab, and glatiramir acetate may be useful. However, in many cases, cure is difficult to achieve (if not impossible) and treatment centers around symptomatic management, such as physical therapy.

Channelopathies

There exist several rare disorders caused by genetic mutations in ion channel subunits or regulatory proteins. As one may expect, this often has significant implications for the integrity of signal transmission (see Genetics Box 2.1 and Pharmacology Box 2.1).

🧬 GENETICS BOX 2.1

Amyotrophic lateral sclerosis (ALS, also called Lou Gehrig disease) is a fatal neurodegenerative disease of upper and lower motor neurons. Three gene groups are associated with ALS: one (e.g., *SOD1*) involved cellular proteostasis, a second (e.g., *TARDBP*) influencing the handling of ribonucleic acid and intracellular transport, and a third (e.g., *TUBA4A*) regulates changes in the cytoskeleton in the motor neuron axon and termini. ALS can be familial and among 25% to 40% of those patients the disease is related to mutations in the *C9ORF72* gene.

💊 PHARMACOLOGY BOX 2.1

Some manifestations of amyotrophic lateral sclerosis (ALS), such as sialorrhea (hypersalivation) can be managed with anticholinergic drugs. Rizulole was the first drug to be approved for the treatment of ALS. It inhibits presynaptic glutamate release, postsynaptic glutamate receptor signaling, and voltage-gated sodium channels.

Given the variety and complexity of these disorders, two representative examples are discussed:
- Erythromelalgia
  - Mutation in the alpha subunit gene (*SCN9A*) of voltage-gated Na^+ channels leads to
  - AP generation at hyperpolarized potentials, which leads to
  - hyperexcitability of nociceptors of dorsal root ganglion and sympathetic ganglion neurons.
    Nociceptor activation $\rightarrow$ perception of burning.
    Sympathetic activation $\rightarrow$ alteration of cutaneous vascular tone.
- Presentation:
    Episodes of erythema, swelling, and burning pain.
    Primarily affects the extremities.
    Common triggers include exercise and heat.

TABLE 2.5 Examples of Demyelinating Disease

Disease	Site	Classification	Mechanism	Symptoms
Multiple sclerosis	CNS	Myelinoclastic	Autoimmune destruction of myelin	Scanning speech, intention tremor, nystagmus, optic neuritis (sudden vision loss), hemiparesis, incontinence
Guillain Barré syndrome	PNS	Myelinoclastic	Autoimmune destruction of Schwann cells surrounding peripheral nerves	Symmetric ascending muscle weakness/paralysis
Krabbe disease	CNS/PNS	Leukodystrophic	Galactocerebrosidase deficiency → build-up of galactocerebroside and psychosine inhibits myelin formation	Peripheral neuropathy, developmental delay, optic atrophy
Charcot-Marie Tooth	PNS	Leukodystrophic	Defective production of multiple proteins involved in myelin sheath	Progressive loss of muscle tissue and touch sensation across body
Central pontine myelinolysis	CNS	Myelinoclastic	Osmotic destruction of pontine white matter following rapid correction of hyponatremia	Acute-onset paralysis, dysarthria, dysphagia, diploplia, loss of consciousness
Tabes dorsalis	PNS	Myelinoclastic	Syphilitic destruction of dorsal columns and roots	Impaired sensation and proprioception worst in lower extremities

CNS, Central nervous system; *PNS*, peripheral nervous system.

- Hyperkalemic periodic paralysis
  - Mutation in the inactivation gate (*SCN4A*) of the voltage-gated Na^+ channel leads to
  - loss of inactivation $\rightarrow$ sustained Na^+ conductance $\rightarrow$ continued muscle contraction.
  - Muscle remains depolarized $\rightarrow$ no communication of further signals $\rightarrow$ paralysis.

- $\uparrow K^+$ worsens symptoms because of the reduction of electrochemical gradient for K^+ efflux, leading to further prolongation of sodium conductance and muscle contraction.
- Presentation:
  Episodic violent muscle twitching and substantial muscle weakness.
  May occur at random or following exercise.

SUMMARY

- Neurons are the basic cellular elements of the nervous system.
- Dendrites receive input from other cells, the axon conducts information, and the release of neurotransmitters at the axon terminals allows information to cross the synapse between a neuron and a target cell.
- Like most cells, neurons possess a resting membrane potential (E_m) owing to the unequal distribution of ions (Na^+, K^+, and Cl^-) between the intracellular and extracellular spaces. The average resting membrane potential of a typical neuron is –60 to –70 mV. The *electrogenic* Na^+,K^+-ATPase pump helps maintain the concentration gradients for Na^+ and K^+.
- The combination of electrical and chemical forces influencing an ion's movement across the cell membrane is called the electrochemical gradient.
- The Nernst equation defines the equilibrium potential of each ion. This Nernst potential is the membrane voltage needed to just balance the concentration gradient of the particular ion.
- Stimuli that depolarize the neuron membrane to or above the threshold value trigger an AP, a limited positive feedback loop of membrane depolarization caused by the sudden increase in Na^+ influx. The repolarization portion of the AP is caused by the increase in K^+ efflux.
- The basis of the AP is the sequential opening, locking, and resetting of voltage-gated Na^+ and K^+ channels.
- The AP propagates down the axon as a regenerating wave of depolarization. In many neurons, the myelin sheath increases the efficiency and the rate of AP conduction. An AP in such a neuron propagates rapidly by electrotonic conduction in myelinated areas and slows down to regenerate at nodes of Ranvier. This mode of transmission is called saltatory conduction.
- At axon terminals, an AP induces an increase in the membrane conductance to Ca^{2+}, which causes neurotransmitter vesicles of the presynaptic cell to fuse with the membrane and release neurotransmitter molecules into the synaptic cleft. The neurotransmitters bind to their receptors on the postsynaptic cell and depolarize it, establishing a new action potential.

REVIEW QUESTIONS

Directions: Each of the numbered items or incomplete statements in this section is followed by answers or by completions of the statement. Select the one lettered answer or completion that is best in each case.

1. A 32-year-old businessman arrives in the emergency department with numbness and paresthesias of the lips and tongue. His symptoms started shortly after finishing dinner, where he had indulged in an expensive Japanese restaurant. He has never had these symptoms in the past. In the middle of sharing his medical history, he suddenly becomes severely nauseous, rapidly progressing to vomiting and diarrhea. He also complains of severe weakness and numbness progressing from his face to his upper extremities. Toxic exposure is suspected.
   Which part of the action potential curve is impaired in this patient? And why?
   A. Resting membrane potential
   B. Depolarization
   C. Repolarization
   D. Hyperpolarization

2. Hyperkalemia is an emergent clinical condition characterized by serum potassium levels greater than the upper limit defined by a given institution, usually around 5.5 mEq/L. For a neuron assumed to only contain K^+ channels, what is the Nernst potential (E_K) when $[K^+]_{intracellular}$ = 150 mEq and $[K^+]^{extracellular}$ = 7 mEq at a temperature of 37° C?
   A. -81.86 mV
   B. -9.77 mV
   C. $+81.86$ mV
   D. -91.00 mV
   E. -78.12 mV

3. In demyelinating diseases, such as multiple sclerosis, the myelin sheath made by oligodendrocytes or Schwann cells is damaged. How will this disease process change the speed of signal propagation (v), the time constant (τ), and the space constant (λ) of the neuron?

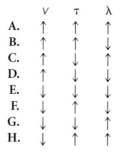

	v	τ	λ
A.	$\uparrow$	$\uparrow$	$\uparrow$
B.	$\uparrow$	$\uparrow$	$\downarrow$
C.	$\uparrow$	$\downarrow$	$\uparrow$
D.	$\uparrow$	$\downarrow$	$\downarrow$
E.	$\downarrow$	$\downarrow$	$\downarrow$
F.	$\downarrow$	$\uparrow$	$\downarrow$
G.	$\downarrow$	$\downarrow$	$\uparrow$
H.	$\downarrow$	$\uparrow$	$\uparrow$

ANSWERS TO REVIEW QUESTIONS

1. **The answer is B.** This man likely consumed *fugu*, or puffer-fish at his dinnertime excursion. Pufferfish contain lethal amounts tetrodotoxin, a potent neurotoxin that binds to an extracellular site of the fast voltage-gated sodium channel. This temporarily disables pore opening for the channel, preventing Na^+ influx, depolarization, and initiation of the action potential. Symptoms generally begin within minutes of ingestion, starting with paresthesias in the lips and tongue and progressing through severe gastrointestinal symptoms, weakness, numbness, and eventually respiratory failure because of paralysis of the diaphragm and intercostal muscles. There is no cure, but early resuscitation airway protection by nasotracheal intubation can be lifesaving until the toxin wears off. Of note, tetrodotoxin is often used in neuroscience experiments given its specific blockade of the fast-gated sodium channels.

2. **The answer is A.** To solve this, one must simply plug in the values stated in the problem into the Nernst equation, assuming $T = 273.15\ °K + 37\ °K = 310.15\ °K$ and $z = +1$. The correct answer is -81.86 mV, which is greater than the K^+ Nernst potential when the extracellular K^+ concentration is normal. Another way to think about this is that the elevated extracellular K^+ concentration decreases the normal electrochemical gradient favoring the efflux of K^+ out of the neuron.

The elevated Nernst potential in the hyperkalemic condition leads to a slight increase or depolarization in the normal resting membrane potential of -90 mV. In the clinical scenario, the cell membrane is more permeable to potassium than sodium at rest, and thus the membrane is depolarized relative to baseline. This brings the membrane potential closer to threshold, which in turn opens some fast voltage-gated sodium channels. However, this low-level activation usually leads to inactivation of the same channels, leading to refractory states and thus impairment of both neuromuscular function (weakness) and cardiac function (ventricular fibrillation and asystole). Thus it is critical to keep a close eye on serum potassium levels in the clinic.

3. **The answer is F.** As discussed in the text, myelination decreases the time constant, so a demyelinating disease would increase the time constant. Because the speed of propagation (v) is proportional to the inverse of the time constant (Eq. 2.8), v will decrease with demyelinating diseases. Because the membrane resistance decreases with demyelinating disease, the length constant will decrease as well (Fig. 2.6). This means that the propagating action potential will not travel as far down the axon before decaying by the same amount before demyelination.

3

Central Nervous System

INTRODUCTION

Because of the development of new research techniques, knowledge of the brain acquired in the past 2 decades has exceeded the amount learned in all previous centuries. Numerous questions remain unanswered:
- "What is consciousness?"
- "What defines our personality?"
- "How can we learn better?"

The central nervous system (CNS) is composed of the brain and spinal cord.
- Integrates information received from the body
- Coordinates and influences activity the body

As previously mentioned, the nervous system is broadly broken down into the CNS and the peripheral nervous system (PNS). Major anatomic differences are summarized in Table 3.1. The differences in regeneration ability are particularly notable:
- PNS
  - The axon is permitted to grow distally from site of injury
  - Portion distal to injury undergoes Wallerian (anterograde) degeneration with preservation of the distal endoneurial tube as a "pathway"
- CNS
  - Damaged tissue forms a glial scar, restricting future regeneration
  - Reduced ability to recover from injury

STRUCTURE AND FUNCTION: THE BRAIN

The brain (Fig. 3.1) is the center of the nervous system. It can be divided into different sections based on developmental origins (Fig. 3.2).

Meninges

In addition to the skull, there are three layers that protect the brain called meninges (Table 3.2).
- Inflammation of these layers is called meningitis.
- These membranes also form several potential and real spaces (Table 3.3) which can become filled with pus, excess cerebrospinal fluid (CSF), or blood during pathologic states (see Clinical Correlation Box 3.1).

Cerebrospinal Fluid

The CSF serves the following roles for the brain:
- Protection against trauma
- Transportation of hormones
- Removal of metabolic waste

Clinical Correlation Box 3.1

Meningitis typically affects the leptomeninges (pia and arachnoid) of the brain and spinal cord. The space between them is filled with cerebrospinal fluid (CSF), aiding in infection spread.

Causes of infectious meningitis include:
- Bacteria
- Viruses
- Fungi
- Tuberculosis (TB)
- Parasites

Common clinical signs include:
- Fever
- Headache
- Photophobia (are the lights switched off when you walk into the room?)
- Nuchal rigidity (inability to flex the neck forward)
- Kernig's sign (while supine, inability to extend the knee while the hip is flexed)
  - Meningeal irritation caused by movement of the spinal cord
- Brudzinski's sign (passive flexion of the neck causes flexion of legs/thighs)
  - As earlier; movement of spinal cord by neck flexion "cancelled out" by hip flexion

To diagnose meningitis, one may perform a lumbar puncture to identify the responsible organism by culture and specific CSF characteristics.

CSF findings in meningitis

	Opening Pressure	Cell Type	Protein	Sugar
Bacterial	↑	↑ polymorphonuclear leucocytes	↑	↓
Fungal/TB	↑	↑ lymphocytes	↑	↓
Viral	Normal/↑	↑ lymphocytes	Normal/↑	Normal

CSF is produced by the ependymal cells of the choroid plexuses of the lateral, third, and fourth ventricles. The flow of CSF through the ventricles is as follows (see also Fig. 3.3):

Right and left lateral ventricles → interventricular foramen (of Monro) → third ventricle → cerebral aqueduct (of Sylvius) → fourth ventricle → lateral foramina (of Luschka) **or** medial foramen (of Magendie) → subarachnoid space → arachnoid villi → superior sagittal sinus (see Clinical Correlation Box 3.2)

Clinical Correlation Box 3.2

If there is an obstruction anywhere in the path of cerebrospinal fluid (CSF) flow, it can lead to hydrocephalus, which is a dilation of the cerebral ventricles (noncommunicating hydrocephalus) or subarachnoid space (communicating hydrocephalus) with CSF.

TABLE 3.1 Anatomic Differences Between the Central Nervous System and Peripheral Nervous System

Embryonic Origin of Collections of Neural Cell Bodies	Neural Tube	Neural Crest Ectoderm
Myelin-forming glia cell	Oligodendrocyte (form parts of myelin for multiple axons)	Schwann cell (form 1 segment on 1 neuron)
Regenerative ability	Practically none	Limited: 1–4 mm/day, may grow back to wrong target or regenerate incompletely

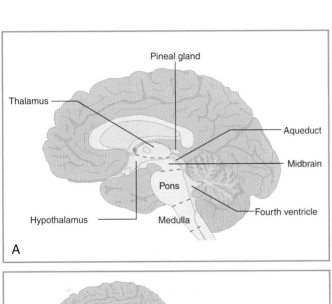

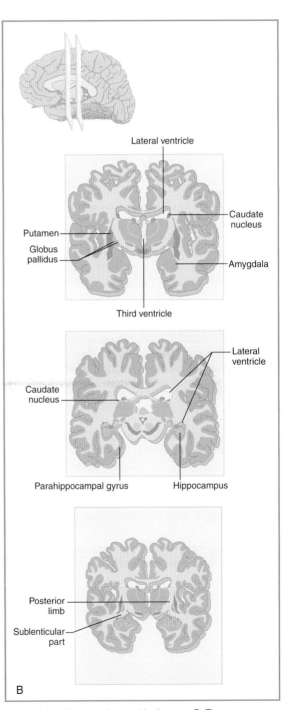

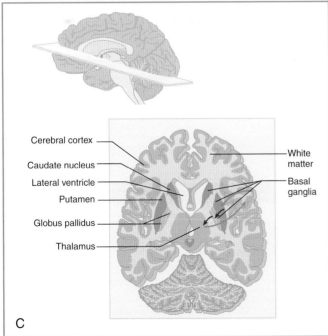

Fig. 3.1 Labeled cross-sections of the brain. A, Major components of the diencephalon and brainstem. B, The amygdala and hippocampus, major components of the limbic system in each cerebral hemisphere, as seen in coronal sections. C, Major components of the basal ganglia in each cerebral hemisphere, and some of their principal connections. (Modified from Nolte J. *Elsevier's Integrated Neuroscience*. Philadelphia, PA: Elsevier; 2007.)

The blood-brain barrier is formed by tight junctions between choroid plexus cells, and the cerebral capillaries have few fenestrations. This has several implications:

- Transport of substances (including immunologic cells and drugs) from the blood to the brain slow and limited.
- Water-soluble, large molecular weight substances cannot cross this barrier, thus protecting the brain from many harmful substances.

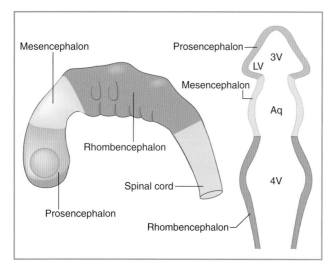

Fig. 3.2 Primary brain vesicles at about the time of neural tube closure (about 4 weeks). *3V, 4V,* Third and fourth ventricles; *Aq,* aqueduct; *LV,* lateral ventricle. (From Nolte J. *Elsevier's Integrated Neuroscience.* Philadelphia, PA: Elsevier; 2007.)

TABLE 3.2 The Three Meningeal Membranes That Surround the Spinal Cord and Brain

Layer	Location	Description
Pia mater	Covers brain and spinal cord surface	Delicate, highly vascular
Arachnoid	External to the pia mater, internal to the dura mater	Delicate, nonvascular, contains *granulations* that absorb cerebrospinal fluid
Dura mater	Exterior layer, tightly adherent to the skull	Dense, tough

Mnemonic: The meninges "PAD" the brain from the inside to the outside.

- Metabolic waste, such as carbon dioxide, however, is lipid-soluble and can easily leave the brain and go into the blood.
- Some circulating peptides (e.g., insulin) and plasma proteins (e.g., prealbumin) can also cross the blood-brain barrier.

Blood Supply

The blood supply to the brain arises from two main routes:

- The internal carotid arteries give rise to the anterior and middle cerebral arteries (ACA, MCA)
- The vertebral arteries unite to form the basilar artery, which then form the posterior cerebral arteries.

These three pairs of cerebral arteries connect to one another via communicating arteries at the base of the brain, forming the circle of Willis (Fig. 3.4). The blood drains out through the jugular veins.

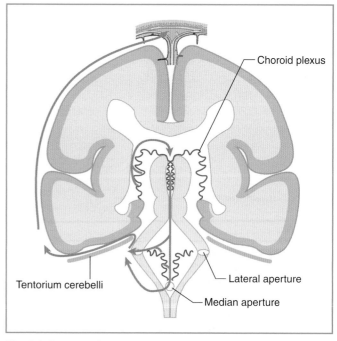

Fig. 3.3 Pathway of cerebrospinal fluid flow. (From Nolte J. *Elsevier's Integrated Neuroscience.* Philadelphia, PA: Elsevier; 2007.)

TABLE 3.3 The Three Meningeal Spaces

Space	Location	Description	Clinical Correlate
Subarachnoid space	Between the pia and arachnoid and terminates at S2 vertebra	Where CSF is produced and contained	Subarachnoid hemorrhage causes the "worst headache of one's life"
Subdural space	Between arachnoid and dura	Contains superior cerebral "bridging veins" from the brain	Ruptured veins cause subdural hematoma, a low-pressure hemorrhage that gradually causes headache and confusion. Appears crescent-shaped on CT scan
Epidural space	Between the dura and skull	Contains meningeal arteries, in the spinal cord it contains fatty areolar tissue, lymphatics, and venous plexuses	Trauma to the temporal region shears the middle meningeal artery and causes an epidural hematoma, a high-pressure hemorrhage that presents with a lucid interval followed by loss of consciousness. Appears lens-shaped on CT scan because of limitation by skull's sutures

CSF, Cerebrospinal fluid; *CT,* computed tomography.
Hemorrhagic blood can accumulate in any of these spaces in pathologic conditions.

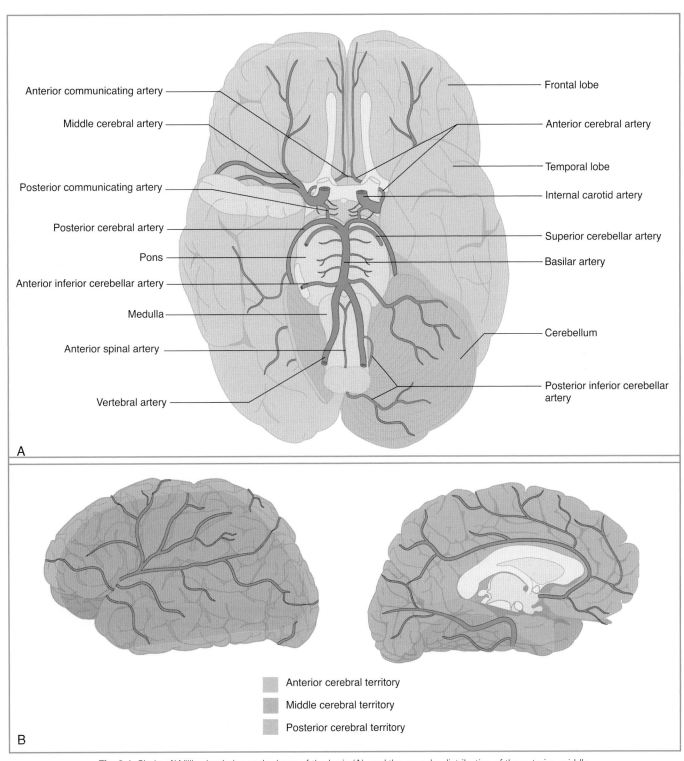

Fig. 3.4 Circle of Willis circulation at the base of the brain (A), and the vascular distribution of the anterior, middle, posterior cerebral arteries (B). (From Nolte J. *Elsevier's Integrated Neuroscience*. Philadelphia, PA: Elsevier; 2007.)

Autoregulation

Blood supply to the brain must be tightly regulated (Fig. 3.5). The brain, which is largely incompressible, is housed inside the rigid skull. The brain is comprised of the brain parenchyma and fluid. Because the volume of the brain is fixed, for one component to expand, the other must compensate if there is no change in pressure, as illustrated by the subsequent equation.

$$V_{intracranial} = V_{brain} + V_{CSF} + V_{blood} + V_{mass\,lesion} \qquad \textbf{(Eq. 3.1)}$$

This is called the Monro-Kellie doctrine, where V represents the volume.

Intracranial volume remains constant in physiologic states.
- V_{brain} represents the amount of volume comprised of brain parenchymal cells, which is also largely constant in the developed brain.

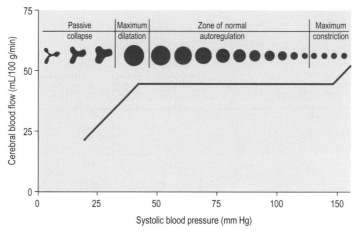

Fig. 3.5 Autoregulation of cerebral blood flow over a range of arterial blood pressures, and corresponding changes in blood vessel diameter. Blood vessel radius is inversely related to the fourth root of vascular resistance by Poiseuille's equation. (From Handy JM, Bersten AD. *Oh's Intensive Care Manual*, 8 Edition. Philadelphia, PA: Elsevier; 2018. Fig. 44.1.5.)

- V_{CSF} is largely homeostatic provided there are no obstructions and under normal physiology.
- $V_{mass\ lesion}$ can be added into the equation during pathologic states (e.g., tumor, hydrocephalus, hemorrhage).
  - Because intracranial volume must remain constant (assuming the skull is intact) another component of equation must decrease.
- V_{blood} is controlled by the body, through blood volume entering the brain.

As volume increases within the confined skull (assuming no brain herniation), intracranial pressure (ICP) must eventually increase. Mean arterial pressure (MAP) also decreases, causing a large decrease in cerebral perfusion pressure (CPP) according to:

$$MAP - ICP = CPP \qquad \textbf{(Eq. 3.2)}$$

CPP is necessary for life because the brain has a very high metabolic demand, but the brain is also very sensitive to over-perfusion. The brain thus maintains proper cerebral blood flow (CBF) and CPP according to:

$$CBF = CPP/CVR \qquad \textbf{(Eq. 3.3)}$$

whereby the cerebral vascular resistance (CVR) controls the other two parameters (see Fast Fact Box 3.1).

Fast Fact Box 3.1

Note that Eq. 3.3 is similar to Ohm's law

$$I = V / R$$

where current (I) is represented as blood flow and voltage (V) is represented as a pressure gradient. R represents a resistance.

To vary the CVR, the cerebral small arteries and arterioles constrict and dilate, changing the CBF so that it remains at approximately 50 mL/100 g /min (see Fig. 3.3).
- CBF is maintained with a MAP between 50 to 125 mm Hg
- Blood flow decreases dramatically at MAP less than 50 mm Hg

- Blood flow increases dramatically at MAP more than 125 mm Hg

The change in vessel size through cerebral autoregulation is thought to potentially work through three different mechanisms:
1. Myogenic regulation: Changes in transmural blood pressure can be detected by vascular smooth muscle in arterioles through mechanical sensors.
2. Neurogenic regulation: Resistance arterioles receive sympathetic innervation from brainstem blood pressure (BP) control centers for vasoconstriction, and para-sympathetic innervation that releases nitric oxide and causes vasodilation.
3. Metabolic regulation: Metabolic demand is balanced with blood flow, such that Increased metabolic activity (inc. PCO_2) leads to vasodilation while excessive oxygen concentrations lead to vasoconstriction to protect against oxygen toxicity (see Clinical Correlation Box 3.3).

Clinical Correlation Box 3.3

Local vasodilation increases blood flow to keep up with metabolic demand, and also to carry away CO_2-rich blood from the brain. This is the basis for measuring the use of different brain regions under functional magnetic resonance imaging (fMRI).

The Cerebrum

The cerebrum controls all voluntary actions in the body and is composed of:
- Two cerebral hemispheres (left and right)
- Four primary lobes of cerebral cortex
  - Frontal
  - Parietal
  - Temporal
  - Occipital
- Several subcortical structures
  - Thalamus
  - Hypothalamus

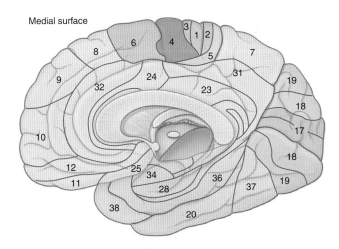

Medial surface

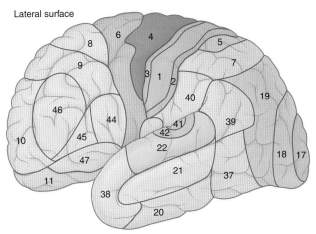

Lateral surface

Fig. 3.6 Various cortical areas of the cerebral cortex. Select Brodmann's areas are shown on the medial surface of the hemisphere (top), and the lateral convex surface of the hemisphere (bottom). (From Mtui E, Gruener G, FitzGerald MJT. *Fitzgerald's Clinical Neuroanatomy and Neuroscience*, 7th Edition. Elsevier; 2016. Fig. 29.4.)

- Basal ganglia
- Hippocampus

Cerebral Cortex

The cerebral cortex is composed of six layers that are largely segregated by their connections with other cortical and subcortical regions of the brain:

- Layers I (molecular layer, contains few neurons), II (external granular layer), and III (external pyramidal layer) are the primary input for corticocortical afferents from the same cerebral hemisphere.
- Layer III is the primary output layer of corticocortical efferents to both ipsilateral and contralateral cortices.
- Layer IV (internal granular layer) is the input for specific ipsilateral thalamic and cortical afferents.
- Layer V (internal pyramidal layer) contains the efferents to subcortical structures (i.e., basal ganglia), the brain stem, and spinal cord.
- Layer VI (multiform layer) contains excitatory and inhibitory efferents to the thalamus.

Columnar layers of the cerebral cortex form characteristic cortical columns that share similar functions or pay attention to the same portion of a particular topographic map. Based on the differences in cortical column organization across the cortex, German anatomist Korbinian Brodmann defined numerous cortical areas that were anatomically similar (Fig. 3.6).

Different topographic maps can largely be separated into sensory, motor, and association areas. These may be visually represented as homunculi (Fig. 3.7).

- Sensory
  - Receive and process information from primary sense modalities from contralateral body.
  - Controlled by:
    Visual cortex (vision)

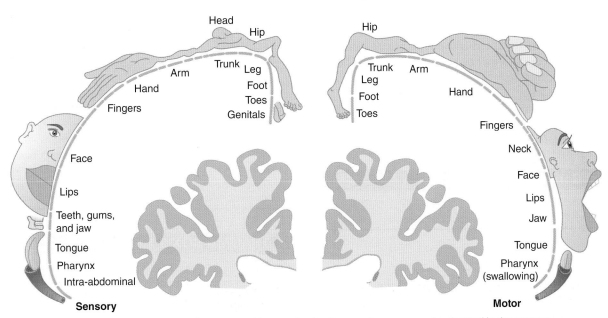

Fig. 3.7 Homunculi representing topographic mapping for the somatosensory cortex, located in the postcentral gyrus in the parietal lobes; and motor cortex, located in the precentral gyrus in the frontal lobe. (From Nolte J. *Elsevier's Integrated Neuroscience*. Philadelphia, PA: Elsevier; 2007: Fig. 9.5.)

Auditory cortex (hearing)

Somatosensory cortex (touch)

Piriform cortex (olfaction)

- Motor
  - Executes voluntary motor movements to contralateral body
  - Controlled by:

    Primary motor cortex

    Supplemental motor area and premotor cortex assist in selecting voluntary movements
- Association
  - Integrate input from various cortical regions into single cortical region.

    Aids in accurate perception of environment.

    Relate information to past experiences to inform future actions.
  - Language processing and production

    For written word, information must travel from primary visual cortex $\rightarrow$ visual association cortex $\rightarrow$ angular gyrus $\rightarrow$ Wernicke's speech area (text/language understanding)

    For vocalization, information must travel from arcuate fasciculus $\rightarrow$ Broca's speech area (motor speech patterns) $\rightarrow$ primary motor cortex (see Clinical Correlation Box 3.4).

Clinical Correlation Box 3.4

The anterior association area, or prefrontal cortex, is essential for planning, executive decision-making, and appropriate social behavior. Famously, an American railroad worker named Phineas Gage reportedly underwent major personality changes (including a tendency toward inappropriate, uninhibited social behavior) after surviving a work accident in which an iron rod was driven completely through his head, destroying most of his left frontal lobe.

Finally, although the right and left cerebral cortex are connected by the corpus callosum (a large tract of corticocortical fibers running across the interhemispheric fissure), there is still functional lateralization of tasks to specific hemispheres.

- Left: Often dominant for speech, writing, language, and algebraic calculation.
- Right: Often dominant for construction and nonverbal ideation, and perceives both sides of visual space (rather than only contralateral side) (see Clinical Correlation Box 3.5).

Clinical Correlation Box 3.5

Left-sided neglect, or inability to see the left visual space, may occur with damage of right hemisphere.

Thalamus

The thalamus (Fig. 3.8) serves several essential functions that are spatially divided:

- Main "relay station" for sensory and motor information between the cerebral cortex (except for olfaction)
  - Ventral anterior (VA) nuclei carry motor signals from cortex to arms.

Also carries motor signals from basal ganglia

- Ventral lateral nuclei carry motor signals from cortex to legs. Also carries motor signals from cerebellum
- Ventral posteromedial nuclei carry sensory signals to cortex from arms.
- Ventral posterolateral nuclei carry sensory signals to cortex from legs.
- Additional key roles in:
  - Emotion (anterior nucleus)
  - Memory (dorsomedial nucleus)
  - Vision (lateral geniculate body)
  - Hearing (medial geniculate body)
  - Integration of sensory and motor systems (pulvinar nucleus)

Given its varied roles as a central signal integrator in the cerebrum, we will discuss the specific thalamic circuits throughout the chapter.

Hypothalamus

As the name implies, the hypothalamus sits just beneath the thalamus (Fig. 3.9). The hypothalamus also serves varied functions in the CNS:

- Regulation of the autonomic nervous system
- Appetite
- Circadian rhythm
- Hormone synthesis and regulation
- Emotion

As with the thalamus, the hypothalamus is divided into several nuclei to serve these functions:

- Anterior nucleus: thermal cooling, parasympathetic tone
- Posterior nucleus: thermal heating, sympathetic tone
- Lateral hypothalamus: stimulates hunger
- Ventromedial nucleus: stimulates satiety
- Suprachiasmatic nucleus (SCN): direct retinal input to regulate circadian rhythm
- Mammillary body: memory (see Fast Facts Box 3.2. Also Trauma Box 3.1, Pharmacology Box 3.1, Development Box 3.1 and Genetic Box 3.1.)

Fast Fact Box 3.2

Orexin is a neuropeptide primarily released by the lateral hypo-thalamic area. When triggered by signals from the suprachiasmatic nucleus, it drives arousal through stimulation of monoaminergic and cholinergic neurons in the brainstem. It is also triggered by ghrelin, a hormone signaling decreased energy stores, and thus increases hunger. Thus hunger indirectly promotes wakefulness, whereas satiety promotes sleep—explaining the phenomenon of "food coma"!

⚡ TRAUMA BOX 3.1

One dramatic aspect of narcolepsy is the "sleep attack," when an affected patient suddenly and unexpectedly falls asleep in the middle of whatever he or she as doing. A related phenomenon is cataplexy, where patients have the abrupt loss of muscle tone in response to strong emotions (laughter, anger, fear, surprise). As you can imagine, these events, leading to the unanticipated loss of consciousness, can be highly dangerous if a patient falls or is operating a motor vehicle or heavy equipment, making catalepsy a major risk for traumatic injury.

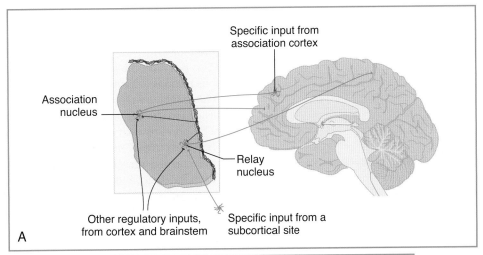

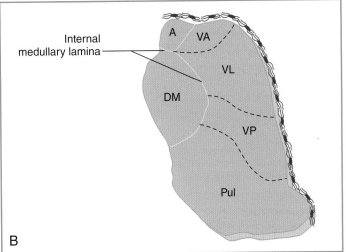

Fig. 3.8 Connections between the thalamus and the cortex (A). The major thalamic nuclei: *A*, Anterior; *DM*, dorsomedial; *LD*, lateral dorsal; *LGB*, lateral geniculate body; *LP*, lateral posterior; *MGB*, medial geniculate body; *P*, pulvinar; *VA*, ventral anterior; *VL*, ventral lateral; *VPL*, ventral posterolateral; *VPM*, ventral posteromedial (B). (Modified from Nolte J. *Elsevier's Integrated Neuroscience*. Philadelphia, PA: Elsevier; 2007. Figs. 5.15 and 5.16.)

PHARMACOLOGY BOX 3.1

Narcolepsy is often treated with stimulants, such as modafinil and armodafinil. These drugs selectively inhibit the reuptake of dopamine and thereby indirectly increase the release of histamine and hypocretins/orexins from hypothalamic neurons. Tangentially related is the observation that first generation anti-histamines often cause somnolence in adults, but may cause hyperactivity in children, indicating that endogenous histamine is important in neural networks involved in sleep wake cycling.

GENETICS BOX 3.1

Narcolepsy is a disease of sleep dysregulation in which affected patients have excessive daytime somnolence, suffer from "sleep attacks" in which they cannot resist the urge to fall asleep, have difficulty sleeping at night and may have vivid dreams, hypnagogic hallucinations, and motor paralysis around transition to sleep. The gene HLA-DQB1*06:02, which encodes peptide presenting proteins on immune cells, is tightly associated to narcolepsy, but how this MHC class II immune system gene is mechanistically related is unclear.

DEVELOPMENT BOX 3.1

Narcolepsy can affect patients of any age, but typically manifests initially in adolescents. Pathologically, there is a loss of hypothalamic neurons that produce hypocretins (also termed orexins) that regulate normal circadian sleep-wake cycles.

Basal Ganglia

The basal ganglia (BG), as their name implies, are located at the base of the forebrain (Fig. 3.10). As with the thalamus and hypothalamus, they are composed of several parts. Known functions include:

- Voluntary motor control (including eye movement)
- Procedural learning

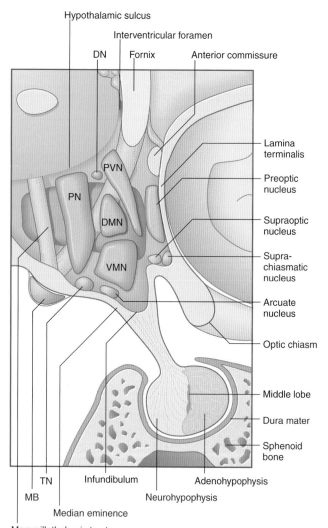

Fig. 3.9 Hypothalamic nuclei and hypophysis, viewed from the lateral side. *DMN*, Dorsomedial nucleus; *DN*, dorsal nucleus; *MB*, mammillary body; *PN*, posterior nucleus; *PVN*, paraventricular nucleus; *TN*, tuberomammillary nucleus; *VMN*, ventromedial nucleus. The lateral hypothalamic nucleus is shown in pink. (From Mtui E, Gruener G, FitzGerald MJT. Fitzgerald's *Clinical Neuroanatomy and Neuroscience*, 7th Edition. Elsevier; 2016. Fig. 26.1.)

The circuits involving the BG are notoriously tricky for students, but it is helpful to replicate the diagrams with special note to the double-negative connections (i.e., inhibition of inhibitors = activation).

The BG assists in initiating voluntary movement through the direct pathway (Fig. 3.11A).

- Initiated by a signal from the cortex (i.e., supplementary motor area).
- This activates the putamen, which in turn inhibits the globus pallidus internus (GPi).
- GPi inhibition releases the inhibitory hold on the thalamus by the GPi, which activates thalamic nuclei, such as VA.
- This promotes excitatory signals travelling to the cortex (i.e., the primary motor cortex).
- Movement is executed.

The BG suppresses unwanted movement through the indirect pathway (Fig. 3.11B).

- Initiated by a signal from the cortex (i.e., supplementary motor area).
- This **activates** the putamen, which in turn inhibits the globus pallidus externus (GPe).
- GPe inhibition releases the subthalamic nucleus (STN).
- The STN activates the GPi, which in turn inhibits the thalamus.
- This prevents excitatory signals from traveling to the cortex (i.e., the primary motor cortex).
- Movement is prevented.

Both the direct and indirect pathways are modulated by dopaminergic projections from the substantia nigra pars compacta to the striatum (caudate and putamen).

- The neurons in the putamen feeding into the direct pathway have primarily D1 receptors.
  - Dopamine (DA) binding $\rightarrow$ D1-R activation $\rightarrow$ excitatory effect on direct pathway $\rightarrow$ promovement
- The neurons in the putamen feeding into the indirect pathway have primarily D2 receptors.
  - DA binding $\rightarrow$ D2-R activation $\rightarrow$ inhibitory effect on indirect pathway $\rightarrow$ promovement

Reward Circuit

DA also plays a key role in reward learning. The parts of the brain that are thought to be involved in reward learning are:

- Nucleus accumbens
- Ventral pallidum
- Ventral tegmental area (VTA)

Note that all three areas are also linked into the limbic system, which regulates emotion.

The primary pathway involved in reward learning is the VTA to nucleus accumbens.

- Dopamine is the key neurotransmitter to "code" rewarding outcomes
- If reality > expectations $\rightarrow$ firing increased
- If expectations > reality $\rightarrow$ firing suppressed (see Clinical Correlation Box 3.6)

Clinical Correlation Box 3.6

Drugs (such as amphetamine and cocaine) that act to upregulate dopamine release or potentiate the neurotransmitter's effects can induce addictive behavior through the reward circuitry.

Although this model helps characterize adaptive learned behavior to immediate rewards, the neural mechanism underlying delayed gratification is not understood via this mechanism.

Memory and the Limbic System

Memory can be classified as declarative or nondeclarative.

- Nondeclarative memory is procedural memory, which can be thought of as "muscle memory," for example, the skills for riding a bike or playing the piano.

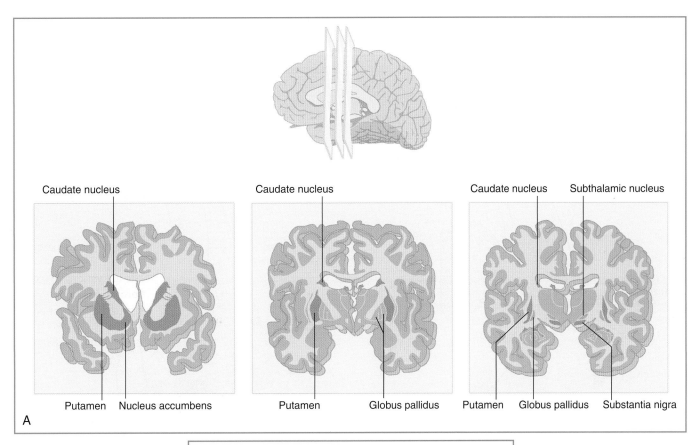

Caudate nucleus

Caudate nucleus

Caudate nucleus   Subthalamic nucleus

Putamen   Nucleus accumbens

Putamen   Globus pallidus

Putamen   Globus pallidus   Substantia nigra

A

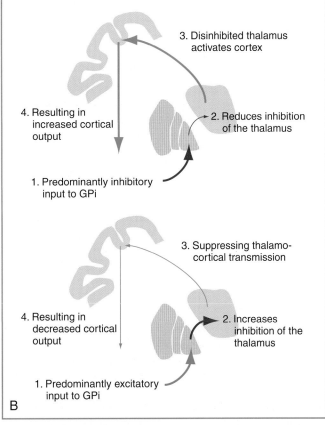

3. Disinhibited thalamus
activates cortex

4. Resulting in
increased cortical
output

2. Reduces inhibition
of the thalamus

1. Predominantly inhibitory
input to GPi

3. Suppressing thalamo-
cortical transmission

4. Resulting in
decreased cortical
output

2. Increases
inhibition of the
thalamus

1. Predominantly excitatory
input to GPi

B

Fig. 3.10 Coronal sections through the brain illustrate the relative anatomic positions of the deep structures of the brain that comprise the basal ganglia (A). Connections between the basal ganglia and the thalamus (B), with *red arrows* indicating inhibitory signals and *green arrows* indicating activating signals. *GPi*, Gobus pallidus internus. (Modified from Nolte J. *Elsevier's Integrated Neuroscience.* Philadelphia, PA: Elsevier; 2007.)

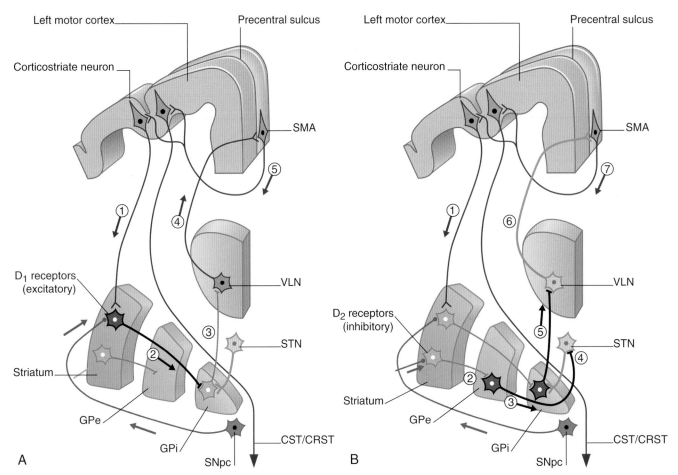

Fig. 3.11 Coronal section through the motor loop. A, The sequence of five sets of neurons involved in the "direct" pathway from sensorimotor cortex to thalamus with final return to sensorimotor cortex via SMA. B, The sequence of seven sets of neurons involved in the "indirect" pathway. The *red/pink* neurons are excitatory utilizing glutamate. The *black/gray* neurons are inhibitory utilizing γ-aminobutyric acid. The *brown*, nigrostriatal neuron uses dopamine which is excitatory via D1 receptors on target striatal neurons and inhibitory via D2 receptors on the same and other striatal neurons. *CST/CRST*, Corticospinal, corticoreticular fibers; *GPe*, globus pallidus externus; *GPi*, globus pallidus internus; *GPL, GPM*, lateral and medial segments of globus pallidus; *SMA*, supplementary motor area; *SNpc*, compact part of substantia nigra; *STN*, subthalamic nucleus; *VLN*, ventral lateral nucleus of thalamus. (From Mtui E, Gruener G, FitzGerald MJT. *Fitzgerald's Clinical Neuroanatomy and Neuroscience,* 7th Edition. Elsevier; 2016. Fig. 33.2.)

- Declarative memory can be further broken down into:
  - Episodic: Ability to reexperience past events
  - Semantic: Knowing facts, or the ability to recognize familiar people
  - Working: Information that one can manipulate in the short-term, for example, remembering a phone number while dialing it.

Episodic memory requires a process of encoding/learning new information (which requires attention and working memory), storage/consolidation of the information, and retrieval of the information.

- Retrieval via recognition: Choosing the right answer on a multiple-choice question.
- Retrieval via recall: Filling in the answer to a free-response question.

Because working memory commonly declines with age, so too can episodic memory, because the initial step of encoding can be impaired. Semantic memory is usually spared by normal aging, but can be affected by a variety of brain pathologies, including viral infections (such as herpes encephalitis), certain strokes, semantic dementia, and Alzheimer disease (AD).

The limbic system tightly couples emotional learning and memory (Fig. 3.12). The primary pathway involved in these processes is the Papez circuit (Fig. 3.13).

- Function: primarily responsible for memory
- Trajectory
  - Hippocampus → hypothalamus → thalamus → cortex → hippocampus

There are some additional structures that feed into this circuit, which are thought to mediate specific behaviors and memory processing.

- The dorsomedial nucleus of the thalamus has reciprocal connections with the hypothalamus and cortex (orbitofrontal

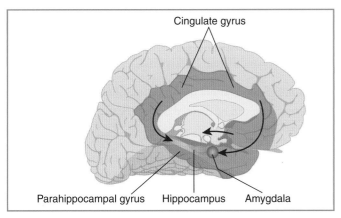

Fig. 3.12 An anatomic schematic of the limbic system, with representative connections. (From Nolte J. *Elsevier's Integrated Neuroscience.* Philadelphia, PA: Elsevier; 2007.)

and prefrontal). It may play a role specifically in affective behavior and memory.

- The amygdala has been implicated in fear and excessive sympathetic stimulation (see Clinical Correlation Box 3.27).

Clinical Correlation Box 3.7

Bilateral lesions to the amygdala can cause Klüver-Bucy syndrome, which elicits placidity, hyperorality (compulsion to examine objects by mouth), hyperphagia or pica (overeating or eating inappropriate objects), visual agnosia (inability to recognize familiar objects/people), and hypersexuality.

Although this model helps explain some aspects of short-term memory storage, the neural basis for long-term storage of explicit memory (including episodic and semantic memory) is not yet understood (see Case Study Box 3.1).

Case Study Box 3.1

A cornerstone of all neuroscience curricula, Henry Gustav Molaison (previously known only as H.M. to protect his identity) has helped scientists understand that working and procedural memory work through different mechanisms than explicit memory formation.

Molaison was a patient who had bilateral surgical removal of the anterior two-thirds of his medial temporal lobes (including the hippocampi and amygdalae) to try to cure his intractable epilepsy. After the surgery, he was no longer able to form new explicit memories and had severe anterograde amnesia (and moderate retrograde amnesia). However, he retained most of his presurgical memories and knowledge, and had functioning working and long-term procedural memory. Even though he could not remember it, he was able to learn and improve on new motor skills.

This was a rare case that gave insights into the development of theories based around cognition and memory, and some major differences between the formation and storage of different types of memory.

The Cerebellum

The name cerebellum is derived from the diminutive form of the Latin word for brain (cerebrum), and thus translates into "little brain." It lies just below the cerebral hemispheres and posterior to the fourth ventricle and brainstem. It functions to coordinate and regulate motor activity. Although less well characterized, it

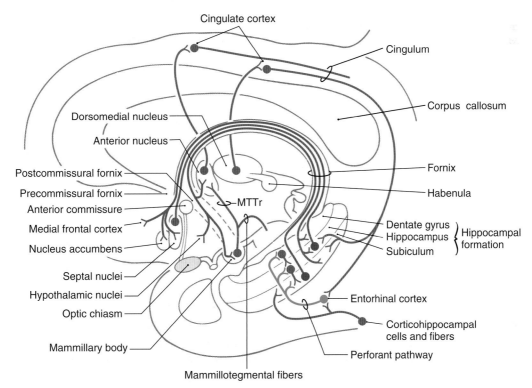

Fig. 3.13 The Papez circuit of the limbic system. *MTTr,* Mammillothalamic pathway. (From Haines DE, Mihailoff GA. *Fundamental Neuroscience for Basic and Clinical Applications,* 5th Edition. Elsevier; 2018. Fig. 31.5.)

has also been suggested that the cerebellum may play a role in cognitive functions, such as language, attention, and regulating fear or pleasure.

Compared with the cerebrum, the cerebellum has several distinct structural features:
- Two hemispheres connected in the middle by cortex called the vermis.
- Small lobe at the posterior border called the flocculonodulus.
- Connection to the brainstem through three pairs of cerebellar peduncles.
  - Superior: Primary output carrying information from cerebellum to thalamus and red nucleus of midbrain
  - Middle: Input from contralateral cerebral cortex
  - Inferior: Input about proprioception from ipsilateral body

Cerebellar Cortex

Unlike the cerebrum, the cerebellar cortex has only three neural layers that are homogeneous across space. From deep to superficial:
- Granular layer: Includes numerous, small granule cell bodies (glutaminergic) and fewer Golgi cells.
  - The excitatory granule cells project up to the molecular layer, forming parallel fibers.
  - The Golgi cells act as local inhibitory feedback on the granule cells.
- Purkinje layer: Composed of the cell bodies of the Purkinje cells and cortical interneurons.
  - The inhibitory projections of the Purkinje cells are the only output of the cerebellar cortex.
  - These axons project through the cerebellar white matter to the deep cerebellar nuclei (there are four: fastigial, globose, emboliform, and dentate) or vestibular nuclei.
- Molecular layer. This layer contains the dendrites of the Purkinje cells, the parallel fibers, stellate cells, and basket cells.
  - Stellate and basket cells both inhibit the Purkinje cells via gamma aminobutyric acid (GABA)ergic synapses.
  - The parallel fibers are axons of the granule cells, which run perpendicular to the dendrites of the Purkinje cells (Fig. 3.14).
    The parallel fibers synapse onto the dendritic projections of thousands of Purkinje cells.
    These excitatory synapses modulate the firing of the Purkinje cells, and potentially play a role in adaptive motor learning.

The microcircuitry of the cerebellum can be simplified into a very simple block diagram (Fig. 3.15). There are only two inputs to the cerebellum, both excitatory to their targets:
- Climbing fibers
  - Arise from the contralateral inferior olivary nucleus of the medulla
  - Travel through the inferior cerebellar peduncle
  - Synapse onto deep nuclei and Purkinje cells
- Mossy fibers
  - Main afferents from all other cerebellar inputs (especially brainstem and spinocerebellar tract)
  - Synapse onto deep nuclei and granule cells (indirectly exciting Purkinje cells)

Just like the cerebral cortex, the cerebellar cortex also contains somatotopic maps (Fig. 3.16) of sensory input and motor output. In this map, the parallel fibers of granule cells are thought to span different body parts.

Functional Subdivisions of the Cerebellum

The cerebellum can be divided into three main functional subdivisions (Fig. 3.17):
1. Vestibulocerebellum
   a. Includes flocculonodulus and fastigial nucleus
   b. Associated with controlling eye movements and posture
2. Spinocerebellum
   a. Includes the vermis, intermediate zone, globose nucleus, and emboliform nucleus
   b. Associated with maintenance of position and posture of the trunk (vermis) and extremity (intermediate zone)
3. Cerebrocerebellum
   a. Includes the cerebellar hemisphere and dentate nucleus
   b. Associated with fine motor control

STRUCTURE AND FUNCTION: THE SPINAL CORD

The spinal cord carries two broad types of communication:
1. Efferent motor neural outputs from the brain
2. Afferent sensory neural inputs to the brain to the body

The spinal cord begins just inferior to the brainstem. In the newborn the spinal cord terminates (conus terminalis) at the body of L3, whereas in the adult the spinal cord only extends to the lower border of L1.

There are 31 pairs of spinal nerves:
- 8 cervical (C1–C8)
- 12 thoracic (T1–T12)
- 5 lumbar (L1–L5)
- 5 sacral (S1–S5)
- 1 coccygeal (Co) nerve pair

Peripheral spinal neurons (not including cranial nerves) enter and exit the spinal cord through intervertebral foramen between adjacent vertebrae. C1 however exits between the occipital bone of the skull and the first vertebra (the atlas).

All branches of spinal nerves contain both efferent motor and afferent sensory fibers:
- Motor fibers travel out through the ventral roots from the anterior horn of the gray matter.
- Sensory fibers travel in through the dorsal roots to the posterior horn of the gray matter.

Somatotopic Organization

Instead of being surrounded by gray matter like the brain, the spinal cord has superficial white matter tracts surrounding the deeper gray matter.

Just like the brain, the spinal cord maintains somatotopic organization within the central gray matter and surrounding white matter tracts (Fig. 3.18).

Although each spinal cord segment may seem to look alike at first, there are many key characteristics that can help differentiate the level of the spinal cord segment.

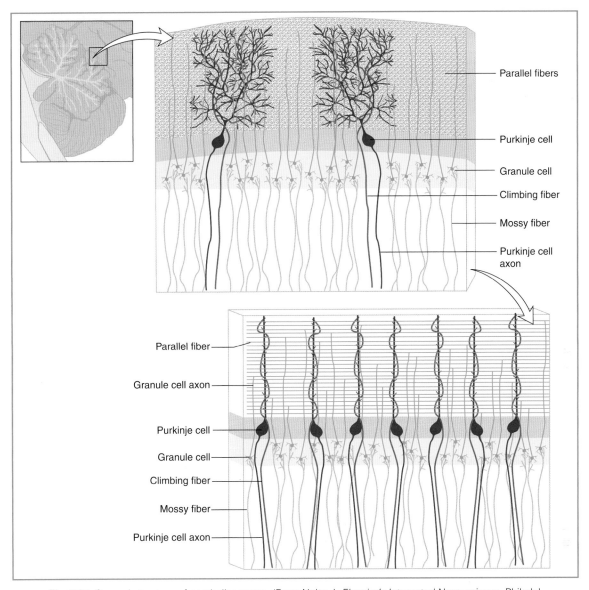

Fig. 3.14 General structure of cerebellar cortex. (From Nolte J. *Elsevier's Integrated Neuroscience.* Philadelphia, PA: Elsevier; 2007.)

- Amount of gray matter versus white matter (Fig. 3.19)
  - White matter decreases rostral to caudal because fewer neurons travel to/from the end of the spinal cord
- Amount of gray matter in anterior horn (see Fig. 3.18)
  - Increase in lateral anterior horn cell mass at level of arms and legs
- Interomediolateral cell column (lateral horn) presence
  - Primarily present from C8 to L3
  - Innervation to viscera

Major Descending Tract

The spinal cord contains many descending tracts that travel from the brain or brain stem to the spinal cord to elicit motor output.

- Most of these tracts contain an upper motor neuron (UMN) that will cross from one side of the body to the other at the level of the brain stem. If all of the nerves in the tract cross together at the same level, this is called a decussation.

- UMN is carried down spinal cord in a white matter tract.
- Close to the level of the spinal cord that it will exit, the UMN will synapse onto a lower motor neuron (LMN) in the anterior horn of the gray matter.
- The LMN will exit the ventral horn and innervate a target muscle.

Therefore each hemisphere of the cerebrum controls the contralateral side of the body. However, if the cerebellum modifies motor control, it usually synapses on an UMN on the contralateral side. Thus the cerebellum controls the ipsilateral side of the body.

There are two main categories of descending pathways: lateral and medial tracts.

- Lateral
  - Lateral corticospinal tract and rubrospinal tract
  - Primarily control distal musculature and activate flexor muscles

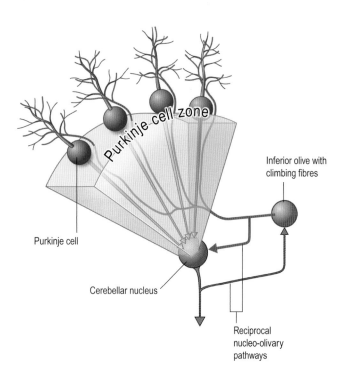

Fig. 3.15 A cerebellar module illustrating the microcircuitry of the cerebellum. Purkinje cell axons and climbing fibers are located in a white matter compartment, shown as a transparent structure in this diagram. (From *Gray's Anatomy*, 41st Edition. Elsevier; 2016. Fig. 22.12A.)

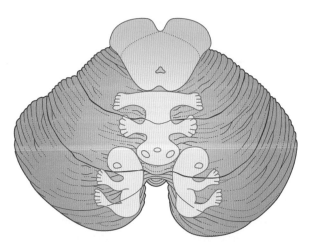

Fig. 3.16 The two somatotopic neural maps of the body projected onto the cerebellar cortex. These maps are primarily associated with the spinocerebellum. (From Mtui E, Gruener G, FitzGerald MJT. *Fitzgerald's Clinical Neuroanatomy and Neuroscience*, 7th Edition. Elsevier; 2016. Fig. 25.7.)

- Medial
  - Vestibulospinal tracts, reticulospinal tracts, and ventral corticospinal tracts
  - Primarily control axial musculature and activate extensor muscles

The primary descending tract we will discuss is the corticospinal tract (Fig. 3.20).

- Involved in voluntary skilled motor activity (primarily of the upper limbs).

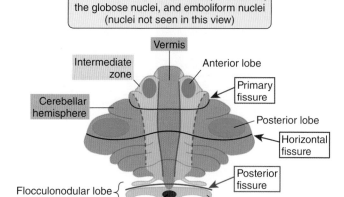

Fig. 3.17 The three functional units of the cerebellum: vestibulocerebellum, spinocerebellum, and cerebrocerebellum. (Modified from Singer HS, Mink JW, Gilbert DL, Jankovic J. *Movement Disorders in Childhood*, 2nd Edition, Elsevier; 2015. Fig. 2.1.)

- Inputs
  - Primary (2/3) $\rightarrow$ motor cortex, premotor cortex, supplementary motor area
  - Minor (1/3) $\rightarrow$ Somatosensory cortex, cingulate gyrus, association areas of parietal lobe
- Pathway
  - Cortex $\rightarrow$ posterior limb of internal capsule $\rightarrow$ brainstem $\rightarrow$ pyramidal decussation at medulla oblongata $\rightarrow$ descent $\rightarrow$ synapse onto LMN in dorsolateral anterior horn $\rightarrow$ alpha motor neuron $\rightarrow$ target muscle

The corticobulbar tract serves a similar role in intentional motor movement for the face and neck. The LMNs for the corticobulbar tract are cranial nerves.

Major Ascending Tracts

The spinal cord also contains many ascending tracts that travel from the spinal cord to the brain or rostral spinal cord. These tracts collect information from different sensory neurons in the PNS and relay this information primarily to the brain for processing and/or monitoring of the external world or intrinsic self.

- Sensory input enters first-order neurons, whose cell bodies lie in the dorsal root ganglion.
- The first-order neurons usually synapse onto ipsilateral second-order neurons.
- The second-order neurons **cross** at or above the level of the first-order neurons.
- Second-order neurons continue to ascend on contralateral side and synapse with third-order neurons in the thalamus.
- Thalamic neurons project the somatosensory cortex (postcentral gyrus).

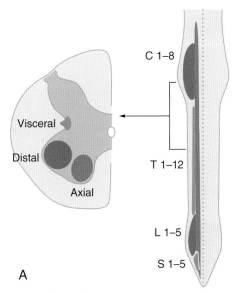

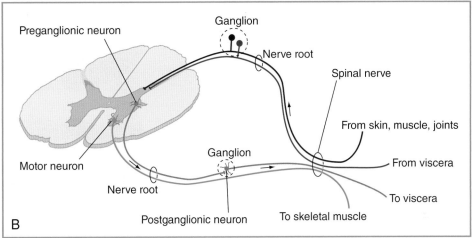

Fig. 3.18 A, An axial section of the spinal cord illustrating the somatotopic organization of the motor neurons in the anterior horn of the grey matter (left). A longitudinal section of the spinal cord to demonstrate the presence of enlarged anterior horns because of the innervation of the arms and legs (*light blue*), and the presence of a lateral horn (interomediolateral cell column) in the thoracic and sacral regions to innervate viscera. B, Schematic view of the origins and terminations of the fibers found in spinal nerves. (B from Nolte J. *Elsevier's Integrated Neuroscience*. Philadelphia, PA: Elsevier; 2007.)

There are two primary ascending pathways: the spinothalamic tract and the dorsal columns (see Fig. 3.19):
- Spinothalamic tract: Carries sensation of pain and temperature
- Dorsal columns: Carries sensation of proprioception (where the body is in space), discriminative touch, and vibration
Their differences are summarized in Table 3.4 (see Fast Facts Box 3.3).

Fast Fact Box 3.3
Because the ascending and descending paths travel in opposite directions through the spinal cord, Wallerian degeneration occurs in opposite directions. Ascending tracts above the lesion will degenerate following spinal cord injury, whereas descending tract below the lesion will degenerate.

Monosynaptic (Myotatic) Spinal Reflex
A reflex is an involuntary action in response to a stimulus.
- Reflexes are primarily controlled by circuits within the spinal cord.
- As reflexes do not require processing by the cerebral cortex, they are usually instantaneous.
- Certain reflexes can be repressed through top-down control of cortical signaling to inhibitory interneurons in the spinal cord.
Reflex arcs can be:
- Autonomic or somatic (affecting muscle tone).
- Highly complex, containing many synapses, or simple with only a single afferent and a single efferent limb that mediates reflexive movement.
  - All reflex arcs must contain at least one afferent and one efferent limb.

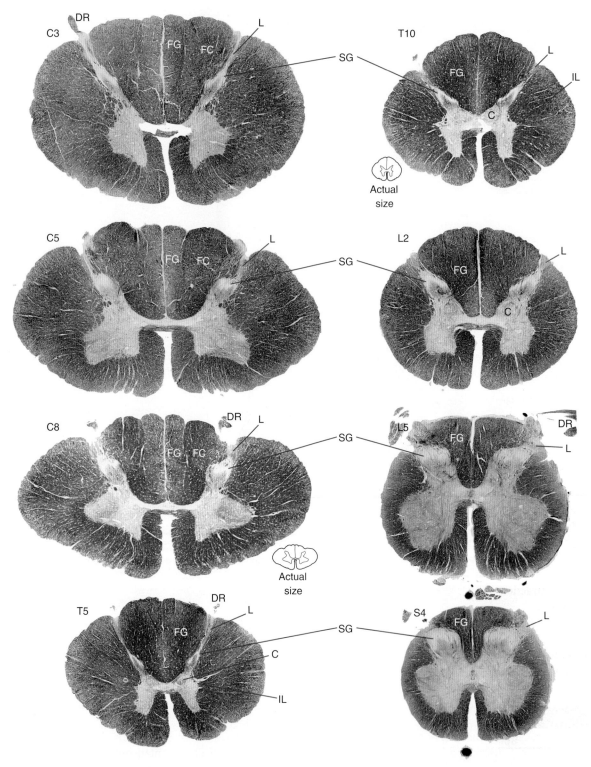

Fig. 3.19 Pathology spinal cord segments depicting how the anatomy of the cord changes from the most rostral segment (top left) to the most caudal segment (bottom right). *C*, Clarke's nucleus; *DR*, dorsal root; *FC*, fasciculus cuneatus; *FG*, fasciculus gracilis; *IL*, intermediolateral cell column; *L*, Lissauer's tract; *SG*, substantia gelatinosa. (From Vanderah TW, Gould DJ. *Nolte's the Human Brain*, 7th Edition. Elsevier; 2016. Fig. 10.8.)

To describe the reflex arc, we will discuss a simple monosynaptic muscle stretch reflex, or myotatic reflex, using the familiar example of the patellar reflex "knee jerk" (Fig. 3.21):

- The muscle possesses intrafusal fibers, composed of muscle spindles sensing muscle proprioception, running parallel to muscle fibers.

- A reflex hammer hits the patellar tendon, causing the quadriceps muscle to elongate.
- When the muscle lengthens, the muscle spindle is stretched and increases firing rate.
- This signal is transmitted to the alpha-motor neurons, which also increase firing rate.

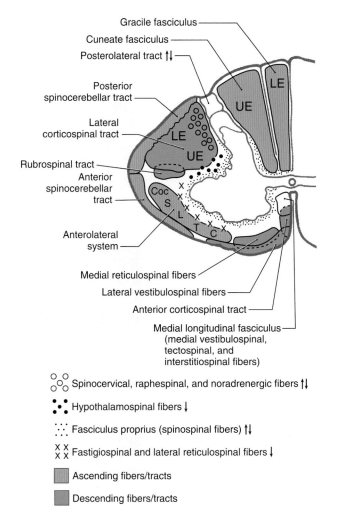

Gracile fasciculus
Cuneate fasciculus
Posterolateral tract ↑↓
Posterior spinocerebellar tract
Lateral corticospinal tract
Rubrospinal tract
Anterior spinocerebellar tract
Anterolateral system
Medial reticulospinal fibers
Lateral vestibulospinal fibers
Anterior corticospinal tract
Medial longitudinal fasciculus (medial vestibulospinal, tectospinal, and interstitiospinal fibers)

Spinocervical, raphespinal, and noradrenergic fibers ↑↓
Hypothalamospinal fibers ↓
Fasciculus proprius (spinospinal fibers) ↑↓
Fastigiospinal and lateral reticulospinal fibers ↓

Ascending fibers/tracts
Descending fibers/tracts

Fig. 3.20 Locations of the ascending and descending tracts of the spinal cord within the white matter. (From Haines DE, Mihailoff GA. *Fundamental Neuroscience for Basic and Clinical Applications*, 5th Edition Philadelphia, PA: Elsevier; 2018. Fig. 9.12.)

- This causes contraction of the quadriceps muscle (and thus knee extension).

Often, the afferent neurons will also synapse onto an interneuron, which synapses onto α motor neurons (αMNs) for the antagonistic muscle to cause that muscle to relax so there is not cocontraction on either side of the joint.

CENTRAL NERVOUS SYSTEM PATHOPHYSIOLOGY

The CNS is our source of conscious and unconscious behavior, and coordinates and integrates motor and sensory signals from the entire body. When a part of the CNS is not functioning appropriately, a wide range of symptoms can occur ranging from mild fatigue and confusion, to the ability to only move the eyes and nothing else.

Cerebral Disease

Dementia encompasses several diseases characterized by cognitive deficits in memory, communication, language, attention, judgment, reasoning, and occasionally visual perception.

Although there are many causes of dementia, the vast majority of cases are caused by AD, especially in patients older than 65 years of age.

- AD is a neurodegenerative disease of cortical neurons, glutamatergic neurons, and cholinergic neurons in the nucleus basalis of Meynert.
- Characterized by cortical atrophy beginning in the temporal lobes.
- On pathology, one finds:
  - Neurofibrillary tangles containing hyperphosphorylated tau protein
  - Amyloid plaques composed of amyloid β (Aβ) protein, with the pathogenic protein comprised of 42 (versus 40) amino acids.
    Aβ-42 is cleaved from amyloid precursor protein (APP), which is encoded by a gene on chromosome 21; thus, patients with Trisomy 21 have an increased genetic risk of AD because of increased APP production.
    The most common cause of early-onset AD is from missense mutations in *presinilin* genes 1 and 2, which increase the production of Aβ-42.

Aphasia is also a broad term, meaning the loss or decreased capacity for communication. Two classic types of aphasia occurring from cortical lesions are:

- Broca's aphasia
  - Broca's area (frontal lobe) controls motor output for speech
  - Lesion causes nonfluent speech with retained comprehension

TABLE 3.4	**Comparison of the Spinothalamic Tract and the Dorsal Columns**	
	Spinothalamic Tract	**Dorsal Columns**
Function	Pain and temperature	Conscious proprioception, discriminative touch, vibration
Receptors	Free nerve endings of fast-conducting A-δ and slow-conducting C pain fibers	Muscle spindles, Golgi tendon organs, Pacinian & Meissner's corpuscles
First-order neuron	Soma in DRG. Project through Lissauer's (dorsolateral) tract	Soma in DRG. Project to gracile or cuneate fascicles and ascend to caudal medulla. Also project to collaterals for spinal reflexes
Second-order neuron	Soma in dorsal horn.	Soma in gracile or cuneate nuclei of caudal medulla
Location of crossing second-order neurons	Ventral white commissure of the spinal cord, at approximately the level of first-order neuron entry. The second-order axon continues to ascend in the contralateral white matter to the thalamus	Internal arcuate fibers in the medulla, that merge to form the medial lemniscus in the medulla. The second-order fibers continue to ascend in the medial lemniscus to the thalamus
Third-order neurons	Soma in VPL nucleus of the thalamus	Soma in VPL nucleus of the thalamus

DRG, Dorsal root ganglion; *VPL*, ventral posterolateral.

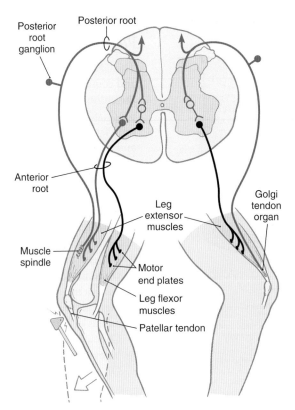

Fig. 3.21 Pathway for the patellar tendon reflex and reciprocal inhibition (left) and autogenic inhibition (right). The inhibitory glycinergic interneurons are represented by the red open cell bodies. (From Haines DE, Mihailoff GA. *Fundamental Neuroscience for Basic and Clinical Applications*, 5th Edition. Philadelphia, PA: Elsevier; 2018. Fig. 9.9.)

- Wernicke's aphasia
  - Wernicke's area (temporal lobe) processes language input
  - Lesion causes nonsensical speech with poor comprehension

Pathology of Deep Brain Structures

Parkinson disease is a degenerative disorder of the substantia nigra and its projections to the striatum.
- Loss of dopaminergic input → suppression of direct pathway and activation of indirect pathway → net antimovement effect (Fig. 3.22)
- Symptoms include a "pill-rolling" tremor at rest, cogwheel rigidity, masked facies (reduced expression), shuffling gait, and bradykinesia (slow movement).
- Dementia occurs in later stages of the disease.

Parkinson disease may be treated with a combination of levodopa (a dopamine precursor able to cross the blood-brain barrier) with carbidopa (does not cross the blood-brain barrier and decreases the amount of levodopa that circulates peripherally). Another treatment is deep brain stimulation, using a probe to inhibit GPi and thus increase promovement circuits.

Wilson disease, or hepatolenticular degeneration, is an autosomal recessive disorder of copper metabolism. Excessive copper deposition leads to pathology involving the following organs:
- Liver, leading to cirrhosis
- Eyes, giving rise to the pathognomonic corneal Kayser-Fleischer rings

- Lentiform nucleus (putamen and globus pallidus) of the basal ganglia leading to:
  - Tremor ("wing-beating")
  - Chorea (dance-like movements)
  - Athetosis (serpentine movements)
  - Rigidity
  - Psychosis

Wilson disease can be treated with penicillamine, a copper chelator, to combat the excess copper deposition.

Posterior Fossa Malformations

In Arnold-Chiari type 1 malformations, the posterior fossa is reduced and causes herniation of the cerebellar tonsils through the foramen magnum at the base of the skull. Symptoms include headache, unsteady gait, and other cerebellar signs.

In the more severe Arnold-Chiari type 2 malformations, the brainstem may also be caudally displaced, resulting in potential paralysis if the descending spinal tracts are affected.

Cerebellar Disease

Chronic alcohol abuse can lead to superior anterior vermis atrophy because of direct toxicity of alcohol to the cerebellum. This disorder is characterized by truncal and lower more than upper limb dystaxia, leading to gait abnormalities. It will stabilize and even improve with cessation of alcohol intake, and worsen with continued abuse.

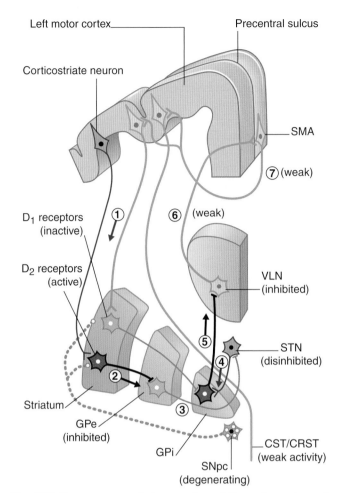

Fig. 3.22 Consequences of degeneration of the pathway from the compact part of the substantia nigra (*SNpc*) to the striatum (S) in Parkinson disease. The effects arise from loss of tonic facilitation of spiny striatal neurons bearing D1 receptors, together with loss of tonic inhibition of those bearing D2 receptors. The direct pathway is disengaged, and the indirect pathway is activated by default. (1) Corticostriate neurons from the sensorimotor cortex now strongly activate those GABAergic neurons (2) in the striatum that synapse upon others (3) in the external pallidal segment (*GPe*). The double effect is disinhibition of the subthalamic nucleus (*STN*). The STN discharges strongly (4) onto the GABAergic neurons of the internal pallidal segment (*GPi*); these in turn discharge strongly (5) into the ventral lateral nucleus (*VLN*) of thalamus, resulting in reduced output along thalamocortical fibers (6) traveling to the supplementary motor area (*SMA*). Inputs (7) from SMA to corticospinal and corticoreticular fibers (*CST/CRST*) become progressively weaker, with consequences for initiation and execution of movements. (From Mtui E, Gruener G, FitzGerald MJT. *Fitzgerald's Clinical Neuroanatomy and Neuroscience,* 7th Edition. Elsevier; 2016. Fig. 33.6.)

Medulloblastoma, the most common pediatric brain tumor, arises from an overproliferation of primitive cerebellar cells. Children often present with a stumbling gait and dizziness, as well as signs of ICP caused by blockage of the fourth ventricle. This tumor is often treated with a triad of chemotherapy, radiation, and surgical resection.

Spinal Cord Lesions

Complete transection of the spinal cord causes complete paralysis and sensory loss bilaterally at and distal to the lesion.

Brown-Séquard Syndrome

Occurs with a partial transection of one-half of the spinal cord. This causes:
- Ipsilateral weakness below the lesion, because of inability of the crossed corticospinal tract to synapse onto the distal αMNs.
- Ipsilateral loss of conscious proprioception below the lesion, because of inability of the uncrossed first-order neurons to ascend in the dorsal columns.
- Contralateral loss of pain and temperature at and below the lesion, because of inability of contralateral second-order fibers of the spinothalamic tract to ascend.
- Ipsilateral loss of pain and temperature at the level of the lesion, because of the loss of the ipsilateral dorsal horn, where all first-order sensory nerves enter.

Babinski Sign

Normally, stroking the inferior lateral edge of the foot across the ball of the foot elicits a reflex causing flexion (plantarflexion) of the toes. However, if it produces extension (dorsiflexion) of the toes, this is termed a "Babinski sign."
- In infants, this is normal. This is because the myelination of the corticospinal tract (promoting flexion) is not complete until 1 to 2 years of age.
- In adults, this is pathologic. It reflects loss of influence of the corticospinal tract, leading to extensor response.

Upper Versus Lower Motor Neuron Diseases

Lesions of the corticospinal tract can occur in:
- UMNs, that is, above the αMN
- LMNS, that is, the αMNs
  In UMN lesions, patients present with:
- Weakness
- Hyperreflexia (because of lack of cortical inhibition of spinal cord reflexes)
- Spasticity/increased tone (because of lack of cortical inhibition)
- Presence of Babinski sign
  In LMN lesions, patients present with:
- Weakness
- Diminished reflexes (because of loss of efferent spinal cord circuitry)
- Atrophy ± fasciculations (small muscle twitches)
- No Babinski's sign

SUMMARY

- The CNS consciously and unconsciously integrates motor and sensory information from the internal and external environments help us understand and interact with the world.
- The CNS has two major components: the brain and spinal cord.
- The brain is protected by the bony skull, three layers of meninges (the pia, arachnoid, and dura mater) and CSF fluid which bathes the brain. A blood-brain barrier also exits around the brain to protect it from harmful metabolites and chemicals circulating in the blood stream.
- The blood supply to the brain arises from the internal carotids and vertebral arteries to form the circle of Willis.
- Cerebral blood flow and cerebral perfusion pressure are carefully autoregulated to ensure that the brain receives adequate nutrients.
- The cortex is a collection of specialized neurons that are heterogeneous in function and space, often with topographic organization representing specific areas of the body.

- The thalamus acts as the main relay station between the cortex and other parts of the brain and spinal cord.
- The basal ganglia and cerebellum are both involved in regulation of movement.
- The spinal cord serves as an afferent and efferent extension of the brain. The main efferent descending pathway of the spinal cord is the corticospinal tract, which controls conscious movement of the body. The main afferent ascending pathways of the spinal cord are the spinothalamic tract, sensing pain and temperature, and the dorsal columns, sensing conscious proprioception, light touch, and vibration.
- The cerebrum tends to control and sense the contralateral side of the body, while the cerebellum tends to control the ipsilateral side of the body.

REVIEW QUESTIONS

Directions: Each of the numbered items or incomplete statements in this section is followed by answers or by completions of the statement. Select the one lettered answer or completion that is best in each case.

1. Which of the following symptoms would help differentiate between a patient with meningitis versus infectious encephalitis/brain abscess?
   A. Fever
   B. Headache
   C. Paralysis in the right hand
   D. Nuchal rigidity
   E. Positive Brudziński's neck sign

2. A healthy 4-year-old boy slipped while running on ice, hitting the right temple region of his head. He was initially lucid, but lost consciousness on his way to the hospital. Which one of the following signs or symptoms was likely not present in the patient when he arrived at the hospital?
   A. Mydriasis of the right eye
   B. Decreased respiratory ability
   C. Weakness of left-sided extremities
   D. Lacunar stroke
   E. No fracture of the temporal bone

3. Which of the following statements is not true?
   A. Epidural hematomas may cross the falx cerebri, but not sutures
   B. Subdural hematomas cross the falx cerebri and tentorium cerebelli
   C. Not all epidural hematomas are arterial in origin
   D. If air is detected in an epidural hematoma, a sinus or mastoid air cell may be fractured

   E. Cerebral edema as secondary brain injury can compress ventricles and efface sulci

4. Which of the following therapies could be used to reduce intracranial pressure?
   A. Hypoventilation
   B. Mannitol therapy
   C. Hyperbaric oxygen with hypoventilation
   D. A and B only
   E. B and C only
   F. All of the above

5. A 66-year-old patient presents with sudden weakness in his face and right arm, but largely preserved leg strength, and no other apparent symptoms. Which vascular distribution is likely affected?
   A. Left anterior cerebral artery (ACA)
   B. Left posterior inferior cerebellar artery (PICA)
   C. Left anterior inferior cerebellar artery (AICA)
   D. Pontine branches of the basilar artery
   E. Left middle cerebral artery (MCA)

6. A 23-year-old known male drug user presents with bradykinesia, akinesia, and rigidity. Which of the following structures likely has neurons with increased firing?
   A. Thalamic neurons projecting to the cortex
   B. Neurons from the putamen projecting to the GPi
   C. Neurons in the STN projecting to the GPi
   D. Dopaminergic neurons projecting from the substantia nigra pars compacta to the putamen
   E. Neurons from the GPe to the STN

ANSWERS TO REVIEW QUESTIONS

1. **The answer is C.** Meningitis occurs with no focal neurologic defects because the meninges are inflamed, not a local portion of the brain. This is different from infectious encephalitis or a brain abscess in which a particular area of the brain is directly affected, thus causing focal neurologic defects, such as paralysis or loss of sensation in parts of the body that correspond to the infected part of the brain. Encephalitis and meningitis can both present with nonspecific symptoms, such as fever and headache. A positive Brudziński's neck sign occurs when a forced flexion of the neck elicits a reflexive flexion of the hips, which "cancels out" the irritation caused by the spinal cord within the meninges when the neck is flexed. Nuchal rigidity and a positive Brudziński's neck sign are also not particularly sensitive for meningitis, and can also be seen in encephalitis, depending on the region of the brain that is infected.

2. **The answer is D.** Lacunar strokes are caused by occlusion of a deep penetrating artery, and are likely caused by atherosclerosis (likely not significant in such a young patient) or lipohyalinosis (small-vessel disease in the brain) because of hypertension (also not likely in such a young patient). This presentation of lucidity followed by a rapid loss of consciousness after trauma to the temporal bone most likely is caused by an epidural hematoma. The hematoma can compress intracranial structures, such as CN III which travels with the parasympathetic fibers (which usually constrict the pupil), leading to a dilated/ "blown" pupil (mydriasis) that is fixed down and out because of unopposed CN IV and CN VI innervation of the superior oblique and lateral rectus, respectively. Uncal (transtentorial) herniation caused by increased ICP can compress the medulla leading to respiratory arrest and death. The effect of increased pressure or mass effect can also lead to compression of the crossed pyramid pathways, causing weakness on the opposite side of the lesion. Children have increased skull plasticity, so epidural hematomas can occur without fracture.

3. **The answer is B.** Subdural hematomas are bounded between the arachnoid and the dura, including the dural reflections, such as the tentorium cerebelli and falx. Because epidural hematomas lie on top of the dura, they are not bounded by dural reflections. Epidural hematomas can be formed from arterial and venous tears.

4. **The answer is B.** Hypoventilation would lead to a buildup in CO_2 in the brain, causing vasodilation and increased ICP. Hypoventilation would also cause inadequate oxygenation, leading to anaerobic metabolism by the neurons, increasing lactic acid production and lowering pH, thus exacerbating the vasodilatory response and increase ICP. If anything, the patient should hyperventilate to reduce CO_2 and decrease ICP. The problem with choice C is that even though hyperbaric oxygen can cause vasoconstriction and potentially decrease ICP, when it is delivered at the same time as CO_2, the vasodilatory effect of CO_2 predominate over hyperbaric oxygen's vasoconstrictive effects, leading to increased delivery of toxic, high oxygen levels to the brain. Intravenously administered mannitol can create hypertonic blood which draws out water from the neurons, reducing fluid inside the intracranial space in the short term (osmotherapy). As a side note, craniotomies can help relieve increased ICP because of the presence of a mass.

5. **The answer is E.** Weakness in several regions of the body implies that there was a lesion somewhere along the corticospinal tract (CST). Because the lesions caused focal neurologic defects in weakness, the vascular lesion likely is affecting the cortex, principally the motor cortex. Recall the homunculus, and that the face and arm are represented along the lateral edge of motor cortex, which is supplied by the MCA (see Fig. 3.1). Because the CST crosses at the pyramids, the left brain (fed by the left MCA) creates motor weakness on the right side. The ACA, however, would supply primarily the portion of the motor cortex that represents the right leg, which is still functional in this patient. A lesion in the PICA causes Wallenberg syndrome, or lateral medullary syndrome, affects both the inferior cerebellar peduncle resulting in ipsilateral (same side as the lesion) cerebellar signs (dysdiadochokinesia, dysmetria, and dystaxia) and affects the lateral medulla. The spinothalamic tract and spinal trigeminal nucleus and tract of CN V are affected, leading to loss of pain and temperature sensation on the contralateral (opposite side from the lesion) side of the body and ipsilateral side of the face, respectively. Descending sympathetic tracts can also be affected leading to Horner syndrome (ptosis, miosis, anhidrosis). If the nucleus ambiguous and glossopharyngeal nerve roots are affected, there can also be a loss of the gag reflex. The AICA makes a small contribution to the cerebellum, but primarily an occlusion to the AICA results in lateral pontine syndrome. This affects the vestibular and cochlear nuclei leading to falling to the side of the lesion and ipsilateral hearing loss or tinnitus, respectively. It also results in damage to the principal sensory nucleus of CN V and facial nucleus leading to ipsilateral loss of sensation of the face and paralysis, respectively. Finally, lesions to the pontine branches of the basilar artery, especially at the base of the pons, affect the anterior basis pontis which carries the corticospinal and corticobulbar tracts bilaterally, leading to quadriparesis. The trochlear and oculomotor nerves, however, are not affected, allowing the patient to move their eyes vertically to communicate. Patients remain conscious.

6. **The answer is C.** This drug user is exhibiting Parkinson-like signs, despite his young age. He likely took MPTP, which is an analog of meperidine (Demerol) which selectively destroys dopaminergic neurons. It was identified as an impurity in the production of the drug MPPP.

4

Peripheral Nervous System and Autonomic Nervous System

INTRODUCTION

The peripheral nervous system (PNS) is the direct extension of the central nervous system (CNS), and it is capable of consciously monitoring and reacting to primarily external stimuli. Dysfunction of this system can lead to an inability of patients to consciously interact with their environment or to receive signals that do not accurately represent their environment.

It can be broken down into two subsystems:

1. The autonomic nervous system (ANS), which is not regulated by conscious control and is involuntary.
2. The somatic nervous system, which contains afferent sensory nerves and efferent motor nerves (which are mostly voluntary) from the CNS.

The ANS generally helps maintain healthy homeostasis, influencing physiology independent of conscious awareness. The ANS receives information from the other body systems (the internal environment) and from the surroundings (the external environment) and automatically adjusts the activity of the sympathetic and parasympathetic nervous systems to match the overall needs of the body. The function of the ANS is critical to adapting to various stimuli, and its dysfunction may have a profoundly negative influence, contributing significantly to disease.

PERIPHERAL NERVOUS SYSTEM STRUCTURE

The PNS is comprised of efferent nerves traveling from the CNS to (primarily) muscle for motor actuation and afferent nerves traveling from (primarily) sensory receptors to the CNS for interpretation.

The PNS is generally differentiated from the CNS in the following ways:

1. It is not contained within the bony confines of the skull and spinal vertebra.
2. It is not protected by the blood-brain barrier. Therefore toxic injury from circulating substances can more easily affect the PNS.

Cranial Nerves

There are thirteen pairs of nerves that exit the brain, called cranial nerves (CNs). We will focus on the twelve clinically relevant CN pairs (Table 4.1) (see Fast Fact Box 4.1).

Fast Fact Box 4.1

One of the cranial nerve (CN) pairs, the nervus terminalis or CN zero (CN 0), serves a controversial role in humans. Originating from the septal nuclei and traveling very close to the olfactory nerves (CN I), this nerve pair is thought to be either a vestigial structure or to sense pheromones. CN 0 will be precluded from further discussion in this text.

Although all the nerves in Table 4.1 are considered CNs, they are not all technically part of the PNS. Neither CN I nor CN II originates in the brainstem and thus is technically part of the CNS.

- CN I feeds directly into the limbic-associated cortex rather than relaying through the thalamus.
- CN II (and the retina) is an extension of the diencephalon.

Note that parasympathetic innervation arises from CN III, VII, IX, and X, whereas sympathetic innervation is primarily from the sympathetic chain ganglion off of the spinal nerves. In addition to the functions listed in Table 4.1, CN V_3, VII and X also innervate the outside of the tympanic membrane, and IX innervates the inner tympanic membrane and the middle ear. CN IX and X also play a key role in baroreception and chemoreception: CN IX carries sensory innervation from the carotid body at the bifurcation of the internal and external carotid arteries, and CN X carries sensory innervation from the stretch receptors in the walls of the aortic arch and from chemoreceptors in the aortic bodies adjacent to the arch.

A major exception to the rule that general and special sensation is carried by afferent fibers and motor outputs are carried by efferent fibers is CN VIII. CN VIII has a special somatic efferent branch that actually carries signals that aid in a special sensation (hearing) from the brain to the cochlea and vestibular end organs.

Spinal Nerves

Spinal nerves originate from the spinal cord. As mentioned in Chapter [3], there are 31 pairs of spinal nerves:

- 8 cervical (C1–C8)
- 12 thoracic (T1–T12)
- 5 lumbar (L1–L5)
- 5 sacral (S1–S5)
- 1 coccygeal (Co)

In general, the cervical nerves provide movement and sensation to the arms, neck, and upper portion of the trunk, and they also control breathing. The thoracic nerves provide movement and sensation to the trunk and abdomen. The lumbosacral nerves provide movement and sensation to the legs, bladder, bowel, and sexual organs.

Spinal nerves can carry sympathetic, parasympathetic, motor, and sensory information.

- The ANS controls the sympathetic and parasympathetic innervations without conscious effort.
- The somatic nervous system consciously controls motor innervations to muscle.
- The somatic nervous system uses specialized receptors to sense the world.

TABLE 4.1   Summary of the Main 12 Cranial Nerve Pairs Along With Anatomy and Function

CN#	Name	Exit From Skull	Nuclei	Role	Function	Example of Clinical Relevance
I	Olfactory	Cribriform plate	Anterior olfactory nucleus (forebrain)	S	• Smell from the nasal cavity	Infection of cells that support olfactory bulb neurons by SARS-CoV-2 virus can cause anosmia (loss of sense of smell) in patients with COVID-19. Strong connections between sense of smell, memory, aggression and other emotions may be related to connections to the amygdala, thalamus, hippocampus, and frontal cortex directly.
II	Optic	Optic canal	Lateral geniculate nucleus (thalamus)	S	• Vision from the retina	CN II is the only location where the CNS can be visualized (through an ophthalmoscope). Blurring of optic disc margins on fundoscopic exam (papilledema) may indicate accelerated hypertension, cerebral edema from increased intracranial pressure, a CNS mass/space occupying lesion. CNS inflammatory diseases (e.g., multiple sclerosis) may present as optic neuritis on fundoscopic exam and may cause blindness.
III	Oculomotor	Superior orbital fissure	Oculomotor nucleus, Edinger-Westphal nucleus	M	• Eye movement, innervates the: superior, medial, and inferior rectus, inferior oblique, and levator palpebrae muscles • Parasympathetic pupillary constriction innervates the sphincter pupillae and ciliary body muscles	Diplopia (double vision) results from dysfunction of the extraocular muscles according to the innervation by the oculomotor nerve. CN III palsy can be seen in diabetic neuropathy, granulomatous neuropathy (sarcoidosis, tuberculosis) or from an aneurysm in the adjacent Circle of Willis such as the posterior communicating artery. If diplopia is acute in an adult, an intracranial hemorrhage may be imminent and must be evaluated immediately. A long history of CN III palsy may be due to migraine. Anisocoria results when dysfunction of one CN III results in pupillary dilation.
IV	Trochlear	Superior orbital fissure	Trochlear nucleus	M	• Depresses, laterally rotates, and intorts the eye: innervates the superior oblique muscle	Diplopia resulting from dysfunction of CV IV is most severe when gazing downward as when a patient is walking down stairs.
V	Trigeminal • V₁: Ophthalmic • V₂: Maxillary • V₃: Mandibular	V₁: Superior orbital fissure V₂: Foramen rotundum V₃: Foramen ovale	Principal sensory trigeminal nucleus, Spinal trigeminal nucleus, Mesencephalic trigeminal nucleus, Trigeminal motor nucleus	B	• Facial sensation • Innervates muscles of mastication masseter, temporalis, medial pterygoid, and lateral pterygoid muscles	Herpes Zoster infection (shingles) can affect the sensory component of CN V. If the tip of the nose has the shingles rash, there is concern for branch V2 and ocular involvement. Muscles of mastication. Cornea reflex (with CN X): touching the cornea may stimulate parasympathetic output from CN X and slow the heart rate, causing syncope. Smelling salts, which contain ammonia, can be detected by patients with defects of CN I function because such compounds are sensed by neurons in CN V.
VI	Abducens	Superior orbital fissure	Abducens nucleus	M	• Eye abduction, innervates the lateral rectus muscle	Esotropia (movement of the affected eye towards the midline) and diplopia. CN VI is the longest of the CNs, crosses the tentorium, and can be affected by Circle of Willis aneurysms.

Continued

TABLE 4.1   Summary of the Main 12 Cranial Nerve Pairs Along With Anatomy and Function—cont'd

CN#	Name	Exit From Skull	Nuclei	Role	Function	Example of Clinical Relevance
VII	Facial	Internal acoustic meatus	Facial nucleus, Solitary nucleus, Superior salivary nucleus	B	• Motor innervation facial expression, posterior belly of digastric, stylohyoid, and stapedius muscles • Taste (special sensation) from anterior 2/3 of tongue • Secretomotor parasympathetic innervation of salivary glands (except parotid) and lacrimal glands	Hyperacusis (increased sensitivity to or pain from sound) may occur when the stapedius muscle is paralyzed. Ramsey-Hunt syndrome is due to Herpes Zoster infection and manifests as shingles rash in the ear and motor weakness of the face. Bell's Palsy is a peripheral CN VII motor neuropathy leading to facial weakness (inability smile, frown, loss of nasolabial fold). When the ipsilateral forehead is affected, the dysfunction is peripheral, but when a stroke affects CN VII centrally, the muscles of the forehead are spared because there is nerve cell cross over (bilateral innervation).
VIII	Vestibulocochlear	Internal acoustic meatus	Vestibular nuclei, Cochlear nuclei	S	• Hearing • Balance: senses rotation and gravity	Vestibular dysfunction. Cold and warm water infusion into the ear of a comatose patient allows the examiner to evaluate the integrity of CN's VIII (afferent branch) and CN's III and VI (efferent branch) by inducing eye movements. A normal response to cold water is movement of both eyes toward the irrigated ear, but if there is a lesion in the reflex arc, the cold water will drive one or both eyes away from the irrigated ear to the contralateral side. Warm water has the reverse effects. The mnemonic for this abnormality is COWS = Cold Opposite, Warm Same.
IX	Glossopharyngeal	Jugular foramen	Inferior salivary nucleus, Solitary nucleus, Nucleus ambiguus	B	• Motor innervation: stylopharyngeus muscle • Taste (special sensation) from posterior 1/3 of tongue and thirst (in conjunction with Hypothalamic response to thirst) • Secretomotor parasympathetic innervation of parotid glands • Sensation from palatine tonsils	Swallowing and dysphagia. Loss of gag reflex.
X	Vagus	Jugular foramen	Dorsal motor vagal nucleus, Solitary nucleus, Nucleus ambiguus	B	• Motor innervation of palatoglossus, and muscles for voice and resonance • Branchiomotor innervation laryngeal and pharyngeal muscles (except stylopharyngeus) • Taste (special sensation) from epiglottis • Parasympathetic innervation: thoracic and abdominal viscera down to splenic flexure	Loss of function of CN X leads to resting tachycardia (increased heart rate). Stimulation of CN X leads to vasovagal response that may be seen in the corneal reflex as well as in response to pain, manifesting as bradycardia (slow heart rate), nausea, and diaphoresis (sweating).
XI	Accessory	Jugular foramen Ascending fibers-foramen magnum	Spinal accessory nucleus, Nucleus ambiguus	M	• Motor innervation: sternocleidomastoid and trapezius muscles	Weakness due to neck or shoulder injury can lead to impaired shoulder shrug.
XII	Hypoglossal	Hypoglossal canal	Hypoglossal nucleus	M	• Motor innervation glossal and tongue muscles (except the palatoglossus) for	Weakness causes the tongue to deviate toward the side with the lesion, which could be due to infection, neoplasia, or trauma. Tongue atrophy seen with chronic CN XII dysfunction.

B, Both motor and sensory role; *M*, purely motor role; *S*, purely sensory role.

Sensory Receptors

The afferent fibers of the spinal nerves carry sensory information including:

1. Light touch
2. Vibration
3. Pain
4. Temperature

The specialized sensory receptors are innervated by several types of sensory nerve fibers including: Aβ (type II), Aδ (type III), and C (type IV) fibers.

- Aβ fibers are thickly myelinated, 6 to 12 μm in diameter, fast (33–75 m/s), and are sensitive to cutaneous mechanoreceptors.
- Aδ fibers are thinly myelinated, 1 to 5 μm in diameter, have a low activation threshold, are moderately fast (5–30 m/s), and are sensitive to temperature and mechanical (free nerve ending receptors) stimuli, and some nociceptors (pain receptors).
- C fibers are unmyelinated, 0.2 to 1.5 μm in diameter, slow (<1 m/s), and carry nociceptors (and some warmth receptors).

General Sensation

To initially measure general sensation, such as light touch and vibration (carried by the dorsal columns), a set of specialized sensory receptors (Table 4.2) are needed in the skin, which convey information to the sensory neuron whose cell body is in the dorsal root ganglion.

- Fig. 4.1 illustrates where many of these sensory receptors are found in the skin.
- General sensation and proprioception are more rapidly adapted for than heat and pain because they are carried on the faster Aβ and Aδ fibers (as opposed to the slower C fibers).

Pain and Temperature Sensation

Pain is a highly subjective phenomenon and can be caused by a variety of pathologies including injury, disease, or even mental suffering.

- First pain is sharp and immediate. It is modulated by intermediately fast Aδ fibers. This type of pain can be thought of as "good" acute pain because it acts as a warning signal to respond to a harmful stimulus (such as placing your hand on a hot stove).
- Second pain is a delayed, diffuse, longer lasting sensation that is modulated by the slower C fibers. This pain is the chronic "bad" pain that is usually associated with pathology or damage that remains even after the stimulus that caused the acute pain is removed (see Clinical Correlation Box 4.1).

Clinical Correlation Box 4.1

Referred pain, or improper sensation of pain in an incorrect region of the body, may occur because of imprecise topographic mapping of multiple afferent inputs to the same dorsal horn neurons *or* mixing of nerve fibers. For example, the pain of a kidney stone may be "referred" to the groin in addition to classic flank pain.

Pain and temperature are not only both carried by the spinothalamic tract into the CNS, but can also be sensed by the same specialized receptors. Extreme heat *or* extreme cold can both trigger the sensation of pain.

Special Sensation

Specialized nerve endings also serve in many of the special senses relayed by the CNs and interpreted by specific topographic maps in the cerebral cortex. These senses include vision, hearing, olfaction, and taste.

Although the specific pathways for each of these special senses is outside the scope of this text, Table 4.3 gives a general overview of the specific receptors that are used to detect these various special senses, as well as the neural pathways these signals traverse and the specialized intermediate neuron types and thalamic nuclei used to transmit the signal to the specialized region of the cortex that interprets the sensory signal.

AUTONOMIC NERVOUS SYSTEM STRUCTURE

The ANS connects to the entire body, collecting information from and distributing instructions to the skin and organs, such as the eyes, and the visceral organs, such as the heart and blood vessels, lungs, gastrointestinal (GI) tract, bladder, and reproductive organs.

The ANS is composed of two divisions:

1. Sympathetic nervous system.
2. Parasympathetic nervous system.

Their distinct structures support different but complementary functions, which are described later. Many consider the complex neuronal network of the GI enteric nervous system (ENS) to be a third division of the ANS because it, too, generally works unconsciously (see Ch. 25 for a description of the ENS).

The ANS shares many basic structural and functional characteristics with the neurologic system involved in the control of skeletal muscle, the motor system. For example, the general structure of a nerve cell and the initiation and propagation of action potentials in the ANS resemble those of the motor system. The primary distinction is that the motor system is under conscious control, whereas the ANS works largely unconsciously. In the

---

TABLE 4.2 Summary of Different Touch Sensory Nerve Endings in Skin

Sensory Nerve Ending	Adaptation Speed	Receptive Field Size	Terminal Location	Type of Sensation
Meissner's corpuscles	Fast	Small	Superficial	Vibration
Merkel's discs	Slow	Small	Superficial	Pressure
Pacinian corpuscles	Fast	Large	Deep	Pressure, vibration
Ruffini ending	Slow	Large	Deep	Pressure

Hair follicles also act as the principle cutaneous receptor of hairy skin. They sense the deflection of hair and are rapidly adapting. Meissner's corpuscles and Merkel's discs are found in glabrous (hairless) skin.

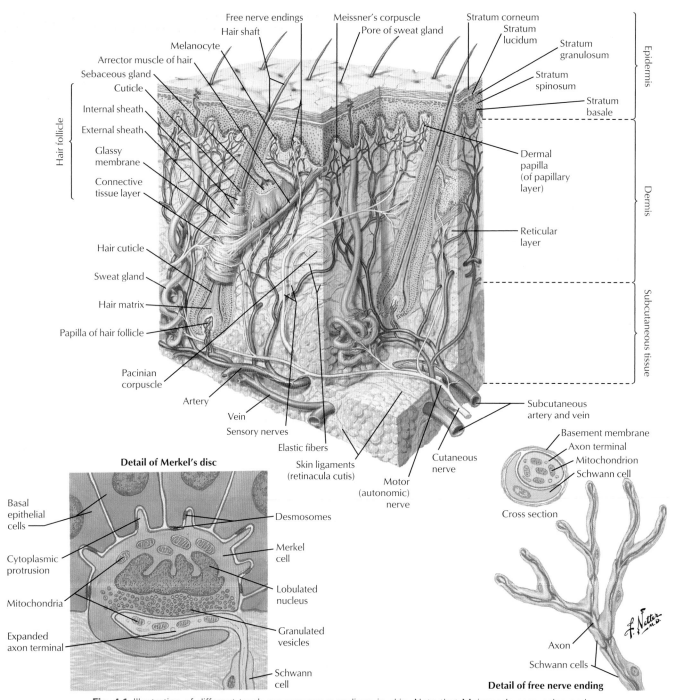

Detail of Merkel's disc

Detail of free nerve ending

Fig. 4.1 Illustration of different touch sensory nerve endings in skin. Note that Meissner's corpuscles and Merkel's discs are found in glabrous (hairless) skin. (Netter illustration used with permission of Elsevier Inc. All rights reserved. www.netterimages.com.)

TABLE 4.3	**Overview of Pain and Temperature Sensation and Special Sensation System Architecture**			
Stimulus	**Light**	**Sound**	**Temperature, Pain Sensation**	**Odor**
Receptor	Rhodopsin	Unknown	Heat: TRPV1/2 Cold: TRPM8, TRPA1	G-Protein coupled olfactory receptors
Primary sensory cell	Photoreceptor	Inner hair cell	Dorsal root ganglion cell	Olfactory sensory neurons
Relay neuron	Bipolar cell	Spiral ganglion cell	Spinal cord neurons	Mitral/ tuft cells
Thalamic nucleus	Lateral geniculate nucleus	Medial geniculate nucleus	Ventral posterolateral nucleus	None, goes straight to cerebrum

following section, it is useful to compare and contrast the structure and function of the ANS with those of the motor system.

Autonomic Nervous System Organization

Recall that like all homeostatic systems, the ANS must monitor the target tissues, transmit information on function back to the CNS via afferent pathways, integrate this information in central control centers, and then instruct the target tissues via efferent pathways.

Target Tissues

The major tissues influenced by the ANS are:
1. Smooth muscles (such as those of blood vessel walls, the alimentary canal, and the urinary bladder);
2. Glands (such as the sweat glands and those of the respiratory and GI tract);
3. Cardiac muscle and cardiac electrical conduction system.

Peripheral Nerves

Specialized endings of afferent ANS nerves gather and communicate information from target tissues including the skin, internal organs, and associated blood vessels.
- Chemoreceptors send signals about variables, such as the pH and partial pressure of oxygen, in their tissues.
- Mechanoreceptors or baroreceptors, measure wall tension and thus pressure in blood vessels and viscera, such as the GI and urinary tracts.
- Nociceptors serve relay signals interpreted as pain when viscera are damaged and/or overdistended, which are notably not unconscious (unlike the rest of the ANS).

ANS afferent neurons have long processes that go from their specialized endings in peripheral tissues to their cell bodies in the dorsal root ganglia of the spinal cord. Information is transmitted to the spinal cord by short axons where it can be processed, integrated with other signals, and acted on via autonomic reflexes of varying complexity.

Once signals are processed and appropriate responses are "decided," they are transmitted via efferent ANS nerves, the most prominent of which is the vagus nerve (CN X).

Peripheral Ganglia

A collection of interconnected ANS neurons is known as a ganglion, and ganglia are found only in the ANS.

The sympathetic nervous system is divided into two sets of ganglia:
- Paravertebral ganglia are arranged in two longitudinal (rostrocaudal) chains, one on either side of the spinal column.
- Prevertebral ganglia are nerve tissue nodes anterior to the spinal column in the midline. They are situated around and take their names from three major branches of the descending aorta (Fig. 4.2):
  - Celiac ganglion, also called the solar plexus, (the celiac trunk)
  - Superior mesenteric ganglion (the superior mesenteric artery)
  - Inferior mesenteric ganglion (the inferior mesenteric artery)

The parasympathetic nervous system is neuroanatomically distinct from the sympathetic nervous system, with ganglia located very near or actually embedded in the walls of its target organs (see Fig. 4.2).

Spinal Cord Levels

Another major neuroanatomic distinction between the sympathetic and parasympathetic nervous systems is in the location of the cell bodies of their respective preganglionic neurons.
- In the sympathetic nervous system, preganglionic neurons originate in the thoracic and lumbar levels of the spinal cord.
- In the parasympathetic nervous systems, preganglionic neurons originate from specific CN nuclei or from the sacral level of the spinal cord.
  - The four CN nuclei are:
    Oculomotor (CN III)
    Facial (CN VII)
    Glossopharyngeal (CN IX)
    Vagus (CN X)

Central Integration Centers

The powerful homeostatic control exerted by the ANS requires the integration of signals indicating the state of target tissues. In addition to the peripheral ganglia and the spinal cord, a number of structures within the CNS are important in this respect.
- The brain stem contains a number of vital centers that coordinate autonomic reflexes involved in the maintenance of homeostasis by influencing variables, such as blood pressure and respiration.
  - Low blood pressure detected by the carotid body baroreceptors stimulates reflex increases in heart rate and contractility.
  - Decreased blood pH detected by the carotid body chemoreceptors stimulates an increased respiratory rate so that the lungs "blow off" CO_2, thus raising blood pH.
- The hypothalamus is a complex collection of neurons called nuclei, located in the diencephalon, just superior to the midbrain and below the thalamus and cerebral hemispheres.
  - The central location of the hypothalamus reflects its primary position in the CNS—receiving information from and sending instructions to other systems.
  - Among the many homeostatic variables it can modify are body temperature, thirst, hunger, and sleep.

Autonomic Nervous System Efferent Neurons

The ANS efferent neurons differ importantly from lower motor neurons of the motor system.
- In the motor system, an upper motor neuron (with its cell body in the motor cortex) sends its axon down the spinal cord, where it synapses on a lower motor neuron (that has its cell body in the ventral horn of the spinal cord), which in turn sends its axon out to the periphery, where it synapses directly on skeletal muscle.
- In the ANS, two neurons exist in series, forming a path from the spinal cord to the effector organs (see Figs. 4.2 and 4.3).
  - The first of these, like the lower motor neuron, has its cell body in the spinal cord, but its axon terminates in one or more (because of branching) ANS ganglia.
  - The second ANS neuron has its cell body in the ganglion, and its axon projects to the periphery, ending near target tissues.
  - The two neurons are therefore called the preganglionic neuron and the postganglionic neuron, respectively.

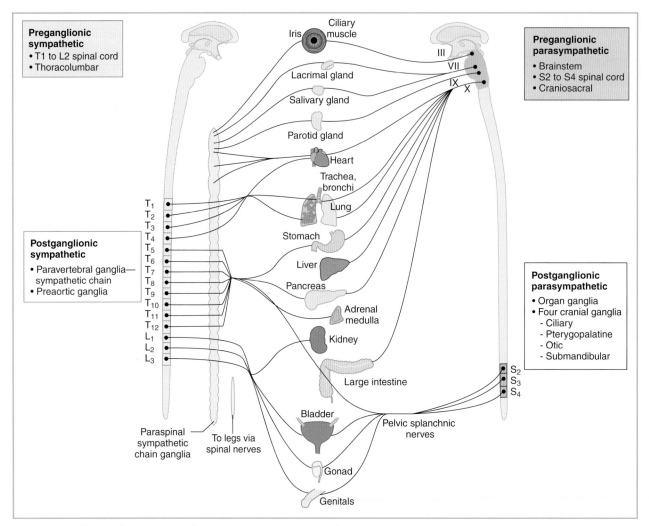

Fig. 4.2 Components of the autonomic nervous system. Sympathetic preganglionic neurons from the thoracic and lumbar levels of the spinal cord send out relatively short axons and synapse either in the paravertebral or prevertebral ganglia. An exception is the neurons that go all the way to the adrenal medulla. The parasympathetic preganglionic neurons have relatively long axons and synapse on ganglia very near or actually embedded in the target organs or tissues. (From Kester M. *Elsevier's Integrated Pharmacology*, Second Edition. Philadelphia, PA: Elsevier. 2011. Fig. 6.2.)

Autonomic Nervous System Neurotransmitters

Among the myriad molecules involved in the functions of the ANS are the neurotransmitters and their receptors. Again paralleling the motor system, ANS neurotransmitters are the chemical signaling molecules released from axon terminals to bridge information-bearing neurochemical signals in the form of an action potential across the synaptic cleft separating a neuron from target cells.

Acetylcholine

Acetylcholine (ACh) is a critical neurotransmitter for both the motor system and the ANS.

- In the motor system, it mediates stimulation at the neuromuscular junction by binding to nicotinic ACh receptors on the sarcolemma, thereby inducing membrane-depolarizing ion fluxes.
- In the ANS, ACh mediates stimulation of both ganglia and peripheral target tissues.
  - ACh can be found within:
    The connections between preganglionic and postganglionic neurons.

The axon terminals of sympathetic postganglionic neurons that end on sweat glands.

The ends of all parasympathetic postganglionic neurons.

- The ACh receptors at ANS ganglia (i.e., on the postganglionic neurons) are nicotinic (though a different subtype than those of the motor system), whereas those on the peripheral target tissues at parasympathetic postganglionic synapses are muscarinic ACh receptors.

Collectively, the receptors that bind ACh are described as cholinergic.

Norepinephrine

Norepinephrine (NE) is an important neurotransmitter found in the vesicles of postganglionic sympathetic neurons (except the ones that terminate on sweat glands).

Epinephrine

Epinephrine (Epi), also called adrenaline, is a powerful neurotransmitter and hormone released by the medulla of the adrenal

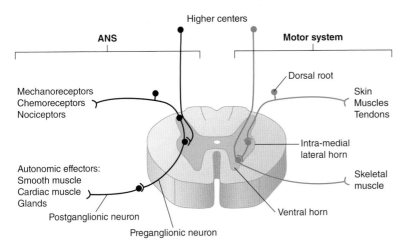

Fig. 4.3 The autonomic nervous system (*ANS*) versus the motor system. The ANS has a two-neuron pathway from the spinal cord to the target tissue, a preganglionic and a postganglionic neuron in series. The relatively high diversification (branching) of the sympathetic neurons is not shown, but it allows one preganglionic cell to synapse on up to 20 postganglionic cells in different ganglia. In the motor system, upper motor neurons from the cerebral cortex send axons down the spinal cord that synapse on lower motor neurons whose axons exit to the periphery and synapse directly on skeletal muscle cells.

glands. Like NE, epinephrine binds to several types of adrenergic receptors.

- The most important adrenergic receptors are α_1, α_2, β_1, β_2, and β_3.
- Their characteristics are described in Table 4.4.

Neuropeptides

A number of larger signaling molecules are also found in the axon terminals of ANS neurons, including:

- Substance P, released by afferent fibers synapsing in the spinal cord in response to nociceptive signals from the periphery.
- Neuropeptide Y, found along with NE in the ends of sympathetic postganglionic neurons innervating blood vessels.
- Vasoactive intestinal peptide (VIP), present in terminal vesicles of parasympathetic postganglionic neurons in saliva glands.

AUTONOMIC NERVOUS SYSTEM FUNCTION

The effects of the ANS on the body can be divided into three basic categories:

1. Coping with a threat of harm (e.g., escaping or combating an attacker).
2. Consuming and digesting food.
3. Reproduction.

Most effector tissues, such as the heart, the GI tract, and the genitourinary system are innervated by both the sympathetic and parasympathetic nervous systems. In some cases, their effects are antagonistic, in that parasympathetic stimulation will drive a physiologic variable one way (e.g., decrease heart rate) whereas sympathetic activation will do the opposite (e.g., increase heart rate).

- Under relatively normal circumstances, there is a baseline activity of the sympathetic system called sympathetic tone.
- Stressful situations (real or perceived) that demand emergency responses precipitate increased sympathetic activity and concomitant decreased parasympathetic stimulation.
- Thus the sympathetic nervous system is responsible for fight-or-flight responses.

However, it would be a mistake to conclude that these systems are always at odds with one another. In fact, they often work additively or synergistically. It is the balance between the activity of the two subsystems at any one time that determines the target value, direction, and magnitude of the shift in a given variable.

Table 4.4 lists the organ specific effects of SNS and PSN stimulation, some of which are detailed later.

Effects on the Cardiovascular System

Sympathetic stimulation, mediated largely by the binding of NE and/or Epi to beta-1 adrenergic receptors, increases heart rate and the force of contractility.

- Both of these changes work to increase blood pressure and cardiac output, providing organs, such as the brain and skeletal muscle, with increased oxygen and glucose for defense (fight) or for escape (flight).

Parasympathetic stimulation slows the heart rate, thereby decreasing cardiac output and blood pressure (see Fast Fact Box 4.2).

Fast Fact Box 4.2

Interestingly, the vagus nerve, which carries peripheral nervous system signals, tonically slows the heart rate, so that the heart normally beats at a lower rate than its intrinsic pacemaker would direct. Disrupting the vagus nerve (as occurs in patients who receive a heart transplant) allows the heart to beat at its higher intrinsic rate.

Effects on the Gastrointestinal System

Sympathetic stimulation decreases peristaltic contractions that propel food in the GI tract, relaxes the gallbladder, and constricts sphincter muscles such as the sphincter of Oddi. Thus digestion is shut down when danger threatens.

Parasympathetic stimulation opposes these actions, increasing smooth muscle contraction to produce peristalsis, inducing contraction of the gallbladder, and relaxing sphincter muscles.

Effects on the Renal System

Sympathetic innervation of the kidney is a critical control center for the regulation of blood pressure, with little input from the parasympathetic nervous system.

- Adrenergic stimulation augments the secretion of renin, leading to the generation of angiotensin II, a powerful vasoconstrictor that elevates blood pressure.
- When pressure is high enough or the demand for increased pressure resolves, sympathetic stimulation decreases, inducing a decrement in renin release.

TABLE 4.4 Effects of Autonomic Nervous System Stimulation on Target Organs

Organ	Function	SNS Effect [Adrenergic Receptor]	PNS Effect
Heart	Rate	Increase [β_1]	Decrease
	Contraction	Increase velocity and force [β_1]	Decrease
Blood vessels			
• Skin and internal organs	Contraction	Increase [α_1]	None
• Skeletal muscle	Contraction	Decrease [β_2]	None
Eye			
• Pupil sphincter	Constriction	None	Increase
• Radial pupil muscle	Dilation	Increase [α_1]	None
• Lacrimal glands	Tearing	Increase	Increase
Lungs	Broncho-constriction	Increase [β_2]	Decrease
Kidney	Renin secretion	increase [α_1, β_1]	None
GI tract			
• Tract walls	Contraction	Decrease [β_2]	Increase
• Sphincters	Contraction	Increase [α_1]	Decrease
• Glands	Secretion of enzymes	Increase mucus [α_1, α_2] and ions	Increase
• Liver	Glycogenolysis	Increase [β_2]	None
GU tract			
• Bladder	Contraction	Decrease [β_2]	Increase
• Trigone Sphincter	Contraction	Increase [β_1]	Decrease
• Penile	Erection	Promotes	
	Ejaculation	Promotes [β_1]	
Adrenal medulla	Epi and NE secretion	Increase [nicotinic AchR]	None
Posterior pituitary	ADH secretion	Increase [β_1]	None

AchR, Acetylcholine receptor; *ADH*, antidiuretic hormone; *GI*, gastrointestinal; *GU*, genitourinary; *NE*, norepinephrine.
From Brunton, LL, Chabner, BA, Knollmann, BC. *Goodman and Gilman's the Pharmacological Basis of Therapeutics*. Twelfth Edition. McGraw-Hill Education / Medical. 2011.

Effects on the Genitourinary System

Micturition is mediated by four key control circuits involving both divisions of the ANS:

1. Sympathetic signals from adrenergic neurons in the lumbar spinal cord cause relaxation of the detrusor muscles of the urinary bladder wall and contraction of the trigone and internal urethral sphincter, thus inhibiting the outflow of urine.
2. Parasympathetic preganglionic neurons in the sacral spinal cord synapse on parasympathetic postganglionic (cholinergic) neurons in the bladder wall, and these promote detrusor contraction and trigone and internal urethral sphincter relaxation.
3. The micturition reflex center in the brainstem receives information on bladder wall tension (and thus bladder pressure) from afferent nerves and, when pressure rises, inhibits sympathetic neurons that prevent voiding.
4. The contraction or relaxation of the external urethral sphincter, which is skeletal muscle under voluntary control with lower motor neurons in the sacral spinal cord.

The regulation of male sexual function is another example of cooperation rather than antagonization between the two divisions of the ANS. The parasympathetic system mediates erection, whereas the sympathetic system controls ejaculation.

Effects on the Dermatologic System

Unlike other systems, the components of the skin, especially its blood vessels and sweat glands, are exclusively under sympathetic influence, without parasympathetic input. Sympathetic activation results in several responses mediating thermoregulation, including:

- Constriction of dermal vessels, shunting blood away from the skin where heat is lost to the environment.
- Secretion by the sweat glands, which help cool the body.
- Contraction of the pilomotor muscles that raise body hair, which conserves heat.
- A separate ANS reaction in the skin is the vasodilator response to injury.
- Afferent ANS neurons near skin areas that suffer traumatic damage release substance P both at the site of injury and in the spinal cord.
- Branches of their axons that innervate blood vessels cause the relaxation of smooth muscle and vasodilation.
- This increases the volume and decreases the speed of blood flow, allowing inflammatory and repair cells from the blood to access the site of damage.

Effects on the Pulmonary System

Sympathetic stimulation, working through beta-2 adrenergic receptors, causes relaxation of the smooth muscle investing the bronchioles, resulting in bronchodilation. This provides greater ventilation during exertion for fight or flight.

Parasympathetic activity opposes this action, causing bronchoconstriction and increased secretion by bronchial glands.

Effects on the Endocrine System

Upon sympathetic stimulation (indicating stress), the hypothalamus releases corticotropin-releasing hormone, which reaches the anterior pituitary and causes the release of adrenocorticotropic hormone (ACTH).
- ACTH reaches the adrenal cortex and induces the production and release of glucocorticoids.
- This cascade has a profound and diverse effects on salt and water balance, immune function, and glucose supply and metabolism (see Ch. 29).

The most rapid and dramatic autonomic endocrine response is sympathetic stimulation of the adrenal medulla. Structurally and functionally, this subsystem is distinct from the rest of the ANS in that the adrenal gland is supplied by preganglionic, not postganglionic, sympathetic neurons.

Sympathetic preganglionic neurons whose axons exit the spinal cord synapse directly on these medullary cells (which resemble postganglionic sympathetic neurons), and activation causes the secretion of potent adrenergic mediators.
- Whereas most sympathetic postganglionic neurons release NE into the limited extracellular space of a target tissue, adrenal neuroendocrine cells release a combination of Epi (80%) and NE (20%) into the bloodstream, in amounts large enough to transiently maintain relatively high serum concentrations.
- These powerful mediators circulate widely, acting like sympathetic hormones (see Clinical Correlation Box 4.1, Trauma Box 4.1, Pharmacology Box 4.1, Development Box 4.1 and Genetics Box 4.1).

⚡ TRAUMA BOX 4.1

Patients with familial dysautonomia have impaired pain perception, which can lead to delay or failure to recognize traumatic injury. Attacks called dysautonomic crises in response to stress (physical and emotional) include vomiting, hypertension, tachycardia, diaphoresis, sialorrhea (hypersalivation), blotching of the skin and a negative change in personality. Traumatic injury can be an effect of the disease and a precipitant of exacerbations. Protecting patients (especially children) from trauma is a major part of therapy.

🖊 PHARMACOLOGY BOX 4.1

Treatment of familial dysautonomia is limited to controlling the manifestations. The medication fludrocortisone can be helpful in limiting episodic hypotension by increasing renal resorption of sodium like aldosterone and thus maintaining a relatively high intravascular volume (See Ch. 9 (Vasculature) and Ch. 19 (Control of blood pressure and extracellular volume)).

🖊 DEVELOPMENT BOX 4.1

Familial dysautonomia typically manifests as children are delayed meeting developmental milestones, such as acquiring a steady gait and fluent speech. They often have spinal curvature, corneal abrasions, and puffy, red hands as well. It first may be suspected when infants 7 months or older do not develop overflow tears when crying.

🧬 GENETICS BOX 4.1

Familial dysautonomia (Riley-Day Syndrome, or Hereditary Sensory and Autonomic Neuropathy 3, HSAN3) is a condition affecting the autonomic nervous system. Affected patients have attacks of sudden changes in parasympathetic and sympathetic activity in the cardiovascular, gastrointestinal, and cutaneous systems (among others). It is caused by mutations in the Elp1/IKBKAP gene, and patients can be tested for such mutations to make the diagnosis, but the pathophysiologic mechanism is as yet unclear.

Integrated Responses

Most of the time, the sympathetic and parasympathetic nervous systems will mediate a given target tissue's homeostasis independent from other organ systems; that is, the demands of a given circumstance may require, for example, decreased heart rate (increased parasympathetic tone) but increased sweating (increased sympathetic tone).

However, two aspects of the sympathetic nervous system suggest the ability for large scale, coordinated activity that organizes many or all of the body systems in response to stress (actual or imagined):
- High degree of divergence in the sympathetic nervous system
  - A single preganglionic neuron may send axon branches to numerous ganglia.
  - This allows multiple end organs or tissues to be activated at the same time.
- The adrenal medullary response (as described earlier)
  - Epi is released and circulates widely, allowing it to agonize adrenergic receptors throughout the body simultaneously.

Such widespread sympathetic activity stimulates a cascade of physiologic changes favorable for escaping danger:
- The heart increases its rate and contraction, and lung bronchioles dilate to provide the oxygen to *supply oxygen to sustain exertion.*
- Vasodilation in the skeletal muscle brings the increased blood flow from the heart to the tissues needed for fight or flight.
- The catabolism of glycogen in the liver and lipids in adipose tissues liberates glucose and fatty acids, the easily used fuels of brain and muscle.

Although such reactions can be lifesaving under some conditions (e.g., when chased by a predator), they can be deleterious under others (see Clinical Correlation Box 4.2).

Clinical Correlation Box 4.2

Many medications selectively target specific adrenergic receptors to minimize unintentional side effects. For example, metoprolol selectively antagonizes the beta-1 adrenergic receptors of the heart to support patients with hypertension and acute MI.
- Beta-1 antagonism → reduced HR, contractility → reduced cardiac output → reduced BP and oxygen demand

BP, Blood pressure; *HR*, heat rate; *MI*, myocardial infarction.

AUTONOMIC NERVOUS SYSTEM PATHOPHYSIOLOGY

When the ANS does not function normally, it can cause organ-specific widespread disruption of homeostasis.

Horner Syndrome

Autonomic innervation of the eye includes both sympathetic and parasympathetic contributions.

- The sympathetic preganglionic neurons send axons up the paravertebral chains where they synapse on cells in the superior cervical ganglion. Postganglionic neurons from here innervate the iris radial muscle that dilates the pupil, the lacrimal glands that produce tears, and the muscles that help raise the eyelids.
- The parasympathetic preganglionic neurons of CN III synapse on cells of the ciliary ganglion, which in turn stimulate the iris pupillary sphincter muscle that constricts the pupil.

When the sympathetic neuron is damaged or inhibited, the affected side has a loss of sympathetic tone, producing excessive parasympathetic tone.

- The decreased pupil dilation, eyelid raising, and tear production leaves the parasympathetic forces inducing constriction unopposed.
- Patients display a triad of *miosis* (small, contracted pupils), ptosis (eyelid drooping), and anhydrosis (decreased tear production) results, a condition called Horner syndrome.

Lesions to the Hypothalamus

When the hypothalamus is damaged, it can affect complex functions, such as appetite and weight control, thirst and osmolality control, and thermoregulation.

Damage to the hypothalamus most often arises from three causes:

- Ischemia (i.e., impaired blood flow, as in a stroke)

- Neoplastic (i.e., cancer)
- Traumatic

The exact manifestations of hypothalamic dysfunction depend on the particular hypothalamic nuclei and/or tracts affected. Some experimental lesions in animals produce dramatic increases in appetite and body weight (hyperphagia), whereas others induce a loss of appetite (anorexia) that can be fatal. Thermoregulation in patients who have suffered hypothalamic lesions can be difficult, as they become hypothermic when their heat-conserving mechanisms fail and body temperature falls toward room temperature.

Vasovagal Episode

The initial response to painful stimuli is often an increase in sympathetic activity that elevates the heart rate, cardiac contractility, and therefore the blood pressure.

Shortly thereafter, the increased blood pressure can trigger baroreceptors in the heart and arteries and lead to a reflex increase in parasympathetic activity that decreases the heart rate and dilates blood vessels to reduce the blood pressure.

When such a compensatory reflex overcompensates and parasympathetic activity is too high, the blood pressure can drop precipitously.

- The low blood pressure during such an excessive parasympathetic reflex is often accompanied by a mixture of ANS effects, including profuse sweating, clammy and pale skin, nausea, and lightheadedness and possibly fainting (syncope).
- Because excessive activity of the vagus nerve (CN X) is responsible for the vasodilation and other cardiovascular manifestations, this group of symptoms is called a vasovagal episode.

SUMMARY

- The PNS can be broken down into two subsystems: the ANS which regulates sympathetic and parasympathetic activity, and the somatic nervous system, which contains afferent sensory nerves and efferent motor nerves from the CNS.
- The PNS is comprised of 13 CN pairs; only 12 are clinically significant. CN II is technically considered part of the CNS.
- There are 31 spinal nerve pairs, which are broken down into cervical, thoracic, lumbar, sacral, and coccygeal.
- Specialized sensory receptors allow the PNS to sense light touch, vibration, pain, and temperature.
- Sensory receptors use three types of sensory nerve fibers: Aβ (type II), Aδ (type III), and C (type IV) fibers (listed from fastest to slowest conduction velocity).
- Light touch information tends to travel on the fastest sensory nerve fibers whereas pain and temperature information travel on the slowest sensory nerve fibers.
- The ANS works largely unconsciously and integrates information from the internal and external environments to maintain total body homeostasis.
- The ANS has two divisions, the sympathetic nervous system and the parasympathetic nervous system.

- The major neurotransmitters of the ANS are acetylcholine (ACh), norepinephrine (NE), and epinephrine (Epi), although a number of neuropeptides and other signaling molecules are important as well.
- Both sympathetic and parasympathetic preganglionic neurons release ACh.
- Because most sympathetic postganglionic neurons release NE and/or Epi, the sympathetic nervous system is also called the adrenergic division of the ANS. Because all parasympathetic postganglionic neurons release ACh, the parasympathetic nervous system is also called the cholinergic division of the ANS.
- Many target tissues are influenced by both the sympathetic and parasympathetic nervous systems, which may work antagonistically or cooperatively.
- Widespread, simultaneous activation of the sympathetic nervous system induces the preparation for the fight-or-flight response.
- Dysfunction of the ANS causes organ-specific or organ system-specific disease. In Horner syndrome, lack of sympathetic tone causes miosis, ptosis, and anhydrosis on the affected side. Excessive parasympathetic activity carried by the vagal nerve (CN X) can cause a vasovagal episode, with hypotension and possible syncope.

REVIEW QUESTIONS

Directions: Each of the numbered items or incomplete statements in this section is followed by answers or by completions of the statement. Select the one lettered answer or completion that is best in each case.

1. A 36-year-old man is exposed to diisopropyl phosphofluoridate (DFP), a biologic toxic agent that blocks the acetylcholinesterase enzyme, which catabolizes ACh at synapses. Which of the following would you expect among his symptoms?
   A. High heart rate (tachycardia) and high blood pressure (hypertension)
   B. Hypersalivation and hyperlacrimation (increased tearing and salivation)
   C. Constipation
   D. Urinary retention
   E. Ejaculation

2. A 28-year-old woman injects cocaine into her bloodstream. This drug causes the accumulation of norepinephrine and would be expected to manifest as
   A. Urinary incontinence
   B. Bowel incontinence
   C. Elevated heart rate and blood pressure
   D. Depressed heart rate and blood pressure
   E. Miosis

3. Which of the following drugs might help a patient with low blood pressure and a slow heart rate?
   A. Metoprolol, a drug that blocks cardiac β–adrenergic receptors
   B. Atropine, a drug that block the cardiac effects of ACh
   C. Acetylcholine
   D. Diisopropyl phosphofluoridate (DFP), a drug that blocks the breakdown of ACh

4. Which of the following is the predominant neurotransmitter at both sympathetic and parasympathetic ganglia?
   A. Epinephrine (Epi)
   B. Norepinephrine (NE)
   C. Substance P
   D. Acetylcholine (ACh)
   E. Vasoactive intestinal peptide (VIP)

5. A 64-year-old man presents to an emergency department with a broken toe. He is accidentally given an injection of atropine, a drug that antagonizes the effects of ACh at muscarinic receptors, instead of an analgesic. Which of the following symptoms do you expect him to have?
   A. Tachycardia (a high heart rate)
   B. Hypertension (high blood pressure)
   C. Cool, clammy, pale skin
   D. Diarrhea
   E. Increased tearing and salivation

ANSWERS TO REVIEW QUESTIONS

1. **The answer is B.** Exposure to DFP causes the accumulation of ACh, which mimics hyperactivity of the parasympathetic division of the ANS. Thus increased salivation and tearing are expected, along with a decrease in the heart rate (bradycardia) and blood pressure (hypotension), increased contraction of the peristaltic and bladder wall muscles (causing defecation and urination), and penile erection.

2. **The answer is C.** Because NE is a major neurotransmitter for the SNS, its overabundance would mimic the fight-or-flight response. Cocaine thus causes tachycardia (increased heart rate) and hypertension (increased blood pressure). All the other symptoms are manifestations of excessive or unopposed parasympathetic activity.

3. **The answer is B.** By inhibiting the parasympathetic neurotransmitter ACh, atropine essentially produces a pharmacologic vagotomy, blocking the parasympathetic break on heart rate and causing the pulse to increase. This in turn, can elevate blood pressure. All the other substances would either inhibit sympathetic tone (metoprolol) or increase parasympathetic signals, which would further decrease the heart rate and blood pressure.

4. **The answer is D.** Both SNS and PNS preganglionic neurons release ACh at synapses with their postganglionic counterparts.

5. **The answer is A.** By inhibiting the actions of ACh on muscarinic receptors, atropine produces a constellation of symptoms that in some organ systems resembles an increase in sympathetic tone. Thus its effects on the heart include an increase in the pulse and blood pressure, which makes this drug useful in patients suffering from hypotension because of a low heart rate. In the GI tract, it decreases motility and impairs salivation. It likewise inhibits lacrimation. In the skin, where sympathetic postganglionic neurons release ACh to induce secretion by sweat glands, atropine does not mimic a hyperadrenergic state. Instead, sweating is decreased and the skin becomes dry, hot, and red. In addition, the antagonization of muscarinic receptors can produce mydriasis (dilation of the pupil) with subsequent difficulty seeing, and toxic doses of the drug can cause profound behavioral changes including delirium, characterized by restlessness and confusion. The clinic picture of atropinism has been encapsulated in the mnemonic: "Fast as a hare, red as a beet, hot as an iron, blind as a bat, and mad as a hatter."

5

The Neuromuscular Junction and Skeletal Muscle

INTRODUCTION

Muscle comes in three varieties:
1. Cardiac
2. Skeletal
3. Smooth

These three types are differentiated based on:
1. Distinct control systems (neuronal, neurohormonal)
2. Anatomic locations
3. Specialized cellular structure, function, and biochemistry.

The major function of skeletal muscle is its role as the effector organ in voluntary movement. It mediates transformation of central nervous system electrical activity into purposeful mechanical actions, such as maintaining posture, moving limbs and digits, and speaking. In addition, it has secondary roles:

- Potential source of metabolic energy. In cases of stress, such as starvation, skeletal muscle tissue can be catabolized (broken down) to provide energy.
- Contributes to body heat generation.

The precise control of muscle activity by the nervous system is necessary for effective reflexive and conscious movement. This chapter focuses on its neuronal control of muscle, whereas the discussion of the molecular basis of the contractile machinery and the distinctions between different types of muscle will be covered in Chapter 6.

SYSTEM STRUCTURE

Three organ systems are involved in movement:
1. Nerves (including the brain and spinal cord)
2. Muscles
3. Bones

This chapter will discuss nerves and their interface with muscles at the neuromuscular junction. Although bones have their own physiologic functions and regulatory systems (see Ch. 33), we will currently only discuss them as scaffolding.

Neuromuscular Organs

Although most conscious movement requires input from the brain, reflexive movements require only the spinal cord and the skeletal muscles.

Central Nervous System

The central nervous system is composed of the brain and the spinal cord.

- Higher areas of the brain generate instructions for purposeful, conscious movements and modify lower systems that carry out unconscious movements and reflexive muscle contractions.
- The spinal cord performs two critical functions:
  - Carries information in two directions: sensory input from periphery to the brain, and movement instructions from the brain to periphery.
  - Simple reflex movements requiring no input from the brain.

Skeletal Muscles

Skeletal muscles are found throughout the body connected to bones via tendons.

Collectively, skeletal muscles make up 45% to 50% of total body mass.

- Skeletal muscles receive variable percentages of cardiac output depending on the activity level.
- Various sizes and shapes of skeletal muscles correlate with their skeletal attachments and motor functions.

Neuromuscular Tissues

Tissues important in the generation and tailoring for movements include specific areas of the brain and spinal cord, as well as the skeletal muscles.

Motor Nerve Tissues

Fig. 5.1A illustrates some of the brain tissues involved in the generation and transmission of motor instructions.

The premotor cortex and supplementary motor area are located in the frontal lobe.

- The premotor cortex receives input from the cerebellum, which provides important signals regulating balance and coordination.
- The supplementary motor area receives input from the basal ganglia, a complex subcortical tissue involved in the prioritization of movement programs and their components.
- In addition, both the premotor cortex and the supplementary motor area are connected to networks of sensory and association neurons that provide information important for planning and executing movements.

The primary motor cortex is a strip of frontal lobe cerebral cortex that receives input from the premotor cortex, the supplementary motor area, the cerebellum, and higher sensory and association areas of the brain. The primary motor cortex is arranged as a modified body map called a homunculus.

The axons of the neurons in the motor areas travel through the internal capsule to reach the brain stem and spinal cord (Fig. 5.1B). A number of spinal cord tracts are involved in the

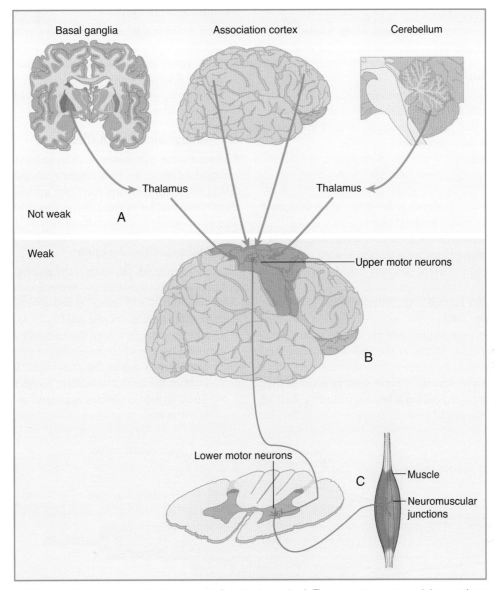

Fig. 5.1 Neural tissues involved in the control of skeletal muscle. A. The premotor cortex and the supplementary motor area are frontal lobe tissues that receive input from the cerebellum and deeper structures, such as the basal ganglia, and transmit information to the primary motor cortex. B. Neurons with their cell bodies in the primary motor cortex send their axons down the internal capsule into the brain stem and medulla. At the pyramidal decussation, the axons cross the midline and enter the spinal cord. C. At a given spinal cord level, the ventral and dorsal roots fuse and synapse on the target skeletal muscle. (From Nolte J. *Elsevier's Integrated Neuroscience*. Philadelphia, PA: Elsevier. 2007. Fig. 14.9.)

transmission of movement instructions to and from higher centers. Among these, the lateral corticospinal tract is critical in voluntary limb movement.

- The cell bodies of neurons of the lateral corticospinal tract are in the primary motor cortex.
- Their axons comprise part of the internal capsule and then constitute part of the lateral column of the spinal cord.
- The axons of many, but not all, motor tract neurons cross the midpoint between their origin and termination, which explains why neurons with cell bodes on the left side of the brain control muscles on the right side of the body and vice versa. Such a crossing of an axon from one side to the other is called a decussation.

The peripheral nerves that control voluntary muscles have their cell bodies in the anterior horn of the spinal cord gray matter (Fig. 5.1C).

- Their axons exit the spinal cord via ventral roots, and fuse with dorsal roots to form spinal nerves.
- These are branched out into peripheral nerves, a large collection of which is called a plexus (e.g., the brachial plexus).
- Peripheral nerves continue to branch out until they reach their target muscles.

Skeletal Muscle Tissue

Skeletal muscle tissue is surrounded by a collagen-containing layer called the epimysium. A block of skeletal muscle tissue is subdivided into bundles of muscle cells by perimysium. A single bundle is subdivided by the endomysium, which insulates individual muscle cells (Fig. 5.2).

Neuromuscular Cells

Three cell types are critical to basic movements.
1. Efferent neurons that carry instructions to skeletal muscles.
2. Afferent neurons that relay information from skeletal muscles to the central nervous system.
3. Skeletal muscle cells.

Nerve Cells

Neurons in higher brain centers such as the lateral corticospinal tract are called upper motor neurons (see Fig. 5.1).

The nervous system cells involved in transmitting instructions for voluntary movements from the spinal cord to skeletal muscles are specialized efferent neurons called lower motor neurons.
- Their cell bodies are located in the anterior horns of the gray matter of the spinal cord.
- Their axons project out sequentially via ventral roots, spinal nerves, and peripheral nerves to the skeletal muscles they innervate.
- Peripheral nerves also contain afferent sensory neurons that relay information from peripheral tissues, including skeletal muscles, back to the spinal cord.

Skeletal Muscle Cells

Skeletal muscles cells, or muscle fibers, are long and cylindrical (Fig. 5.3).
- They result from the fusion of numerous precursor cells during development.
- Skeletal muscle is described as striated because cells appear striped under the light microscope.

Neuromuscular Organelles

Like most other cells, motor neurons and skeletal muscle cells have a number of organelles, including one or more nuclei, endoplasmic reticulum, ribosomes, and the Golgi complex. Although each of these is essential for proper cell function, the following discussion focuses on those organelles critically involved in movement.

The Neuromuscular Junction

The neuromuscular junction is the meeting point between the peripheral nervous system and skeletal muscle. The neuromuscular junction is a chemical synapse between a lower motor neuron and a skeletal muscle cell (Fig. 5.4).
- On the presynaptic side of the neuromuscular junction is the terminal bouton of the lower motor neuron axon.
  - Synaptic vesicles in the presynaptic lower motor neuron contain the neurotransmitter acetylcholine (ACh).
  - These synaptic vesicles aggregate at specific sites called active zones.

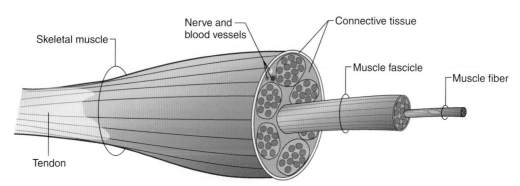

Fig. 5.2 Skeletal muscle subdivisions. The epimysium is the external covering layer of the entire skeletal muscle. The perimysium separates groups of muscle fibers. The endomysium divides individual muscle fibers from one another. (Modified from Carroll R. *Elsevier's Integrated Physiology*. Philadelphia: Mosby Elsevier; 2007. Fig. 5.2.)

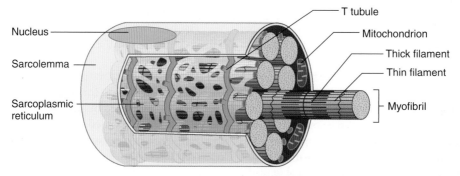

Fig. 5.3 A skeletal muscle fiber. Skeletal muscle fibers are long, cylindrical cells. Because they result developmentally from the fusion of many precursor cells, they have numerous nuclei. The prominent stripes are called striations. (Modified from Carroll R. *Elsevier's Integrated Physiology*. Philadelphia: Mosby Elsevier; 2007. Fig. 5.2.)

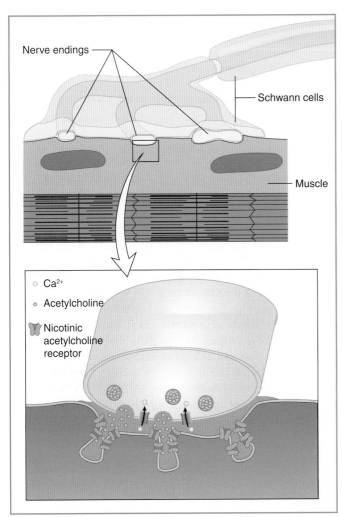

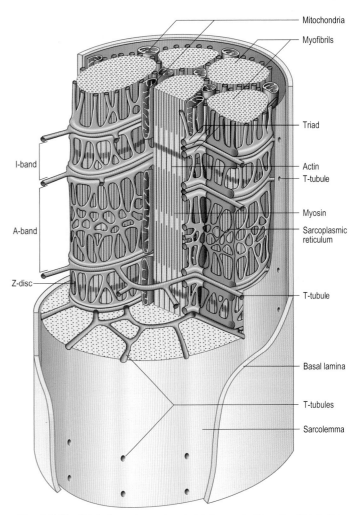

Fig. 5.4 The neuromuscular junction. The terminal bouton has numerous neurotransmitter vesicles that contain acetylcholine (ACh). The vesicles aggregate at active zones. The terminal bouton does not touch its target muscle cell—it is separated from the muscle fiber by the synaptic cleft. The muscle cell membrane, or sarcolemma, apposed to the terminal bouton has numerous synaptic folds where ACh receptors are present in high density. The segment of the sarcolemma with such synaptic folds is known as *the motor end plate*. (From Nolte. J *Elsevier's Integrated Neuroscience*. Philadelphia, PA: Elsevier. 2007. Fig. 14.2.)

Fig. 5.5 The T tubule system of a skeletal muscle fiber. The T tubules are complex invaginations of the sarcolemma. (From Standring S. *Gray's Anatomy*, 41st Ed. Philadelphia: Elsevier; 2016. Fig. 5.42.)

- The nerve and muscle cells are separated by a narrow gap called the synaptic cleft, a complex, amorphously structured extracellular space containing carbohydrates and enzymes.
- On the postsynaptic side of the neuromuscular junction is the muscle cell.

The Sarcolemma and T Tubules

The muscle cell membrane is called the sarcolemma.

- At the points where lower motor neurons synapse with muscle fibers, the sarcolemma forms a shallow depression, or synaptic trough, into which the terminal button fits.
- At the trough, the sarcolemma invaginates into synaptic folds, forming pits which are located directly under the active zones and are studded with numerous ACh receptors. This area is referred to as the motor end plate.

The sarcolemma also has a system of deep invaginations that topologically extend the extracellular space into the muscle fiber. By means of this system of T tubules, subcellular structures even in the center of the muscle fiber are not far from the extracellular space (Fig. 5.5).

The Sarcoplasmic Reticulum

Along with the T tubules, the skeletal muscle fiber contains a structurally and functionally specialized endoplasmic reticulum called sarcoplasmic reticulum (SR), a system of closed membrane pouches (i.e., they do not open to the extracellular space).

- These membrane-enclosed spaces are longitudinal in the middle and have lobulated ends called terminal cisternae.
- The SR has a high internal concentration of calcium.

When a muscle fiber is viewed under an electron microscope, each T tubule invagination is flanked on either side by a terminal cisterna.

- Together, a T tubule and the two terminal cisternae are called a triad.
- Triads occur at regular intervals along the long axis of the muscle fiber.

Myofibrils and Sarcomeres

Striated muscle appears striped when viewed under the microscope because of the regular arrangement of its contractile components, which are made up of specialized protein aggregates.

A longitudinal section through a muscle fiber reveals many closely packed parallel myofibrils with alternating light and dark bands or cross striations.

- Myofibrils are long, tubular structures with longitudinal axes parallel to the longitudinal axis of the whole muscle cell (Fig. 5.6A).
- Myofibrils have five main components (Fig. 5.6B):
  - An I band is the light cross striation (cylindrical).
  - A Z line is a dark line in the center of an I band (disc-shaped).
  - An A band is the dark cross-striation (cylindrical).
  - An H band is a lighter cross-striation in the center of the A band (cylindrical).
  - A M line is a dark line in the center of the H band (disc-shaped).

A sarcomere, a portion of a myofibril between two consecutive Z lines, is the basic functional contractile unit of skeletal muscle. As mentioned earlier, triads occur at regular intervals along the length of the muscle fiber. Each sarcomere has two associated triads, one at each of the I band and A band borders.

Molecules

Several unique molecules are responsible for the electrochemical events that transmit instructions for movement down a nerve cell axon and across the synaptic clefts that separate upper motor neurons from lower motor neurons and lower motor neurons from skeletal muscle cells. In addition, the molecules of skeletal muscle cells constitute the contractile machinery ultimately responsible for movement.

Motor Neuron Molecules

Motor neurons have many proteins embedded in their cell membranes. Among the most important membrane proteins for neuronal control of skeletal muscle contraction are the channels and ion pumps.

Each synaptic vesicle of a motor neuron terminal contains approximately 10,000 molecules of ACh, the fundamental neuromuscular neurotransmitter that activates skeletal muscle. ACh receptors (AChRs) are found in high concentrations on the sarcolemma, clustered around the mouths of the synaptic folds (see Fig. 5.4).

- The AChR is a complex protein pentamer embedded in the lipid bilayer of the sarcolemma.
- Each receptor has five subunits (two α and one each of β, γ, and δ) that combine to form a central ion channel.
- Because the α subunit has the ACh binding site, each ACh receptor can accommodate two neurotransmitter molecules. The five subunits combine to form a central ion channel.

The enzyme acetylcholinesterase (AChE) is associated with the extracellular surface of the sarcolemma via hydrophobic interactions. It is therefore an inhabitant of the synaptic cleft.

Skeletal Muscle Proteins

Like motor neurons, skeletal muscle cells have a number of molecules essential for motor function. The most important of these are the proteins that combine to form the contractile machinery and are responsible for the striated appearance of skeletal muscle fibers. Thin filaments and thick filaments comprise the primary two divisions of the contractile protein machinery.

Thin Filaments

The light I bands of the sarcomere are composed of protein polymers called thin filaments. Thin filaments have three subcomponents, each of which is bound to the Z line by minor proteins (Fig. 5.7A):

- Actin polymers
- Tropomyosin polymers
- Troponin complexes
  G-actin is the monomeric (globular) form of the protein actin.
- G-actin monomers are polarized, having a plus end and a minus end.
- G-actin monomers polymerize into double helical strands of F (filamentous)—actin. Seven consecutive G-actin monomers constitute a single turn of the F-actin double helix.
- Because the constituent G-actin monomers are polarized, F-actin polymers are also polarized and "point" out from the Z line to which they are attached.
- Each Z line thus has thin filaments anchored upon it, projecting out in both directions, that is from both its sides (left and right in a longitudinal view, front and back in a transverse view).

The F-actin double helix has a groove on either side, which is occupied by a thin supercoiled double helix protein called

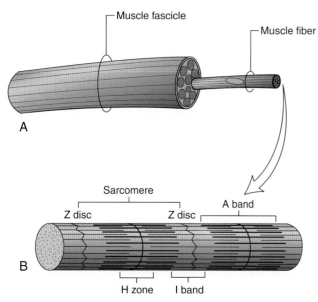

Fig. 5.6 Myofibrils and sarcomeres. A. A skeletal muscle fiber is composed of numerous myofibrils—closely packed, parallel cylindrical structures. B. A single myofibril is a series of alternating dark and light bands. The sarcomere is the basic unit of the myofibril and extends from one Z line to the next. The sarcomeres of a given myofibril are in register with those of adjacent myofibrils, accounting for the striations of a skeletal muscle cell. (Modified from Carroll R. *Elsevier's Integrated Physiology.* Philadelphia: Mosby Elsevier; 2007. Fig. 5.2.)

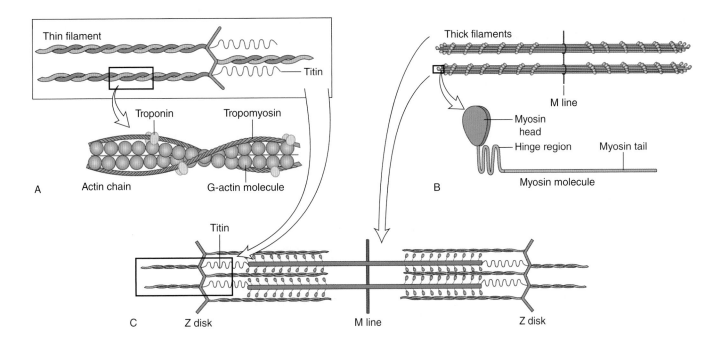

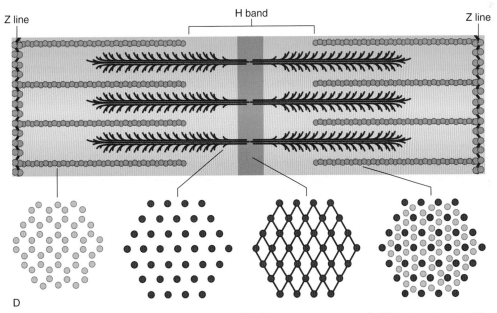

Fig. 5.7 Component proteins of the sarcomere. A. Thin filaments are composed of G-actin polymerized into a double helix of F-actin, tropomyosin, and the three-part regulatory troponin complex. The three proteins of the troponin complex are TnT, TnI, and TnC. B. Thick filaments are composed of myosin. Each myosin monomer has a long tail, a neck, and a head. The tails of two myosin monomers form a double helix. Multiple myosin helices comprise a thick filament. The bare zone in the center of the thick filament lacks myosin heads. C. Thin filaments protrude from Z lines and interdigitate with thick filaments. Minor proteins keep adjacent filaments in register. The bare zones of thick filaments make up the sarcomere's H band. D. Sections through different parts of the sarcomere may show only thin filaments, only thick filaments, or the crystalline array where they overlap. (Modified from Carroll R. *Elsevier's Integrated Physiology*. Philadelphia: Mosby Elsevier; 2007. Fig. 5.2.)

tropomyosin. Each tropomyosin molecule extends the length of seven G-actin monomers on an F-actin polymer.

Each tropomyosin molecule has associated with it a three-part regulatory protein complex called troponin. These three constituents of the troponin complex are called troponin T (TnT), troponin I (TnI), and troponin C (TnC) on the basis of their respective regulatory functions (see later).

Thick Filaments

The dark A bands contain another protein polymer essential to the molecular basis of muscle contraction. This second polymer is called the thick filament, and it is composed primarily of the protein myosin.

A single myosin molecule has a long, straight double-helical "tail" and a double "head" portion at one end (Fig. 5.7B).

- Between the long tail and the head is a point of flexion or the "neck." The arrangement of the neck can be likened to two golf clubs wrapped around each other and then bent near the two heads.
- Myosin molecules aggregate with their tails together to form thick filaments.
- The head of the individual myosin molecules projects out from the cylindrical mass of tails at regular intervals and angles.

Like the F-actin polymers of thin filaments, thick filaments are polarized.

- The center of each thick filament is a bare zone, with only myosin tails and no heads jutting out. This bare zone constitutes part of the central, lighter H band of the A band.
- Polarized thick segments protrude out from either side of the bare zone. Minor proteins in the bare zone help keep parallel thick myosin filaments aligned, and these minor proteins constitute the central M line of the A band.

A fundamental property of skeletal muscle structure and function is that thin filaments of the I band overlap with thick filaments of the A band (Fig. 5.7C). The sarcomere thus has the following molecular structure as one "reads along" its length:

- A Z line at one end has thin filaments projecting from it, forming the I band.
- The thin and thick filaments begin to overlap, interdigitating as the I band ends and the A band starts.
- The thin filaments at one end terminate, leaving only thick filaments, with a central bare zone (H band) at the center of the sarcomere (M line).
- After the bare zone, thick filaments are oriented in the opposite direction from those before the bare zone (the other half of the H band).
- Thick and thin filaments again interdigitate, making a new A band. As with the thick filaments, this second set of thin filaments is oriented in the opposite direction from the first set.
- The A band ends and the second I band starts.
- Finally, the thin filaments of the second I band end by anchoring in the other Z line that defines the single sarcomere.

Neuromuscular Cations

If skeletal muscle proteins constitute the contractile machinery, cations are the battery power of the electrochemical events of motor neuron and skeletal muscle cell function. Although anions, such as chloride (Cl^-), are important in nerve cell and muscle cell physiology, three cations deserve particular attention:

- Sodium (Na^+)
- Potassium (K^+)
- Calcium (Ca^{2+})

Sodium and Potassium

As described in Chapter 2, there is a large concentration gradient favoring the influx of Na ions into the nerve and a second concentration gradient favoring the efflux of K^+ out of the neuron.

- The differential distribution of the charged ions across the nerve cell membrane produces a neuron membrane potential of approximately -60 to -70 mV.

- The situation is similar with the muscle fiber, which has a resting membrane potential of -90 mV.

Calcium. Both lower motor neurons and muscle fibers depend on the presence of a Ca^{2+} ion gradient.

- The Ca^{2+} concentration outside lower motor neurons is much greater than that in the nerve cell cytoplasm.
- In conjunction with the negative resting membrane potential of the lower motor neuron, there is a large electrochemical gradient favoring the influx of Ca^{2+} into the nerve cell.

The situation is more complex with the muscle fiber. Whereas there is still a large electrochemical gradient promoting the influx of Ca^{2+} from the extracellular fluid into the cytoplasm, the more important gradient is the one favoring the efflux of Ca^{2+} from the lumen of the SR (which has a high relative Ca^{2+} concentration) into the cytoplasm.

SYSTEM FUNCTION

Skeletal muscle is arguably the organ system with the tightest relationship between structure and function. The activity of motor neurons and skeletal muscle cells is the direct result of the orderly movement of their components.

Neuromuscular Cations and the Action Potential

As detailed in Chapter 2, an action potential is a wave of membrane depolarization, turning a negative resting membrane potential into a brief positive membrane potential. Changes in membrane permeability and conductance of ions are responsible for the generation and spread of action potentials in both nerves and muscle cells.

In a lower motor neuron, action potentials, caused by increased membrane permeability and conductance to Na^+, propagate down the axon to the many nerve terminals.

- At the terminal, depolarization increases membrane permeability and conductance of Ca^{2+}, which subsequently enters the nerve terminal down its electrochemical concentration gradient.
- Ca^{2+} influx results in the release of ACh from the nerve terminal.

On the other side of the synapse, muscle fiber depolarization triggered by ACh is mediated by increased sarcolemma permeability.

- This leads to increased conductance of Na ions into the cell, and subsequent increased K ions permeability and conductance out of the cell.
- The depolarization propagates across the entire sarcolemma and spreads via the T tubule system into the muscle fiber.
- The action potential triggers Ca^{2+} efflux from the terminal cisternae into the cytoplasm.

After an action potential has passed, membrane cation permeabilities and conductances return to their previous levels and the membrane potential repolarizes, going back to its resting negative value. Neurons and muscle fibers restore electrochemical gradients by extruding Na and taking in K^+ by means of ion pumps, such as the Na^+,K^+-ATPase.

Neuromuscular Molecules

The cations and molecules of excitable cells such as motor neurons and skeletal muscle have a reciprocal relationship.

- An action potential is the result of the function of molecules, such as the ion pumps and channels in the membrane of motor neurons and skeletal muscle cells.
- The release of neurotransmitters and the activation of the contractile proteins are the result of changes in the intracellular cation concentrations brought about by the action potential.

Excitation Contraction Coupling

Excitation contraction coupling is the process by which electrical events (action potentials) are transformed into mechanical events (muscle contractions).

Calcium is the ion essential to the function of sarcomere contractile molecular machinery, and is the means by which electrochemical events (the action potentials of the motor neuron and the muscle fibers) are converted into mechanical events (muscle contraction). Thus the essential step in excitation contraction coupling is the opening of voltage-gated Ca^{2+} channels.

Acetylcholine

ACh is the neurotransmitter molecule responsible for "ferrying" the neuronal action potential across the synapse and initiating a new action potential on the muscle fiber sarcolemma.

When an action potential arrives at a motor neuron terminal, the transient increase in the membrane conductance of Na^+ and Ca^{2+} leads to an influx of Na^+ and Ca^{2+} down their respective electrochemical gradients that causes vesicle fusion with the nerve terminal membrane and the release of ACh into the synaptic cleft.

Once released from the presynaptic neuron, ACh diffuses across the synapse and two molecules of ACh bind to each ACh receptor, resulting in transformation of the neuronal action potential into a muscle fiber action potential by way of a chemical signal.

- ACh soon diffuses from the receptor binding sites and is cleaved by synaptic AChE into acetate and choline, thus inactivating the neurotransmitter signal.
- Approximately 50% of the choline thus produced is taken up by the nerve terminal and recycled into new ACh.

How does ACh engender a new action potential in the sarcolemma?

- The binding of two molecules of ACh to an AChR leads to a conformational shift in the AChR, with the opening of the ion channel and an increase in the sarcolemma permeabilities and conductances for Na^+ and K^+.
- This allows Na to enter the muscle fiber down its electrochemical concentration gradient, and the sarcolemma is depolarized.
- The action potential propagates along the sarcolemma and via T tubules into the muscle fiber.
- Depolarization is transmitted from the T tubules to the membrane of sarcoplasmic reticulum, which has numerous voltage-gated Ca^{2+} channel proteins on its surface:
  - L-type calcium channel, involved in slowly activated sustained conductance

- Dihydropyridine (DHP) receptor, which acts as a voltage sensor that relays the stimulus to release calcium from the SR.
- With depolarization, the SR channels open, releasing Ca^{2+} from the SR into the cytoplasm.

Calcium release from the SR stores is mediated by membrane protein receptors known as ryanodine-sensitive calcium release channels (RyR).

- The RyR is one of two types of calcium-release channels important in excitation-contraction coupling.
- The other channel, more abundant in smooth muscle, is the inositol 1,4,5-triphosphate-stimulated channel (IP3).

Crossbridge Cycling

Contraction depends upon the binding of thick filament myosin heads to thin filament F-actin at specific binding sites.

- In the resting (uncontracted) state of the sarcomere, myosin heads are blocked from binding to actin because tropomyosin occupies the F-actin double-helical groove and sterically inhibits such binding.
- When Ca^{2+} becomes available, it binds troponin C, which triggers a conformational change in TnC.
- TnC thus inhibits TnI, leading the entire troponin-tropomyosin complex to shift away from the F-actin groove.
- This unmasks the previously blocked myosin crossbridge binding site on actin, allowing myosin crossbridges to bind to actin and contraction ensues by means of crossbridge cycling.

Crossbridge cycling is the sequence of molecular events underlying muscle contraction (Fig. 5.8A).

- The myosin head is both an enzyme and a motor. It contains an enzymatic active site that binds the energy molecule adenosine triphosphate (ATP) and cleaves it into adenosine diphosphate (ADP) Pi (Pi is inorganic phosphate).
- In the relaxed state, the myosin head binds a molecule of ATP and has a low affinity for actin.
  - The myosin head then cleaves the ATP into ADP + Pi, which remain in the myosin head active site.
  - This mechanism temporarily stores in the myosin head the chemical energy of the cleaved high-energy phosphate bond and gives the myosin head a high affinity for actin.
- When the actin crossbridge binding site is unmasked, the myosin head binds to the thin filament.
- The ADP and Pi are then released from the active site and the myosin head undergoes a conformational change called the power stroke.
  - The power stroke reduces the angle the myosin head makes with the thick filament from 90 to 45 degrees.
  - The thin actin filament is pulled a short distance by the myosin crossbridge power stroke.
- After the power stroke, a new molecule of ATP then binds to the empty active site on the myosin head, causing it to separate from the thin filament binding site.
- The process of binding and cleavage of the new ATP "resets" the myosin head to its 90-degree angle and restores its high affinity for actin, preparing the system for another round of this crossbridge cycling.

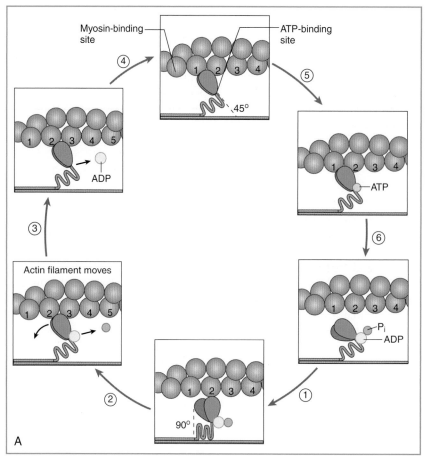

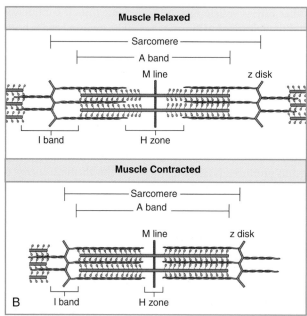

Fig. 5.8 A. Muscle movement is caused by conformational of changes in the myosin motor protein. Ca^{2+} entry exposes the actin-binding sites. The contraction process is initiated (1) by the binding of the myosin head to actin. Release of inorganic phosphate (Pi) (2) initiates the power stroke, moving the myosin heads to a 45-degree angle, and shortening the sarcomere. (3) Following the power stroke and dissociation of adenosine diphosphate (*ADP*), (4) myosin is tightly bound to actin at a 45-degree angle in a rigor complex. (5) Binding of adenosine triphosphate (*ATP*) to myosin breaks the actin-myosin bond. Hydrolysis of ATP moves the myosin head to a 90-degree angle, where it can again bind to actin, returning to (1). Following the power stroke, the process repeats provided that there are sufficient stores of ATP and that Ca^{2+} keeps the actin-binding sites exposed. B. Consecutive crossbridge cycles by many myosin heads cause the thin and thick filaments to slide over one another, shortening the sarcomere. (From Carroll R. *Elsevier's Integrated Physiology.* Philadelphia: Mosby Elsevier; 2007. Figs. 5.6 and 5.7.)

Sliding Filaments

The sliding filament model explains muscle contraction at a molecular level (Fig. 5.8B). How does crossbridge cycling translate into muscle contraction?

- Crossbridge cycling leads to the dragging of thin filaments by the myosin head power stroke.
- This causes thin filaments to slide over thick filaments, increasing the overlap between thick and thin filaments.
  - Z lines at either end of the sarcomere are pulled toward each other.
  - The I band (where thin filaments do not overlap with thick filaments) and the H band (where thick filaments do not overlap with thin filaments) progressively narrow as many sequential rounds of crossbridge cycling take place.
  - The width of the A band is unchanged throughout contraction.

The length of the filaments remains the same, but because their overlap increases, the entire sarcomere shortens. In fact, the degree of filament overlap is directly proportional to (and one of the major determinants of) the force a muscle can generate.

Contraction Cessation

The cessation of contraction is as critical for muscle function as contraction itself. How do the motor neuron and muscle shut off?

- Several key processes lead to the "resetting" of the neuron and muscle cell.
  - Voltage-gated Na channels inactivate, ending the neural action potential.
  - AChR channels inactivate after ACh diffuses away, ending the muscle cell action potential.
  - The electrogenic Na^+,K^+-ATPase ion pump in both the neuronal membrane and the sarcolemma restores the electrochemical gradients by transporting three Na^+ cations out of the cell in exchange for two K^+ cations.
  - Increased cell membrane permeability and conductance to K^+ additionally aids in repolarizing the membrane.
- As such, crossbridge cycling is a self-limiting process as well.
  - Once an action potential in the muscle cell ends, the Ca^{2+} channels in the SR close.
  - Powerful Ca^{2+} pumps in its membrane rapidly move Ca^{2+} from the cytoplasm back into the SR lumen.
  - Decreased availability of Ca^{2+} leads to the diffusion of Ca^{2+} from TnC.
  - This allows the troponin-tropomyosin complex to move back into F-actin groove where the interaction of myosin crossbridge heads with their actin binding sites is inhibited.
  - With the cessation of myosin head binding and crossbridge cycling, contraction ends and passive relaxation occurs (see Clinical Correlation Box 5.1).

Clinical Correlation Box 5.1

Malignant hyperthermia is a clinical condition associated with overactivity of calcium release in relation to reuptake, in which the muscles are rigid and produce muscle damage and excessive lactic acid production.

- Malignant hypothermia can be triggered by certain inhaled anesthetics.
- It is caused by mutations in the ryanodine receptor, which regulates calcium release from the sarcoplasmic reticulum.
- A drug called dantrolene can inactivate that abnormal calcium release by binding to the ryanodine receptor and inhibiting calcium release.

Adenosine Triphosphate, Creatine Phosphate, and Creatine Kinase

If skeletal muscle proteins are the contractile machinery and cations are the battery power, ATP is the energy "fuel" of the muscle fiber.

- When crossbridge cycling takes place, ATP is rapidly hydrolyzed.
- Without a reserve of high-energy phosphate bonds, rapid depletion of the available ATP pool with subsequent inhibition of muscle contraction would result.
  - The molecule creatine is produced in muscle fibers and is phosphorylated to creatine phosphate.
  - When crossbridge cycling starts to hydrolyze the available ATP to ADP + P_i, creatine phosphate can donate a high-energy phosphate to ADP, restoring it to ATP. This is catalyzed by the enzyme creatine phosphokinase (CPK).
  - A clinically important metabolite of creatine is called creatinine (see Clinical Correlation Box 5.2).

Clinical Correlation Box 5.2

Creatinine and Creatine Phosphokinase

Apart from the importance of the creatine system for maintaining adenosine triphosphate supplies and muscle function, this system has two extremely important clinical roles.

The first involves creatinine (Cr), a metabolite of creatine and creatine phosphate.

- Creatinine is produced by and secreted into the bloodstream from skeletal muscle at a roughly regular rate.
- Because it is freely filtered from the blood by the kidney and is excreted in the urine, the Cr serum level is a marker of renal function.
- When a patient's renal function is impaired, the kidney's glomerular filtration rate falls and the serum Cr concentration typically rises. The higher the serum Cr concentration, the worse the glomerular filtration rate.

The second clinical role is the measurement of serum levels of the enzyme creatine phosphokinase (CPK). Distinct isoforms of CPK are found in different tissues.

- Skeletal muscle has a CPK isoform called MM, whereas cardiac (heart) muscle has an isoform called MB.
- When one of these tissues is damaged and cells are lysed (broken apart), there is a release of the tissue-specific CPK isoform from the cells into the bloodstream.
- Measurement of the specific CPK isoform serum concentration allows for the assessment of specific tissue damage.
  - An elevated CPK-MM concentration may indicate skeletal muscle trauma or necrosis (cell death and lysis) from disorders, such as polymyositis and rhabdomyolysis.
  - Elevated CPK-MB are diagnostic of myocardial infarction (or heart attack, the death or infarction and subsequent necrosis of cardiac muscle cells).

Anaerobic glycolysis and oxidative phosphorylation are the two main metabolic pathways for ATP production in skeletal muscle. They both use glucose as their main fuel.

- Anaerobic glycolysis does not require oxygen and generates only two new ATP for each molecule of glucose.
- Oxidative phosphorylation requires oxygen and produces 38 ATP molecules per glucose molecule.

Dystrophin

Dystrophin is a large structural protein found on the cytoplasmic side of the sarcolemma.

- It binds the muscle fiber cytoskeleton to the sarcolemma, so that myofibril shortening with contraction is transmitted to the sarcolemma.

Neuromuscular Organelles

The movements of two organelles are essential for skeletal muscle function.

- Motor neuron synaptic vesicles must move to release ACh into the synaptic cleft.
- Muscle fiber sarcomeres maintain relatively fixed positions within the cell but must shorten.

Motor Neuron Vesicle Fusion

As discussed earlier, a single nerve terminal depolarization leads to an increased neuron cytoplasmic Ca^{2+} concentration that causes the fusion of approximately 60 ACh-containing vesicles with the nerve terminal cytoplasmic membrane and exocytosis of the neurotransmitter. The subsequent depolarization of the muscle cell membrane is called an end-plate potential (EPP).

The large EPP is actually the sum of discrete small depolarizations called miniature end-plate potentials (MEPPs) (Fig. 5.9A).

- Each MEPP has an amplitude of 0.4 mV and correlates to the fusion of one synaptic vesicle and the release of a single quantum or packet of ACh.
- At rest, there is a random release of one or a few vesicles, with generation of MEPPs of different integer multiples of 0.4 mV (Fig. 5.9B).

Sarcomere Shortening

The molecular events of crossbridge cycling and the sliding filament model discussed earlier explain the shortening of a single sarcomere.

- When the effect of a small shortening of one sarcomere is multiplied by the many sarcomeres in series in a single myofibril, the shortening of a single myofibril is considerable.
- When many myofibrils shorten, the whole muscle fiber likewise shortens.
- The shortening of many muscle fibers manifests as contraction of the entire muscle, with change in muscle length and the generation of force.

Neuromuscular Cells

Although the previous discussion detailing the structure and function of the skeletal muscle system on the subcellular level

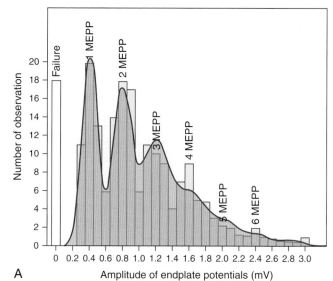

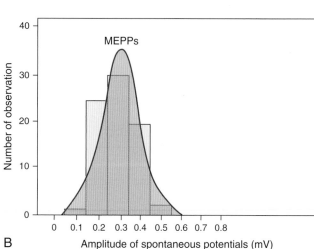

Fig. 5.9 End-plate potentials (EPP) and miniature end-plate potentials (*MEPP*). A. Stimulating a lower motor neuron with low level electrical shocks induces a depolarization known as an end-plate potential of the associated skeletal muscle. The histogram shows the frequency of EPP of different magnitude and demonstrates that the most common EPP are multiple of 0.4 mV. Each 0.4 mV depolarization is defined as a miniature end-plate potential and corresponds to the fusion of a single lower motor neuron synaptic vesicle and release of its ACh. A physiologic EPP corresponds to 60 MEPPs. B. Even at rest, spontaneous MEPPs occur as single neurotransmitter vesicles release their contents into the synapse.

has treated the constituent cells generically, there is significant variability among motor neurons and among skeletal muscle cells. The differences among these cells are anatomic, structural, and functional.

Functional Heterogeneity of Lower Motor Neurons

Lower motor neurons are heterogeneous.

- Type I lower motor neurons are small diameter nerves that typically conduct an action potential at a high speed and are easily triggered. Such small nerves synapse on only a few muscle fibers.

- Type II lower motor neurons are large-diameter nerves that have even higher action potential conductance rates, but require greater stimulation to be triggered. These large nerves synapse on many muscle fibers.

Functional Heterogeneity of Skeletal Muscle Fibers

Like motor neurons, skeletal muscle fibers vary, and their names reflect differences in their structure, biochemistry, function, and (gross or microscopic) appearance.

- Type I fibers are also referred to as "slow," "oxidative," and "red."
  - They produce slow, sustained, powerful contractions for functions, such as weight bearing and posture.
  - They do not fatigue easily, and depend upon oxidative phosphorylation for energy production.
- Type II fibers are "fast," "glycolytic," and "white" (because of fewer mitochondria).
  - They produce faster, shorter contractions and use glycolysis for ATP generation.

Neuromuscular Tissues

To produce physiologically useful contractions, the functions of skeletal muscle cells need to be coordinated in both space and time. There are two types of coordination:

- Coordination within cells during a single contraction.
- Coordination within cells during a series of contractions.

Motor Units

A single lower motor neuron branches out and synapses on numerous muscle fibers (Fig. 5.10A). This provides the first type of coordination, which operates among cells.

- In large muscles that are responsible for powerful, gross contractions, a single lower motor neuron may synapse on over a thousand muscle fibers.
- In small muscles that mediate very precise movements, a single neuron may synapse on as few as two or three muscle fibers.

Any given muscle fiber is innervated by only one motor neuron. A single lower motor neuron and all of the muscle fibers it innervates is termed a motor unit, the functional contractile unit of skeletal muscle.

- Type I motor units are composed of a small nerve synapsing on a few muscle fibers and generating a small force in muscles used for precision movement, such as the muscles of the eye.
- Type II motor units have large nerves that synapse on numerous muscle cells and produce large, gross forces in strength muscles, such as the quadriceps (Table 5.1).
- Because the type and function of the lower motor neuron determine the type of muscle cell, all the muscle fibers in a single motor unit are the same type.

Because different motor unit types are present in a single muscle, a random sample of a tissue demonstrates a checkerboard appearance of differently staining muscle fibers (Fig. 5.10B).

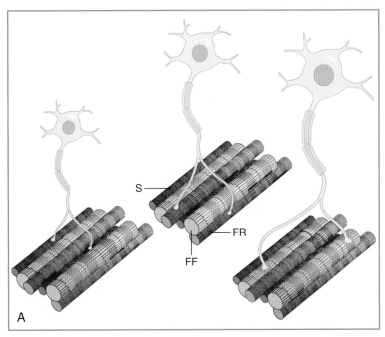
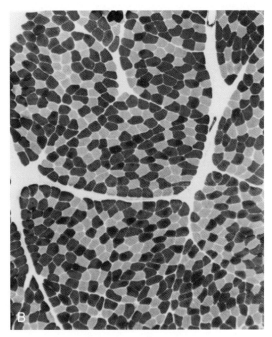

Fig. 5.10 The motor unit. A. A lower motor neuron generally synapses on more than one muscle fiber. A single lower motor neuron and all the muscle fibers on which it synapses constitute a motor unit, the basic physiologic unit of skeletal muscle contraction. B. A single muscle is comprised of numerous motor units. Because the type of lower motor neuron determines some of the biochemical features of its associated muscle fibers, a sample of skeletal muscle has a checkerboard appearance, with type I (*lightly stained white*) and type II (*darkly stained*) muscle fibers mixed together. *FF*, fast twitch, fatigable; *FR*, fast twitch, fatigue resistant; *S*, slow twitch. (A, From Nolte J. *Elsevier's Integrated Neuroscience*. Philadelphia, PA: Elsevier. 2007. Fig. 14.7. B, From Amato A. Disorders of skeletal muscle. In: *Bradley's Neurology in Clinical Practice*. 2016: p. 1915–1955.e5. Fig. 110.2.)

TABLE 5.1	Types of Skeletal Muscle Motor	
	Type I	Type II
Lower Motor Neurons		
Cell diameter	Small	Large
Rate of action potential	Fast	Very fast
Conduction		
Excitability	High	Low
Skeletal Muscle Cells		
Alternate names	Slow, oxidative, red	Fast, glycolytic, white
Rate of myosin ATPase	Slow	Fast
Oxidative capacity	High	Low
Glycolytic capacity	Low	High
Examples of function	Posture	Limb movement

ATPase, Adenosine triphosphatase.

Twitch and Tetanus

A single action potential causes the release of sufficient SR calcium ions to produce a transient muscle contraction. Because the Ca^{2+} is rapidly pumped back into the SR, however, the contraction from a single action potential is a small twitch, which generates a force and a lengthening less than the maximum the muscle can achieve (Fig. 5.11).

- If a series of action potentials stimulates contraction, but the time interval between action potentials is long enough to allow complete relaxation of the muscle tissue, the result will be a series of twitches.

    However, if the time interval between action potentials is shortened so that the SR cannot recollect all of the Ca^{2+} that it released into the cytoplasm before the next action potential arises, complete relaxation does not take place before the next contraction occurs.
- In this case, the new contraction starts with a partially contracted muscle, and contractile forces "stack" onto each other.
- If the frequency of action potentials is high enough, twitches fuse together in a process called summation and the muscle achieves tetanus, a state of maximum contractile force and shortening.

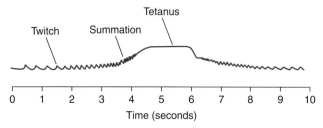

Fig. 5.11 Twitch and tetanus. If a skeletal muscle is stimulated with a brief electrical shock, a single twitch occurs. If a series of electrical shocks is used but the frequency of stimulation is low enough, each twitch resolves as the muscle relaxes completely between stimulations. However, if the frequency is increased, summation occurs and individual twitches stack onto one another, leading to the sustained maximal muscle contraction known as tetanus.

- Tetanus provides the second type of coordination, which operates within cells during a series of contractions.

Skeletal Muscle Organs

The integrated function of many neuromuscular tissues gives rise to the gross behavior of skeletal muscles. Although skeletal muscles play important roles in the metabolism of protein, fat, and glucose, and the generation of body heat, the present discussion focuses on the physiology of muscle contraction.

Length-Stress Relationships

As shown in Fig. 5.12, a muscle can be attached by its two ends to a device that keeps its length fixed and measures the stress it generates before and during stimulation by an electric shock. This allows for the measurement of two types of stress (see Fig. 5.12):

- Passive stress, the stress in the system before the muscle is stimulated.
- Total stress, the stress measured when the stretched muscle is stimulated. The total stress is the sum of the passive stress and the active stress caused by contraction.

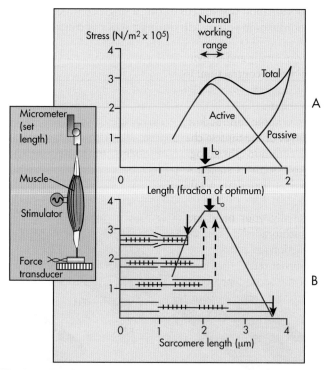

Fig. 5.12 The force of contraction is dependent on the length of the sarcomere. The inset shows the experimental setup, with a micrometer used to adjust muscle length and a force transducer to measure isometric tension. A. The force of contraction at a given length is calculated by subtracting the passive tension from the total tetanic tension. The force of contraction is then plotted as a function of sarcomere length. Contractile force is maximal at sarcomere lengths between 2 and 2.5 mm but gradually decreases at sarcomere lengths above or below this range. B. The overlap of the thick and thin filaments at the various muscle lengths explains this length dependence of contractile force. (From Levy M, Koeppen B, Stanton B. *Berne & Levy Principles of Physiology*, Fourth Edition. Elsevier, Mosby. 2005. Fig. 12.10.)

As the muscle is stretched increasingly farther from its relaxed state, the elastic components of the contractile machinery and cytoskeleton generate the passive stress of the muscle.

- Passive stress is directly proportional to stretch.
- Total stress initially increases with stretching; it then achieves a maximum, after which more stretching of the muscle results in less than maximum total stress.
  - This decrease in total tension must result from a decrease in active stress with stretching of the muscle beyond an optimal point.

The sliding filament model of muscle contraction explains this phenomenon (see Fig. 5.12).

- When the muscle is unstretched and is at a length less than the optimum, the thick and thin filaments overlap so much that they may interfere with each other when crossbridge cycling takes place.
- As the muscle is stretched and reaches the optimum length (L_O in Fig. 5.12), the overlap between thick and thin filaments is optimized, and the resulting active stress generated is at its maximum.
- When stretched even farther, however, the filaments overlap less as the thin filaments are too far away for some myosin heads to reach and bind to thin actin filaments. This results in less-than-maximal force generation, and the total stress therefore decreases.

Isometric and Isotonic Contractions

Experimentally and in living physiology, muscles are capable of two types of contraction: isometric and isotonic.

- An isometric contraction generates a force while the length of the muscle is unchanged.
- An isotonic contraction generates a constant force while the length of the muscle changes.

In common physiologic movements, both types of contraction occur in stages. As an example, consider picking up a glass of water on a table and bringing it to your lips to drink.

- Initially, your hand grasps the glass and your biceps and brachioradialis muscles start to contract. This initial contraction generates an isometric force, and the muscles do not shorten yet.
- In the second phase, an isotonic contraction starts, as the force generated by your muscles overcomes the gravitational and inertial forces keeping the glass on the table. The glass starts to rise as your muscles shorten and your elbow bends, and the force generated by your muscles as the glass is moving is constant.

The shape and connections of a muscle are related to its gross function, so that the forces transmitted to the skeleton are not wasted.

- Most muscles are anatomically arranged so that their resting length is at or near the optimum length, where filament overlap and active force generation are maximized.
- In addition, many muscles cross over joints so that a small change in muscle length at the proximal end of a limb produces a small change in joint angle that translates into a large movement in the distal limb.

- Growth and exercise may alter the maximum force and/or velocity with which a skeletal muscle contracts (see Clinical Correlation Box 5.3).

Clinical Correlation Box 5.3

Growth and Exercise

Lengthening of muscle fibers occurs with normal growth, so that skeletal muscle can keep pace with skeletal growth.

- Lengthening results from the addition of new sarcomeres in series with old sarcomeres, so that myofibrils, muscle fibers, and the entire muscle are longer.
- The muscle can increase its shortening velocity, although it does not increase force generation.

With exercise (training and repeated use), a muscle fiber increases in diameter because of the production of new myofibrils in parallel to old ones.

- This enlargement of the muscle is called hypertrophy, and a hypertrophic muscle cell is able to generate greater forces.
- In contrast to hypertrophy, hyperplasia is the appearance of new muscle cells from cell division. Mature muscle cells have a limited ability to divide.

PATHOPHYSIOLOGY

Diseases involving skeletal muscle are characterized by issues with movement, strength, or both.

- Paralysis, the inability to make a voluntary movement, may occur because of dysfunction anywhere along the path from impulse generation in the motor cortex of the brain, down the axons of upper motor neurons in the spinal cord to the lower motor neurons, along the lower motor neuron axon, across the synapse, or in the muscle fibers themselves.
- Paresis is weakness of voluntary muscle contraction.

Denervation, Hypersensitivity, and Renervation

If a lower motor nerve is cut or destroyed, the muscle cells of the motor unit no longer receive stimulation in the form of ACh.

- The result is flaccid paralysis, in which the muscle lacks normal tone and is flabby.
- Reflex arcs are disrupted, and a patient may have decreased or absent reflexes in the involved muscle.
- The muscle fibers, starved for stimulation, adapt by increasing their production of ACh receptors; the denervated muscle is thus hypersensitive to ACh.

If a lower motor neuron axon regrows and synapses again on the muscle fibers, there can be a return of function.

- In some instances, when multiple axons are damaged and regrowing, the new axon and synaptic terminals are of a different type than the original.
- The result is a change of muscle fiber type, and microscopic examination of a sample of such muscle reveals an abnormal homogeneity of muscle fiber types and a loss of the normal checkerboard intermingling of cell types. This condition is called fiber type grouping.

Fasciculations and Fibrillations

Fasciculations are visible twitches of single motor units.

- Commonly appear in lower motor neuron diseases, such as damage to the anterior horn cell bodies, characteristic of

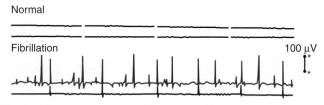

Fig. 5.13 Electromyogram (EMG) showing fibrillation of muscle compared to normal EMG.

amyotrophic lateral sclerosis (ALS), polio, and West Nile virus.
- Clinically, they look like brief ripples under the skin. Fibrillations are spontaneous contractions of single muscle fibers.
- Unlike visible fasciculations, fibrillations are invisible to the eye but can be identified by electromyography, a technique that measures electrical activity in muscle cells (Fig. 5.13).

Botulism

Clostridium botulinum is a gram-positive rod-shaped bacterium that produces a potent protein toxin.
- Patients can contract *C. botulinum* infection through a contaminated skin wound or ingesting the bacterium's preformed toxin in spoiled foods.
- Botulinum toxin enters motor nerve terminals and inhibits the release of ACh, leading to flaccid paralysis, impairing crucial muscles, such as in Fig. 5.14.
- It is one of the most potent toxins known, and as little as 1 mcg can be deadly to a person.

Contractures and Atrophy

If a limb is immobilized for long periods by paralysis or physical restraint, the process of growth is reversed.
- Sarcomeres are removed in series from the myofibrils, resulting in a shortening of muscle called a contracture.
- Patients with paralyzed limbs must therefore have physical therapy so that contractures do not occur.
  With denervation, muscle cells shrink in size, the process of atrophy.
- Over months, atrophic cells can degenerate completely and be replaced by fat or connective tissue.
- Atrophy is also classically seen in conditions with lower motor neuron damage.

Muscular Dystrophy

The dystrophin protein mentioned earlier is one of many cytoskeletal proteins that link the contractile machinery of the muscle cell to the sarcolemma and to other cells. Dystrophin is encoded by a very large gene on the X chromosome, leaving it prone to mutations.

If this gene is mutated so that no dystrophin is produced, Duchenne's muscular dystrophy (DMD), a congenital X-linked hereditary disorder, results.
- DMD manifests as progressive muscle weakness.
- It is present in one out of every 3500 male newborns and is fatal by age 20 to 30 years from events, such as respiratory muscle failure and/or aspiration pneumonia.

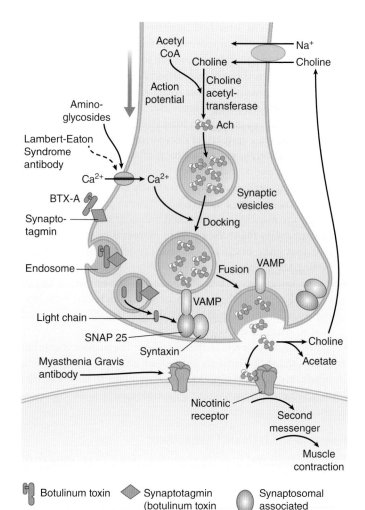

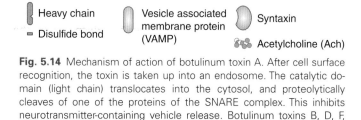

Fig. 5.14 Mechanism of action of botulinum toxin A. After cell surface recognition, the toxin is taken up into an endosome. The catalytic domain (light chain) translocates into the cytosol, and proteolytically cleaves of one of the proteins of the SNARE complex. This inhibits neurotransmitter-containing vehicle release. Botulinum toxins B, D, F, and G cleave proteins of the vesicle-associated membrane protein (VAMP) family while botulinum toxins A, C, and E cleave synaptosomal associated protein (SNAP)-25. Botulinum toxin C can also cleave syntaxin. (From Huang W, Foster JA, Rogachefsky AS. Pharmacology of botulinum toxin. *J Am Acad Dermatol* 2000;43:249–259.)

A less severe form of the disease, called Becker's muscular dystrophy, is caused by a different mutation in the gene that results in a decreased amount or abnormal size of the dystrophin molecule.

Rigor Mortis

With death, there is eventual depletion of the muscle fiber's pool of ATP.
- Without new ATP to fill the active site of the myosin head, the crossbridge cannot release from its actin binding site (see Fig. 5.8A).
- This causes a stiffening of the muscle, a freezing in midcontraction known as *rigor mortis* ("the stiffness of death").

Myasthenia Gravis

Myasthenia gravis is an autoimmune disorder of the neuromuscular junction that manifests as progressive skeletal muscle weakness and fatigability.

The defect in myasthenia gravis is a depletion of AChR and a distortion of the synaptic folds.

- In myasthenia gravis, as in other autoimmune disorders, the body's immune system misidentifies a normal protein (in this case, the AChR) as a foreign or dangerous one and attempts to eradicate it by producing anti-AChR antibodies.
- These antibodies bind to the AChR and interfere with neuromuscular function in three ways
  - Augmenting the rate of AChR endocytosis and destruction.
  - Steric hindrance of the ACh binding sites.
  - Precipitating the formation of the immune system's membrane attack complex, which then damages the muscle cell membrane.

The paucity of AChRs on the surface of the muscle fibers means that there are fewer ACh binding sites when an action potential arrives at the lower motor neuron terminal and subsequently releases ACh.

- With fewer open AChRs, there is less depolarization of muscle fibers, and many fibers that would normally reach threshold and contract do not have an action potential.
- Repeated stimulation leads to progressive neuromuscular fatigue and manifestly poorer performance as the nerve terminal is depleted of ACh with each subsequent stimulation. Symptoms include:
- Generalized proximal limb weakness and fatigability with repeated activity; these symptoms subside with rest.
- Drooping of the eyelids (ptosis) and double vision (diplopia) occur with weakness of the lid and extraocular muscles, respectively.
- If facial muscles suffer, a flattened smile or a snarl when attempting to smile may occur.
- Patients may have difficulty chewing and swallowing.
- "Mushy" or nasal speech may develop, and there may be weakness with neck extension.
- Difficulty breathing, sometimes severe enough to require hospitalization and mechanical ventilation—referred to as a crisis—can result if the diaphragm is affected.

There are two general categories of treatment

- Use of inhibitors of AChE, so that the ACh released from nerve terminals into the synapse is not rapidly catabolized, but can bind to the remaining AChRs for a longer time. A short-acting AChE inhibitor (edrophonium) is used to diagnose myasthenia gravis by demonstrating an improvement in muscle weakness with the inhibitor.
- Direct targeting of the immune system.
  - Surgical resection of the thymus.
  - Use of immunosuppressive agents (i.e., corticosteroids).
  - Removal of anti-AChR antibodies from the blood via plasmapheresis.
  - Use of intravenous immune globulin, an injection of other antibodies to block the anti-AChR antibodies by a poorly understood mechanism.

Treatments have significantly reduced the mortality of the disease, but in most cases, patients require lifelong medical therapy (see Development Box 5.1, Pharmacology Box 5.1 and Genetics Box 5.1).

DEVELOPMENT BOX 5.1

Primary carnitine deficiency can be screened for in newborns. If it is not detected and treated, patients present between 3 and 24 months with lethargy, irritability, and poor feeding. Because carnitine is important for fatty acid metabolism and energy generation, untreated disease leads to encephalopathy, cardiomyopathy, myopathy, and other metabolic abnormalities, such as hypoglycemia. These energy limitations damage neuromuscular tissues that depend heavily on adequate adenosine triphosphate.

 PHARMACOLOGY BOX 5.1

Pharmacologic replacement of L-carnitine can prevent permanent damage to the brain, heart, and skeletal muscles.

 GENETICS BOX 5.1

Primary carnitine deficiency arises from mutations in the SLC22A5 gene, which encodes the OCTN2, a renal epithelial cell transporter that allows dietary carnitine to be retained by the kidneys rather than being lost in the urine.

SUMMARY

- There are three types of muscle: skeletal muscle (under voluntary control), smooth muscle (involuntary), and cardiac or heart muscles.
- The organs essential for voluntary movements are the brain, the spinal cord, and the skeletal muscles.
- Upper motor neurons start in the primary motor cortex of the brain and send their axons down the spinal cord. Lower motor neurons start in the anterior horn of the spinal cord, synapse on muscle fibers, and propagate action potentials by means of the neurotransmitter acetylcholine (ACh).
- When ACh is released from the terminals of lower motor neurons, it diffuses across the synapse and binds to ACh receptors embedded in the muscle cell membrane. This

binding leads to the opening of the ACh receptor ligand-gated ion channel and triggering of an action potential in the muscle cell.

- Muscle cell myofibrils are the microscopic cross-striations of skeletal muscle. A sarcomere, the distance between two Z lines, is the basic contractile unit of a skeletal muscle cell.
- Each sarcomere is an arrangement of overlapping thin and thick filaments. The thin filaments are composed of F-actin, tropomyosin, and the three-part troponin complex. The thick filaments are composed of myosin.
- The sarcoplasmic reticulum (SR) is a skeletal muscle organelle comprised of membrane-bound spaces that store relatively large amounts of calcium ions.

- Excitation contraction coupling is characterized by an action potential that causes the release of calcium ions from the SR, which allows myosin heads to bind to actin.
- The complete sequence of myosin binding, power stroke, releasing, and resetting is known as crossbridge cycling.
- A single lower motor neuron and all associated muscle fibers constitute a motor unit.
- A twitch is the contraction of skeletal muscle in response to a single lower motor neuron action potential. Tetanus is the "stacking" of sequential muscle cell contractions from depolarizations temporally close enough together so that complete relaxation cannot occur between them.
- An isometric contraction of a muscle is one in which stress increases while the length of the muscle is constant. An isotonic contraction is one in which the length of the muscle decreases while the stress is constant.
- Diseases affecting the skeletal muscle system may interfere with any step from action potential generation through sarcomere shortening. Paralysis is the inability to move. Paresis is weakness of movement.

REVIEW QUESTIONS

Directions: Each of the numbered items or incomplete statements in this section is followed by answers or by completions of the statement. Select the one lettered answer or completion that is best in each case.

1. Which of the following ions is stored in the sarcoplasmic reticulum (SR)?
   A. Na^+
   B. K^+
   C. Ca^{2+}
   D. Cl^-
   E. HCO_3^-

2. A 27-year-old woman presents to the emergency department with progressive weakness, drooping eyelids (ptosis), double vision (diplopia), and appears to snarl when asked to smile. She most likely has antibodies directed against which of the following?
   A. Acetylcholine
   B. AChE
   C. Presynaptic voltage-gated Ca^{2+} channels
   D. Postsynaptic ACh receptors
   E. Dystrophin

3. A 54-year-old man with amyotrophic lateral sclerosis has spontaneous movements of his tongue that are visible to the naked eye. Such movements are called:
   A. fibrillations
   B. fasciculations
   C. tetanus
   D. palsies
   E. twitches

4. A 64-year-old man comes to the emergency department with chest pain. His electrocardiogram (ECG) indicates he has had a myocardial infarction (heart attack). Which of the following would you not expect to be greatly elevated in his blood?
   A. Actin
   B. Troponin I
   C. Troponin T
   D. CPK-MB isoform

ANSWERS TO REVIEW QUESTIONS

1. **The answer is C.** The sarcoplasmic reticulum is a major storage site for Ca^{2+}. When an action potential travels along the sarcolemma to the T tubules, it triggers voltage-gated Ca^{2+} channels on the SR to open and release the stored Ca^{2+}. Although other ions may be contained in the SR, Ca^{2+} is the most prominent and important for skeletal muscle contraction.

2. **The answer is D.** This patient has symptoms consistent with myasthenia gravis, an autoimmune disease characterized by the production of antibodies directed against the receptor for ACh. A disease with a distinct but somewhat similar presentation is Eaton Lambert syndrome, in which antibodies directed against the presynaptic Ca^{2+} channel interfere with ACh release from the terminals of lower motor neurons. Unlike myasthenia gravis, Eaton Lambert syndrome often occurs in patients with lung cancer. Dystrophin is the protein whose gene is mutated in muscular dystrophy.

3. **The answer is B.** Fasciculations are contractions of the muscle fibers in a single motor unit and are visible to the naked eye. Fibrillations are depolarizations resulting from one or a few vesicles of ACh being release by a presynaptic neuron. They may be detected by electromyography but are not visible to the naked eye. Tetanus is the achievement of maximal muscle contraction by means of "stacking" muscle fiber depolarizations on one another without full recovery in between successive stimulations. A palsy is dramatic, uncontrolled movements of the body. Twitch is a term generally reserved for electrical stimulation of muscle fibers and corresponds to the skeletal muscle contraction induced by a single action potential.

4. **The answer is A.** Muscle fiber necrosis results in the release of a number of muscle specific proteins. The CPK, troponin I, and troponin T proteins are routinely used to diagnose cardiac muscle cell death, the definition of a myocardial infarction or heart attack. All of these would be expected to be elevated in this patient. Actin is not routinely measured in such situations.

6

Smooth Muscle

INTRODUCTION

Like skeletal muscle (see Ch. 5), the primary function of smooth muscle is contraction. However, although skeletal muscles often attach to bones and cross joints so that contraction produces limb movement, smooth muscle typically forms tissues within organ systems (e.g., vascular, respiratory, gastrointestinal [GI]) to regulate the movement of liquids (blood), gases (air), and/or solids (food) within hollow tubular structures (e.g., blood vessels, bronchi, alimentary tract). Smooth muscle also has synthetic functions that are important physiologically.

SYSTEM STRUCTURE

Just as skeletal muscle function requires the integration of three organ systems (nervous system, skeletal muscle system, and skeletal system), smooth muscle function requires three components:
- Neural input
- Smooth muscle
- Target organ systems

Smooth Muscle in Organs

With the possible exceptions of the urinary bladder and the uterus, there are no true smooth muscle organs. Instead, smooth muscle is a component of many organ systems.
- Often, these organ systems are hollow, and smooth muscle is a component of the walls of the constituent organs.
- Smooth muscle thus serves a contractile tissue that, like connective tissue, serves a roughly consistent function in many anatomic locations.

Smooth Muscle Tissues

Smooth muscle is present in the following tissues:
- The walls of arteries, veins, and lymphatic ducts of the cardiovascular system (Fig. 6.1)
- The walls of bronchi of the respiratory tract (Fig. 6.2)
- The walls of the esophagus, stomach, small intestine, and colon of the GI tract (Fig. 6.3)
- The ureters and urinary bladder of the genitourinary tract
- The myometrium of the uterus
  Smooth muscle cells form sheets and layers (Fig. 6.4). In longitudinal section, the individual cells appear tightly packed in a staggered array (see Fig. 6.4). This staggering means that in transverse section, the single plane of section "catches" different

cells at different points along the longitudinal axis—some at one end, others in the middle (see Fig. 6.4).

Smooth Muscle Cells

Both the muscle cells and the nerve cells with which they are physically associated differ between the skeletal muscle system and the smooth muscle system. Their histologic differences are the basis of functional differences among these cells.

Innervation

Skeletal muscle cells and lower motor neurons make up the neuromuscular junction, or synapse, discussed in Chapter 5. Smooth muscle cells are often associated with neurons as well, but these nerve cells are part of the autonomic nervous system (see Ch. 4).
- Many smooth muscle tissues have dual innervation from both the sympathetic and parasympathetic branches of the autonomic nervous system.
- Instead of terminal boutons, the axons of these autonomic nerves end in dilated structures called varicosities.
- Although these varicosities are closely approximated to the cell membrane of smooth muscle cells, they do not form neuromuscular junctions (Fig. 6.5).

Histology

When relaxed, a single smooth muscle cell is fusiform, or long and tapered at both ends.
- The staggered arrangement of cells allows for close packing: the thickest middle portion of one cell typically is surrounded by the smaller ends of adjacent cells, and vice versa (see Fig. 6.4A).
- These cells are called "smooth" because, unlike skeletal muscle cells, they have no striations. They have a homogeneous appearance under the light microscope.

Smooth Muscle Organelles

When examined by electron microscopy, a number of organelles are visible in smooth muscle cells.
- They contain a single large, centrally located nucleus.
- For synthetic function, they often possess ribosomes, rough endoplasmic reticulum (ER), and Golgi apparati.
- However, the organization of myofilaments is especially characteristic of smooth muscle cells.
  Like skeletal muscle, smooth muscle contains myofilaments, both thick and thin.
- Skeletal (striated) muscle is highly organized into sarcomeres, producing the striations (Fig. 6.6A and B).

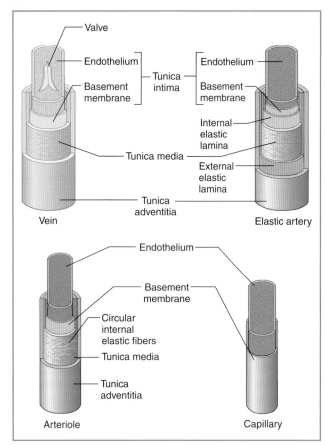

Fig. 6.1 Smooth muscle layers in the wall of peripheral blood vessels. Longitudinal sections of an artery and an arteriole reveal the smooth muscle tissue layer beneath the endothelium. Note that smooth muscle cells are oriented circularly around the vessel lumen, so that even slight contraction will cause important changes in the radius of the lumen. The thickness of the smooth muscle layer is greater in arteries than in veins. Capillaries lack a smooth muscle layer. (From Carroll RG. *Elsevier's Integrated Physiology.* Elsevier; 2006. Fig. 8.1.)

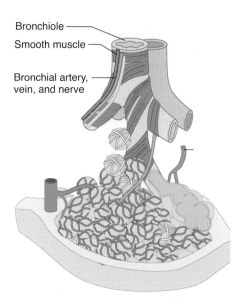

Fig. 6.2 Smooth muscle in the walls of bronchi and bronchioles. Strips of smooth muscle beneath the respiratory mucosa wind obliquely down the airways of the lung. (Modified from Carroll RG. *Elsevier's Integrated Physiology.* Elsevier; 2006. Fig. 10.2.)

- The absence of such striations in smooth muscle cells is a direct consequence of the different arrangement of thick and thin filaments.
  - Smooth muscle cells have no sarcomeres and no regularly ordered association or ratio between the different contractile protein polymers (Fig. 6.6C and D).
  - Instead of the skeletal muscle ratio of 2:1 thin to thick filaments, there is a looser ratio of approximately 10:1 thin to thick filaments.

Whereas sarcomeres in skeletal muscle are connected in series to form myofibrils parallel to the long axis of the muscle fiber, the contractile machinery of smooth muscle cells, lacking sarcomeres, is not limited to this one alignment but is often oriented obliquely.

Smooth muscle cells also have intermediate filaments that interconnect various components of the cytoskeleton (Fig. 6.7A).

- Dense bodies are protein-anchoring structures to which thin filaments attach (analogous to skeletal muscle Z lines).
- Dense bodies may be entirely within the cytoplasm, or they may be bound to the inner aspect of the cell membrane.

Skeletal and smooth muscle cells both have sarcoplasmic reticulum (SR), a collection of closed membranes that store Ca^{2+}.

- Smooth muscle cell SR is not as well developed as that of skeletal muscle.
- As in skeletal muscle cells, the smooth muscle cell membrane is called the sarcolemma and the cytoplasm is called the sarcoplasm.

Although skeletal muscle fibers are the result of the fusion of numerous precursor cells, smooth muscle cells remain distinct. However, in different anatomic and functional contexts, these individual smooth muscle cells may be more or less interconnected.

- Gap junctions, desmosomes, and other structures can mechanically, electrically, and chemically couple adjacent smooth muscle cells (see Fig. 6.7A and B).
- Although smooth muscle cells lack the T tubules of skeletal muscle, they do possess sarcolemma invaginations called caveolae, which perform a similar function (Fig. 6.8).

Smooth Muscle Molecules

As in skeletal muscle, thick filaments in smooth muscle are composed of myosin. However, the smooth muscle isoform is different from that of skeletal muscle. Thin filaments also contain actin and tropomyosin but lack the troponin regulatory complex seen in skeletal muscle. Extensive extracellular connective tissue networks contain elastin, collagen, and reticulin.

Smooth Muscle Cations

As in skeletal muscle cells, there are three cations differentially distributed between the intracellular and extracellular spaces:

- Sodium (Na^+)
- Potassium (K^+)
- Calcium (Ca^{2+})

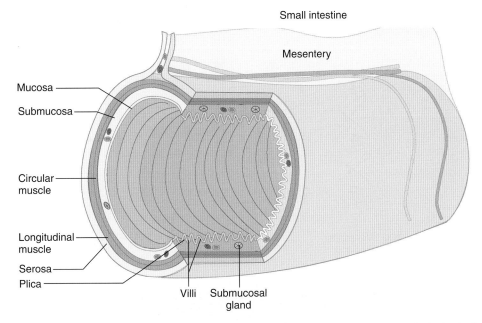

Fig. 6.3 Smooth muscle in the walls of the gastrointestinal (GI) tract. Note that there are both circular layers, which alter the lumen radius according to Poiseuille's law, and longitudinal layers which facilitate the movement of GI contents (peristalsis). In addition, the muscularis mucosae allows the mucosal layer of the GI tract to move. The submucosal (Meisner's) and myenteric (Auerbach's) plexuses are collections of autonomic neurons that modulate smooth muscle contraction. (Modified from Carroll RG. *Elsevier's Integrated Physiology.* Elsevier; 2006. Fig. 12.1.)

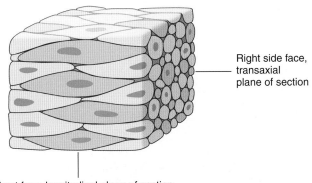

Fig. 6.4 Sheets and layers of smooth muscle cells. Smooth muscle cells are packed tightly together and are staggered in a block of tissue. A longitudinal plane of section (front face of the block) displays the fusiform shape of the cells and how the thicker central part of a given smooth muscle cell is often apposed to the thinner ends of adjacent cells. A transverse or transaxial plane of section (right side face of the block) catches different cells in different places along their long axis.

The electrochemical gradients driving these cations are identical between skeletal and smooth muscle cells:

- The electrochemical gradient for Na^+ greatly favors its influx into a smooth muscle cell.
- The opposite is true for K^+, which exits the cell when K^+-specific ion channels open.
- The cytoplasm of a smooth muscle cell normally has low concentration of Ca^{2+} relative to the extracellular space and the lumen of the SR, so that a large electrochemical gradient favors the entry of this cation into the sarcoplasm.

SYSTEM FUNCTION

Like skeletal muscle, the main function of smooth muscle is contraction. However, unlike skeletal muscle, smooth muscle contraction is largely under unconscious control by the autonomic nervous system. As with their structures, the contractile mechanisms of skeletal and smooth muscle are similar on many scales but differ importantly and reflect their distinct physiologic roles.

Smooth Muscle Cations

As in other excitable cells, such as skeletal muscle cells and neurons, the movement of cations via their electrochemical gradients can cause and result from changes in the cell membrane electrical potential. The relationship between changes in the membrane potential and contraction in smooth muscle cells, however, is not as rigid as that of excitation contraction coupling in skeletal muscle cells.

Smooth Muscle Membrane Electrical Potential

For skeletal muscle, an action potential is absolutely necessary for contraction. However, there is no consistent relationship between changes in smooth muscle membrane potential and contractility. There is great variability from one smooth muscle subtype to another.

- Some smooth muscle cells manifest regular, intrinsic, sinusoidal alterations in membrane potential that are unaccompanied by a change in contractile state (Fig. 6.9A).
- Other smooth muscle cells are activated by an action potential. These cells often exhibit contractile summation and tetanus like skeletal muscles if action potentials "stack" in rapid succession (Fig. 6.9B).

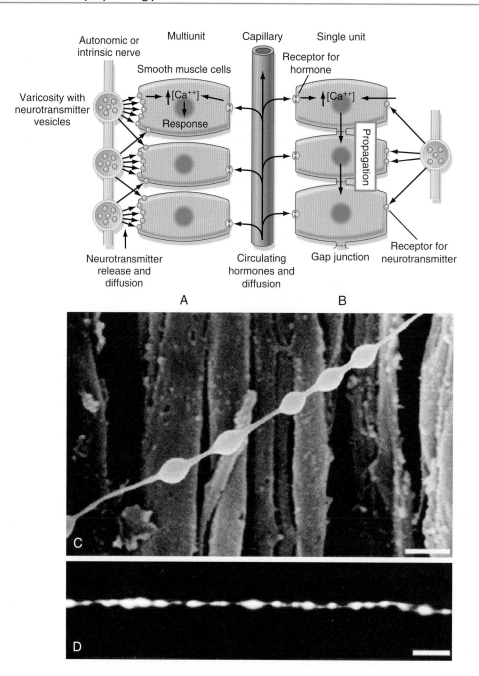

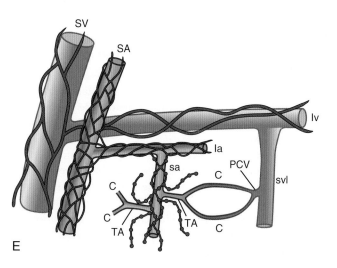

Fig. 6.5 Autonomic neuron endings near smooth muscle cells. Unlike the arrangement between skeletal muscle cells and lower motor neurons, there is no synapse between smooth muscle cells and autonomic neurons. Instead, multiple terminal varicosities (A and D) or single varicosities (B) of autonomic or intrinsic nerves that contain neurotransmitter laden vesicles are closely apposed to the smooth muscle cell membrane (C). In (E), the sympathetic innervation of vascular structures is shown. *C, capillaries; la,* large arterioles; *lv,* large veinules; *PCV,* post capillary veinules; *SA,* small arteries; *sa,* small arterioles; *SV,* small veins; *svl,* small veinules; *TA,* terminal arterioles. (From Koeppen BM, Stanton BA. *Berne and Levy Physiology.* Elsevier; 2018: p. 280–299. Fig. 14.6.)

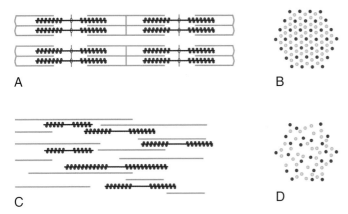

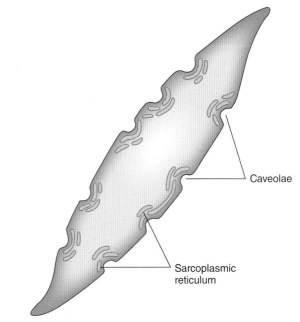

Fig. 6.6 Thick and thin filaments in skeletal and smooth muscle. A, In skeletal muscle, thick and thin filaments are arranged into sarcomeres. B, A transverse section of a sarcomere is characterized by an almost crystalline regularity of filaments and demonstrates the 1:2 ratio of thick to thin filaments in this type of muscle. C, Smooth muscle cells have thick and thin filaments but lack this highly organized pattern of sarcomeres. D, A transverse section of smooth muscle reveals a ratio of thick to thin filaments of approximately 1:10. Nevertheless, the contractile machinery and sliding filament model are largely the same in both types of muscle cells.

Fig. 6.8 Depiction of caveolae.

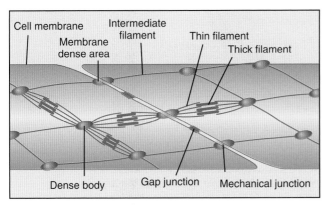

Fig. 6.7 Dense bodies serve as rivet-like anchoring points for thin filaments during contraction. (From Levy MN, Koeppen BM, Stanton BA. *Berne & Levy Principles of Physiology*, 4th Edition. Elsevier; 2005. Fig. 14.2.)

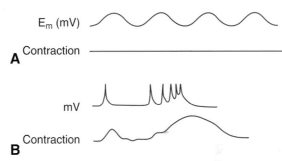

Fig. 6.9 The relationship between electrical activity and contraction in smooth muscle. A, Unlike excitation-contraction coupling in skeletal muscle, spontaneous, periodic membrane depolarization may not cause contraction in some smooth muscle cells. B, In other smooth muscle tissues, a depolarization must reach or exceed a threshold value to cause contraction and rapid sequences may generate tetanus. Various stimuli may induce contraction or relaxation in smooth muscle from different anatomic locations. The critical factors determining a given smooth muscle cell's response to an agent are the type and number of cell surface receptors and their associated signal transduction mechanisms.

As with many cell types, the smooth muscle cell's resting membrane potential is the function of the variable permeability to and different intra- and extracellular concentrations of sodium, potassium, chloride, bicarbonate, and other ions. Ion pumps and membrane channels similar to those in skeletal muscle maintain electrochemical gradients.

Calcium

Skeletal and smooth muscle contraction and relaxation share dependence on changes in the intracellular Ca^{2+} concentration. Influx and efflux of Ca^{2+} into the sarcoplasm determine the sarcoplasmic Ca^{2+} concentration, but the sources of Ca^{2+} vary from one type of smooth muscle cell to another.

Some Ca^{2+} enters from the extracellular pool by means of sarcolemmal ion channels.

- These sarcolemmal Ca^{2+} channels are often voltage-gated or ligand-gated, but others simply remain open for long periods ("leak" channels).

- There are also mechanically-gated Ca^{2+} channels that respond to stretch by allowing influx of Ca^{2+}.
  Other smooth muscle cells have significant Ca^{2+} caches in SR.
- When smooth muscle is stimulated, the entry of extra-cellular Ca^{2+} may trigger the release of sarcoplasmic stores through calcium-gated calcium channels.
- In other cells, stimulatory ligands may activate receptors and generate second messengers, such as inositol triphosphate (IP3) and diacylglycerol (DAG) (see appendix on signal transduction) which may liberate sarcoplasmic Ca^{2+}.
- Whatever the mechanism, stimulation increases the intracellular Ca^{2+} concentration (Fig. 6.10A1-3).

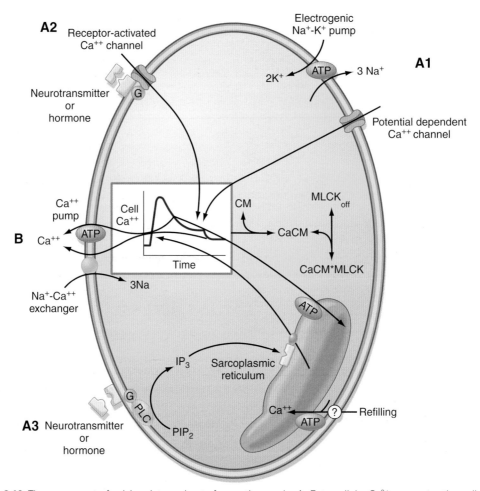

Fig. 6.10 The movement of calcium into and out of smooth muscle. A, Extracellular Ca^{2+} may enter the cell through voltage-gated (*A1*) or ligand-gated channels (*A2*) in the sarcolemma. Leak Ca^{2+} channels open independent of membrane voltage changes or the binding of ligand and spend a relatively large amount of the time open, allowing Ca^{2+} to enter the cell. Ca^{2+} itself, or second messengers, such as inositol triphosphate (*IP3*), may induce the release of Ca^{2+} from the sarcoplasmic reticulum. B, Specialized ion pumps in the sarcolemma remove Ca^{2+}, extruding it into the extracellular space. Some of these use the energy liberated by the cleavage of adenosine triphosphate (*ATP*), while others use the energy of the steep electrochemical gradient favoring the influx of Na^+. Other ATP-requiring Ca^{2+} pumps sequester Ca^{2+} in the sarcoplasmic reticulum. *MLCK*, Myosin light-chain kinase. (Modified from Koeppen BM, Stanton BA. *Berne and Levy Physiology.* Elsevier; 2018: p. 280-299. Fig. 14.10.)

Smooth Muscle Molecules

A number of molecules are important in smooth muscle contraction and relaxation. Among them are regulatory mediators, contractile proteins, kinases, and phosphatases that modulate the contractile proteins, channels and pumps that control the movement of cations, and the small molecules that fuel contraction.

Regulatory Mediators

A number of well-characterized regulatory mediators influence smooth muscle contractility; those that promote and those that inhibit contraction depend on the particular smooth muscle subtype. These mediators include:
- Epinephrine and norepinephrine
- Endothelial derived relaxing factor (EDRF; later identified as nitric oxide, NO)
- Prostacyclin (PGI₂)
- Acetylcholine (ACh)

- Serotonin
- Histamine
- Bradykinin
- Adenosine diphosphate (ADP)
- Estrogen and progesterone
  Like neurons, smooth muscle cells receive both stimulatory and inhibitory signals.
- Stimulatory signals may be in the form of mediators that depolarize the smooth muscle cell and/or increase sarcolemmal permeability to Ca^{2+}.
- Inhibitory signals may hyperpolarize the cell and/or decrease sarcolemmal permeability to Ca^{2+}. Inhibitory signals may prevent contraction and may also promote relaxation in smooth muscle cells.
- A mediator that stimulates a certain type of smooth muscle cell may have an inhibitory effect on smooth muscle in another location.

Contraction

Although skeletal and smooth muscle both depend on Ca^{2+} for regulation of contraction and relaxation, the resemblance is somewhat superficial. Although increases in skeletal muscle sarcoplasmic Ca^{2+} initiate contraction by binding to troponin and exposing the myosin binding site on actin filaments, smooth muscle cells lack troponin and possess a different Ca^{2+}-sensitive contraction and relaxation control mechanism.

When stimulation of smooth muscle leads to an increase in sarcoplasmic Ca^{2+}, four Ca^{2+} ions bind to a regulatory protein called calmodulin.

- The Ca^{2+}-calmodulin complex activates myosin light-chain kinase (MLCK).
- MLCK phosphorylates (and thereby activates) the smooth muscle thick filament myosin light chain.
- Phosphorylation of myosin leads to crossbridge cycling with actin, and thereby contraction (Fig. 6.11).

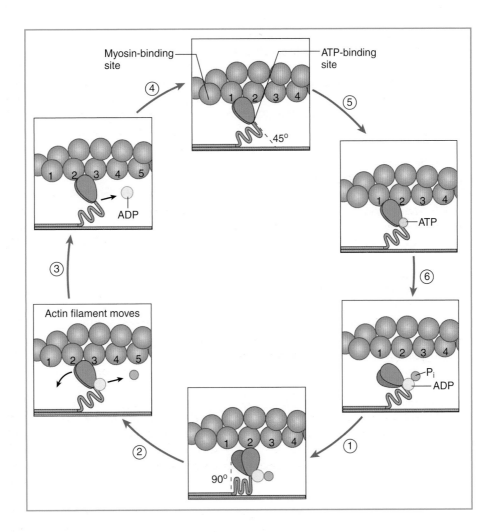

Fig. 6.11 The role of Ca^{2+} in smooth muscle contraction. The myosin heads of smooth muscle progress through four chemical reactions similar to those in skeletal muscle. Reaction 1, in which the myosin head is neither phosphorylated nor bound to actin, depends on Ca^{2+} binding to calmodulin. This complex then activates the enzyme myosin light-chain kinase (MLCK), which adds a phosphate group taken from adenosine triphosphate (*ATP*) to myosin. This greatly increases the affinity of myosin for actin and the rate of reaction 2, crossbridge cycling, thus augmenting contraction. Myosin phosphatases can remove the phosphate group from myosin, whether the myosin is bound to actin (reaction 3) or not (the reverse of reaction 1), returning it to its lower cycling rate. Note that when the unphosphorylated myosin head is bound to actin and is associated with adenosine diphosphate (*ADP*) + P_i, it produces the latch bridge state responsible for smooth muscle tone. In reaction 4, substitution of an ATP for ADP + P_i resets the myosin head by decreasing its affinity for actin. Any stimulus that increases intracellular concentrations of cyclic adenosine monophosphate (cAMP) will activate protein kinases that phosphorylate MLCK, decreasing its affinity for the Ca^{2+}-calmodulin complex and thus inhibiting contraction. (From Carroll RG. *Elsevier's Integrated Physiology.* Elsevier; 2006. Fig. 5.6.)

Crossbridge cycling in smooth muscle is similar to that in skeletal muscle, although the rate of smooth muscle crossbridge cycling is much lower than that of skeletal muscle. Recall that this process entails:
- Attachment of the myosin head to an actin binding site
- Power stroke
- Release of ADP and inorganic phosphate
- Binding of a new adenosine triphosphate (ATP) molecule
- Release of myosin itself
- Resetting of the myosin head for a new power stroke by splitting the terminal high-energy phosphate bond of the ATP molecule

As in skeletal muscle, contractile filaments have different states, with four such states in smooth muscle. The myosin head may be phosphorylated or unphosphorylated, and it may be bound to actin or unbound (see Fig. 6.11).
- In the unphosphorylated state, the rate of myosin crossbridge cycling is very low.
- In the phosphorylated state, the rate is much higher, although it is still much lower than the skeletal muscle rate.

Similar to skeletal muscle, crossbridge cycling and numerous ion pumps in smooth muscle consume ATP. Note, however, that activated MLCK also uses ATP to phosphorylate myosin and thus regulate the rate of crossbridge cycling.

When smooth muscle stimulation decreases, sarcolemma and SR membrane transporters pump Ca^{2+} out of the cell and into the SR, respectively.
- This decreases the sarcoplasmic Ca^{2+} concentration.
- Ca^{2+} dissociates from calmodulin, which inactivates MLCK.
- A separate enzyme called myosin phosphatase removes phosphate groups from the myosin light chain.

However, although the dephosphorylated myosin has a lower rate of crossbridge cycling, it also has a lower rate of detachment from actin than does the skeletal muscle isoform.
- It thus enters a latch bridge state, where it stays attached to the thin filament, maintaining contraction for prolonged periods despite low sarcoplasmic Ca^{2+} concentrations and with minimal ATP consumption.
- This is what allows smooth muscle cells to maintain a state of prolonged partial contraction known as tone.
- Tone becomes particularly important in processes, such as regulation of blood pressure or maintaining the competence of sphincters in the urinary or digestive systems.

Relaxation

In time, in the setting of a low sarcoplasmic Ca^{2+} concentration, the dephosphorylated myosin heads do detach from actin, and the contractile filaments relax.

In addition, mediators that bind to sarcolemma receptors that activate the adenylate cyclase-cyclic adenosine monophosphate (cAMP) second messenger system (see appendix on signal transduction) will activate protein kinases that phosphorylate MLCK, which decreases its affinity for the Ca^{2+}-calmodulin complex, so that it remains relatively inactive (see Fig. 6.11).
- Example: binding of epinephrine to the beta-2-adrenergic receptor, which relaxes vascular smooth muscle and causes vasodilation.

- In addition, mediators that increase intracellular concentrations of cyclic guanosine monophosphate (cGMP) will also activate protein kinases that promote relaxation by modulating the activity of Ca^{2+} ion pumps (see Fig. 6.10B).

These kinases increase the activity of myosin light chain phosphate (see Fig. 6.11) and modulate the activity of Ca^{2+} ion pumps, increasing the extrusion and/or sequestration of Ca^{2+}, decreasing the sarcoplasmic Ca^{2+} concentration and thereby promoting relaxation (see Fig. 6.10B).

Finally, hyperpolarization of the sarcolemma may close voltage-gated Ca^{2+} channels, decreasing the influx of Ca^{2+} and allowing the tonically contracted smooth muscle to relax (Fig. 6.12).

Adenosine Triphosphate

Smooth muscle uses significantly less ATP than skeletal muscle.
- Although ATP is expended in the regulation of smooth muscle contraction, the latch bridge mechanism allows smooth muscle to generate and sustain significant forces with a net saving of ATP over skeletal muscle.
- This economy lets smooth muscle function at a low metabolic rate, and oxidative phosphorylation is sufficient for producing the necessary ATP.

Smooth Muscle Organelles

As in other cells, mitochondria produce ATP via oxidative phosphorylation. Ribosomes, rough ER, and the Golgi apparatus are important in the production and secretion of collagen, elastin, proteoglycans, and other extracellular matrix components by smooth muscle cells. Thus smooth muscle cells have synthetic and secretory abilities similar to those of fibroblasts.

Smooth Muscle Cells

When a smooth muscle cell contracts, the outer membrane wrinkles and the nucleus takes on a "corkscrew" appearance (Fig. 6.13). Contraction in smooth muscle pulls the cell inward from all directions, as opposed to skeletal muscle, in which contraction generally just shortens the longitudinal dimension of the cell. Smooth muscle contractions are of two distinct patterns depending on the functional requirement:
- Vascular and sphincter smooth muscle cells maintain tone.
- Contraction of smooth muscle in the GI and genitourinary tracts is intermittent, or phasic, to propel materials (food, feces, urine, etc.) forward.

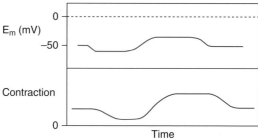

Fig. 6.12 Relaxation of smooth muscle in response to membrane hyperpolarization. Among the many stimuli that can induce smooth muscle relaxation, hyperpolarization of the sarcolemma may close voltage-gated Ca^{2+} channels in some smooth muscle cells. The resulting decrease in cytoplasmic Ca^{2+} allows such cells that are tonically contracted to relax.

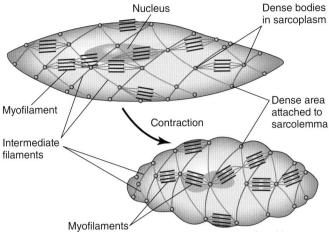

Fig. 6.13 Morphologic changes in smooth muscle cells with contraction. Because the contractile proteins of smooth muscle cells are arranged obliquely instead of in parallel sarcomeres, contraction induces a dramatic shape change in the cell. The sarcolemma wrinkles, and the nucleus takes on a corkscrew-shaped appearance. These changes are reversible with relaxation.

Smooth Muscle Tissues

To induce changes of sufficient magnitude, a single smooth muscle cell must coordinate its contractile activity with several other cells. There are two mechanisms that allow such co-ordination of distinct smooth muscle cells into organized smooth muscle tissues.

- The chemical and mechanical interconnection of cells
- The regulation of contraction by soluble mediators that harmonize the responses of an individual smooth muscle cell with others in a tissue.

Unitary Versus Multiunit Tissues

Some smooth muscle tissues are characterized by a high degree of electrochemical coupling between adjacent cells, owing to the presence of numerous gap junctions.

- In such tissues, the stimulation of one cell will cause contraction in the group of connected cells, known as a syncytium.
- These are called unitary tissues and are found in the sphincters of the GI and genitourinary tracts (Fig. 6.14A).

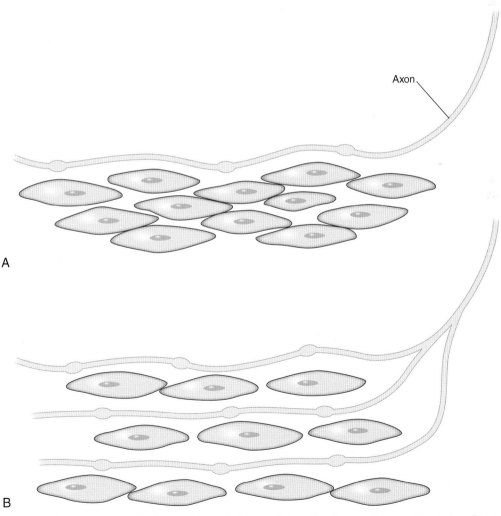

Fig. 6.14 Unitary versus multiunit smooth muscle tissues. A, In unitary tissues, the smooth muscle cells are electrochemically linked into a single syncytium. B, Multiunit tissues are composed of cells that act separately and must be individually stimulated to contract or relax. Note the different arrangement of autonomic nerve cell neurotransmitter-containing vesicles between the two tissues.

Other smooth muscle tissues, such as those of the vas deferens and the iris, are called multiunit tissues because of the relative paucity of electrochemical cell-cell interconnections.

- Each cell in such a tissue must be stimulated independently to contract (Fig. 6.14B).
- Often, the cells of multiunit tissues are controlled by neural and endocrine factors.

The degree of cell-cell interconnection is actually a graded phenomenon; unitary and multiunit tissues are two ends of a spectrum.

- In general, smooth muscle tissues that maintain tone (vascular, sphincters) are closer to the unitary end and do not exhibit action potentials.
- Smooth muscle tissues requiring phasic contraction, such as the iris, are more likely to have action potentials and are closer to the multiunit end (see Fast Fact Box 6.1)

Fast Fact Box 6.1

Cell-cell interconnection in a given tissue may change over time, as gap junctions are dynamic structures. Neuro hormonal influences can increase or decrease their number. For example, the uterus, which generally has a multiunit structure, demonstrates a great increase in gap junctions and movement toward the unitary end of the spectrum at the end of pregnancy in anticipation of labor.

The Control of Contraction

Smooth muscle contraction is involuntary, unlike skeletal muscle, which is under conscious control. This presents a unique challenge in regulation.

- Smooth muscle in vessels and sphincters must maintain tone, but they must be able to adjust how much tone is present.
- Tissues that contract phasically must be able to modify the frequency and the strength of such intermittent contractions.

The various stimuli that cause and/or influence smooth muscle contraction reflect the heterogeneity of different smooth muscle tissues. Smooth muscle contraction is often independent of neurons, and some smooth muscle has no neural input at all.

Smooth muscle contraction is often modified by both sympathetic and parasympathetic inputs. However, the specific response to a given stimuli is different from cell to cell, and may even differ depending on the concentration of a given neurotransmitter.

- Example 1: GI smooth muscle contracts in response to parasympathetic stimuli and decreases contraction in response to sympathetic stimuli. However, vascular smooth muscle increases contraction in response to sympathetic stimuli.
- Example 2: The amount of epinephrine influences its effect on vascular contractility.
  - In low concentrations, stimulation of β_2-adrenergic receptors (via the cAMP pathway) leads to relaxation of smooth muscle and subsequent vasodilation.
  - In higher concentrations, α_1-adrenergic receptors are activated, leading to smooth muscle contraction and vasoconstriction (via the phospholipase [PLC]-IP$_3$-DAG pathway).

Endocrine factors can also have differential effects on smooth muscle.

- Estrogen and progesterone alter uterine phasic contraction.
  - Estrogen induces phasic hyperpolarizations in the sarcolemma.
  - Progesterone hyperpolarizes it nonphasically.
- Angiotensin II is a potent mediator that increases vascular tone.
  - Inhibiting angiotensin II generation or action with medications, such as angiotensin-converting enzyme (ACE) inhibitors or angiotensin II receptor antagonists, is an important means of correcting high blood pressure and treating kidney disease, respectively.

Many smooth muscle tissues are influenced by the paracrine factors of nearby or adjacent cells other than neurons. These factors include NO, bradykinin, and histamine. The best example of this is the effect of endothelium on vascular smooth muscle:

- If an isolated vascular smooth muscle tissue is exposed to ACh, activation of the PLC-IP$_3$-DAG second messenger system results in contraction.
- However, a sample of vascular smooth muscle with an intact endothelium will relax when exposed to ACh.
- This paradoxical reaction occurs because the ACh binds to endothelial receptors and promotes the production of NO. The NO diffuses from endothelial cells and increases smooth muscle cell cGMP levels, resulting in relaxation.

Local metabolites, such as adenosine, carbon dioxide, and protons (H$^+$), can also influence smooth muscle.

- As tissues increase their metabolic rate (demand) or suffer decreased blood flow (supply), the local concentrations of these mediators increase.
- Often, these markers of increased metabolic activity promote vascular smooth muscle relaxation to induce vasodilation and increase local tissue blood flow to meet metabolic demand.
- This action, in turn, corrects the demand-supply imbalance and "washes out" the metabolites, diluting the stimuli for smooth muscle relaxation and vasodilation.
- Thus the contractile state of the vascular smooth muscle is constantly modified to match the metabolic needs of the tissues.
- This is an important example of a homeostatic mechanism (see Ch. 1).

Finally, mechanical forces, such as stretch, can stimulate smooth muscle contraction. This is another important homeostatic mechanism.

- In tonically contracted smooth muscle tissues, such as the vascular system, this response is a critical component of blood pressure autoregulation.
  - Increased blood pressure stretches the smooth muscle in the walls of blood vessels.
  - If the smooth muscle relaxes and the vessels dilate, the resistance to blood flow decreases, thereby lowering the blood pressure.
- In phasically contracting tissues, such as in the GI and genitourinary systems, stretch is a stimulus to increase activity, facilitating the movement and digestion of food and the removal of waste products.

Smooth Muscle and Organ Functions

Changes in the state of contraction of smooth muscle tissues have organ-specific effects that depend on both the physical arrangement of the smooth muscle tissues in the particular organ and on the material contained in that organ.

- The smooth muscle in blood vessel walls is typically in a state of partial contraction.
  - Limited contraction of vessel wall smooth muscle tends to increase blood vessel diameter and increase blood flow.
  - Excessive relaxation may cause stasis of blood.
  - Excessive contraction can obstruct blood flow entirely.
- In the GI tract, the rate of phasically contracting smooth muscle tissue regulates the movement of food and feces.
  - Slowing the rate leads to stasis $\rightarrow$ constipation.
  - Increasing the rate leads to augmented motility $\rightarrow$ diarrhea.

Smooth Muscle Orientation

The arrangement of smooth muscle tissues within different organs reflects the function of the tissue in that particular organ.

- In blood vessels, smooth muscle is circumferentially arranged so that contraction will decrease the radius of the vessel lumen (see Fig. 6.1).
- In the GI tract, different orientations of distinct smooth muscle layers within the walls allow mixing and peristalsis, the propulsion of the luminal contents (see Fig. 6.3; and Ch. 25).

Resistance in Tubular Structures

Recall that Ohm's law describes the relationship among the flow of something (electrons, fluids); the gradient that drives this flow (potential difference, pressure differences); and the resistance to this flow (see Ch. 9.)

In many tissues, smooth muscle regulates resistance. This is especially true in the vascular and respiratory systems, where changes in smooth muscle contractility alter tube caliber and therefore the resistance to the flow of materials.

In the cardiovascular system, Ohm's law takes this form:

$$BP = CO \times TPR$$

where BP is blood pressure, CO is cardiac output, which is the product of heart rate and stroke volume, and TPR is total peripheral resistance. In conjunction with Poiseuille's law, we can rearrange this relationship and express it in this way:

$$TPR = 8\eta l / \pi r^4$$

where η is the viscosity of the fluid (blood), l is the length of the tube (vessel), and r is the radius of the tube (vessel). This equation quantifies the exquisite sensitivity of the resistance to the vessel radius.

- Smooth muscle contraction decreases this radius and dramatically increases TPR.
- Conversely, relaxation decreases TPR by allowing the vessel radius to increase.

Length-Stress Relationships

Smooth muscle manifests length-stress relationships qualitatively akin to those of skeletal muscle.

- Total stress generation is the sum of passive and active stress.
- Active stress generation follows a parabolic curve with a central maximum, representing optimum overlap between thick and thin filaments.

However, smooth muscle contraction occurs over a broader range of lengths than skeletal muscle (Fig. 6.15A and B). The maximal shortening velocity of skeletal muscle is many times greater than that of smooth muscle, although smooth muscle can generate forces equal to or greater than skeletal muscle (Fig. 6.15C).

Smooth muscle typically exhibits viscoelastic or (plastic) homeostatic properties, defined as follows:

- In hollow tubular structures, smooth muscle tone determines the baseline pressure exerted on the luminal contents.
- When a stimulus stretches the muscle, it initially resists this stimulus and a counterstress is generated, thereby increasing the pressure inside the tube.
- In time, the muscle relaxes and takes on a new (greater) resting length to return to its original internal pressure.

The faster the development of the stretching stimulus, the greater the transient counterstress generated, and the higher the brief increase in content pressure, but the faster the "decay" to a new resting length and return to the baseline stress and pressure. A stretching stimulus that evolves more slowly produces a smaller counterstress and increase in pressure, but it decays to baseline more slowly (Fig. 6.15D).

An opposite stimulus causes the reverse of these changes.

- A decrease in luminal contents brings about a decrease in luminal pressure and wall stress.
- The smooth muscle shortens and increases its degree of contraction to restore the baseline force and maintain luminal pressure (Fig. 6.15E) (see Development Box 6.1 and Genetics Box 6.1).

🧬 GENETICS BOX 6.1

Alpha actin 2 (ACTA2) is the most common isoform in smooth muscle of a family of important contractile proteins, and missense mutations in the ACTA2 gene are associated with the rare disease multisystemic smooth muscle dysfunction syndrome, a disease characterized by abnormal smooth muscle contractility in the cardiovascular, genitourinary, gastrointestinal, and other systems.

🧬 DEVELOPMENT BOX 6.1

Neonates with multisystemic smooth muscle dysfunction syndrome present with dilated, fixed pupils that do not respond to light, and a widely patent ductus arteriosus, reflecting smooth muscle dysfunction. Patients have hypoperistalsis and decreased bladder contraction. As patients age, they can develop large arterial aneurysms as impaired vascular smooth muscle contraction allows the progressive stretching of the vessel wall by blood pressure. Rupture of such dilated vessels can be fatal, so often they must be corrected surgically.

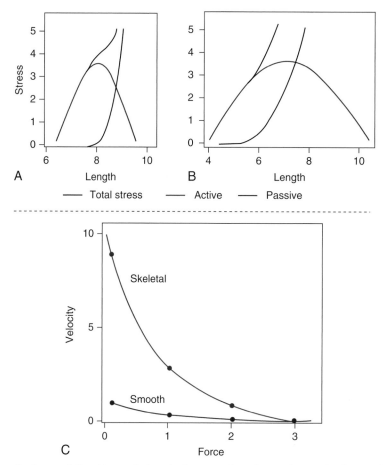

Fig. 6.15 Length-stress relationships and viscoelastic properties of smooth muscle tissues. A, In skeletal muscle, total stress generation is the sum of passive stress and active stress. B, Smooth muscle behaves in a qualitatively similar manner but can generate active stress over a broader range than skeletal muscle can. As a smooth muscle cell is stretched, the overlap of thick and thin filaments is at first improved, then optimized, but then falls away from the optimum length. Active stress generation is maximal when the degree of filament overlap is optimal. C, Although smooth muscle can generate stress and force equal to those generated by skeletal muscle, the velocity of shortening of smooth muscle is significantly lower than that of skeletal muscle.

PATHOPHYSIOLOGY

Disease states resulting from problems with smooth muscle can affect any of the organ systems in which smooth muscle functions.

- Disorders in contractile function typically occur when smooth muscle contracts too much or too little, often producing a pathologic alteration in the resistance to flow in hollow tubular structures.
- Pathologic smooth muscle synthetic function may also contribute to disease.

Cardiovascular

Because of its prominent structural and functional roles in blood vessels, smooth muscle dysfunction has dramatic consequences for cardiovascular homeostasis.

- Alterations in blood pressure are often because of changes in the contractile state of smooth muscle.
- In some clinical situations, using pharmacologic agents acting on smooth muscle can be used therapeutically to alter blood pressure. (see Clinical Correlation Box 6.1).

Clinical Correlation Box 6.1

A number of pharmacologic agents can be used to alter blood pressure.

In hypertension, where blood pressure is pathologically elevated, several agents can be used to lower blood pressure in the short or long term. One such group of agents is the nitrates.

- Nitrates are metabolized to nitric oxide (NO), which enters the cytosol of smooth muscle cells and activates the enzyme guanylate cyclase.
- This leads to the conversion of guanosine triphosphate (GTP) to cyclic guanosine monophosphate (cGMP).
- Increased concentration of cGMP leads to phosphorylation of: (1) myosin light-chain kinase (MLCK), inactivating it, and (2) myosin light chain phosphatase, activating it.
- These two changes together lead to dephosphorylation of myosin, causing smooth muscle relaxation and lowering of total peripheral resistance.

In hypotension, where blood pressure is pathologically low, agents known as vasopressors can be used to raise blood pressure.

- Certain agents, such as dobutamine, increase the contractility of the heart (and thereby stroke volume) via beta-1 adrenergic stimulation.
- Other agents, such as phenylephrine, lead to contraction of vascular smooth muscle via alpha-1 adrenergic stimulation.
- Many agents, such as epinephrine/norepinephrine, lead to increased blood pressure via diverse mechanisms.

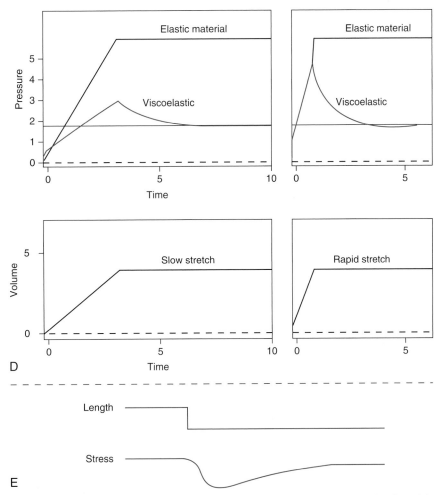

Fig. 6.15 cont'd D, Smooth muscle displays viscoelastic properties. In a three-dimensional model system, smooth muscle in the wall of a hollow tube exerts a tonic pressure on the contents of the tube. Stretching the smooth muscle slowly results in a small increase in the pressure that decays slowly to baseline, whereas stretching the smooth muscle rapidly produces greater pressure that decays more quickly. E, In a linear model of the reverse process, shortening a smooth muscle results in an early loss of stress followed by a gradual recovery toward baseline as the muscle adapts to the new length.

Septic Shock

In serious infections, the release of endogenous and exogenous chemical mediators during the inflammatory response may cause the relaxation of smooth muscle in many vascular beds, lowering peripheral resistance to blood flow as many blood vessels dilate.

- As predicted by Ohm's law, the blood pressure decreases, sometimes precipitously and to dangerously low levels, a condition known as shock.
- Because of the infectious basis, this type of reaction is known as septic shock.

Treatment typically involves restoration of volume, early antibiotic administration, and administration of vasopressors, such as norepinephrine to maintain vascular tone.

Cardiogenic Shock

Because cardiac output is the product of stroke volume of blood ejected per cardiac contraction and heart rate (contractions per minute), any serious impairment in cardiac contractility, such as a severe heart attack, will reduce the stroke volume and thus the cardiac output. A decrease in heart rate may do the same.

In either situation (or when the two concur), a life-threatening decrease in blood pressure known as cardiogenic shock may ensue.

- In response to the low blood pressure (hypotension), the homeostatic systems of the body attempt to maintain the blood pressure by increasing peripheral resistance.
- This is accomplished by increased vascular smooth muscle tone.
- The result is a patient whose skin is cool and sometimes blue (cyanotic) from arterial constriction in the skin that slows down the flow of deoxygenated blood.

Treatment revolves around supporting contractility, controlling preload (as the pump cannot effectively move blood forward), and reducing afterload (to reduce the resistance to blood flow) with pharmacologic and even mechanical supports.

Raynaud Phenomenon and Prinzmetal Angina

Vascular smooth muscle occasionally spasms inappropriately. In peripheral tissues, this may lead to a deprivation of blood flow that brings oxygen and nutrients and washes out metabolic wastes. This situation is called ischemia.

- When ischemia occurs in a place in the extremities (fingers and toes) in response to minor cold exposure, it is known as Raynaud phenomenon, and it can threaten the viability of the involved digits.
- If this smooth muscle spasm occurs in the coronary arteries of the heart, it is known as Prinzmetal angina. If prolonged, the spasm may lead to heart tissue death (myocardial infarction, or a heart attack).

  Both disorders may be treated (carefully) with nitrates and calcium channel blockers, which aid in vasodilation to combat spasm.

Thermoregulation

Although thermoregulation is a physiologic homeostatic mechanism for maintaining core body temperature, numerous pathologic conditions can alter the balance between heat generation and heat dissipation.

- In patients in fever or heat stroke, the body promotes peripheral arterial dilation to "dump" heat into the environment, leading fair-skinned patients to appear flushed.
- In patients exposed to excessive cold, peripheral artery vasoconstriction shunts blood away from the skin and minimizes heat loss. In such cases, light-skinned individuals may appear pale (decreased blood flow to the skin) or even blue (stasis of deoxygenated blood in the skin).

Orthostatic Hypotension

When sympathetic neurons that regulate arterial smooth muscle tone are lost (because of diabetic neuropathy, infiltrate diseases, such as amyloid, or normal aging), smooth muscle relaxation and loss of reflexive constriction can occur.

- In such patients, changes of position from lying to sitting and sitting to standing are no longer accompanied by reflexive vascular smooth muscle contraction, which increases peripheral resistance to blood flow and maintains blood pressure.
- Instead, there is a gravity-mediated pooling of blood and decreased venous return to the heart, with a subsequent decrease in cardiac stroke volume and loss of blood pressure.
- Known as orthostatic hypotension, this disorder can manifest as lightheadedness (presyncope) or even frank fainting/loss of consciousness (syncope).

Atherosclerosis

Most heart attacks, many strokes, and much peripheral vascular disease are the result of progressive arterial wall damage and inflammation called atherosclerosis. Smooth muscle cells, along with endothelial cells, platelets, and monocyte-macrophages, as well as myriad inflammatory mediators, growth factors, and cholesterol, are believed to be the major effectors of this process.

An atherosclerotic area of an artery is essentially a complex sore (or lesion) on the inner aspect of the vessel wall.

- Smooth muscle cells in such an area have been observed to alter their appearance and migrate from the vessel media through the fenestrations in the elastic lamella and into the intima (Fig. 6.16A and B).

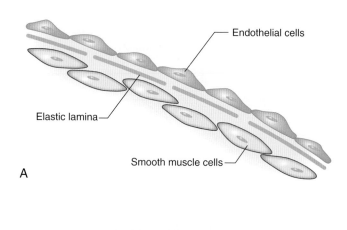

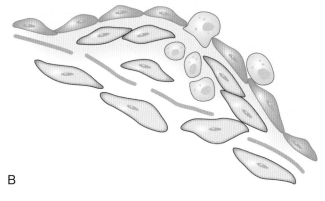

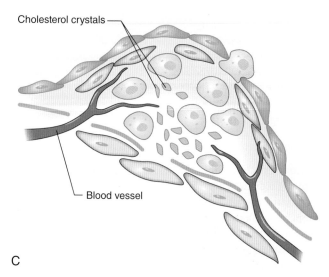

Fig. 6.16 The role of smooth muscle cells in atherosclerosis. A, In the wall of a healthy artery, the smooth muscle cells have a contractile phenotype and occupy a place in the media, beneath the endothelium that rests on the elastic lamella. B, As vessel walls are damaged by such stimuli as high blood pressure and toxic cholesterol metabolites, the smooth muscle cells change from a contractile to a proliferative, synthetic phenotype, and move into the vessel intima through fenestrations in the elastic lamella. C, There, colluding with dysfunctional endothelial cells, macrophages, and platelets, they elaborate inflammatory mediators and contribute to the formation of a lesion called an atheromatous plaque. Smooth muscle cells in atheromas are thought to have a pathologic, rather than physiologic, role in the progression of atherosclerotic disease.

- As they do so, they activate or augment numerous synthetic and proinflammatory mechanisms.
- In fact, some researchers refer to the change in function in smooth muscle cells a shift from the "contractile" to the "synthetic phenotype."

The response to injury hypothesis postulates that recurrent or consistent mechanical and chemical insults cause the vessel wall to undergo changes, including intimal thickening, fatty streak formation, and finally development of an atheromatous plaque (Fig. 6.16C).

- The slowly growing plaque gradually occludes the artery lumen and limits blood flow to tissues.
- In the heart, this arterial narrowing causes cardiac ischemia, which may manifest as angina and/or cardiomyopathy with heart failure.

The rupture of a plaque results in blood clot formation (thrombosis), which occludes the vessel lumen.

- When this occurs in a coronary artery, a heart attack ensues.
- In the central nervous system, such an event results in damage to and/or death of part of the brain—a stroke.

Pulmonary

Just as the dysfunction of smooth muscle tissue profoundly affects blood pressure and blood flow systemically, it can do so in the pulmonary vascular tree as well. For example, pulmonary hypertension results from the dysregulation of smooth muscle contraction in the blood vessels of the lungs and is extremely difficult to manage, often prompting lung transplant in advanced cases.

However, much more common is excessive contraction and hypertrophy of the smooth muscle tissues of the bronchi in diseases, such as asthma, which can cause impairment of airflow and therefore of gas exchange.

- Smooth muscle contraction in respiratory passages increases resistance to airflow (again in accordance with Ohm's law).
- Excessive airway smooth muscle contraction in response to such trigger stimuli as allergens, cold air, and exercise may cause attacks of asthma, a disease characterized by intermittent airflow obstruction accompanied by reversible bronchoconstriction.
- The bronchi of people with asthma are termed "hyperresponsive" because smooth muscle constriction with profound resistance to airflow occurs on exposure to relatively low concentrations (compared with nonasthmatics) of stimuli.
- During an attack of airway bronchoconstriction, a patient may have shortness of breath (called dyspnea), coughing, chest tightness, and turbulent airflow in the contracted bronchi and bronchioles that often produces audible wheezing (Fig. 6.17).

An acute attack of asthma may be temporarily ameliorated by the patient inhaling a β_2-adrenenic receptor agonist medication that induces smooth muscle relaxation and bronchodilation. Inflammation of the airways is thought to contribute to smooth muscle hyperresponsiveness, and the most effective long-term treatment for asthma are antiinflammatory drugs, such as inhaled steroids.

Gastrointestinal

Because smooth muscle tissues are components of the GI tract from the esophagus to the end of the colon, increased contraction or decreased contraction can affect almost any part of the tract. In addition, because the contraction of smooth muscle tissue in the walls of the GI tract is phasic and effective peristalsis depends on the orderly sequence of contractions in segments of the tract, any disorder in contraction can disrupt the movement of food and/or feces.

Achalasia

The lower esophageal sphincter is composed of smooth muscle. In the condition known as achalasia, inappropriate tonic contraction of this muscle inhibits the normal passage of food and fluid beyond a sphincter that cannot relax. Patients may experience difficulty swallowing and may have chest pain as well.

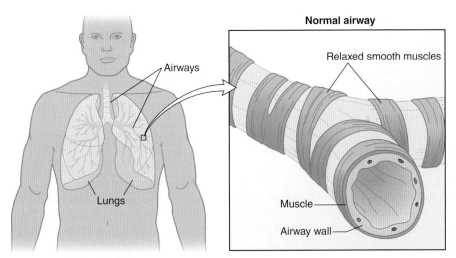
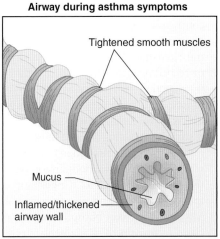

Fig. 6.17 Contraction of smooth muscle is dysregulated in conditions, such as asthma, resulting in narrowing of the airway and impaired breathing because of increased resistance to air flow.

Diabetic Peripheral Autonomic Neuropathy and Gastroparesis

Diabetic peripheral autonomic neuropathy in the GI system can result in decreased esophageal and gastric motility and emptying.
- This impairment in stomach motility is known as gastroparesis.
- Patients may experience nausea, vomiting, and acid reflux when the alimentary tract contents do not move along normally because normal peristalsis does not occur.

Hirschprung Disease

The failure of neural crest cells to migrate to the distal colon during development results in an absence of ganglion cells (Meissner's and Auerbach's plexuses, portions of the parasympathetic-enteric nervous system; see Fig. 6.3).
- Without these neurons, smooth muscle in the distal colon cannot relax, producing an obstruction to the movement of feces.
- The result is tremendous dilation of the normal colon that is proximal to the segment lacking autonomic ganglia, a syndrome called Hirschprung disease (also known as congenital megacolon).

Genitourinary

Like smooth muscle tissues in the GI tract, those in the genitourinary tract, such as in the wall of the urinary bladder, depend on autonomic neurons to regulate the passage of organ contents.
- Any irritation of the bladder wall, such as that inflammation which accompanies a urinary tract infection (also called cystitis), may induce spasms of bladder wall smooth muscle and thus urinary incontinence.
- Conversely, inhibition of or damage to the parasympathetic neurons that increase bladder contraction can impair bladder emptying.

Diabetic Peripheral Autonomic Neuropathy and Bladder Dysmotility

Just as diabetic peripheral autonomic neuropathy may affect vascular and GI smooth muscle, it may also affect bladder contractility.
- Patients suffer from urinary retention when para sympathetic neurons are lost because smooth muscle in the bladder wall does not generate sufficient contractile force to empty the bladder.
  - As more and more urine fills the bladder, the smooth muscle is increasingly stretched and moves to that portion of the length-stress curve where active force generation is impaired.
  - Eventually, the overstretched bladder is almost unable to contract, establishing a vicious cycle in which urinary retention begets more urinary retention.
- The loss of sympathetic neurons, which normally cause bladder wall smooth muscle relaxation, can cause the opposite problem, with inappropriate contraction causing bladder spasms that result in urinary incontinence.

These two problems of insufficient and excessive bladder contractility may coincide in a single patient, a condition known as bladder dysmotility.

SUMMARY

- Smooth muscle is a component of the walls of many hollow or tubular organs, including blood vessels, bronchioles, the GI tract, and the genitourinary tract.
- Smooth muscle contraction is modulated by autonomic neurons. Therefore smooth muscle, unlike skeletal muscle, is generally not under voluntary control.
- Although smooth muscle, like skeletal muscle, has thin filaments made of actin and thick filaments made of myosin, smooth muscle does not have a regular arrangement of these contractile proteins into sarcomeres.
- Numerous mediators can alter the contractile state of smooth muscle tissue. Whether a given mediator causes contraction or relaxation depends on the receptor and associated signal transduction machinery in a given cell. Different smooth muscle tissues are very heterogeneous in their responses to different regulatory mediators.
- A stimulus inducing smooth muscle contraction increases the intracellular concentration of Ca^{2+}. The Ca^{2+} binds to calmodulin, and the Ca^{2+}-calmodulin complex binds to and activates the enzyme MLCK. MLCK phosphorylates the light chain of myosin thick filaments, increasing crossbridge cycling.
- Myosin light chain phosphatase dephosphorylates the light chain of myosin thick filaments, decreasing crossbridge cycling. Dephosphorylated myosin is still able to bind to thin actin filaments, inducing the latch bridge state that allows smooth muscle to maintain prolonged contraction known as tone.
- Like skeletal muscle contraction, smooth muscle contraction depends on ATP, but smooth muscle uses significantly less ATP than skeletal muscle.
- The contractile activity of distinct smooth muscle cells are coordinated by intercellular chemical and mechanical connections and by regulatory mediators.
- In tubular structures, such as blood vessels and the GI tract, the contraction of circumferentially oriented smooth muscle tissues leads to a decrease in the lumen of the tube and an increase in resistance to the flow of material in accordance with Ohm's law and Poiseuille's law. In the GI tract, longitudinally oriented smooth muscle tissues with phasic contraction generate peristalsis.
- Smooth muscle tissues display viscoelastic homeostatic properties in response to stretch.
- Pathophysiologic conditions can arise from either contractile or synthetic problems in smooth muscle.
- Excessive smooth muscle contraction may affect blood vessels (Raynaud phenomenon, Prinzmetal angina) causing ischemia, pulmonary bronchi (asthma), and the esophagus (achalasia).
- Insufficient smooth muscle contraction may affect blood vessels (septic shock).

- Diabetic peripheral autonomic neuropathy damages the nerve cells that regulate smooth muscle contraction in the cardiovascular system, the GI tract, and the genitourinary tract, producing orthostatic hypotension, gastroparesis, and bladder dysmotility, respectively.

- Smooth muscle cells have numerous synthetic functions, as well as the ability to contract. Dysregulation of some of these synthetic functions contributes to the process of atherosclerosis.

REVIEW QUESTIONS

Directions: Each of the numbered items or incomplete statements in this section is followed by answers or by completions of the statement. Select the one lettered answer or completion that is best in each case.

1. In smooth muscle, contraction depends on the binding of Ca^{2+} to:
   A. Calcineurin
   B. Calmodulin
   C. Tropomyosin
   D. Troponin
   E. Myosin light-chain kinase

2. A 74-year-old man with poorly controlled type II diabetes for over 20 years, but no other medical problems might be expected to have each of the following except:
   A. Dizziness and near fainting when rising up out of bed too quickly
   B. Nausea and regurgitation or vomiting after large meals
   C. Bronchial hyperresponsiveness and intermittent dyspnea and wheezing
   D. Difficulty urinating

3. Which of the following is not caused by excessive smooth muscle contraction?
   A. Achalasia
   B. Prinzmetal angina
   C. Raynaud phenomenon
   D. Asthma
   E. Septic shock

4. An 88-year-old man has a severe heart attack and goes into cardiogenic shock. You would expect his peripheral vascular smooth muscle contraction to be _____ and his peripheral resistance to blood flow to be _____.
   A. decreased; decreased
   B. increased; decreased
   C. decreased; increased
   D. increased; increased

ANSWERS TO REVIEW QUESTIONS

1. **The answer is B.** In smooth muscle, Ca^{2+} from the extracellula space and/or the sarcoplasmic reticulum binds to calmodulin. The Ca^{2+}-calmodulin complex then activates myosin light-chain kinase, which phosphorylates the myosin head, increasing crossbridge cycling. Smooth muscle, unlike skeletal muscle, lacks troponin.

2. **The answer is C.** A patient with long-standing diabetes may have peripheral neuropathy. The nerve dysfunction results in loss of smooth muscle tone. When this occurs in the peripheral blood vessels, orthostatic hypotension ensues, with low blood pressure because of gravity-mediated blood pooling that is not compensated for. In the GI tract, loss of normal peristalsis results in gastroparesis with nausea and regurgitation after a large meal. When the bladder is affected, the ability to urinate completely may be impaired. Asthma, however, is characterized by excessive smooth muscle contraction in response to stimuli, such as allergens, cold air, and exercise.

3. **The answer is E.** Septic shock occurs when a serious infection is accompanied by high concentrations of inflammatory mediators that cause widespread vascular smooth muscle relaxation and therefore vasodilation, decreased peripheral resistance, and low blood pressure. All the other conditions are characterized by inappropriate smooth muscle contraction causing blockage of the esophagus (achalasia), coronary vessels (Prinzmetal angina), peripheral vessels (Raynaud phenomenon), or airways in the lung (asthma).

4. **The answer is D.** In this situation where the heart is damaged and not pumping blood well (decreased stroke volume, therefore decreased cardiac output), the homeostatic mechanism (the baroreceptor reflex) invoked to maintain blood pressure is peripheral arterial smooth muscle contraction to increase peripheral resistance.

Musculoskeletal Physiology

A.R. is a 30 year-old high-school teacher who presented to her primary care provider with "weakness" and trouble seeing.

PRESENTATION

When asked to elaborate on her symptoms, A.R. reported that the weakness began 2 months ago. The weakness mainly affected her facial muscles, with jaw fatigue during chewing and difficulty swallowing. She has also experienced weakness in her upper arms, and noted that it acutely worsened following her usual daily gym routine. In general, she remarked that the symptoms are mild or absent in the morning, but worsen as the day goes on. Furthermore, she has new-onset diplopia (double vision) that seems to worsen in the evening after correcting a few of her students' papers.

On physical examination, A.R. was found to have ptosis (eyelid drooping, see Fig. 6.1.1) of both eyes, with worsening noted following repeated blinking. On visual testing, she is initially able to follow a finger with ease, but as testing continued, her eye movements become disconjugate (uncoordinated). When asked to smile, she produces a strange, "horizontal" smile with furrowed brows. Motor strength in bilateral upper limbs was initially normal, but deteriorated on repeated testing. When allowed to recover for several minutes, her arm strength returned to baseline. No fasciculation (small, visible jerks in the muscle) was noted. Muscle tone, reflexes, and sensation were normal.

Blood testing was within normal limits except for high levels of an antiacetylcholine receptor antibody in her plasma. Electromyographic testing—a technique used to study the electrical activity produced by skeletal muscles—revealed progressive weakness and decreased amplitude of contraction of the distal arm muscles following repeated stimulation of the ulnar and median nerves. When given an intravenous administration of edrophonium, an acetylcholinesterase inhibitor, both her symptoms and electromyographic findings disappeared within 40 seconds. Chest x-ray and computed tomography scan demonstrated an enlarged thymus for her age.

DISCUSSION

When considering weakness, such as that affecting A.R., one must recall that "weakness" may emerge from an insult at any point along the chain of neural command—from the muscle itself, to the neuromuscular junction, up to the cerebral cortex. To localize the origin of weakness, we must ask the following questions:

Is the weakness symmetric or focal? Was the onset slow or sudden? Systemic illness, such as that associated with metabolic or genetic abnormalities, tends to present as nonfocal and gradual, whereas a cerebrovascular accident (stroke) affecting the motor cortex and/or descending motor pathways will be focal and acute.

Has there been a change in muscle tone and/or reflexes? Damage to the lower motor neurons (i.e., originating at the anterior gray column) will decrease reflexes and muscle tone, in addition to causing muscle fasciculations. Conversely, damage to upper motor neurons causes weakness associated with hyperreflexia and increased muscle tone because of decreased inhibitory spinal input to peripheral neurons.

Is the weakness proximal (closer to the heart) or distal (closer to the fingertips and toes)? Diseases of the muscle will often present with proximal weakness. Diseases of the peripheral nerves will preferentially affect longer nerves, and thus commonly will present with distal sensory and motor deficits.

Is the weakness constant? Diseases of the neuromuscular junction are characterized by weakness that comes and goes.

In A.R.'s case, note the symmetric, gradual-onset weakness with preserved muscle tone and reflexes, affecting cranial nerves and proximal muscles, and intermittent in nature. This suggests a disorder in the neuromuscular junction.

Myasthenia gravis (MG), literally "grave muscle weakness," is an autoimmune disorder in which the body produces antibodies against acetylcholine (ACh) receptors at the neuromuscular junctions of skeletal muscle. Recall that in normal physiology, action potentials in the motor neuron stimulate release of ACh into the neuromuscular junction, which binds to postsynaptic ACh receptors and leads to contraction of the skeletal muscle. Antibody binding, on the other hand, leads to ACh receptor inactivation, preventing additional ACh in the synapse from triggering depolarization and subsequent contraction of the skeletal muscle cell. As more and more ACh receptors are inactivated, skeletal muscle progressively loses response to stimulation. This leads to an exaggerated fatigue response: with fewer ACh receptors, it is more difficult to achieve threshold potential for contraction.

Clinically, patients complain of weakness worsening with activity. In two-thirds of patients diagnosed, the initial symptoms are related to the eye: (1) ptosis caused by weakness of the levator palpebrae superioris; and/or (2) diplopia arising from weakness of the extraocular muscles and subsequent inability to "conjugate" (match) eye movements. Weakness of muscles of mastication and facial expression are also common, leading to difficulty eating and speaking, as well as an odd "snarl" expression. As the disease progresses, weakness spreads from the face

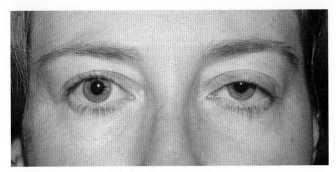

Fig. 6.1.1 Ptosis. (From Tyers AG, Collin JRO. *Colour Atlas of Ophthalmic Plastic Surgery,* 4th Edition. Ch. 9: p. 175-231. Fig. 9e)

to the upper limbs and—more seriously—muscles of respiration, including the diaphragm. Paralysis of the respiratory musculature necessitates assisted ventilation to survive. The disease course is frequently marked by exacerbations and remissions, but the remissions usually do not return the individual to prior levels of normal functioning.

Of note, abnormalities in the thymus are seen in 10% of patients with MG, and it is thought that this may lead to incorrect "instructions" from T cells to B cells to produce autoantibodies. However, thymectomy generally is not a cure.

TREATMENT AND SUBSEQUENT COURSE

A.R. was treated with pyridostigmine bromide, which is a long-acting anticholinesterase drug similar to edrophonium. Both medications bind to and disable acetylcholinesterase, the enzyme responsible for degrading ACh, and thus allow ACh to build up in the neuromuscular junction and bind more effectively to the remaining ACh receptors. She was also started on a corticosteroid, which suppresses the immune system and prevents further production of anti-AChR antibodies. A few weeks following diagnosis, she suffered an acute exacerbation of her symptoms and had difficulty breathing—a myasthenic crisis. She was intubated and underwent plasmapheresis, a procedure in which a portion of the patient's plasma is removed and replaced with fresh plasma containing no autoantibodies. After stabilization, she underwent thymectomy with significant improvement, although not remission, of her symptoms. She has been able to resume working and exercise as before, although she continues to take an anticholinesterase medication and visits for frequent follow-ups with her neurologist to assess for symptom recurrence.

Circulatory Physiology

7

Blood and Hemostasis

INTRODUCTION

Blood is a specialized type of connective tissue that performs several key functions required for the viability of all other organs:
- Major transportation route via the circulatory system.
- Brings oxygen and nutrients (i.e., glucose), as well as endocrine hormones.
- Removes carbon dioxide and waste products for disposal.
- Maintains body temperature.
- Provides defense against infection.

SYSTEM STRUCTURE

The structure of blood differs in two important aspects from that of other organ systems:
1. Blood is liquid under normal conditions rather than solid.
2. Blood circulates throughout the body.

These features are essential to the functions blood performs, and loss of either can result in serious pathophysiology.

Gross Anatomy of the Circulatory System

A healthy adult normally has approximately 5 liters (female) to 6 liters (male) of blood within the circulatory system. In brief, the circulatory system is constructed as follows (Fig. 7.1):
- Blood cells are produced in bone marrow.
- Blood circulates via blood vessels.
- The heart serves as the central pump of the circulatory system.
- Arteries carry blood from the heart to capillary beds of peripheral tissues and organs, where it exerts its main effects.
- Veins return blood to the heart.
- Lymphatic vessels return extracellular fluid to the circulatory system.

Components of Blood

Blood consists of two components:
1. Formed elements: includes red blood cells, white blood cells, and platelets.
2. Plasma: the aqueous medium that contains a variety of proteins, small molecules, and ions.

These two components can be separated by centrifugation (Fig. 7.2).
- The hematocrit, or percentage of blood volume consisting of red blood cells, is calculated by measuring the height of the packed red cells and dividing by the height of the total blood in the tube. If a small volume of blood is prevented from clotting and the red blood cells are allowed to sediment on their own based on their density, one can both calculate the hematocrit and the rate at which the cells sediment in mm/hr. This rate is known as the erythrocyte sedimentation rate (ESR) and is a general measure of inflammation. The increased ESR in inflammatory states is due to increased erythrocyte density due to the adhesion of proinflammatory proteins to the red blood cells. The blood is also less viscous in inflammatory states, allowing erythrocytes to sediment faster. A commonly used formula is that the ESR $= 200 -$ ($2*$hematocrit).
- The hematocrit constitutes 40% to 50% of the blood volume in a normal adult.

Blood Cells and Organelles

Blood cells are produced in bone marrow by hematopoietic stem cells (HSCs).
- HSCs are undifferentiated cells.
- They can either divide (via mitosis) to produce additional stem cells or differentiate into specialized cells.

When differentiated cells reach a sufficient degree of maturity, they exit the bone marrow to circulate in the vasculature. The number and morphology of different blood cells within the circulatory system may be assessed by peripheral blood smears (Fig. 7.3).

There are several different blood cell types found in peripheral blood (Table 7.1), each specialized for different functions.

Erythrocytes (Red Blood Cells)

- Most numerous of the formed elements with about 4 to 6 million erythrocytes per µL of blood.
- Biconcave discs with no nucleus, mitochondria, or ribosomes (Fig. 7.4).
  - Lack of organelles facilitates transit through circulatory system.
  - Large surface-to-volume ratio facilitates gas exchange.
- Eosinophilic (pink) staining on peripheral smears because of high protein content.
  - Contain mainly hemoglobin.
- Immature erythrocytes, or reticulocytes, normally comprise around 1% of circulating red blood cells (RBCs).
  - Also lack nuclei.
  - Basophilic (blue) staining because of ↑ ribonucleic acid (RNA) content reflecting ongoing protein synthesis.
  - Marker of ↑ erythroid proliferation (see Fast Fact Box 7.1).

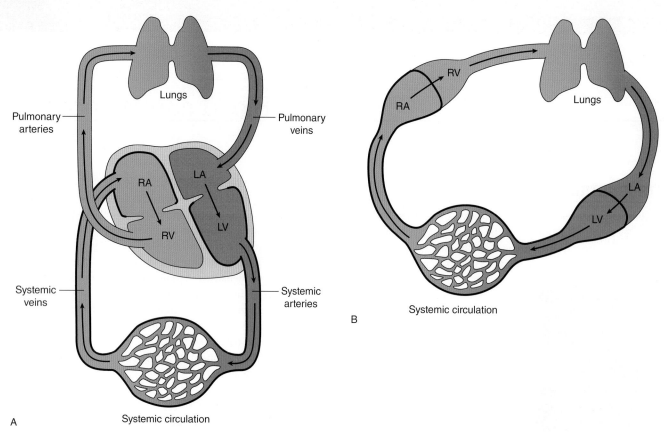

Fig. 7.1 Simplified diagram of the circulatory system. While the volumes of blood in the arterial and venous systems appear roughly equal, the greater capacitance of the venous system compared to the arterial system results in a greater volume of blood being in the veins than in the arteries. Note the lymphatic system is not pictured. *LA*, Left atrium; *LV*, left ventricle; *RA*, right atrium; *RV*, right ventricle.

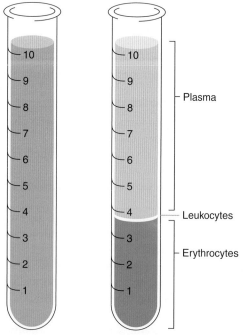

Fig. 7.2 Hematocrit tubes before and after centrifugation. Blood from a patient is collected in a test tube. Before centrifugation (*left*), the blood appears to be homogeneously red from the abundance of erythrocytes. After centrifugation (*right*), the red cells fall to the bottom of the tube, the white cells form a small band called the buffy coat, and the plasma remains on top.

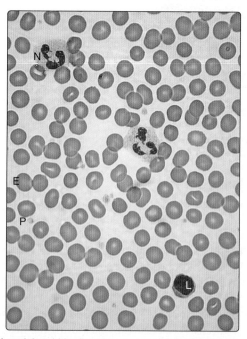

Fig. 7.3 A peripheral blood smear. A drop of normal blood is smeared onto a glass slide, dried, stained, and examined under a light microscope. Note the shapes, relative numbers, and relative sizes of erythrocytes (*E*), neutrophils (*N*), lymphocytes (*L*), and platelets (*P*). (From Howard M, Hamilton P. *Haematology: An Illustrated Colour Text*, 4th Edition. Philadelphia, PA: Elsevier. 2013. Fig. 9.2b.)

TABLE 7.1 The Formed Elements of Blood

Cell	Diameter (μm)	Number[a]
Erythrocytes	6.5–8	Males: $4.1–6 \times 10^6/\mu L$
		Females: $3.9–5.5 \times 10^6/\mu L$
Leukocytes		4,000–10,000/μL
Neutrophils	12–15	60%–70%
Eosinophils	12–15	2%–4%
Basophils	12–15	0%–1%
Lymphocytes	6–18	20%–30%
Monocytes	12–20	3%–8%
Platelets	2–4	$1.5–4.5 \times 10^5/\mu L$

[a]Some sources give these values per cubic millimeter (mm³). Microliters and cubic millimeters are identical units.

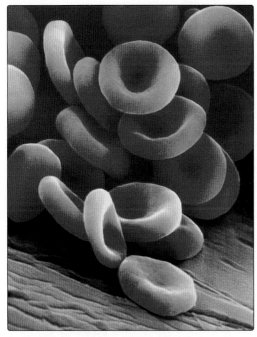

Fig. 7.4 A scanning electron micrograph of typical erythrocytes. Note especially the biconcave-disc shape of the cells and their lack of a nucleus. During development, red cell precursors eject their nucleus, making them lighter and thus easier for the heart to pump throughout the circulatory system. The cytoplasm is filled largely with hemoglobin for carrying oxygen. (From Howard M, Hamilton P. *Haematology: An Illustrated Colour Text*, 4th Edition. Philadelphia, PA: Elsevier. 2013. Fig. 2.1. (Copyright Dennis Kunkel Microscopy Inc.))

Fast Fact Box 7.1

During tissue staining, pathologists employ the dyes hematoxylin and eosin for a basic H&E stain. Hematoxylin, which is a base and positively charged, binds to negatively charged/acidic substrates, such as DNA/RNA. It stains them blue/violet. Eosin, which is acidic and negatively charged, stains positively charged/basic substrates, such as positively-charged amino acid side chains (lysine, arginine). It stains them pink/red.
Basic Binds Basophilic Becoming Blue
Acidic Attaches Acidophilic Appearing Auburn
DNA, Deoxyribonucleic acid; *H&E*, hematoxylin and eosin; *RNA*, ribonucleic acid.

Leukocytes (White Blood Cells)

- White blood cells (WBCs) are roughly twice the size of RBCs.
- Less numerous with 4000 to 10,000 per μL of peripheral blood.
- There are several different types of leukocytes, classified according to their nuclear shape and the presence and type of granules in their cytoplasm (Fig. 7.5):
  - Granulocytes (contain cytoplasmic granules).
    Neutrophils (polymorphonuclear leukocytes [PMNs]).
      Account for 60% to 70% circulating WBCs.
      Nuclei with 2 to 5 lobes linked by fine chromatin threads.
      Larger primary granules (lysosomes) and smaller secondary granules containing several mediators.
      Immature neutrophils ("band forms") have a nonsegmented nucleus and serve as a marker for ↑ myeloid proliferation.
    Eosinophils
      2% to 4% of circulating WBCs.
      Bilobed nuclei that appear as "sunglasses."
      Numerous large, eosinophilic granules containing major basic protein (MBP), histamine, and other mediators.
    Basophils
      Less than 1% of leukocytes.
      Irregular multilobulated nuclei.
      Numerous large, basophilic granules containing histamine, heparin, and leukotrienes.
  Mononuclear granulocytes (nongranule containing, nonlobulated nuclei).
    Monocytes.
      Largest blood cell diameter (12–20 μm).
      Kidney-shaped nucleus.
      Precursors of macrophages in peripheral tissues.
        May also develop into mast cells when they enter tissues such as the skin and gastrointestinal (GI) tract.
    Lymphocytes.
      Approximately the size of an erythrocyte but grow when activated.
      Characterized by a spherical, deeply basophilic nucleus surrounded by a very thin rim of cytoplasm.
      The different subclasses of lymphocytes, including B cells and T cells, are described in Chapter 8.

Platelets (Thrombocytes)

- 150,000 to 450,000 per μL in normal blood.
  - Note: One-third of total platelet pool is stored in the spleen!
- Small, anucleate cell fragments with a diameter of 2 to 4 μm.
- Essentially membrane-enclosed sacs of cytoplasm that pinch off from large cells called megakaryocytes, which remain in the bone marrow.
- Contain dense granules (calcium, adenosine diphosphate) and alpha-granules (von Willebrand factor, fibrinogen).
- Possess a number of cell surface glycoprotein adhesion molecules called "integrins" that mediate attachment to a blood vessel wall when endothelium is damaged or dysfunctional.

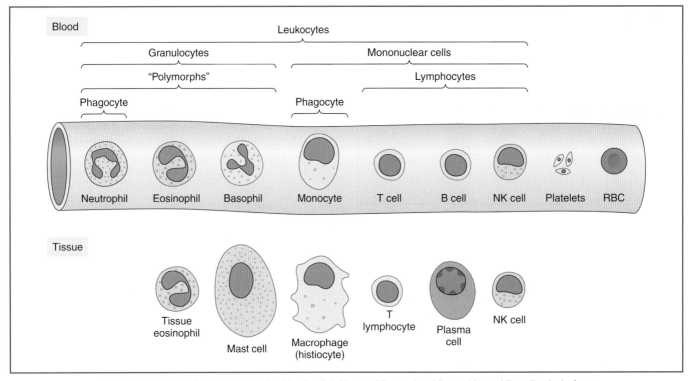

Fig. 7.5 Five types of leukocytes (white blood cells). Neutrophils, eosinophils, and basophils collectively form the granulocytes, or granule-containing leukocytes. Monocytes can transform into macrophages and travel to sites of inflammation. Lymphocytes circulate between the blood, peripheral tissues, and the lymphatic and lymph node system. There are two subtypes of lymphocytes, T cells and B cells, but they cannot be differentiated from one another by light microscopy alone. *NK*, Natural killer; *RBC*, red blood cell. (From Actor JK. *Elsevier's Integrated Review: Immunology and Microbiology*, 2nd Edition. Philadelphia, PA: Elsevier. 2011. Fig. 2.1.)

TABLE 7.2 The Molecular Constituents of Plasma	
Proteins	**6.0–8.0**
Albumin (g/dL)	3.4–5.0
Total globulin (g/dL)	2.2–4.0
Transferrin (mg/dL)	250
Haptoglobin (mg/dL)	30–205
Hemopexin (mg/dL)	50–100
Ceruloplasmin (mg/dL)	25–45
Ferritin (mcg/L)	15–300
Nonproteins	
Cholesterol (mg/dL)	140–250
Glucose (mg/dL)	70–110
Urea nitrogen (mg/dL)	6–23
Uric acid (mg/dL)	4.1–85
Creatinine (mg/dL)	0.7–1.4
Iron (mcg/dL)	50–150

The role of platelets in hemostasis, the control of bleeding, is described later in this Chapter.

Blood Molecules

Plasma contains over 100 different proteins, as well as numerous other molecules, listed in Table 7.2. Blood proteins can be classified as extracellular or intracellular.

Extracellular (Plasma)

- Total plasma protein.
  - Normal range of 6.0 to 8.0 g/dL.
  - Functions of numerous proteins as carriers, clotting factors, immunoproteins, hormones, or enzymes are detailed below for the coagulation cascade and in subsequent chapters for the immunoproteins and hormones.
- Albumin is the principal plasma protein.
  - Normal range of 3.4 to 5.0 g/dL of plasma protein.
  - Accounts for nearly two-thirds of total plasma protein mass.
- Globulin consists of several groups of proteins (α-, β-, and γ-globulin).
  - Normal range of 2.2 to 4.0 g/dL (see Fast Fact Box 7.2).

Fast Fact Box 7.2

The proteins in plasma can be separated using a technique known as protein electrophoresis, in which proteins exposed to an electrical field move through a solid gel based on their size and charge. Different proteins are distinguished by their respective mobility in the gel.

Intracellular

- Hemoglobin.
  - Principal intracellular protein of RBCs.
  - Molecular weight of 68,000 kDa.
  - Tetrameric protein consisting of:
    Two α and two β polypeptide chains (the "-globin" part of hemoglobin).

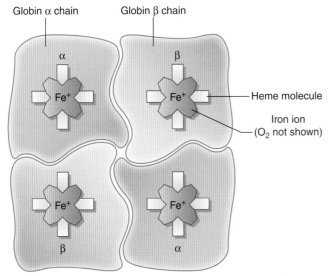

Fig. 7.6 The structure of hemoglobin. Hemoglobin, the main oxygen-carrying molecule in erythrocytes, is composed of four protein chains: two α chains and two β chains. Each chain wraps around a heme molecule. Each heme molecule has a central coordinated iron atom (Fe), critical to binding molecular oxygen (not shown). Because each Fe atom can bind one oxygen (O_2) molecule, a single molecule of hemoglobin can bind four molecules of O_2.

Heme moieties (the "hemo-" part of hemoglobin), a planar molecule that contains a central iron ion capable of reversibly binding a molecule of oxygen (O_2) (Fig. 7.6).
- Often affected in several significant inherited diseases. Two genes encoding the β chain (one from each parent). Four genes encoding the α chain (two from each parent) (see Clinical Correlation Boxes 7.1–7.3.)

Myoglobin

Similar to a monomer of hemoglobin that does not have the same oxygen carrying physiology as hemoglobin (see the pulmonary section).

Present in skeletal muscle and released into the peripheral blood when muscle cells are disrupted and easily filtered by the kidney and can cause acute kidney injury.

Clinical Correlation Box 7.1

In adults, the most common type of hemoglobin is hemoglobin A (HbA; $\alpha_2\beta_2$). However, human infants have a different type of hemoglobin called hemoglobin F ($\alpha_2\gamma_2$) until about 6 months of age. This form of hemoglobin has much greater affinity for O_2. In disorders affecting HbA such as sickle cell disease, upregulation of HbF (via hydroxyurea) can thus lessen patient symptoms.

Clinical Correlation Box 7.2

The coordination of iron into the heme moiety makes blood appear bright red when well oxygenated (as in an artery) and bluish-purple when poorly oxygenated (as in a vein). Conversely, the catabolism of heme moiety in degenerating red blood cells produces the green, brown, and black colors of bile (biliverdin, bilirubin), stool (stercobilin), and bruises (methemoglobin), respectively.

Clinical Correlation Box 7.3

Sickle cell anemia is caused by a point mutation in the beta chain gene producing a valine (rather than the normal glutamate) in the sixth amino acid position. This altered hemoglobin is known as HbS, compared with normal adult hemoglobin HbA. Patients may be heterozygous ("sickle cell trait") or homozygous for the disease allele, with only the latter presenting significant pathology. Whereas HbS initially forms normally, states of deoxygenation, dehydration, and/or acidosis lead to polymerization and precipitation of HbS aggregates. This distorts the normal biconcave shape of the RBCs, leading them to collapse on themselves and "sickle." This morphology leads to:
- Destruction (hemolysis)
- Adherence to endothelial cell walls and each other, producing obstruction to flow (vasoocclusion).

There are several clinical consequences of increasing sickling:
- Vasoocclusive crises
  - Restriction of blood flow to organs leading to ischemia, pain, necrosis, and organ damage.
    - Acute chest syndrome (most common cause of death)
    - Stroke
    - Dactylitis (painful finger swelling)
- Autosplenectomy
  - Spleen is usually infarcted before the end of childhood, leading to susceptibility to encapsulated bacteria.
- Anemia
  - Chronic, but may be acutely worsened in aplastic crisis (caused by parvovirus B19 infection) and hemolytic crisis.
- Renal papillary necrosis (because of low O_2 content in renal medulla)

Patients are generally managed chronically with hydroxyurea (increases fetal hemoglobin, or HbF), high-dose folic acid, and penicillin (to fend off infections following autosplenectomy). For crises, patients receive hydration, pain medication, and blood or exchange transfusions. Supplemental oxygen given to patients can reverse the HbS polymerization process. Sickling of affected RBCs increases blood viscosity and thus decreases ESR. Finally, while bone marrow transplantation is currently the only known cure for sickle cell disease, it requires a matched donor. An exciting development that holds the promise that bone marrow transplant may not be the only possible cure is the gene editing technology known as CRISPR. This technique won the 2020 Nobel Prize in Chemistry.

Besides proteins, plasma also contains:
- Cholesterol, lipids, carbohydrates, and amino acids.
- Degradation products of metabolism, such as urea, uric acid, and creatinine.

Blood Small Molecules and Ions

Plasma also contains dissolved electrolytes, as well as molecular oxygen (O_2), nitrogen, and carbon dioxide. Table 7.3 lists the major ionic constituents of plasma.

SYSTEM FUNCTION

As mentioned in the introduction section, functions of the blood include:
- The absorption and delivery of oxygen and nutrients.
- The removal of metabolic wastes.
- The transport of communication molecules between or among cells.
- Immunologic defense.
- Thermoregulation.

TABLE 7.3 Ionic Constituents of Plasma

Cations	
Sodium (mEq/L)	134–146
Potassium (mEq/L)	3.5–5.0
Calcium (mg/dL)	8.0–10.4
Magnesium (mg/dL)	1.6–3.0
Hydrogen (pH)	7.36–7.44
Anions	
Chloride (mEq/L)	92–109
Bicarbonate (mEq/L)	24–31
Lactate (mEq/L)	1.0–1.8
Sulfate (mEq/L)	1.0
Phosphate (mg/dL)	2.6–4.6

Blood Ions

The concentrations of different cations and anions in the plasma are essential for providing a milieu compatible with cell function. In particular, ionic composition determines:

- Plasma osmolality, which is approximately 280 to 290 mOsm/kg.
- Ionic electrochemical gradients across cell membranes (as described in Part I).
- Hydrogen ion concentration, reflected by the blood pH, buffered into a narrow range of 7.36 to 7.44.
  - The acid-base balance is maintained principally by the bicarbonate buffering system, although phosphates contribute as well.
  - Calcium is an essential ion in the coagulation cascade.

Blood Molecules

The various proteins in blood perform many specialized functions.

Intracellular

In RBCs, the main protein of interest is hemoglobin, which carries oxygen from the alveoli of the lungs to the capillaries of tissues for aerobic respiration.

- In pulmonary capillaries, the partial pressure of oxygen (or oxygen tension) is high → each molecule of hemoglobin binds four oxygen molecules (one O_2 for each of the four heme units).
- In peripheral tissue capillaries, oxygen tension is low, and the oxygen is released from hemoglobin and diffuses into tissue cells.
- Chapter 14 further describes the details of gas exchange in the lungs and oxygen transport to the periphery (see Genetics Box 7.1 and Development Box 7.1).

GENETICS BOX 7.1

Hereditary spherocytosis is a disease of erythrocytes caused by mutations in at least five distinct genes, with autosomal dominant and recessive versions of the condition. Most patients have a lesion in the ANK1 gene that encodes the structural protein ankyrin-1, which contributes to red cell flexibility. Affected erythrocytes have rigid membranes that suffer damage when they navigate capillaries, and loss of cell membrane by repeated cellular trauma results in spherical cells instead of the biconcave discs of unaffected people.

DEVELOPMENT BOX 7.1

At birth, those affected with Hereditary Spherocytosis typically have severe anemia because of red cell destruction, but this tends to improve with age. Patients of any age can develop splenomegaly, likely related to the clearance of damaged erythrocytes by splenic phagocytes leading to engorgement of the spleen. With chronic red cell destruction and the release of hemoglobin that is metabolized by the liver into bilirubin, some patients develop gallstones. Some patients have bone abnormalities, short stature, and delayed sexual development.

The numerous intracellular proteins of WBCs perform many functions, in contrast to the relative simplicity of RBCs. Table 7.4 lists some of the proteins and enzymes within the granules of leukocytes. These include mediators of microbial killing and inflammation, which are described in more detail in Chapter 8.

Briefly, the killing of invading microbes can be accomplished by several strategies, including:

- Enzymatic damage.
- Oxidative damage.
- Sequestration of essential nutrients.

TABLE 7.4 Leukocyte Granule Contents

Cell	Specific Granules	Azurophilic Granules
Neutrophils	Alkaline phosphatase	Acid phosphatase
	Collagenase	α-Mannosidase
	Lactoferrin	Arylsulfatase
	Lysozyme	β-Galactosidase
		β-Glucuronidase
		Cathepsin
		5′ Nucleotidase
		Elastase
		Collagenase
		Myeloperoxidase
		Lysozyme
		Acid mucosubstances
		Cationic antibacterial proteins
Eosinophils	Acid phosphatase	
	Arylsulfatase	
	β-Glucuronidase	
	Cathepsin	
	Phospholipase	
	RNAse	
	Eosinophilic peroxidase	
	Major basic protein	
Basophils	Eosinophilic chemotactic factor	
	Heparin	
	Histamine	
	Peroxidase	

The WBCs thus contain several proteins to execute these specific functions:

- Lysozyme damages bacterial cell walls.
- Elastase and collagenase degrade connective tissue (allowing antimicrobial cells and molecules to get access to invaders).
- Nucleotidase degrades nucleic acids (destroying the deoxyribonucleic acid and ribonucleic acid of microbial invaders).
- Mannosidase and galactosidase degrade carbohydrates critical to the function of some microbial glycoproteins.
- Oxidative enzymes, such as myeloperoxidase, cause a "respiratory burst" that leads to the formation of chemically reactive and highly destructive compounds, such as hydrogen peroxide, superoxide, hydroxyl radicals, and hypochlorite radicals.
- Lactoferrin is a protein that sequesters iron, a nutrient essential for bacterial metabolism.

Extracellular

Plasma proteins can be divided functionally into several groups:

- Carrier proteins
- Clotting proteins
- Immunoproteins (see Ch. 8).
- Hormones (see Endocrine Section)
- Enzymes

Albumin is the major source of intravascular oncotic pressure because it cannot diffuse out of the vessels into the interstitial space (described further in Ch. 9). Albumin also binds and transports many compounds, such as drugs, bilirubin, and fatty acids (see Clinical Correlation Box 7.4).

Clinical Correlation Box 7.4

Hypoalbuminemia is a medical condition in which the blood levels of albumin are abnormally low. It can be caused by various conditions, including liver failure, nephrotic syndrome, chronic malnutrition, loss in the GI tract, or chronic inflammatory states. Because of its role as an oncotic regulator, hypoalbuminemia can lead to generalized edema because of a decrease in oncotic pressure. In some situations of chronic hypoalbuminemia, increased synthesis of other blood extracellular proteins can partially compensate for the low concentration of albumen and increase the low oncotic pressure towards normal.

Other binding and carrier proteins include:

- Transferrin for iron transport.
- Ferritin for iron storage.
- Ceruloplasmin for copper transport.
- Haptoglobin for binding hemoglobin.
- Hemopexin for binding free heme.
- Transcobalamin for transporting cobalamin (vitamin B_{12}).
- Specific hormone binding proteins.
- Apolipoproteins for cholesterol and lipid transport (see Clinical Correlation Box 7.5).

Clinical Correlation Box 7.5

Ceruloplasmin is reduced in Wilson's disease, an autosomal recessive disorder in which copper accumulates in several tissues, including the liver, basal ganglia, eyes, kidneys, and heart.

◆ PHARMACOLOGY BOX 7.1

Pharmacologic antagonists of the coagulation cascade include the direct factor Xa inhibitors such as apixaban and rivaraoxaban. Dabigatran is a direct thrombin (factor IIa) inhibitor. Warfarin interferes with vitamin K dependent gamma carboxylation of factors II, VII, IX, and X (as well as proteins C and S). Heparin increases the activity of antithrombin III against thrombin and factors Xa and IXa by approximately 1000-fold. Low molecular weigh heparins include daltaparin and enoxaparin.

Platelet antagonists include aspirin, which irreversibly acetylates and thus inactivates the cycloxygenase enzyme platelets depend on to generate lipid mediators such as thromboxane A2 and prostacycline from arachidonic acid. Clopidogrel irreversibly binds the platelet P2Y12 receptor for ADP. Inhibitors of the platelet GPIIb-IIIa receptor include the monoclonal antibody abciximab and the peptide eptifibatide.

Thrombolytic agents or "clot busters" include recombinant tissue plasminogen activator (rtPA, alteplase).

Clotting proteins include clotting factors and control enzymes that lead to the formation of fibrin plugs to control bleeding.

The body faces a challenge with respect to blood. For its normal physiologic function, blood must remain a liquid. But it must rapidly transform to a solid locally (but not systemically) when there is vascular wall damage in order to prevent uncontrolled bleeding. The process of hemostasis involves platelets and the coagulation cascade. Plasma clotting factors are the central proteins in the coagulation cascade. They are all synthesized in the liver, except for a portion of factor VIII that is synthesized in endothelial cells and megakaryocytes. Many of the clotting factors are proenzymes that are activated by proteolytic cleavage.

To limit clotting in space and time, plasma also contains anticoagulant proteins that keep the coagulation process under control. These include antithrombin III, protein C, protein S, and tissue factor pathway inhibitor.

Once a clot forms and vessel wall damage is repaired, the clot must be deconstructed, a process called fibrinolysis.

Coagulation factors II, VII, IX, and X, as well as protein C and protein S are synthesized in the liver and require a unique vitamin K-dependent carboxylation reaction that converts specific glutamate residues to gamma-carboxyglutamate. This process is inhibited by the medication warfarin.

The clotting cascade is a series of biochemical reactions involving the plasma clotting factors. Factors may have more than one name as well as a numeric designation. Inactive proenzymes have a Roman numeral while proteolytically cleaved, enzymatically active factors have a lower case a appended to the Roman numeral. Thus, for example, prothombin, also called factor II, is cleaved into the active enzyme thrombin, also called factor IIa.

The proteolytic cascade is triggered by endothelial disruption and culminates in the conversion of fibrinogen (factor I) into the cleavage product fibrin (factor Ia). Fibrin molecules polymerize, producing a fibrin plug that stops bleeding ("hemorrhage") from a damaged blood vessel.

All the coagulation factors involved circulate normally in the plasma but are inactive, and are activated by either conformational changes or limited proteolytic cleavage. Activation of the chain of events leading to coagulation can occur by two pathways, termed the **extrinsic pathway** and the **intrinsic pathway**, which ultimately converge to form a **common pathway** ending in the production of fibrin (See Fig. 7.7).

Amplification of the system is important: each activated coagulation cascade molecule may enzymatically cleave and activate tens, hundreds, or even thousands of substrate molecules.

The extrinsic pathway is thought to be the predominant method of activating the clotting cascade *in vivo*. Damaged tissue or endothelial cells expose a membrane-associated protein called tissue factor (TF), also known as thromboplastin, to the circulating plasma clotting factors. It complexes with factor VII, and the TF/VII complex in the presence of Ca^{2+} and a phospholipid membrane slowly enzymatically cleaves factor X to its active form Xa. Factor Xa, in turn, cleaves factor VII to VIIa, turning the TF/VIIa complex into an efficient enzyme that rapidly cleaves X to Xa, resulting in amplification of the Xa production.

The intrinsic pathway is triggered when factor XII, also known as Hageman factor or contact factor, encounters a negatively charged surface, such as a site of endothelial injury with exposed subendothelial collagen or a foreign surface such as the glass of a test tube. This causes factor XII to undergo a conformational change and become its active form XIIa. XIIa cleaves factor XI to form XIa, and XIa converts factor IX to IXa. IXa, in turn, associates with the accessory factor VIII, calcium ions, and a phospholipid surface, and converts factor X to Xa.

The extrinsic and intrinsic pathways converge in a common pathway. Both pathways produce a "ten-ase" enzyme that converts factor X to Xa. Xa then associates with the accessory factor V, calcium ions, and a phospholipid surface, and converts factor II (prothrombin) to factor IIa (thrombin), which is a highly reactive enzyme.

Thrombin is the key enzyme of the clotting cascade, activating platelets, activating factors V and VIII to accelerate the cascade, converting factor XIII to XIIIa, and cleaving fibrinogen to fibrin. Fibrin polymerizes to form an initial clot, a meshwork of fibrin strands that is subsequently cross-linked and stabilized by factor XIIIa.

Serum is the term for plasma that has been cleared of clotting factors.

Coagulation is potentially harmful if it leads to inappropriate or excessive clotting. Anticoagulant mechanisms inhibit the clotting cascade at a number of points. Antithrombin III is a protease inhibitor that binds and inactivates thrombin (factor IIa), and factors IXa, Xa, XIa, and XIIa. Its action is greatly potentiated by endothelial surface proteoglycans as well as the anticoagulant drug heparin.

Proteins C and S inactivate factors V and VIII. Protein C is activated by a complex of thrombin bound to thrombomodulin on endothelial cell surfaces. Thrombomodulin transforms thrombin from a procoagulant molecule that cleaves fibrinogen into an anticoagulant molecule by redirecting thrombin's enzymatic activity toward protein C. Activated protein C combines

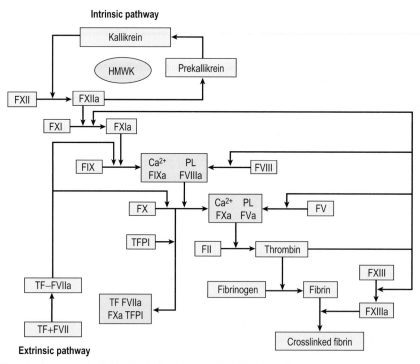

Fig. 7.7 The clotting cascade. In the intrinsic pathway, stimuli such as foreign or activated platelet surfaces, high-molecular-weight kininogen, prekallikrein, or collagen, can activate factor XII. In the extrinsic pathway, thought to be the dominant one in vivo, the release of tissue factor from damaged cells initiates the cascade. Note that in either the extrinsic or the intrinsic pathway, Ca^{2+} and phospholipid surface (PL) are required cofactors for activating factor X, the first step of the common pathway, and that the same cofactors are required for the activation of factor II (prothrombin to thrombin). (From Laffan MA, Bain BJ, Bates I, Eds. Dacie and Lewis Practical Haematology, Twelfth Edition. Philadelphia: Elsevier, 2017. Fig. 18-1)

with protein S, calcium ions, and a phospholipid surface to form a complex that inactivates factors V and VIII, slowing the coagulation cascade. Tissue factor pathway inhibitor (TFPI) binds and inactivates factors Xa and VIIa.

Once vessel damage has been repaired, clots must be removed. The fibrinolytic system dissolves clots, competing with procoagulant systems. Plasminogen is cleaved by plasminogen activators produced by endothelial cells to form plasmin. Plasmin cleaves fibrin into fibrin split products (FSPs), thus degrading clots. Plasmin, like the activated protein C and S system, also degrades factors V and VIII, giving it anti-coagulant properties as well as fibrinolytic ones. Since plasmin is potentially capable of causing severe hemorrhage, it has its own inhibitors. alpha-2-antiplasmin inhibits plasmin directly, and type 1 plasmin activation inhibitor (PAI-1) inhibits the conversion of plasminogen to plasmin.

Many clotting cascade enzymatic reactions require Ca^{2+} as a cofactor (e.g., activation of factors X and II). Chemicals such as Ethylene-Diamine-Tetraacetic Acid (EDTA) which chelate free Ca^{2+} effectively prevent coagulation. EDTA is used in some test tubes into which blood is collected so that contact of the blood with the glass does not precipitate coagulation.

Immunoproteins include complement proteins and antibodies (also known as immunoglobulins) that constitute the large γ-globulin spike in protein electrophoresis (described further in Ch. 8).

Finally, numerous specific hormones, enzymes, and enzyme inhibitors circulate in the plasma. In particularly high concentration are $α_1$-antitrypsin and $α_2$-macroglobulin.

- Important in deactivating the potentially destructive proteases liberated by neutrophils and other leukocytes in response to microbial invaders.
- Prevent excessive damage to the healthy cells and tissues of the body during the fight against infection. Deficiency of alpha1 antitrypsin is a genetic disorder that in some patients causes liver cirrhosis and in some patients lung damage leading to emphysema.

Blood Cells and Organelles

The functions of the cells in blood are based on their major protein components.

- Erythrocytes, with limited organelles and packed with hemoglobin, are the oxygen-carrying cells of the blood.
  - Arise from precursor cells in bone marrow, live about 120 days, normally never leave the circulation, and are degraded by the reticuloendothelial systems of the spleen and liver.
  - Carry oxygen from the lungs and deliver it to all tissues engaging in aerobic metabolism.
- Leukocytes perform multiple functions in the inflammatory and immune responses (see Ch. 8).
  - Neutrophils live only about 6 to 8 hours in the blood and travel to sites of acute inflammation, constituting a principal defense against bacteria.
    Engulf (phagocytose) bacteria and kill them by fusing the phagosome (the intracellular, membrane-enclosed vesicle containing the engulfed invader) with lysosomes and specific granules. This system

restricts the pathogen and the antimicrobial molecules to a small intracellular space, preventing damage to healthy cells.
    Liberate other granule-based mediators into their environments, thus damaging extracellular bacteria and host tissues by oxidative species and specific enzymes.
  - Eosinophils specifically defend against parasites and helminths (worms).
  - Basophils mediate allergic immune reactions.
  - Monocytes exit the vasculature and develop into tissue macrophages that are particularly suited to phagocytosis of foreign bodies and invading pathogens.
  - Mast cell precursors leave the circulation and develop in tissues such as the skin, respiratory tract, and GI tract, where as mature mast cells they mediate allergic reactions and host defense in local tissues.
  - Lymphocytes generate and maintain specific (also called adaptive) immune responses against particular pathogens.
- Platelets function with the coagulation system to control bleeding when blood vessel integrity is breached.
  - Platelets adhere to areas of denuded endothelium and release their granule contents, which causes platelet aggregation, as well as activation of the coagulation system.

Disrupted endothelium exposes subendothelial collagen, which rapidly binds circulating von Willibrand factor (vWF), a protein stored in and secreted by endothelial cells. Platelets express the surface glycoprotein receptor gp 1b/IX that specifically binds vWF. By means of gp1b/IX and vWF, platelets bind to the surface denuded of endothelium, are activated, and degranulate, releasing the contents of their alpha and delta granules.

ADP and serotonin enhance platelet degranulation and aggregation.

Lipid mediator thromboxane A2 (TXA2) produced from platelet arachidonic acid greatly augments their activation and aggregation.

The result is the primary hemostatic plug, an aggregate of platelets that achieves initial hemostasis.

Next, activation of the coagulation system provides fibrin that cements together the platelets of the hemostatic plug. Negatively charged subendothelial connective tissue and tissue factor activate the clotting cascade and activated platelets expedite this process. Platelets express the glycoprotein receptor gpIIb/IIIa that binds fibrinogen, and the cell membrane of the platelets provides the phospholipid surface on which the coagulation reactions occur.

Platelet degranulation also releases procoagulant mediators such as Ca^{2+}, factor V, platelet factor 4 (which neutralizes antithrombin III), and thrombospondin (which also binds fibrinogen). The production and cross-linking of fibrin binds platelets together, forming the secondary (definitive) hemostatic plug (see Fig 7.8).

The heparin-antithrombin III and proteins C and S mechanisms rapidly check the coagulation system. In addition, adjacent endothelial cells secrete prostacyclin that limits coagulation to the site of endothelial injury and plasminogen activators that activate the fibrinolytic system, which eventually degrades and

A. VASOCONSTRICTION

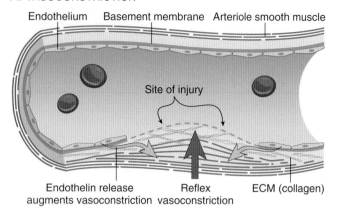

B. PRIMARY HEMOSTASIS

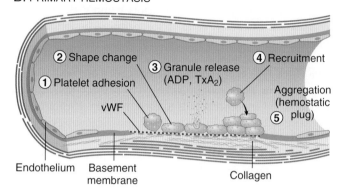

C. SECONDARY HEMOSTASIS

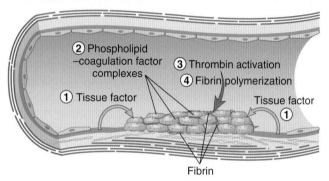

D. THROMBUS AND ANTITHROMBOTIC EVENTS

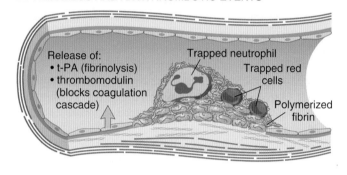

Fig. 7.8 Normal hemostasis. (A) After vascular injury, neurohumoral factors induce transient vasoconstriction. (B) Platelets bind via glycoprotein Ib (*GpIb*) receptors to von Willebrand factor (*vWF*) on exposed extracellular matrix (*ECM*) and are activated, undergoing a shape change and granule release. Released adenosine diphosphate (*ADP*) and thromboxane A_2 (*TxA₂*) induce additional platelet aggregation through platelet GpIIb-IIIa receptor binding to fibrinogen, and form the primary hemostatic plug. (C) Local activation of the coagulation cascade (involving tissue factor and platelet phospholipids) results in fibrin polymerization, "cementing" the platelets into a definitive secondary hemostatic plug. (D) Counterregulatory mechanisms, mediated by tissue plasminogen activator (*t-PA*, a fibrinolytic product) and thrombomodulin, confine the hemostatic process to the site of injury. (From Kumar V, Abbas AK, Aster JC, eds. Robbins and Cotran pathologic basis of disease. 10th ed. Philadelphia: Elsevier; 2021. Fig. 4.4.)

remodels the clot as endothelial cells and fibroblast proliferate and repair the injured area.

Blood Tissues

Bone marrow is the site of hematopoiesis, the production of new blood cells (Fig. 7.9).

- Pluripotent stem cells are undifferentiated bone marrow cells that can divide and whose progeny can develop into all cell lineages.
- Erythroid precursors develop into erythrocytes.
- Myeloid precursors develop into granulocytes and monocytes.
- Lymphoid precursors develop into lymphocytes.
- Megakaryocytes produce platelets.

These processes are tightly regulated by a large number of control proteins called growth factors and cytokines that are produced according to the body's need for these cells. Key factors include:

- Thrombopoietin: hormone growth factor that increases platelet production.

- Erythropoietin (EPO): Hormone growth factor that increases erythrocyte production.
  - Low oxygen concentration → triggers EPO production from the kidney → travel via blood to bone marrow → augmentation of erythrocyte production → correction of oxygen deficiency.
  - High oxygen concentration → EPO release inhibited (see Fast Fact Box 7.3 and 7.4).

Fast Fact Box 7.3

Because the renal medulla operates at low oxygen tension and participates in the filtration of the blood, it is an excellent tissue for sensing and regulating the oxygen-carrying capacity of the blood. Because most of the oxygen carried by blood is bound to hemoglobin inside erythrocytes, the production of red blood cells is the logical variable for the kidneys to control to affect the oxygen concentration of the blood.

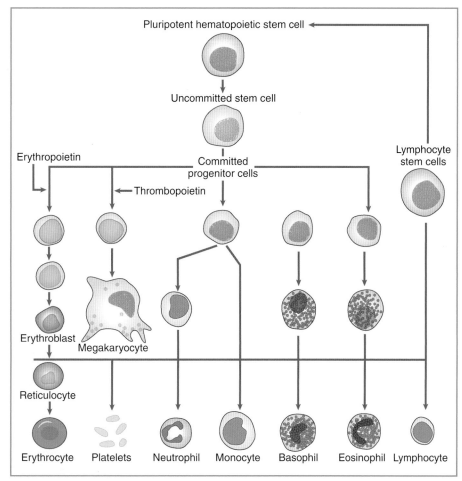

Fig. 7.9 The process of hematopoiesis. Pluripotent stem cells in the bone marrow divide by mitosis and give rise to progeny that commit to one of four basic developmental pathways. The erythroid pathway results in red blood cells. The phagocytic pathway produces monocytes that mature further into macrophages, granulocytes (neutrophils, eosinophils, or basophils), or mast cells. Stem cells that enter the megakaryocytic pathway remain in the bone marrow, while fragments of their cytoplasm pinch off as platelets that leave the marrow to circulate with other blood cells. The lymphoid pathway leads to the production of T cells and B cells. (From Carroll R. *Elsevier's Integrated Review: Physiology.* Philadelphia, PA: Elsevier. 2011. Fig. 6.2.) Erthropoetin and Thrombopoetin are growth factors that augment production of erythrocytes and platelets, respectively. Similar but distinct growth factors regulate the production of various leukocytes. Many of these growth factors are used clinically to treat low cell counts.

Fast Fact Box 7.4

Erythropoiesis-stimulating agents (ESAs) have historically been used as blood doping agents in endurance sports, such as cycling, running, and rowing. This allows athletes to increase oxygen delivery to muscles, which leads to a direct improvement in endurance exercise. However, increased red cell mass beyond natural levels also increases blood viscosity, which carries the danger of thrombosis and vascular occlusion (stroke). For this reason—as well as the obvious ethical concerns—these agents are strictly banned in all athletic events.

The capillary microcirculation is the network of interconnecting capillaries that serves a small volume of tissue. A diagram of a typical tissue microcirculation is shown in Fig. 7.10. Briefly:

- An incoming arteriole gives rise small capillaries whose diameters are only slightly larger than an erythrocyte (10 μm).

- Precapillary sphincters dilate and contract in response to metabolic needs of the tissues, as well as to neural and hormonal mediators, regulating flow to the capillary beds.
- The exchange of nutrients, wastes, gases, and fluid occurs in the tissue capillaries.
- Capillaries then drain into a venule that returns the blood to the venous system.

Occasionally, an arteriovenous shunt brings some arterial blood directly into the venous system, bypassing the capillary bed.

Variations on this general picture of microcirculation occur in each organ system, all of which have their own distinguishing features described in focused chapters:
- The alveolar capillaries of the lungs (Part V).
- The glomerular and peritubular capillary systems of the kidneys (Part VI).
- The portal capillies draining the GI tract (Part VII).
- The myocardial capillaries of the heart (Part IV).

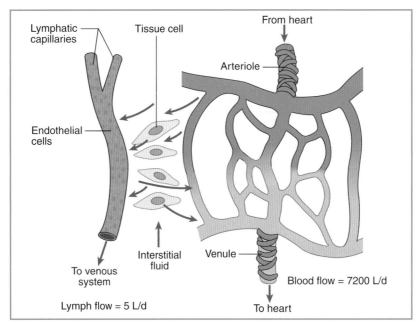

Fig. 7.10 The capillary microcirculation. Small arteries branch into arterioles that have smooth muscle and sphincters that control the flow of blood. Capillaries, blood vessels with walls only one cell thick, constitute a three-dimensional net, carrying nutrients into and wastes out of tissues. Eventually, blood that travels through capillaries rejoin to bring the blood into the venous circulation, where it can travel back toward the heart and lungs to be reoxygenated and then recirculated. (From Carroll R. *Elsevier's Integrated Review: Physiology*. Philadelphia, PA: Elsevier. 2011. Fig. 8.3.)

- The vasa vasorum of arterial walls (Part IV).
- The vasa nervosum of large nerves (Part II).
- The tissue capillaries of muscle and skin (Part II).

PATHOPHYSIOLOGY

Pathology of the blood is manifested by an impairment of the essential functions described in this chapter, such as the delivery of oxygen and nutrients, the removal of waste products, adequate defense, and effective homeostasis.

Essentially, all pathophysiology may be described as quantitative or qualitative problems with any of the formed elements or plasma proteins, or distributive problems in circulating these cells and proteins to the appropriate tissues.

Quantitative Disorders

When considering quantitative issues, one must ask if the deficit exists in production or peripheral destruction. Note that these problems may coexist.

Many disorders are marked by abnormally low concentrations of specific formed elements (Table 7.5). This pathology may be caused by multiple factors:

- Decreased rate of production.
- Increased rate of blood cell loss and/or destruction.
- Hemodilution, as when a patient receives large volumes of cell-free intravenous fluid. This generally affects all cell lines.

The loss of a given cell type leads to predictable effects based on its usual function:

- Anemia leads to pallor (a loss of color in the skin and mucous membranes resulting from loss of pigmented

TABLE 7.5 **Basic Terminology for Quantitative Disorders of Blood Elements**		
Cell Type	↓	↑
Erythrocytes	Anemia	Polycytosis
Leukocytes	Leukopenia	Leukocytosis
Platelets	Thrombocytopenia	Thrombocytosis
All cell lines	Pancytopenia	—

hemoglobin) and lethargy. Anemia may even precipitate damage to the heart and brain because of inadequate oxygen delivery (ischemia).

- Leukopenia may lead to recurrent infections.
- Thrombocytopenia may lead to excessive bleeding secondary to inadequate blood clotting.

Other pathologic conditions are marked by abnormally high concentrations of formed elements (see Table 7.5). As with disorders of low concentrations, high concentrations may also be caused by a number of factors:

- Increased rate of production.
- Decreased rate of blood cell loss and/or destruction.
- Hemoconcentration, as when a patient has lost a significant volume of vascular fluid without losing formed elements (i.e., dehydration).

Pathologically increased concentrations of formed elements may cause distributive problems (see later) as blood vessels are obstructed by clumps of cells. Thrombocytosis commonly leads to vascular occlusion secondary to inappropriate blood clotting.

Qualitative Disorders

In these disorders, the number of formed elements is normal, but there is dysfunction of a given element. These are myriad, but a few examples include:
- Defects in hemoglobin formation → erythrocytes are unable to carry oxygen as effectively as normal cells.
- Defects in immunoreceptors → leukocytes are unable to recognize pathogens.
- Defects in platelet receptors → platelets are unable to initiate/complete their role in coagulation, and thus the patient is at risk for excessive bleeding.

Of note, qualitative disorders may also pathologically increase the normal function of a given cell element. For example, deficits in leukocyte functioning may lead to autoimmunity and destruction of normal host tissue.

Distributive Disorders

In these disorders, blood is unable to travel to a specific location. This involves the scope of occlusive vascular disease, in which blood cells function adequately, but they are unable to reach the capillary microcirculation of a tissue or organ.

The consequences of oxygen and nutrient deprivation, combined with the buildup of metabolic wastes, are localized to a particular organ and often lead to cell death known as necrosis.
- Coronary artery occlusion → myocardial infarction.
- Cerebral artery occlusion → cerebrovascular accident (stroke).

Types of Anemia

One of the most common types of blood disorder is anemia, or reduced erythrocyte concentration relative to age-matched individuals.

The causes are numerous, but a helpful initial approach is to measure the mean corpuscular volume (MCV), which usually resides between 80 and 100 fL. This represents the size of erythrocytes.
- Microcytic (MCV <80 fL).
- Normocytic (MCV 80–100 fL).
- Macrocytic (MCV >100 fL).

From here, a more specific algorithm may be determined to further narrow the differential diagnosis of anemia (Fig. 7.11). Let us now focus on a couple specific examples of anemia.

Iron Deficiency Anemia

This is the most common type of anemia and is caused by a decrease in iron stores (recall: iron is a component of the heme moiety in hemoglobin and directly binds oxygen).

Iron deficiency can arise from:
- Insufficient dietary intake.
  - Adult males require about 1 mg of iron per day to maintain iron stores in the face of obligate losses from the GI tract and skin.
  - Rapidly growing children, menstruating women, and pregnant women require significantly more dietary iron.
- Impaired absorption (malabsorption).
  - Occurs with a variety of GI diseases.
- Excessive loss of iron.

- Occurs with any condition that causes bleeding, such as from the upper (esophagus, stomach, duodenum) or lower (colon) GI tract, the uterus (during menstruation), and trauma (see Fast Fact Box 7.5).

Fast Fact Box 7.5

Normally, senescent red blood cells are degraded by macrophages in the reticuloendothelial system of the liver and spleen, and their iron is recycled by complexing it with transferrin or ferritin. However, if blood cells exit the body, the lost iron must be replenished by the diet to avoid iron deficiency. Thus during iron deficiency, transferrin receptor production will increase while ferritin production decreases.

A deficiency of iron stores leads to an inability to incorporate sufficient iron into heme, and thus an inadequate production of functional hemoglobin. Because of insufficient hemoglobin, erythrocyte production is reduced in addition to bearing lower amounts of hemoglobin than normal per cell. Ultimately, this limits oxygen-carrying capacity.

Because of reduced hemoglobin, the erythrocytes have a large area of central pallor (hypochromic) and are smaller than normal (microcytic), resulting in a hypochromic microcytic anemia. Furthermore, they may irregularly shaped (Fig. 7.12, compare to Fig. 7.3).

In addition, there is laboratory evidence of decreased iron levels in the blood, decreased ferritin (reflecting decreased iron stores), and increased transferrin. The transferrin concentration is also called the total iron binding capacity (TIBC) and its elevation in iron deficiency anemia reflects the body's attempt to mobilize as much iron as possible.

The clinical manifestations of iron deficiency anemia reflect the function of the defective red blood cells:
- Low oxygen → limited cellular respiration → weakness, fatigue, and lethargy.
- Low hemoglobin → pallor.
- Extremely limited oxygen delivery → ischemia → signs of respiratory, cardiac, renal, or neurologic dysfunction.
- Miscellaneous effects of iron deficiency.
  - Dermal atrophy.
  - Brittle nails that become "spooned" (koilonychia).
  - Smooth, sore tongue (glossitis).
  - Pica, the desire to eat ice, dirt, and other nonnutritional substances.

The treatment of choice is iron supplementation and treatment of underlying disease (such as GI disorder or chronic bleeding).

Anemia of Chronic Renal Failure

As previously mentioned, erythropoietin drives the production of erythrocytes from erythroid progenitors. However, what if the kidneys are severely damaged, as in the chronic renal failure resulting from long-standing diabetes or hypertension (high blood pressure)?

In such cases, the production of erythropoietin is greatly impaired, resulting in anemia. Recombinant human erythropoietin can correct the hematocrit and often dramatically improve the symptoms of anemia in such patients.

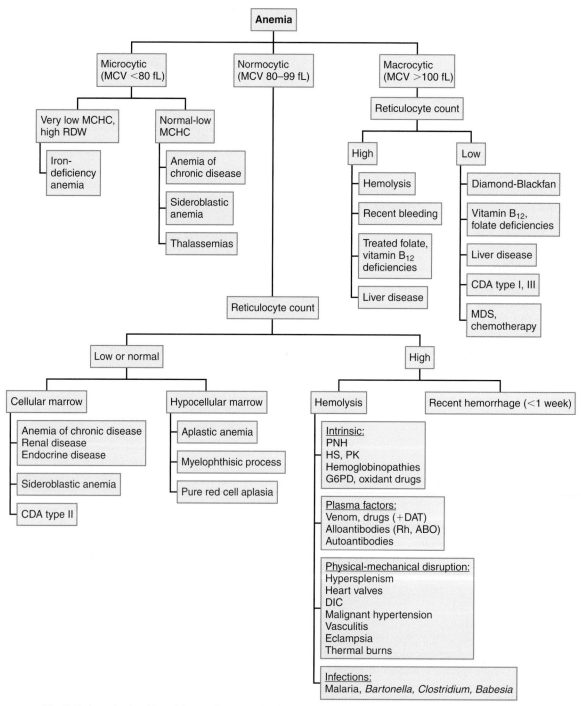

Fig. 7.11 Anemia algorithm. Mean cell volume (*MCV*) is based on adult values; reference ranges must be considered for pediatric patients. *CDA*, Congenital dyserythropoietic anemia; *DAT*, direct antiglobulin test; *DIC*, disseminated intravascular coagulation; *G6PD*, glucose-6-phosphate dehydrogenase; *HS*, hereditary spherocytosis; *MCHC*, mean cell hemoglobin concentration; *MDS*, myelodysplastic syndrome; *PK*, pyruvate kinase deficiency; *PNH*, paroxysmal nocturnal hemoglobinuria; *RDW*, red cell distribution width. (From Wilson CS, Vergara-Lluri ME, Byrnes RK. Evaluation of anemia, leukopenia, and thrombocytopenia. *Hematopathology.* 2017:195–234.e5. Fig. 11.1.)

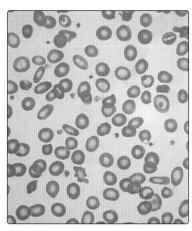

Fig. 7.12 A peripheral blood smear of iron deficiency anemia. Note that the erythrocytes in this smear are microcytic and hypochromic because they contain less hemoglobin than normal red blood cells. (From Howard M, Hamilton P. *Haematology: An Illustrated Colour Text,* 4th Edition. Philadelphia, PA: Elsevier. 2013. Fig. 12.4.)

Disorders of Hemostasis
Hypofunction

Results in hemorrhage. may occur with major trauma where damage to one or more blood vessels can lead to life-threatening low blood pressure and failure to perfuse vital organs if enough blood volume is lost, called hypovolemic shock.

Significant bleeding can occur without major trauma if the components of the hemostatic response are absent or dysfunctional. Such bleeding diatheses include hemophilia (e.g., insufficient factor VIII), liver failure (insufficient production of multiple clotting factors), von Willibrand's disease (insufficient vWF), and thrombocytopenia (insufficient platelets).

Hyperfunction

Results in thrombosis. Thrombosis in the iliac and femoral veins is deep venous thrombosis (DVT), dangerous if the clot breaks off and travels to the lungs as a pulmonary embolus. Hypercoaguable states include deficiencies of natural anticoagulants, such as protein S, protein C, or antithrombin III deficiencies; a mutation called factor V Leiden that makes factor V resistant to enzymatic inactivation by activated protein C, and states such as malignancy and sepsis that involve the production of mediators that inappropriately activate the clotting cascade.

Three general conditions that predispose to thrombosis are 1) endothelial damage/dysfunction, 2) hypercoaguable states, and 3) blood stasis. These three constitute Virchow's triad.

SUMMARY

- The primary function of the blood is to transport substances and cells from one organ to another.
- Oxygen and nutrients are brought to cells while metabolic wastes are removed, maintaining tissue metabolism and respiration.
- Hematopoietic stem cells in bone marrow give rise to all blood cells.
- The primary blood cell types include erythrocytes, which carry hemoglobin to transport oxygen; leukocytes, designed to fight microbial invaders; and platelets, the anucleate cell fragments of megakaryocytes that are involved in blood clotting.
- Among the leukocytes are the granulocytes (neutrophils, eosinophils, and basophils), monocytes, and lymphocytes (T cells and B cells).
- Blood gases are exchanged at the lungs and the peripheral tissues, dietary nutrients are absorbed at the GI tract and delivered to tissues, and metabolic wastes are taken from peripheral tissues and removed by the lungs and kidneys.
- Blood transports hormones and other mediators throughout the body. Many such hormones are bound to carrier proteins, such as albumin.
- The hormone erythropoietin is produced by kidney cells and stimulates the production of erythrocytes by the bone marrow. Other cytokines and growth factors expedite the maturation of megakaryocytes and the various white blood cells.
- The blood supply is essential for the viability of each individual organ, as well as for the communication, homeostasis, and integration of the individual tissues and systems into a whole organism.
- Disorders of blood cells may be quantitative, qualitative, or distributive. In quantitative disorders, the concentration of one or more cell lineages is too high or too low. In qualitative disorders, the concentration of a cell lineage is within the normal limits, but the cells are unable to perform one or more functions. In distributive disorders, the blood cannot be delivered to the target organ.
- Anemia, or low concentration of erythrocytes and/or hemoglobin, is one of the most common blood disorders.
- In iron deficiency anemia, a hypochromic microcytic anemia is observed. Symptoms relate primarily to impaired delivery of oxygen to tissues. In chronic renal failure, decreased production of erythropoietin leads to anemia that can be treated with injections of recombinant human erythropoietin.

REVIEW QUESTIONS

Directions: Each of the numbered items or incomplete statements in this section is followed by answers or by completions of the statement. Select the one lettered answer or completion that is best in each case.

1. An 8-year-old male patient arrives in your clinic with a 3-month history of diarrhea, weight loss, and shortness of breath. He has no past medical history, including no recent infections, travel, or daycare exposure. His mother does note, however, that he sometimes eats dirt when no one is watching carefully. On physical examination, he has wheezing in bilateral lung fields and a mildly distended, nontender abdomen. Laboratory studies reveal marked eosinophilia (60% eosinophils). What is the most likely class of pathogen afflicting him?
   A. Bacteria
   B. Virus
   C. Helminth
   D. Spirochete
   E. None of the above

2. A 20-year-old man with a history of a "blood disorder" arrives in the emergency department with acute onset shortness of breath, cough with sputum production, and fever to 101° F. A pulse oximetry reading from his right index finger returns with a value of 85% (low). What is the most accurate description of the pathophysiology of his disorder?
   A. Sickling of red cells causing vasoocclusion in the pulmonary vasculature
   B. Smooth muscle constriction in the bronchioles
   C. Infection of the upper respiratory tract
   D. Massive degranulation of mast cells
   E. Abnormal accumulation of air in the space of the chest cavity

3. An 84-year-old woman with a history of poorly controlled hypertension for the last 30 years and one heart attack has smoked one pack of cigarettes per day since she was 20 years old. She has felt tired and "washed out" in the past year. Four months ago, she was told she might need to start dialysis soon. On physical examination, her skin and mucus membranes are pale. She has a hematocrit of 24%. Which of the following is a likely component for her anemia?
   A. Lung disease from smoking impairing the uptake of oxygen by her red blood cells
   B. Kidney disease from high blood pressure reducing the production of erythropoietin
   C. Heart disease from high blood pressure and the heart attack impairing her ability to pump blood through her arteries and veins
   D. Bone marrow disease from her age, reducing the production of erythrocytes
   E. Autoimmune disease, in which her own immune system mistakenly destroys her red blood cells

4. Which of the following patients would be expected to have total iron binding capacity and % transferrin saturation in the normal range?
   A. An 80-year-old man with colon cancer that causes lower (colonic) gastrointestinal bleeding
   B. A 28-year-old woman, pregnant with twins, who hates taking prenatal vitamins
   C. A 29-year-old woman nursing the twins recently born via Caesarian section with significant blood loss during the procedure
   D. A 32-year-old woman with heavy periods that last 8 to 10 days for the last year
   E. A 24-year-old man with low blood pressure and significant blood loss from trauma in a motor vehicle accident

5. Which of the following committed stem cell and fully differentiated cell matches is not correct?
   A. Erythroid; erythrocyte
   B. Phagocytic; monocyte
   C. Phagocytic; granulocyte
   D. Megakaryocytic; platelets
   E. Lymphoid; neutrophil

ANSWERS TO REVIEW QUESTIONS

1. **The answer is C.** This is a typical case of ascariasis, caused by the parasitic roundworm *Ascaris lumbricoides*. It is acquired through ingesting soil contaminated with *Ascaris* eggs, which proceed to hatch in the intestines, travel through the gut wall, and migrate (via blood) to the lungs to be coughed up and swallowed. Adult worms then inhabit the intestines, causing malabsorption manifesting as malnutrition, weight loss, and chronic diarrhea. During helminth infections, eosinophils are released more rapidly from the bone marrow (within 1 hour of stimulation), resulting in peripheral eosinophilia. It is thought that the numerous cytotoxic granules contained within eosinophils (including major basic protein, reactive oxygen species, elastase, and more) aid in the immunologic response against helminthes, although this may also lead to significant host pathology. Patients with ascariasis may be treated by albendazole, mebendazole, and pyrantel pamoate, which are all antihelminth agents.

2. **The answer is A.** This patient has sickle cell disease, and is presenting in the emergency department with (most likely) acute chest syndrome. Acute chest syndrome is often precipitated by a lung (i.e., lower respiratory tract) infection. Inflammation and loss of oxygen saturation lead to sickling of red cells, thus leading to a terrible cycle of pulmonary and systemic hypoxemia, worsening sickling, and vasoocclusion. If untreated, patients can perish; acute chest syndrome is in fact the most common cause of death in sickle cell patients.

3. **The answer is B.** This patient with long-standing hypertension has been told that she may soon need dialysis because she very likely has significant kidney disease. Severe damage to the kidneys reduces the production of erythropoietin, the

hormone that stimulates the bone marrow to make red blood cells. If she had lung disease severe enough to impair the uptake of oxygen by her red blood cells, normal kidneys would detect this and increase their production of erythropoietin, resulting in an increase in the hematocrit, a condition known as polycythemia, which is essentially the opposite of anemia. Heart disease and age alone would not produce anemia independently. Autoimmune destruction of red blood cells certainly occurs, but it is a separate disease from the kidney failure that she has. Replacing erythropoietin during dialysis may significantly improve the anemia.

4. **The answer is E.** The patient who suffered the traumatic accident likely has a low hematocrit because of acute blood loss and dilution of the remaining red cells by the intravenous fluids. Given the recent onset of his anemia and its mechanism, he probably has a low to normal transferrin and, because he has lost both transferrin and serum iron (and both have been diluted), he probably has a normal transferrin saturation. The more chronic blood loss of the patient with colon cancer, the woman with heavy menstruation, and the increased demands for serum iron owing to pregnancy and breastfeeding are likely to result in iron deficiency anemia, characterized by increased transferrin (and therefore increased total iron binding capacity) and a low percentage iron saturation of transferrin.

5. **The answer is E.** The erythroid pathway results in red blood cells or erythrocytes. The phagocytic pathway produces monocytes that mature further into macrophages, granulocytes (neutrophils, eosinophils, or basophils), or mast cells. Stem cells that enter the megakaryocytic pathway remain in the bone marrow, while fragments of their cytoplasm pinch off as platelets that leave the marrow to circulate with other blood cells. The lymphoid pathway leads to the production of T cells and B cells.

8

The Lymphatic System and the Immune System

INTRODUCTION

The lymphatic system plays two essential roles in the human body:
1. Absorbs fluid from interstitial space and returns fluid to intravascular space.
   a. Transports lymph filtration fluid that enters the interstitial space from the capillaries.
2. Functional connection of blood and endothelium to the immune system.
   a. Transport of immune cells and products.

LYMPHATIC SYSTEM STRUCTURE

The lymphatic system plays an essential role in fluid transport:
- Capillary endothelium provides a semipermeable barrier between intravascular and extravascular interstitial space.
- Fluid crosses into the interstitial space as arterial blood passes through capillaries.
- Most fluid is reabsorbed at the venous end of the capillary, but a small fraction remains.
- This excess, acellular fluid containing solutes and proteins collects as lymph.
- The lymphatic system then returns lymph to systemic circulation.

The Extracellular Fluid

Total body water, or TBW, is composed of approximately two-thirds intracellular fluid (ICF) and one-third extracellular fluid (ECF) (Fig. 8.1). ECF occupies two compartments:
- 25% of the ECF is within blood vessels as intravascular fluid (plasma).
- 75% is within tissues as extravascular interstitial fluid.

These two ECF compartments are dynamic, with water molecules, ions, and macromolecules moving between them according to physical forces.

The Interstitial Space

The interstitial compartment surrounds tissue cells and forms their immediate environment. It is composed of:
- Collagenous framework filled with a gel-like solution containing negatively charged glycosaminoglycans (GAGs) and proteoglycans.
  - GAGS are long unbranched polysaccharides consisting of a repeating disaccharide unit.
    Examples: Heparin, chondroitin, dermatan, keratan, and hyaluronic acid.
- Proteoglycan consist of "core proteins" attached to one or more GAGs.
- Salts
- Water
- Plasma-derived proteins (e.g., albumin)

The particular composition varies greatly among different tissues. The skin, for example, has denser or "tighter" interstitial spaces with relatively high concentrations of collagen, hyaluronic acid, and albumin, whereas lung tissue has a "looser" matrix.

Lymphatic System Components

To efficiently return fluid from the interstitial space to systemic circulation, the lymphatic system extends small vessels into almost all tissues. This network of vessels is interrupted by lymph nodes, where the immune surveillance is carried out.

Lymphatic System Gross Anatomy

The lymphatic system consists of:
- Lymphatic vessels (lymphatics), a network of tubules connecting the entire system (Fig. 8.2).
  - The largest lymph vessel is the thoracic duct, which feeds into the left subclavian vein to reconnect lymph and systemic circulation.
  - Most lymphatics feed into the cisterna chyli, a large lymph sac feeding into the thoracic duct.
  - Certain lymph vessels drain instead into the right lymphatic duct → right subclavian vein (the right upper extremity, half of thorax, half of head)
- Lymph, fluid contained within the lymphatics.
- Lymph nodes, small swellings linked by lymphatics, are sites of immune cell trafficking.
  - Distributed unevenly throughout the body, particularly numerous in the neck, axillae, and inguinal areas.

Other important organs of the lymphatic system, such as the spleen, thymus, tonsils, and Peyer's patches, are discussed in the context of the immune system (see Clinical Correlation Box 8.1).

Clinical Correlation Box 8.1

Virchow's node, or the "signal node," is a lymph node that sits above the left clavicle and drains the lymph vessels from the abdominal cavity. Swelling of this node is strongly associated with cancer in the abdomen, especially gastric cancer.

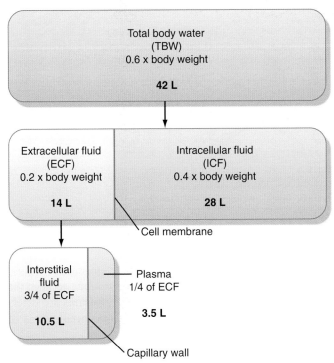

Fig. 8.1 Division of total body water (*TBW*) into extracellular and intracellular fluid compartments (*ECF* and *ICF*). The volumes listed are calculated for a 70-kg person. The ECF is further subdivided into interstitial fluid bathing body cells outside the vascular space and plasma, the ECF volume in the vascular space. (From Koeppen BM, Stanton BA. *Berne & Levy Physiology*, 6th Updated Edition. Elsevier; 2009. Fig. 2.1.)

Lymphatic System Tissues and Cells

Lacteals are lymphatic capillaries embedded within the interstitial space (Fig. 8.3):
- Thin, blind-ended channels lined by a single layer of endothelial cells.
  - In contrast with vascular capillary endothelium (see Ch. 9 and the appendix on endothelial function), lacteal endothelium has no fenestrations, no tight junctions, and virtually no basal lamina.
- Contain bileaflet valves to prevent backflow of lymph. Lymph contains very few cells normally:
- Red blood cells do not ordinarily leave the vasculature and thus are not found in normal lymph.
- White blood cells, on the other hand, can exit (or extravasate) from the postcapillary venules by the process of diapedesis and enter tissues.

Lymph nodes are kidney bean shaped collections of tissue cells and leukocytes, such as macrophages and lymphocytes (Figs. 8.4 and 8.5):
- On the outer (convex) surface, one or more afferent lymphatic vessels "plug into" the node, penetrating the capsule.
- The deeper node is divided into an outer cortex and an inner medulla.
  - Outer cortex
    Subdivided by connective tissue trabeculae, contains dynamic collections of immune cells called follicles.
    The arrangement of these resident immune cells into follicles and zones expedites their communication (described later).

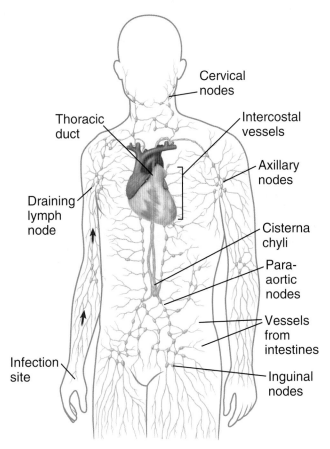

Fig. 8.2 Gross anatomy of the lymphatic system. Although lymph nodes are found throughout the body, note their relatively high frequency in the neck, axillae, and inguinal regions. Lymphatic vessels often follow the general direction of large blood vessels. The majority of lymphatic vessels connect to the cisternae chyli and on into the thoracic duct, but lymphatics from the right side of the body lead to the right lymphatic duct. They all lead back to the venous circulation. (From Abbas A. *Cellular and Molecular Immunology*, 9th Edition. Elsevier; 2018. Fig. 2.13.)

- Inner medulla
- The node's hilum is the area on the inner (concave) surface where efferent lymphatic vessels exit and where a feeding artery and a draining vein "plug into" the node.

LYMPHATIC SYSTEM FUNCTION

The Starling Forces

The process of fluid moving from the vascular space of the capillary into the interstitial tissue is known as transudation.

The three main determinants of filtration of fluid across a capillary membrane into the interstitial space are:
1. The net hydrostatic pressure
2. The net oncotic pressure
3. Capillary filtration

These three variables determine the direction and magnitude of fluid flux between the vascular space of a capillary and the interstitial space.

The hydrostatic and oncotic pressures are called Starling forces and are related to the capillary wall permeability and fluid flux by the Starling equation, described later.

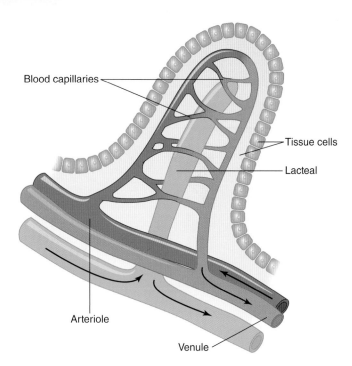

Fig. 8.3 Lymphatics vessel components. Small lymphatic capillaries called lacteals are embedded in tissues. Lymph enters the sealed end and travels out of the tissue (*arrow*). Also shown is a nearby arteriole, blood capillary, and venule, with the flow of progressively deoxygenated blood indicated.

Hydrostatic Pressures

There are two hydrostatic pressures:

1. Capillary hydrostatic pressure (Pc) is the force per unit area of the capillary endothelium that pushes fluid out of the capillary and into the interstitial space.
   a. Determined by systemic blood pressure and the specific resistances of the local arterioles and venules.
      i. Systemic blood pressure is a function of total intravascular salt and water volume, pumping forces generated by the heart, and total vascular resistance (see Part IV).
   b. Pc is approximately 32 mm Hg at the arteriolar end but decreases along the length of the capillary, reaching approximately 15 mm Hg at the venous end of a typical capillary.
2. Interstitial hydrostatic pressure (Pi) opposes Pc.
   a. Thought to be determined by:
      i. Imbalance of opposing mechanical forces exerted by hyaluronan and collagen.
      ii. Affinity of hyaluronan for water
   b. Pi is slightly negative, approximately –3 to 0 mm Hg.
      i. This causes it to "suck" fluid from the capillary into the interstitial space – in the same direction as Pc.

The difference between these pressures represents the net driving hydrostatic pressure for filtration. Note that because Pi is negative, the net driving hydrostatic pressure exceeds Pc.

- Arteriolar end: Pc – Pi = 32 mm Hg – (–3 mm Hg) = 35 mm Hg
- Venous end: Pc – Pi = 15 mm Hg – (–3 mm Hg) = 18 mm Hg

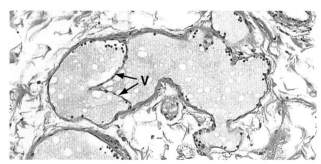

Fig. 8.4 Microscopic view of a lymphatic vessel. Note the thin wall of endothelium and the bileaflet valve, which ensures that lymph flows unidirectionally (*arrows*). (From Young B, O'Dowd G, Woodford P. *Wheater's Functional Histology*, 6th Edition. Elsevier; 2013. Fig. 8.25.)

Oncotic Pressures

Similarly, there are two opposing oncotic pressures. Because there are no large differences in salt concentrations between the interstitium and the plasma, the oncotic pressures are determined entirely by the differences in protein concentrations of the two compartments.

1. Capillary oncotic pressure (IIc) is defined as the colloid osmotic pressure, the component of the total osmotic pressure that is contributed by plasma proteins.
   a. The capillary endothelium allows essentially free diffusion of small solutes, but severely restricts filtration of protein into the interstitial space.
   b. High relative protein content.
   c. IIc is approximately 25 mm Hg.
2. Interstitial oncotic pressure (IIi) is the colloid osmotic pressure exerted by the osmotically active proteins in the interstitium.
   a. Low relative protein content as discussed.
   b. IIi is approximately 0 to –5 mm Hg.

Thus the difference between these pressures represents the net driving oncotic pressure for filtration. In normal conditions, it is positive and thus favors fluid reabsorption.

Fig. 8.6 shows the direction of the vectors for the two hydrostatic and two oncotic pressures.

- At the arteriolar end of the capillary, the hydrostatic forces for filtration exceed the oncotic forces for resorption, and the net effect is fluid filtration.
- At the venous side of the capillary (because of hydrostatic pressure reduction), the oncotic forces exceed hydrostatic forces and the net effect is fluid reabsorption.

In most tissues, the volume of fluid that leaves the capillary and enters the interstitial space exceeds the volume of fluid that is resorbed from the interstitial space back into the capillary. Thus there is a net loss of fluid from the vascular space into the extravascular tissue space. If this fluid is not resorbed and returned to the circulatory compartment by the lymphatic system, it accumulates in tissues and causes swelling called "edema." The compliance of the extracellular space is relatively high, so it takes a considerable volume of fluid to start increasing tissue pressure. This increased interstitial hydrostatic pressure opposed capillary hydrostatic pressure and limits further accumulation of fluid, and it promotes fluid flow into the lymphatic system, both of which are mechanisms of escape from edema.

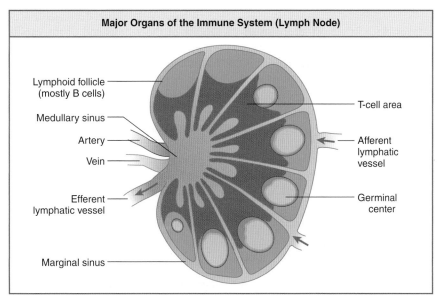

Major Organs of the Immune System (Lymph Node)

Fig. 8.5 Structure of a lymph node. Lymph enters through afferent lymphatic vessels on the convex side of the node. Lymph then percolates through the node and exits via an efferent vessel at the node's hilum on the concave side. The hilum is also the point at which blood enters the node through an afferent arteriole and exits the node via an efferent value. (From Actor JK. *Elsevier's Integrated Review: Immunology and Microbiology*, 2nd Edition. Elsevier; 2012. Fig. 2.5.)

The Capillary Filtration Coefficient

The third factor important in fluid flow across the capillary is capillary filtration, or the volume of fluid filtered from the intravascular to interstitial spaces. It is directly proportional to:
- Capillary wall permeability: the intrinsic hydraulic permeability of the endothelium and the other structural components of the capillary wall.
- Total surface area of the capillaries supplying a local area of tissue.
  The capillary filtration coefficient (K_f) is a quantitative measure of these two parameters.
- Units: milliliters of fluid transported per minute per 1 mm Hg pressure per 100 g of tissue.

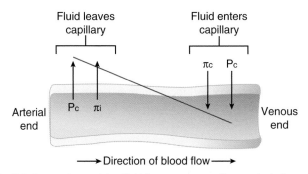

Fig. 8.6 Forces determining fluid flux across a capillary endothelium. As blood flows from the arteriolar end of the capillary toward the venous end, the capillary hydrostatic pressure, Pc, decreases. The interstitial hydrostatic pressure (Pi), the capillary oncotic pressure (Πc), and the interstitial oncotic pressure (Πi) are also shown. At a critical point, the balance of forces shifts from favoring the efflux of fluid from the capillary lumen into the interstitium (transudation) to favoring the resorption of fluid from the interstitium back into the capillary (resorption). Filtration exceeds resorption, but the lymphatics maintain fluid homeostasis in the interstitium by absorbing the excess fluid.

- Independent of hydrostatic and oncotic pressures and depends on the microscopic structure of the vessels and tight junctions between the endothelial cells (see Clinical Correlation Box 8.2)

Clinical Correlation Box 8.2

If the capillary wall is damaged by toxins or inflammatory stimuli, then it becomes much more permeable and K_f increases. Thus, more plasma enters the interstitial space (transudation). Likewise, if the smooth muscle of small arterioles relaxes, opening (or recruiting) previously closed capillaries in a tissue bed, the total capillary surface area rises. This also leads K_f (and thus transudation) to increase.

The Starling Equation

The relationship among hydrostatic pressures, oncotic pressures, and the K_f can be expressed in a compact form known as the Starling equation:

$$Q = (K_f) \times [(Pc - Pi) - \sigma (\Pi c - \Pi i)]$$

The Starling equation states that the overall flow of fluid, Q, expressed in units of volume per time in a given mass of tissue (mL of fluid transported per minute per 100 g tissue) is equal to K_f multiplied by the differences between the hydrostatic and oncotic forces between the capillary lumen and interstitial space.
- The reflection coefficient, σ, a correction factor that varies from 0 to 1 to simulate the decreased contribution of the oncotic pressure gradient to the net driving force. This correction is sometimes necessary to simulate small protein leakage in many body capillaries.

A positive value for Q indicates fluid filtration from the vasculature into the tissues (transudation), whereas a negative value for Q indicates fluid resorption.

The magnitude of Q indicates the quantity of fluid flow.

The Flow of Lymph

The production of lymph takes place in almost all major organs. Lymph does not flow via a pump (such as with the cardiovascular system), but rather by a combination of extrinsic and intrinsic forces. Overall, the net force favors drainage of fluid from the interstitium to the terminal lymphatics.

- Extrinsic forces lead to the generation of tissue compressive or suction forces.
  - Active striated muscle contractions, particularly limb movements during periods of standing and walking.
  - Rhythmic changes of intraabdominal and intrathoracic pressure because of respiration, peristalsis, and arterial pulsation.
- Intrinsic forces occur because of intrinsic contractility of the lymphatic vessels.
  - Individual segments between valves accumulate fluid, which leads to distension and then contraction.
  - This propels fluid upstream in a peristaltic fashion.

LYMPHATIC SYSTEM PATHOPHYSIOLOGY

Any processes in lymph physiology, including filtration, resorption, or lymph flow, can become dysfunctional and result in disease. The aberrant accumulation of fluid in the interstitial space leads to edema.

Edema occurs most commonly by one of four possible mechanisms:

1. Increased intravascular hydrostatic pressure
2. Decreased intravascular oncotic pressure
3. Increased capillary permeability
4. Lymphatic obstruction

Increased Intravascular Hydrostatic Pressure

Increased intravascular hydrostatic pressure (Pc) occurs in:

- States of generalized increased intravascular plasma volume, such as total fluid overload.
- Localized obstruction (increased pressure occurs proximal to the obstruction).

In congestive heart failure (CHF), impaired pumping function of the heart's left ventricle leads to increased pressure in the pulmonary venous circulation as blood backs up, leading to dangerous fluid accumulation in the lungs called pulmonary edema.

In cirrhotic liver disease, obstruction to flow in the portal venous system owing to the destruction of liver parenchyma leads to portal hypertension (elevated Pc) and fluid accumulation in the abdominal cavity called ascites.

Decreased Intravascular Oncotic Pressure

Decreased intravascular oncotic pressure (P_c) occurs in states of hypoproteinemia, usually measured as hypoalbuminemia, a low concentration of albumin in the blood. This condition occurs in cases of:

- Reduced protein intake, as in cases of malnutrition.
- Reduced ingested dietary protein absorption, as in gastrointestinal (GI) malabsorption.
- Reduced albumin production, as in liver failure.
- Increased albumin urinary losses, as in nephrotic syndrome.

Whatever the cause, decreased oncotic pressure impairs the ability of the venous end of the capillary to resorb fluid. Initially, the excess interstitial fluid is returned to the systemic circulation by the lymphatics, but once the volume of fluid exceeds the capacity of the lymphatics, edema results.

Increased Capillary Filtration Coefficient

Increased capillary permeability, expressed quantitatively as an increased capillary filtration coefficient (CFC), occurs when the capillary endothelium is damaged. Examples include:

- Burns, in which connective tissue is destroyed.
- Local inflammation, in which inflammatory stimuli loosen the tight junctions between endothelial cells.
- Toxic damage, in which endothelial cell dysfunction occurs, as in sepsis, pancreatitis, and inhalation injuries (e.g., damage from inhaling smoke).

Lymphatic Obstruction

Lymphatic obstruction occurs in any disease in which lymphatic vessels or nodes are blocked.

- Invasion of neoplastic cells in cancer may invade and disrupt lymphatic channels.
- Surgical removal of lymph nodes.
- Certain parasitic infections, such as filariasis, where small worms penetrate the system and obstruct lymph flow.

In all cases, the resultant edema is localized to the area drained by the affected nodal group.

INTRODUCTION

The many diverse structures and functions of the immune system can be imagined as a great war carried out by the cells of the immune system in defense of the body.

- Immune system cells are the soldiers.
- Immune system molecules are their tools and weapons.
- Immune system responses are the tactical moves.

The immune system primarily exists to protect the body from infection (the invasion of the body by pathogenic microbes).

- Immune system cells sample the matter contacting the body's borders, looking for invaders.
- If detected, the immune system activates and responds to destroy or drive out the enemy.

Note this chapter will focus on broad principles; there is an enormous amount of subtlety in the immunology, as well as frequent, exciting new research insights.

INNATE VERSUS ADAPTIVE IMMUNITY

The body's immune defense has two distinct but highly interrelated subsystems.

The first, the innate immune system, is a nonspecific, immediate immune response. It is multitiered:

- Anatomic barriers
  - Mechanical: skin, mucus, sweat, coughing/sneezing.
  - Chemical: saliva (lysozyme, phospholipase A2), gastric acid, defensins, vaginal secretions.

- Microbial: commensal flora ("good bacteria").
- Inflammation
  - Definition
    Influx of immune cells, fluid, and blood proteins into an area of the body that has been injured and/or infected.
    Prevents infection spread and promotes healing.
  - Acutely inflamed tissue typically shows:
    Rubor (redness)
    Dolor (pain)
    Calor (heat)
    Tumor (swelling)
    Functio laesa (loss of function)
- Cellular response
  - Certain white blood cells (i.e., macrophages, neutrophils, and eosinophils).
  - Detect microbes by means of cell-surface receptors called pattern recognition receptors (PRRs)
    PRRs are generally glycoproteins that bind to specific structures (called pathogen-associated molecular patterns [PAMPs]).
    Found in microbes, but not humans.
    PRRs binding → innate immune cell activation → inflammatory response.
- Plasma protein systems
  - Complement cascade (discussed later)

The innate immune system is rapid and somewhat specific because of the dependence on PAMPs, but PRRs are encoded by invariant genes and cannot adapt. It is also involved in tissue repair following trauma and help contain injurious agents, such as foreign bodies.

If the innate immune system cannot eradicate an invader, then the adaptive immune response is invoked. It differs importantly from innate immunity in several ways (Table 8.1)

The major cells of adaptive immunity are lymphocytes: T cells and B cells.
- The cell-surface receptors of T and B cells recognize particular structures of microbes, produced by a dramatic reshuffling of genes (plasticity).
- Adaptive immune memory cells persist in the circulation (memory).
  - Primary response: The first interaction particular microbe and a human host will produce disease as the host's adaptive immune system responds.
  - Secondary response: On reexposure to the same pathogen, the adaptive immune response is almost instantaneous.

- If the pathogen is eliminated so quickly as to avoid disease symptoms, this is called immunity.
  Differentiates "self" (the human host, in this case) from "nonself."
  Protects the body by triggering a powerful response to neutralize and destroy pathogens, proteins, or cells that are nonself.

The lines of defense are highly intertwined and interdependent. Innate immune cells detect invaders and signal adaptive immune cells about a threat. When in turn the adaptive immune system marshals its forces, it conscripts innate immune cells to do much of the fighting.

IMMUNE SYSTEM STRUCTURE

Immune System Organs and Tissues

The organs of the immune system may be divided in three main categories of function:
- Physical barriers
- Production and "education" of immune cells
- Headquarters or outpost for immune cells in a given anatomic location
  - Spleen screens the bloodstream
  - Lymph nodes screen the lymph
  - Lymphoid organs screen border regions (i.e., GI tract and the upper airways)

Skin and Epithelia

The barriers representing the first line of defense include:
- Skin (primary)
  - Keratinocytes in the epidermis adhere to one another, preventing microbes from freely entering the internal environment of the body.
  - Breaches (burns, punctures, and other wounds) allow pathogens to enter.
- Epithelial linings of the alimentary canal and respiratory tract

Bone Marrow

As discussed in Chapter 7, all blood cells start life in the bone marrow, the flexible tissue on the interior surface of the bones marrow (Fig. 8.7).
- Certain niches within the bone marrow host hematopoietic stem cells.
- When stem cells undergo mitosis, some daughter cells remain stem cells and others differentiate (see Fig. 7.7).
- These differentiated cells then enter systemic circulation via the delicate vessels tracing through the bone (see Clinical Correlation Box 8.3 and Clinical Correlation Box 8.4).

TABLE 8.1 Essential Differences Between Innate and Adaptive Immune System				
	Time	**Specificity**	**Plasticity**	**Memory**
Innate	Minutes to hours	Relatively nonspecific	None	None
Adaptive	Days	Highly specific	Yes	Yes

Clinical Correlation Box 8.3

Inherited or acquired dysfunction of the bone marrow leads to profound, possibly deadly deficits in the immune system functioning. Such so-called immunodeficiency leaves the affected individual more susceptible to infections, as well as malignancy

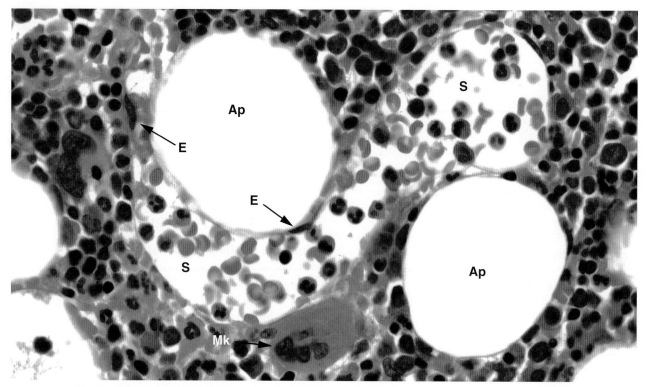

Fig. 8.7 A light micrograph of bone marrow. *Ap,* Adipocytes; *E,* endothelial cells; *Mk,* megakaryocytes; *S,* sinusoids. (From Young B, O'Dowd G, Woodford P. *Wheater's Functional Histology,* 6th Edition. Elsevier; 2013. Fig. 3.3.)

Clinical Correlation Box 8.4

The site of hematopoiesis is not constant throughout human development. In fetuses, the yolk sac is the first site of hematopoiesis! This responsibility shifts to the liver, the spleen, and then finally the bone marrow. Occasionally, in states of extreme hematopoietic stress (such as extensive red blood cell lysis in sickle cell anemia and thalassemia), the spleen and liver—as well as unusual bones—will take on their old role. This results in hepatosplenomegaly, as well as characteristic bony deformities.

The Thymus

The thymus, a lymphoid organ in the mediastinum, is critical to the "education" of the T cells of the adaptive immune system. The thymus is most prominent in infants and children, and it withers away as we age.

The Spleen

Located in the left upper quadrant of the peritoneal cavity, the spleen is the circulation's largest lymphoid organ.
- Histologically, the parenchyma is divided into red pulp and white pulp.
  - Red pulp: connective tissue ('the cords of Billroth') and blood-filled sinuses.
  - White pulp: local hyperplasia of adenoid (lymphatic) tissue.
- Trabecular arteries penetrate the splenic parenchyma (Fig. 8.8)
  - White pulp surrounds the central arterioles.
    A periarteriolar lymphoid sheath (PALS) directly surrounds the central arteriole.
      Rich in T cells.

Adjacent are germinal centers and B cell coronae.
      Rich in B cells.
- Blood eventually flows into trabecular veins and away from the spleen.
  The spleen functions primarily in immune surveillance of the bloodstream.

Lymph Nodes and Other Lymphoid Tissues

The numerous lymph nodes scattered throughout the body are important headquarters through which adaptive immune cells:
- Screen lymph
- Receive and process information
- Communicate with one another
- Reproduce
  The gross structure is presented in Fig. 8.5. As in the spleen, there is a distinct division between the different lymphocytes:
- Paracortical areas are rich in T cells
- Follicles are rich in B cells
  Lymphoid tissues, such as the tonsils of the pharynx and the Peyer's patches of the GI tract, are structurally and functionally similar to lymph nodes.
- Function to screen border areas (GI tract, upper respiratory tract).

Immune System Cells

Innate Immune Cells

- Function
  - Constitute early defense systems of the body.

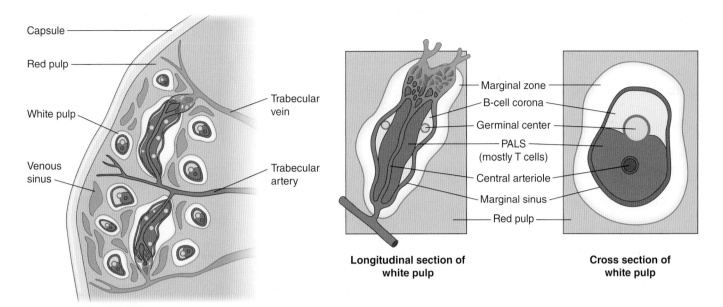

Fig. 8.8 The structure of the spleen. The parenchyma is divided into red pulp and white pulp. Central arteries are surrounded by periarteriolar lymphoid sheaths (*PALS*) populated largely by T cells. Germinal centers, where stimulated immune cells reproduce, and B cell coronae are also components of the white pulp.

- Alert, direct, and carry out orders from adaptive immune cells.
- Location
  - Some circulate through the bloodstream, entering extravascular tissues only when needed to fight an invader.
  - Others reside in tissue "outposts," leaving these tissues only to carry information to adaptive immune cells in lymph nodes.
  Fig. 7.5 shows the major innate immune cells.

Granulocytes

As discussed in Chapter 7, granulocytes have numerous intracytoplasmic granules and fight for the innate immune system. Granulocytes circulate in the bloodstream until they are recruited to tissues.

Mast Cells

Mast cells resemble basophils in having numerous intracytoplasmic granules. Mast cells are powerful effector cells in the tissue, and function particularly in the allergic response.

Monocytes and Macrophages

Monocytes are innate immune cells that have a single, bean-shaped nucleus.
- When circulating monocytes exit the bloodstream and enter tissues, they mature into macrophages.
- Macrophages, stimulated by the presence of an invader or activated by molecular signals of inflammation, may differentiate into:
  - Epithelioid cells
  - Multinucleate giant cells (two or more macrophages fuse)

Dendritic Cells

Immature dendritic cells reside in peripheral tissues, where they have long projections and a central, oval nucleus.
- Act as important innate immune system "border guards," sampling the tissue environment.
- When a pathogen is detected, they migrate to a nearby lymph node and mature.
- Communicate with cells of the adaptive immune system, thereby fulfilling their function as antigen-presenting cells (APCs; see later).

Adaptive Immune Cells

The adaptive immune cells are collectively called lymphocytes because they are the predominant cells found in lymph. However, they join other leukocytes in circulating in the blood as well.
- Viewed under the light microscope, all mature, resting lymphocytes appear similar.
  - Central, round nucleus
  - Small volume of surrounding cytoplasm
  Fig. 7.5 shows the adaptive immune cells.

B Cells and Plasma Cells

B cells are named for the bone marrow, where they are produced.
- Different B cells are designed to respond to different stimuli.
- Once a given B cell encounters its specific stimulus, it is activated and reproduces.
  - Creates a population (or clone) of identical daughter cells that all respond to the same specific stimulus.
  - Some daughter cells undergo further maturation to become plasma cells.
  Larger than resting B cells

Cytoplasm with prominent Golgi apparatus and endoplasmic reticulum

"Nucleus" that resembles a clock face

T Cells

T cells also originate in the bone marrow, but migrate to the thymus (for which they are named) to complete their early development.

* Like B cells, different T cells are also designed to different stimuli.
* There are two main types of T cells (discussed later):
  * Helper T cells (CD4+)
  * Killer T cells (CD8+)

Immune System Molecules

Immune system cells gather, process, and respond to matter on the molecular level. The important molecules of the immune system fall into three broad categories:

* Nonself molecules detected by the immune system indicating the presence of an invader
* Self proteins used to detect nonself molecules
* Molecules used by the immune system to fight invaders

Antigens

An antigen is any substance that provokes an immune response (i.e., immunogenic).

* May be a peptide or a protein, a lipid, a carbohydrate, or some combinations of these.
* An epitope is a region of an antigenic molecule that is specifically recognized by antibodies or T cell receptors (Fig. 8.9A).
* Small monomers (i.e., amino acids, nucleic acids, and single sugars) may be too small to be effective antigens.
  * These may become effective immunogens when bound to a normally inert host protein, also known as haptens (see Fig. 8.9B) (see Fast Fact Box 8.1).

Fast Fact Box 8.1

An important example of a combination antigen is lipopolysaccharide (LPS), a component of the cell wall of certain pathogenic bacteria. A molecule of LPS has a fatty acid-containing lipid A region bound to polysaccharide regions and is a powerful immunogen.

Major Histocompatibility Complexes

* Located on human chromosome 6.
* Encoded by human leukocyte antigen (HLA) genes.
* Code for two sets of cell-surface receptors.
  * Each holds protein fragments (peptides)
  * Presents antigens to cells of the adaptive immune system
  * Allows recognition of the peptide antigens as self or nonself

The extracellular portion of the major histocompatibility complex (MHC) molecules has a groove into which a peptide can fit (Fig. 8.10).

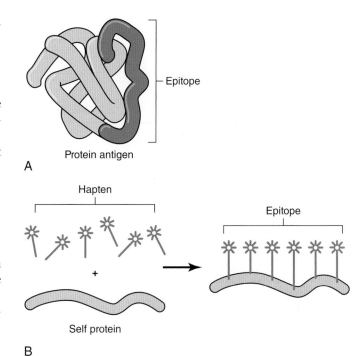

Fig. 8.9 Antigens, epitopes, and haptens. A, An antigen is a substance that elicits an immune response. The protein antigen shown here has a region on the right side, an epitope that is specifically recognized by T cell or B cell receptors. B, Small molecules called haptens are not immunogenic on their own, but when bound to a host protein do constitute an effective antigen.

There are two important subtypes of MHC molecules, outlined in Table 8.2.

The human genome encodes a number of MHC molecules, each able to accommodate a modest number of structurally related peptides.

* Individuals with different MHC genes may differ in their ability to respond to a given antigen.
* If a person lacks all MHC genes encoding molecules that can accommodate a given peptide, he or she may not be able to mount an effective adaptive immune response against that peptide.

Antibodies

Antibodies are proteins secreted by B cells that bind antigen.

* These proteins are recognized as products of the immune system, and as such are deemed immunoglobulins (Igs).
* There are five major isotypes of Ig: IgA, IgD, IgE, IgG, and IgM.
  Immunoglobulin monomers consist of two heavy chains and two light chains, arranged in a Y shape (Fig. 8.11).
* The two branches of the antibody are called the Fab (antigen binding fragment) region.
  * Each branch formed by light chain and the variable region of the heavy chain (V_H).
  * The heavy chains and light chains of a given antibody molecule are identical.
    Thus each branch binds same antigen
* Determines idiotype (unique antigen binding specificity).

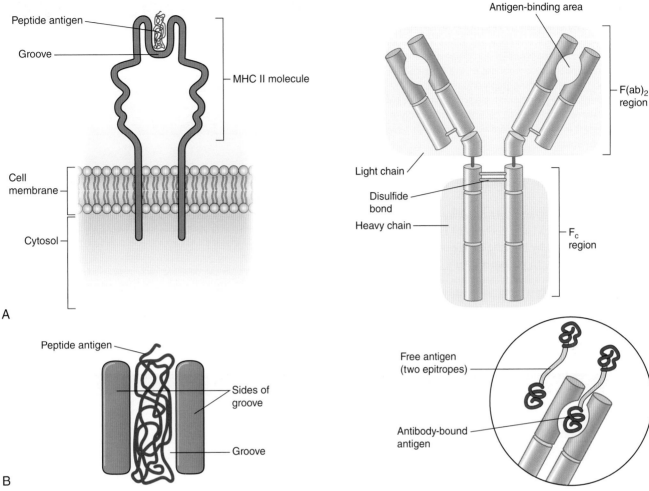

Fig. 8.10 A major histocompatibility complex (*MHC*) II molecule binding a peptide. A, Viewed from the side, the peptide is nestled in the groove of the MHC II molecule. B, Viewed from above, the walls of the MHC molecule and the fit between the peptide and the MHC II are appreciated from the perspective of cells, such as T cells.

Fig. 8.11 Antibodies. An antibody monomer, with identical antigen-binding areas formed by the ends of the heavy and light chains representing the Fab (antigen binding fragment) region and the other ends of the heavy chains, bound together by disulfide bonds, making up the Fc region (see Table 8.3).

- The stem of an antibody molecule is called the Fc (constant fragment) region.
  - Formed by the constant regions of the heavy chains.
  - Determine isotype of the antibody and thus effector function (IgM, IgD, etc.) (see Fast Fact Box 8.2).

Once secreted by B cells or plasma cells, different antibody isotypes are directed to different locations in the body.
- IgG and IgM circulate in the blood.
- IgE circulates in the blood as well, but some binds to the surface of mast cells and basophils, waiting to activate these cells when antigen is encountered.

TABLE 8.2   Differences Between Major Histocompatibility Complex I and Major Histocompatibility Complex II

	Major Histocompatibility Complex I	Major Histocompatibility Complex II
Genes encoding	HLA-A, HLA-B, HLA-C	HLA-DR, HLA-DP, HLA-DQ
Binding	TCR and CD8+	TCR and CD4+
Expression pattern	All nucleated cells	Only on antigen-presenting cells
Antigen type	Presents antigens from *inside* the cell (endogenous)	Presents antigens from *outside* the cell (exogenous)
Example target pathogens	Viruses	Bacteria, protein vaccines
T cell partner	Killer T cell (CD8+)	Helper T cell (CD4+)

HLA, Human leukocyte antigen; *TCR*, T-c II receptor.

Fast Fact Box 8.2

To clarify: two different antibodies of the same isotype (e.g., an immunoglobin [Ig]G_1 antibody that binds to an epitope of the bacterium *Streptococcus pneumoniae* and an IgG1 antibody that recognizes a component of the Epstein-Barr virus) differ in Fab (antigen binding fragment) regions but by definition have the same Fc portion. It is also possible for two antibodies of different isotypes to have the same antigen specificity; that is, they have different Fc portions but essentially identical Fab regions.

- IgA is secreted at the mucosal surfaces, such as the GI tract

In addition, IgG, IgE, and IgD circulate as monomers, IgA exists as a dimer, and IgM as a pentamer (Table 8.3).

Antibodies function by binding antigens to neutralize them and bind to pathogens to opsonize them, "tagging" them for destruction by innate immune systems, such as the complement cascade (see Genetics Box 8.1, Pharmacology Box 8.1, Development Box 8.1, and Oncology Box 8.1).

GENETICS BOX 8.1

Common variable immunodeficiency (CVID) is a syndrome of impaired antibody production by B cells. In some patients, this is caused by a mutation in TN-FRSF13B, a gene that encodes a B cell receptor called TACI. TACI is expressed on the B cell surface and binds the ligand BAFF (the product of TNFSF13B). Activation of TACI by BAFF leads to the promotion of B cell maturation, survival, and antibody production. At least 12 other genes have been found to be mutated in patients with CVID.

PHARMACOLOGY BOX 8.1

The two most important pharmacologic interventions for patients with common variable immunodeficiency (CVID) are antibiotics (sometimes used prophylactically) for bacterial infections, such as pneumonia and periodic immunoglobin (Ig)G infusions using purified antibodies from healthy blood donors. The IgG replacement infusions can be either intravenous or subcutaneous. Together, antibiotics and IgG replacement can greatly reduce the frequency and severity of infections.

TABLE 8.3 **Human Antibody Isotypes**

Isotype of Antibody	Subtypes (H Chain)	Plasma Concentration (mg/mL)	Serum Half-Life (days)	Secreted Form	Functions
IgA	IgA1,2 (α1 or α2)	3.5	6	Mainly dimer; also monomer, trimer	Mucosal immunity
IgD	None (δ)	Trace	3	Monomer	B cell antigen receptor
IgE	None (ϵ)	0.05	2	Monomer	Defense against helminthic parasites, immediate hypersensitivity
IgG	IgG1-4 (γ1, γ2, γ3, or γ4)	13.5	23	Monomer	Opsonization, complement activation, antibody-dependent cell-mediated cytotoxicity, neonatal immunity, feedback inhibition of B cells
IgM	None (μ)	1.5	5	Pentamer	Naive B cell antigen receptor (monomeric form), complement activation

Ig, Immunoglobulin. (From Abbas A. *Cellular and Molecular Immunology*, 9th Edition. Elsevier; 2018. Table 5.2.)

DEVELOPMENT BOX 8.1

Common variable immunodeficiency (CVID) can manifest in children and older adults, but more often does so in the late teens and twenties. Two major causes of morbidity are: (1) accumulated damage to respiratory tract tissues because of recurrent infections, leading to airway structural changes called bronchiectasis, further increasing the risk of infection, and (2) the development of autoimmune diseases, such as arthritis that impair patient mobility and quality of life. Some patients develop splenomegaly, autoimmune hemolytic anemia, or immune thrombocytopenia.

ONCOLOGY BOX 8.1

Patients with common variable immunodeficiency (CVID) have an increased risk of developing non-Hodgkin lymphoma and gastric cancer.

Antigen Receptors

The exquisite specificity of the adaptive immune response resides in the precise binding of antigen receptors on B cells and T cells to specific epitopes.
- Given B cell or T cell produces antigen receptors of single specificity (epitope).
  - Determine the narrow range of substances to which the cell can respond.
- Pro: Infinite possibilities because of random generation of receptors.
- Con: Necessary to trial B cells and T cells to produce the "right" antigens.
  - Many of which produce nonfunctional receptors or receptors directed against antigens the host may never encounter.

B Cell Receptors

The antigen-specific receptors on B cells are essentially antibodies bound to the B cell surface (Fig. 8.12A). A given B cell produces antibody of one specificity (idiotype), but may change the isotype of that antibody over time.

Early in development, the antigen specificity of a particular B cell is determined. Briefly:
- The immature B cell produces a membrane-bound IgM of a particular idiotype, acting as the initial B cell receptor.
- Activated by the presence of its specific epitope in the body:
  - Produces antibodies, secreted protein of its antigenic specificity.
    Thus the B cell receptor is the cell-surface version of antibody or, seen from the other perspective, antibody is the secreted/soluble version of the B cell receptor.
  - May switch to produce antibody of another isotype (i.e., IgM → IgG)
    Directed by cytokines, inflammatory molecules.
- Effective protection from myriad pathogens requires myriad B cells of different specificity.

T Cell Receptors

T cell receptors resemble B cell receptors in their ontogeny but differ from them in their structure and function (Fig. 8.12B).
- T cell receptors remain bound to the cell surface and are not secreted.

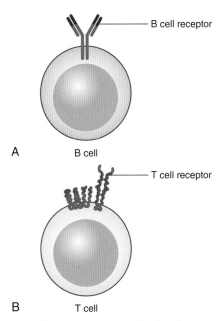

Fig. 8.12 B cell and T cell receptors. A, The B cell receptor is a membrane-bound version of an antibody. It has the same antigen specificity as the antibody the B cell secretes. B, The T cell receptor does not have a secreted counterpart.

- As with B cells, the receptors of a given T cell have the same antigenic specificity.
  - Undergo positive (ability to bind MHC) and negative (weed out under-, over-, and self-reactive cells) selection during development.
  - Need high affinity for nonself antigens to survive.
- As with B cells, effective protection from myriad pathogens requires myriad T cells of different specificity.

Cytokines, Chemokines, and Their Receptors

As in the nervous system, communication between and among cells is critical to the function of the immune system.
- Instead of electrochemical "language" of neurons, the language of the immune system is largely encoded by a large group of messenger molecules called cytokines.
- Cells secrete these molecular "words" in regulated ways and often in complex combinations simultaneously or in temporal sequence.
- However, just as spoken language requires a speaker and a listener, cytokines can have their effects only on cells equipped with appropriate receptors.

One particularly important subset of cytokines is a group of mediators that induce movement in target cells. Such chemotactic cytokines are called chemokines.
- Different chemokines draw leukocytes with the appropriate receptor to specific tissue sites.
- Other chemotactic molecules include bacterial products, complement components (such as C5a), and certain leukotrienes (such as LTB_4).

Adhesion Molecules

How do cells enter exit the circulation and reach peripheral tissues? The molecules involved in this critical and complex process include a group of cell surface proteins called adhesion molecules (Fig. 8.13):

- Margination and rolling
  - Mediated by selectins.
  - Leukocyte appears to "slow down" in bloodstream and roll along vessel wall.
- Tight-binding
  - Mediated by members of the immunoglobulin superfamily (ICAM-1/VCAM-1) and integrins.
  - Leukocyte adheres to vessel wall.
- Diapedesis
  - Mediated by members of the immunoglobulin superfamily (PECAM-1).
  - Leukocyte "squeezes" between endothelial cells and exits vessel (diapedesis).

Effector Molecules

Effector molecules are the armamentarium of molecules released by immune cells to defend the body, once attracted to the front line of battle.

- Vasoactive mediators promote vasodilation and vascular permeability.
  - Mediator Types
    Histamine, serotonin, complement, certain cytokines (interleukin-1 and tumor necrosis factor), prostaglandins, leukotrienes, thromboxane, bradykinin, and nitric oxide.
  - Cause smooth muscle relaxation and changes in epithelial cells that facilitate the passage of fluid, proteins, and cells from the circulation into tissues.
  - By increasing the diameter of the blood vessel and recruiting more capillaries, velocity of blood flow decreases and also expedites diapedesis.
  - Manifest physically as signs of inflammation.
  - If concentrations of vasoactive substances are high enough, these effects may extend from local to systemic (see Clinical Correlation Box 8.5).

> ### Clinical Correlation Box 8.5
>
> When infection and/or traumatic tissue damage is widespread, the immune response may produce high concentrations of vasoactive mediators. As potent vasodilators increase the radius of the vessel lumen, the resistance to laminar flow drops. In accordance with Ohm's law, decreased resistance → decreased blood pressure. Thus patients with severe bacterial blood infections may develop systemic inflammatory response syndrome (SIRS). Clinically, this is identified by four criteria:
> - Heart rate >90 beats per minute (compensatory tachycardia)
> - Temperature >38° C (100.4° F) or <36° C (96.8° F) (autonomic dysregulation)
> - Respiratory rate >20 breaths per minute or $PaCO_2$ <32 mm Hg (impaired gas exchange)
> - WBC >12,000/mm^3 or <4000/mm^3 or >10% bands (evidence of acute immune response or impaired immune system predisposing to infection)
>
> Patients must meet two out of four criteria to qualify for SIRS. If a source is known or suspected, this is termed sepsis. If there is evidence of organ dysfunction or hypoperfusion (i.e., rising lactic acid), this is termed severe sepsis. Finally, if the patient's blood pressure drops (hypotension) and cannot be restored despite proper fluid administration, the patient is in septic shock.
>
> Treatment relies on correcting the underlying problem (i.e., antibiotics) and maintaining intravenous fluids and/or "pressors" (drugs that constrict vessels) to maintain perfusion.
>
> Note: Patients may develop SIRS without infection, such as in anaphylaxis or severe pancreatitis.

$PaCO_2$, Arterial partial pressure of carbon dioxide; WBC, white blood cell.

Once activated, leukocytes are in the heat of battle:
- Release chemicals that damage pathogenic invaders, including:
  - Degradative enzymes that catabolize proteins (proteases), lipids, or nucleic acids
  - Oxygen free radicals
  - Proteins that puncture pathogen membranes
- These effector molecules may also be destructive to host cells. Neutrophils are especially important because of the "oxidative burst" phenomenon (Fig. 8.14):
- Nicotinamide adenine dinucleotide phosphate (NADPH) oxidase produces highly reactive oxygen species.

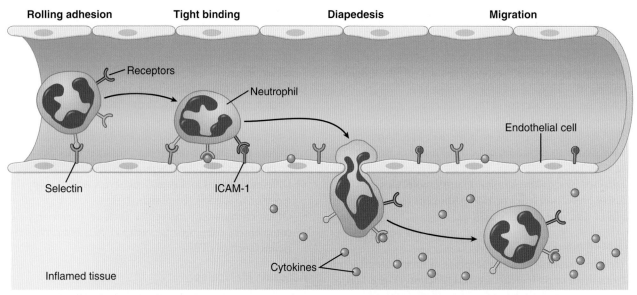

Fig. 8.13 Leukocytes exit from blood vessels into tissue via: (1) margination and rolling; (2) tight-binding; and (3) diapedesis. (From *Guyton AC, Hall JE. Guyton and Hall Textbook of Medical Physiology*, 13th Edition. Elsevier; 2015. Fig. 34.6.)

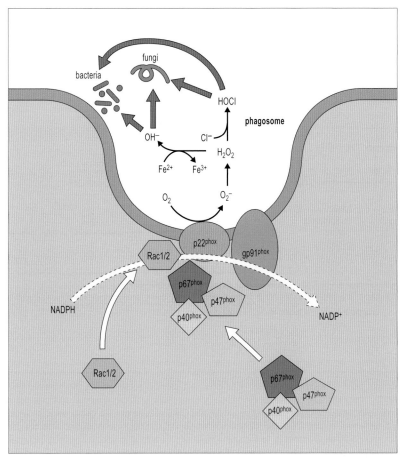

Fig. 8.14 Mechanism of oxidative burst. (From Male D. *Immunology*, 8th Edition. *Elsevier*; 2013. Fig. 16.w1.)

- Converts O_2 to O_2^- (superoxide) and H_2O_2 (hydrogen peroxide).
- Myeloperoxidase, then converts H_2O_2 to HOCl (the hypochlorite radical), which is particularly toxic to bacteria.

The Complement System

The complement system is a cascade of bloodborne innate immune system proteins analogous to the coagulation cascade (see Ch. 7).
- Most complement proteins (designated C1, C2, C3, etc.) are inactive plasma proenzymes under normal conditions.
- The complement proteins at the "top" of the cascade can be activated in three ways:
  - Classical pathway: bind antigen-bound antibodies (Fc regions)
  - Alternative pathway: bind microbe surfaces (PAMPs)
  - Lectin pathway: bind specific microbe protein (mannose)
- Upon activation, complement proteins enzymatically cleave other components and active them.
- Sequential activation of complement components results in two types of effector molecules.
  - Small fragments of some complement proteins (e.g., C4a, C3a, and C5a, in the order of their production) attract and activate immune system cells to the area of inflammation.
  - Larger "terminal" complement proteins (C5b to C9) combine to form a channel (or pore) called the membrane

attack complex, which inserts into the cell membrane of an invader, causing potentially lethal damage to the microbe by cell lysis (Fig. 8.15).

IMMUNE SYSTEM FUNCTION

To effectively defend the body against threats, the immune system must:
- Response to active threats.
- Produce and "train" cellular troops to detect pathogens
- Distinguish between self and nonself.
- Prevent and limit invasion by maintaining fixed barriers, by stationing cells at tissue outposts, and by sending cells to patrol the body.

Thus even in the complete absence of an active infection, the immune system is highly active.

Production of Immune Cells

Innate and adaptive immune system cells originate in bone marrow, derived from hematopoietic stem cells.
- Granulocytes are released in circulation as mature cells.
- Mast cells, monocytes, and dendritic precursor cells must enter tissues to complete maturation.
- Adaptive immune cells must undergo a more complex development in either the bone marrow (B cells) or thymus (T cells).

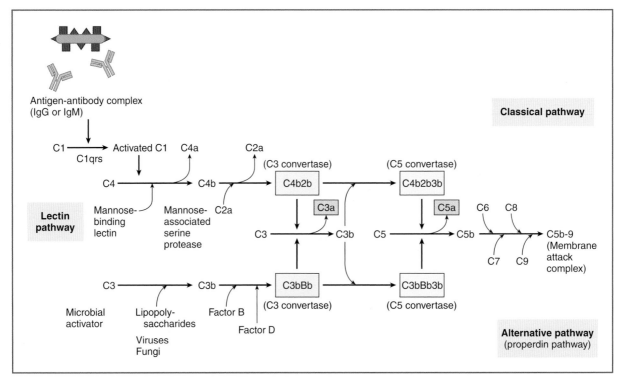

Fig. 8.15 Complement activation pathways. Complement can be activated via the classical, alternative, or lectin pathway by antibodies, microbes, or mannose-binding lectins, respectively. In all three pathways, cleavage of complement proteins (C3 is cleaved into C3a and C3b) results in C3b being deposited on the foreign microbe (C3b cleaves C5 into C5a and C5b) and triggering multiple subsequent effector functions. For example, C3a and C5a are involved in leukocyte activation; C3b is involved in microbe phagocytosis; C5b, C6, C7, C8, and C9 are involved in formation of the membrane attack complex (*MAC*) which inserts into the membrane of the invading microbe and causes its lysis. (From Actor JK. *Elsevier's Integrated Review: Immunology and Microbiology*, 2nd Edition. Elsevier; 2012. Figs. 6.6 and 6.7.)

Functional Classes of Immune Cells

Functional classes of immune cells include (Fig. 8.16):
- Innate cells that are expert at engulfing pathogens (phagocytosis)
- APCs that specialize in presenting antigen to T cells
- T cells that assist B cells and macrophages in fighting pathogens
- T cells that are adept at destroying host cells coopted by invaders

Phagocytes

Phagocytes are cells that take up material by phagocytosis (literally, "cell eating")
- Cell types
  - Dendritic cells, macrophages, and neutrophils
- Function
  - All possess cell-surface receptors that can bind to extracellular material
  - Binding activates a complex program of cytoskeletal rearrangement, culminating in the engulfment of the material into the cell in a membrane-enclosed vesicle called an endosome.
  - Endosomes fuse with lysosomes, membrane-enclosed packets of digestive enzymes, leading to intracellular incarcerated.
- Overall role
  - Neutrophils: combat pathogens and clean up the debris.

- Dendritic cells and macrophages: use antigen processing for presentation.

Antigen-Presenting Cells

Although many cells can process and present antigens to T cells under certain circumstances, there are three types of APCs specialized to do so (and therefore called "professional" APCs):
1. Dendritic cells
2. Macrophages
3. B cells
   Each one can take up materials in the immediate environment, digest them, and load fragments, such as peptides into the groove of MHC II molecules.
- Form close cell-to-cell connections called immunologic synapses with T cells.
- Only those T cells whose receptor can bind to the peptide in the MHC II groove will be activated and stimulated to multiply.
  - This culminates in a population of daughter T cells, each with the same antigen specificity.
- To find the right match, an APC searches through myriad T cells of different specificities, often in an anatomic location, such as a lymph node.
  Although the innate APCs (dendritic cells and macrophages) take up a broad range of materials in only a semispecific way, the

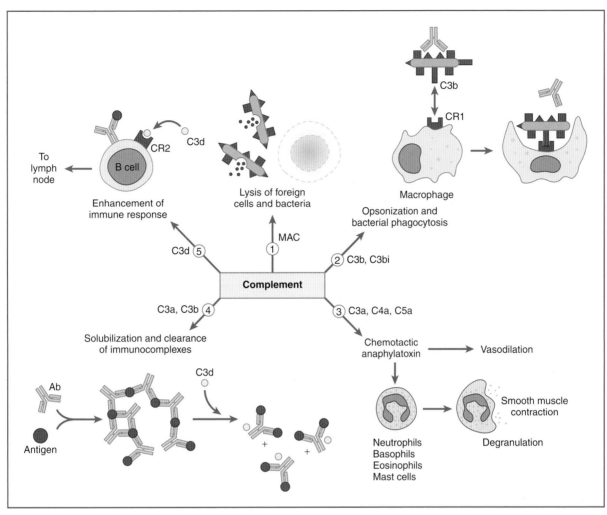

Fig. 8.15 cont'd

B cell is highly restricted in what it can take up and process because its antigen uptake receptor is the specific B cell receptor.

Helper T Cells

Helper T cells expedite the function of B cells and macrophages/dendritic cells.

- Triggered by matching of specific T-cell receptor (TCR) and the peptide in the groove of an MHC II molecule on the surface of an APC.
- After activation, the T cell releases cytokines to direct the activity of APCs:
  - B cell: Produces more antibodies against foreign antigen.
  - Macrophage/dendritic cells: "Fortified" to intensify chemical barrage against invaders in its endosomes (see Fig. 8.16A).

Cytotoxic T Cells

The other subset of T cells consists of those that kill infected host cells and are therefore termed cytotoxic T cells.

- Triggered by matching of specific TCR and the peptide in the groove of an MHC I molecule (see Fig. 8.16B).
  - Signals presence of intracytoplasmic pathogen (i.e., virus).
- Because MHC I molecules are expressed by all nucleated body cells, any nucleated host cell may act like an APC to cytotoxic T cells.

- Once stimulated, the cytotoxic T cell executes a highly regulated program to release cytotoxic mediators:
  - Perforin that puncture the infected cell's membrane
  - Granzymes and granulosins that enter the infected cell through these membrane perforations and initiate a sequence of cell "suicide" called apoptosis.

The virally infected cell thus gives up its life for the collective good of impeding the virus.

The Production of Adaptive Immune Cell Antigen Receptors

As already mentioned, a critical feature of the adaptive immune system is the specificity of T cell and B cell receptors for a given antigen.

- However, the genome is not nearly large enough to encode the myriad of possible B and T cell receptors necessary for defense.
- In addition, the adaptive immune response requires adaptation to combat rapidly evolving pathogens.

The solution to this problem is a set of genes encoding different portions of a B cell receptor or T cell receptor.

- A given cell randomly chooses a particular gene for each of the segments.
- It then strings them together into a cohesive and complete instruction code.

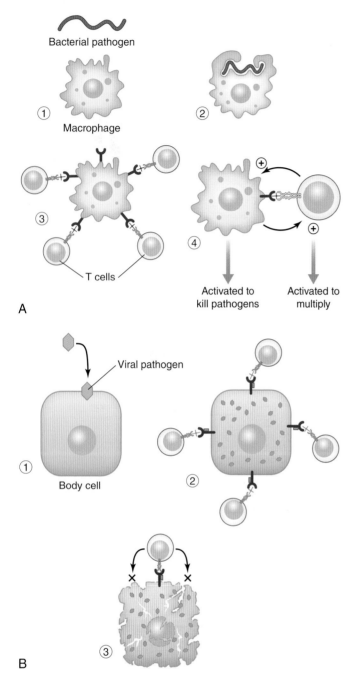

A

B

Fig. 8.16 Antigen-presenting cells, phagocytosis, helper T cells, and cytotoxic T cells. A, An extracellular pathogen, such as a bacterium is bound (1) and phagocytosed (2) by a macrophage. The bacterium, is digested, and peptides are loaded into the clefts of MHC II molecules and expressed on the cell surface. Helper T cells gather around the macrophage, seeking a good fit between their T cell receptors and the pathogen peptide (3). Most cells do not match (x), but eventually one or more does (!). Once the match is made (4), the macrophage stimulates the helper T cell, which divides, stimulating itself and the macrophage. B, An intracytoplasmic pathogen such as a virus (1) infects a nucleated body cell. The infected cell loads some major histocompatibility complex (MHC) I molecules with peptides derived from the virus and expresses them on its surface. Cytotoxic T cells gather around the infected cell, seeking a good fit between their T cell receptors and the pathogen peptide (2). Most cells do not match (x), but eventually one or more does (!). Once the match is made (3), the cytotoxic T cell releases mediators that induce apoptosis (programmed cell death or cell "suicide") in the infected cell.

For example, take the B cell receptor:
- There are four segments to the heavy chain of a B cell receptor (V, D, J, and C segments).
  - The genome encodes for not one but for *65* V, *27* D, *6* J, and *9* C genes.
  - Each one must be combined with one D gene, one J gene, and one C gene to form a functional heavy chain gene.
  - The combinatorial possibilities are enormous.
- A similar gene structure and therefore potential for diversity exists for the light chain of the B cell receptor and both chains of the T cell receptor.
- Unlike other body cells, adaptive immune cells actually cut out of their copy of the genome "instruction manual" the unselected genes, leaving only the selected genes "stitched" or "pasted" together in a neat format (Fig. 8.17).

This system of genetic rearrangement introduces two new problems:
1. A given cell may fail to produce readable genetic instructions. Such cells generally undergo apoptosis.
2. A given cell may produce a genetic instruction that encodes a receptor that will bind to a self-epitope.

Overcoming these problems is the function of adaptive immune cell education.

The Education of Adaptive Immune Cells

Once T cell precursors have rearranged their receptor genes, they are "educated" in the thymus, where they are "tested" for the ability of their T cell receptor to bind to the host's MHC molecules.
- Positive selection
  - If a T cell creates receptor completely unable to recognize the host MHC, that T cell is useless no matter what peptide (self or nonself) it carries.
  - Such cells are deleted or inactivated.
- Negative selection
  - T cells whose receptors bind too strongly to the host MHC and cause activation even when the peptide in the MHC groove is a benign self epitope will needlessly activate the immune system and cause unwanted damage.
  - These, too, are deleted or inactivated.

The "Goldilocks" cell is the ideal: T cells selected to survive and circulate, looking for their antigens, are those that recognize the host's MHC molecules but will bind tightly only if there is a foreign peptide in the groove (see Fast Fact Box 8.3).

Fast Fact Box 8.3

The part of the adaptive response involving bloodborne molecules (primarily antibodies) is called the humoral immune response (think: bodily "humors" in old medical literature). The part of the adaptive response involving antigen-specific T cells is called the cellular response.

Immunologic Memory

Another critical facet of the adaptive immune system is its ability to retain information from an encounter with a given pathogen and recall that information to guide responses to subsequent encounters with that same pathogen.

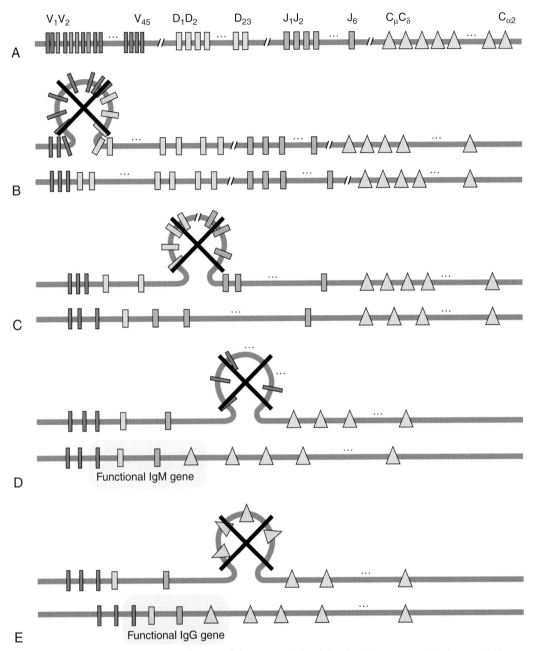

Fig. 8.17 Genetic events in the production of the heavy chain of the B cell receptor and isotype switching. The various segments of the B cell receptor heavy chain that contributes to the F(ab')2 region are called *V, D,* and *J.* The heavy chain C genes encode the different Fc regions of the antibodies that define isotypes (e.g., IgM, IgG, IgA). The human genome encodes 65 V genes, 27 D genes, and 6 J genes, and different B cells use different V, D, and J segments, stitching one of each of them together and deleting intervening deoxyribonucleic acid (DNA) sequences to create a functional gene that encodes the F(ab') region of the antibody heavy chain. There are also V and J gene segments for the light chain, which further contributes to the enormous repertoire of possible antibodies. A, The intact genome with all the possible V, D, and J genes, as well as all nine C genes. B, In a highly regulated process, the DNA bends, breaks, and reseals, randomly bringing one V and one D gene together. C, The process repeats to join the previously juxtaposed V and D genes with a randomly selected J gene. D, Once this process is completed, the antibody specificity of the B cell is established and fixed, and the B cell produces membrane-bound IgM as its receptor by deleting unselected J genes and juxtaposing the selected VDJ genes with the gene encoding the constant region of IgM (CM). E, After this B cell is stimulated, it can bend the DNA again and delete one or more constant region C genes to bring the VDJ gene into apposition with a different C gene; in this example, CG, which leads to the production of a new isotype (here, IgG). Because the VDJ gene is un-changed, the new IgG has the same antigenic specificity as the IgM. This gene rearrangement process is irreversible; deleted DNA cannot be pasted back in, so the alterations can only go forward, not backward. There is similar diversity in the B cell/immunoglobulin light chains and in the two chains of the T cell receptor.

Immunologic memory is affected when, in the course of an adaptive response and the successful eradication of the invader, certain long-lived antigen-specific T and B cells called memory cells are produced.

- Spend the subsequent years patrolling the body, looking for evidence that their old nemesis (the same pathogenic invader) has reappeared.
- If they detect such a reinfection, they quickly marshal adaptive immune forces to stop the bacteria before disease occurs.

The disease-free route to immunity is immunization: protection from infection by means of controlled exposure to either killed of disabled (attenuated) pathogen.

- Example: defective viruses for hepatitis B, mumps, rubella, or smallpox
- Allows adaptive immune system to form antibodies and train memory B and T cells specific for the pathogens.
- If the vaccinated host later encounters the pathogen, the previously formed antibodies and memory cells prevent disease by quickly apprehending and neutralizing the invader.

IMMUNE SYSTEM PATHOPHYSIOLOGY

There are three basic types of immune system dysfunction:
1. Underactivity
2. Overactivity (including autoimmunity)
3. Allergy (targeting harmless nonself antigen)

Immunodeficiency

Immunodeficiency is a broad term indicating insufficient function of one or more components of the immune system.

- Several inherited and acquired causes
- Share general consequence of increased susceptibility to infection
- Type and severity vary depending on mechanism and immunologic subsystem involved

Inherited immunodeficiencies (Fig. 8.18) often result from dysfunction at the level of the genes.

- Affect the production or proper function of any innate or adaptive cell or protein.
- Include deficiencies in:
  - Production or enzymatic activity of complement proteins and in cytokines
  - Cell-surface receptors
  - Signal transduction machinery
- Loss of functional T cells and B cells is called severe combined immunodeficiency (SCID) and can be fatal without bone marrow transplantation or other interventions that restore adaptive immunity.

Equally complex and dangerous are acquired immunodeficiencies, often from environmental exposures.

- Causes include
  - Insufficient nutrition

- Exposure to radiation or chemotherapeutic drugs
- Severe infection
- May include deficiencies along all of the same pathways.

One of the best-known acquired immunodeficiency is acquired immunodeficiency syndrome (AIDS), which results from infection by the human immunodeficiency virus (HIV).

- Target a number of immune cells, especially helper T cells (CD4+).
- Exploits the fact that T cells are essential for response to rapidly reproducing and evolving pathogen.

Autoimmunity

As mentioned earlier, genetic rearrangement during B cell and T cell receptor production can result in receptors that recognize host proteins.

- Under normal conditions, these self-reactive cells undergo apoptosis or are silenced (anergy).
- When protective measures failure, autoimmunity results.

Autoimmunity is an immune response by the host against the host, or inflammation in the absence of infection.

- Autoreactive cytotoxic T cells may attack and kill healthy host cells.
- Helper T cells may promote inflammation where none is needed.
- B cells may produce autoantibodies that bind to self structures.

Examples include rheumatoid arthritis and systemic lupus erythematosus, in which inflammation in the joints, skin, and other locations occurs. Therapies for such diseases currently rely on medications that suppress the immune system. Although these treatments diminish inflammation, they carry the obvious danger of immunosuppression.

Allergy

The exact pathogenesis of allergy is not completely understood. In the simplest terms, allergy is a case of mistaken identity. The immune system somehow mistakes a common, benign component in the environment, such as cat dander, for something dangerous that has to be eradicated.

Allergy is closely related to atopy, a predisposition to produce IgE antibodies.

- These antibodies bind to mast cell and basophil receptors via the Fc region of the molecule, leaving their Fab regions "waving in the wind," waiting to bind their antigen.
- When the antigen reenters the body, it binds to the IgE on the surface of these cells.
- This stimulates them to release chemical mediators, such as histamine and leukotrienes.

Allergic symptoms include itching, sneezing, and even symptoms of asthma, such as wheezing and shortness of breath.

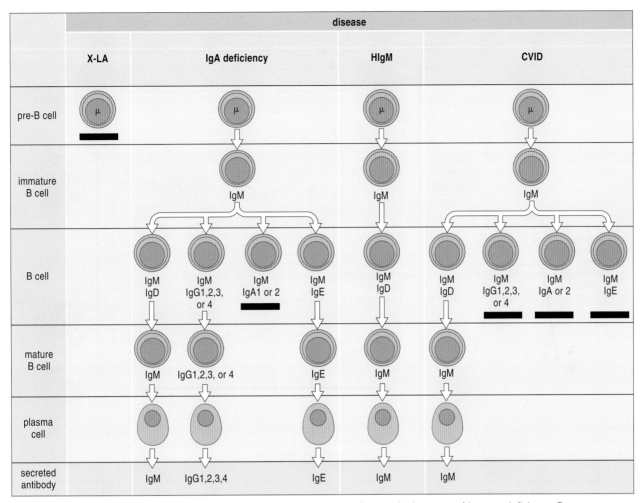

Fig. 8.18 Congenital blockage of B and T lymphocyte maturation results in states of immunodeficiency. Patients with severe combined immunodeficiency are usually affected by severe bacterial, viral, and fungal infections because of loss of functional T and B cells. The other congenital immunodeficiency states also result in a greatly increased susceptibility to infection. (From Male D. *Immunology*, 8th Edition. Elsevier; 2013. Figs. 16.2 and 16.6.)

SUMMARY

- The lymphatic system resorbs the excess fluid filtering across capillaries, screens it for pathogenic invaders, and returns it to the systemic circulation.
- The Starling equation quantifies the flux of fluid across the capillary wall by multiplying the CFC by the difference of the net hydrostatic pressure and the net oncotic pressure.
- Dysfunction of the lymphatic system may result in the accumulation of fluid in peripheral tissues, known as edema. Edema generally results from one or more of four mechanisms: (1) increased capillary hydrostatic pressure; (2) decreased capillary oncotic pressure; (3) increased capillary permeability; and (4) lymphatic vessel obstruction.
- The immune system protects the body from threats, such as infection by pathogenic microbes (viruses, bacterial, fungi, and parasites).

- The innate immune system acts rapidly but relatively nonspecifically to protect the host by using PRRs that bind to the PAMPs of microbes.
- The adaptive immune system of B cells and T cells is a delayed but highly antigen-specific response system that has plasticity and memory. An antigen is any substance that elicits an immune response. A hapten is a nonself molecule too small to be immunogenic by itself, but which, when combined with a self-protein, can be an antigen. An epitope is a region of an antigen specifically recognized by B cells and/or T cells.
- APCs present peptide antigens in the groove of MHC II molecules to helper T cells. All nucleated cells can present peptide antigens in the grooves of MHC I molecules to cytotoxic T cells.

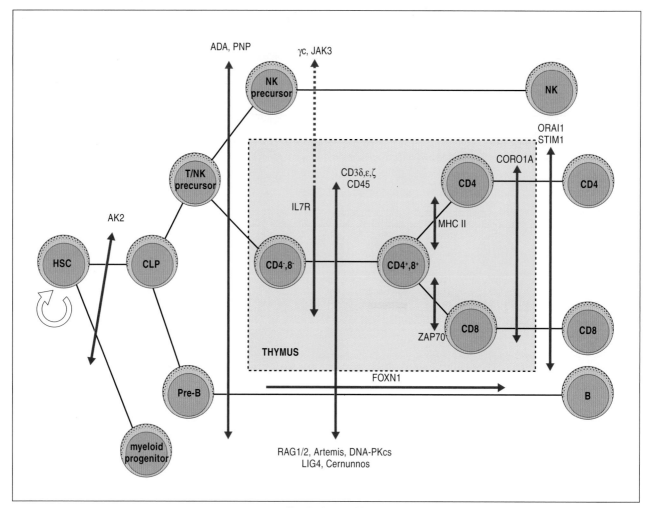

Fig. 8.18 cont'd

- Antibodies are soluble versions of the B cell antigen receptor. The Fab region of the antibody binds to the antigen, while the Fc region determines the isotype (IgA, IgD, IgE, IgG, or IgM) of and the cellular response to the antibody.
- B cell and T cell antigen receptors are produced by a complex process of gene shuffling and deoxyribonucleic acid editing.
- Vaccination can impart immunity by intentionally exposing the host to an attenuated pathogen unable to cause disease but able to stimulate the immune system and create immunologic memory.
- Insufficient immune system function results in immunodeficiency, which may be inherited or acquired (such as AIDS). Immune responses mistakenly directed against self antigens result in autoimmunity and manifest as inflammatory diseases, such as rheumatoid arthritis. Immune responses mistakenly directed against benign nonself antigens result in allergy.

■ REVIEW QUESTIONS

Directions: Each of the numbered items or incomplete statements in this section is followed by answers or by completions of the statement. Select the one lettered answer or completion that is best in each case.

1. A 68-year-old woman has a number of lymph nodes surgically removed from her right axilla because of breast cancer. Which of the following is a likely cause for her subsequent right arm swelling?
   A. Decreased lymph removal

   B. Decreased lymph production
   C. Increased lymph protein content
   D. Decreased lymph cell counts
   E. Increased susceptibility to infection

2. A 36-year-old man is feeling well and has no evidence of illness. Which of the following cells would you expect to find in his lymph?
   A. Neutrophils
   B. Macrophages

C. Eosinophils
D. T cells
E. Liver cells

3. A 44-year-old man is infected with a virus. Which of the following molecules is the most likely to present antigenic epitopes from the virus on the surface of an infected cell?
    A. A B cell receptor
    B. An MHC I molecule
    C. An integrin molecule
    D. A T cell receptor
    E. A cytokine molecule

4. Which of the following is not a function of antibodies?
    A. Opsonization of invaders

B. Inhibiting the entry of pathogens into tissues or cells
C. Binding toxins
D. Presenting antigen to T cells
E. Activating the complement cascade

5. Which of the following is not an effector function of complement activation?
    A. Formation of MAC complex
    B. Macrophage activation
    C. Leukocyte recruitment
    D. Phagocytosis of microbe
    E. Heavy chain isotype switching

ANSWERS TO REVIEW QUESTIONS

1. **The answer is A.** The removal of a number of lymph nodes impairs the drainage of lymph from the affected limb, allowing the accumulation of edema fluid in the interstitial space. None of the other answers, except an increased susceptibility to infection, would result in fluid accumulation in the area. Although areas swollen because of lymphatic dysfunction may indeed be more susceptible to infection, the cause-and-effect relationship in this case is less likely that immunodeficiency from the loss of a few lymph nodes leads to swelling than the reverse.

2. **The answer is D.** Lymphocytes, T and B cells, are the ones most commonly encountered in the lymphatics of healthy individuals. As these cells circulate from blood into tissues and lymph nodes, they enter the lymph and return to the central circulation. Although neutrophils, macrophages, and eosinophils are immune cells, they are not lymphocytes and would not be expected to be found in large numbers in the lymph of a healthy person. Liver cells (hepatocytes) do not normally leave the liver to circulate in the lymphatic vessels.

3. **The answer is B.** When intracellular, intracytoplasmic pathogens, such as viruses infect cells, the infected cells load

MHC I molecules with viral peptides and present them to cytotoxic T cells. B cell and T cell receptors "look" for antigen, and T cell receptors can detect antigen only when it is in the cleft of an MHC molecule. Integrins and cytokines do not bind antigenic epitopes for presentation to T cells. If an APC had phagocytosed some extracellular virus and digested it, peptide epitopes might have been loaded into MHC II molecules for presentation to helper T cells, but this was not a choice in this question.

4. **The answer is D.** Antibodies opsonize, inhibit movement, neutralize toxins, and precipitate complement. Although the B cell receptor is essentially a membrane-bound antibody on the surface of B cells, its function there is to detect extracellular antigen and facilitate its uptake by the B cell. The MHC I and II molecules are important for antigen presentation to T cells.

5. **The answer is E.** Complement results in macrophage and leukocyte recruitment and activation, as well as in phagocytosis and membrane attack complex formation (MAC) via C5b, C6, C7, C8, and C9. Isotype switching is not a direct result of complement activation.

Blood and Lymph

Note: This case will be presented in a slightly different format, to facilitate our discussion of the sequence of the "normal" immune response.

A.P. is a 69-year-old man with hypertension (well controlled, on medications), hypercholesterolemia, and osteoarthritis of the right knee who presents with a cough, sore throat, muscle aches, and low-grade fever (100° F). On history, he remarks that he visited his grandchildren a few days before symptom onset, and that the youngest child had been suffering from a likely respiratory virus.

INTRACELLULAR PATHOGEN RESPONSE: VIRUS

Recall that many pathogens may be evaded through the first-line "barrier defenses" in the respiratory mucosa, such as intact epithelium, mucus production, and the beating of cilia. However, viral particles in respiratory droplets have succeeded in infecting cells in A.P.'s respiratory tract. Some infected cells die, releasing products normally sequestered intracellularly and alerting the cells of the innate immune system. Among these, macrophages are prominent, as they clean up the debris from dead cells.

The macrophages are activated, releasing inflammatory mediators, such as interleukin-1 (IL-1). However, the virus continues to spread. Infected cells load some viral peptides into major histocompatibility complex (MHC) I molecules and display them on their surface, essentially sending out "red flags." In addition, the infected cells may secrete mediators called interferons that induce a relative state of viral resistance in the neighboring cells most at risk for infection by the spreading virus (thus interfering with the viral life cycle). Eventually, cytotoxic T cells with receptors that recognize the viral antigens in the MHC I molecules displayed by infected cells arrive at the scene and kill off these compromised body cells. The infection is thus brought under control as the virus is eliminated.

Interferons and related signaling molecules, such as IL-1, have systemic effects causing fever, loss of appetite, weakness, and muscle aches. Additionally, local inflammation leads to sore throat and cough because of irritation of respiratory tract receptors.

RECOVERY... OR IS IT?

Despite initially feeling better, A.P. soon returns to his physician with a complaint of recurrent symptoms, now including sputum production, high-grade fever (>101.5° F), malaise, and shortness of breath.

EXTRACELLULAR PATHOGEN RESPONSE: BACTERIA

A.P.'s recovery from the viral illness involved the demise not only of the virus but also of infected cells of the respiratory epithelium. This results in a state of impaired first-line defense. This weakness in his living mucosal armor is exploited by a respiratory bacterial pathogen, *Streptococcus pneumoniae*. Unlike the intracellular viral pathogen, *S. pneumoniae* is extracellular.

Macrophages, neutrophils, and dendritic cells stationed in or patrolling the area bind onto the bacteria by means of pattern recognition receptors that recognize pathogen-associated molecular patterns in the bacterial cell wall. These phagocytic cells engulf some of the bacteria and destroy them.

In addition, complement proteins, recognizing the foreign surface of the bacteria, initiate the complement cascade, which performs at least three important functions: (1) the chemotactic fragments C5a, C3a, and C4a (in order of decreasing potency) attract and activate more innate inflammatory cells; (2) complement proteins, such as C3b deposited on the pathogen surface act like knobs onto which phagocytes can grab more efficiently, a process called opsonization; and (3) the formation of the "membrane attack complex" opens holes in the bacterial cell wall, damaging the pathogens (see Fig. 8.15).

Neutrophils release degradative enzymes and oxygen radicals that kill bacteria. Many of the activated neutrophils die along with the bacteria. The resultant mass of liquefied dead bacteria and cells is macroscopically recognized as *pus*, which, because of the metal content of some of the enzymes called metalloproteinases, is yellow to green.

This is evident when A.P. starts to cough up purulent phlegm (sputum) and redevelops fever, malaise, and muscle and joint aches. However, the patient also starts feeling short of breath as the pus and the increasing number of bacteria and inflammatory cells pouring into the lung alveoli impair gas exchange. Thus the patient is now suffering from pneumonia. If A.P.'s blood was tested, there might be an increase in the number of white blood cells, as they are recruited to fight the infection. A microscopic examination of a sputum sample would reveal bacteria, neutrophils, and debris.

COMMUNICATION AMONG IMMUNE CELLS: INITIATION OF THE ADAPTIVE RESPONSE

The innate immune response was mobilized rapidly and effectively, but it could not keep up with the high rate of bacterial reproduction. However, it has successfully delayed bacterial proliferation enough for the adaptive immune response to be brought into play. Antigen-presenting cells (APCs), such as dendritic cells and macrophages, busy phagocytizing and degrading *S. pneumoniae*, load bacterial peptides into MHC II molecules and migrate to lymph nodes. Here, they encounter helper T cells and start the process of trying to find a match between the peptide epitopes of *S. pneumoniae* and helper T cell receptors.

At the same time, B cells are likewise trying to bind bacteria and/or the products of their degradation by means of their receptors. When B cells that can bind *S. pneumoniae* do so, they too process the antigenic proteins and present them to helper T cells. When appropriate matches are made, the helper T cells release mediators, such as IL-2. They then proliferate and provide assistance to cells such as macrophages and B cells. In the latter case, helper T cells stimulate the B cells whose receptors bind *S. pneumoniae*, inducing them to

mature into plasma cells that secrete large amounts of antibody against the pathogen.

RECOVERY

A.P. recovers from pneumonia caused by *S. pneumoniae*, either with or without the assistance of antibiotics (drugs that assist the immune system by poisoning bacteria). A year later he inhales respiratory droplets containing the same strain of bacteria, but this time the response will likely be unnoticed (i.e., the infectious microbes will be destroyed subclinically). In fact, both cellular and humoral immune responses will be invoked again, but much more rapidly and intensely than during the first infection, thus enabling the patient to defeat the bacteria without reexperiencing severe illness. This indicates the success of immunological memory producing effective immunization against this particular strain of *S. pneumoniae*.

Cardiovascular Physiology

9

The Vasculature

INTRODUCTION

The cardiovascular system serves as the principal transportation and distribution network of the body, allowing:

- Delivery of several essential substances (e.g., glucose and oxygen) to the tissues
- Removal of by-products of metabolism (e.g., carbon dioxide, lactate, and heat)

In its simplest formulation, the system is composed of three parts:

1. Pump (the heart)
2. Series of distributing and collecting tubes (the arterial and venous systems)
3. Transport medium (the blood)

The physiology of the vasculature may be understood as blood flow through the vessels, on blood pressure in various parts of the vascular network, and on vascular resistance to flow.

- The relation between these three variables is expressed in an analogy to Ohm's law.

Further discussion of the regulation of systemic blood pressure appears in one of the renal physiology chapters (see Ch. 19) because the renal and cardiovascular systems govern the blood pressure in concert. Chapters 10 and 11 discuss the mechanical action and electrophysiology of the heart. Chapter 12 discusses cardiovascular adaptations to exercise.

SYSTEM STRUCTURE

The heart is comprised of two hollow muscular pumps in series, dividing the circulation into pulmonary and systemic components (Fig. 9.1).

- The right ventricle propels deoxygenated blood from the systemic veins → the pulmonary arteries and on to the lungs.
- Exchange of oxygen and carbon dioxide in the pulmonary capillaries, and the pulmonary veins return the oxygenated blood to the heart via the left atrium.
- The left ventricle propels oxygenated blood received from the pulmonary veins to the remaining tissues of the body through the aorta and its branches.
- Deoxygenated blood eventually returns to the heart in the vena cava via the right atrium.

The circuit from left ventricle to right atrium is the systemic circulation. The circuit from the right ventricle to the left atrium is the pulmonary circulation.

In systemic circulation, the organ systems are connected in parallel, allowing arterial blood flow to shunt between vascular beds based on moment-to-moment need (see Fig. 9.1).

Regurgitant flow (backward flow) in the heart is prevented by a series of unidirectional cardiac valves that guard the entrance and exit of each cardiac ventricle.

- The valves will be discussed in further detail in Chapter 10.
- The slamming shut of the cardiac valves create the "lub-dub" sound heard through the stethoscope over the precordium (the area of the chest over the heart).

Types of Vessels

In the cardiovascular circuit, different vessels are adapted to transport blood at different pressures. The differences between the two main types, arteries and veins, are summarized in Table 9.1, as well as Figs. 7.1 and 9.2.

- Arteries
  - ↑ elastic tissue and smooth muscle.

    Arterial pressure is created not only by the heart but also by smooth muscle in the walls of the arteries, which squeezes the arterial blood.

    This squeezes blood into the high-capacity veins, leaving only around 20% of total blood volume in systemic arteries at any given time.

    The high proportion of elastin in the walls of large arteries gives them elastic recoil, the tendency to shrink back down once stretched.
  - Under high pressure.
  - Relatively low compliance.
- Arterioles
  - Smallest branches of arteries.
  - Highest total resistance in the vascular system.
  - Arterioles are critical for the control of blood pressure and blood flow.

    By constricting some or all of the body's arterioles, the vasculature can direct the flow of blood to the organs that most need it, or it can elevate blood pressure throughout the cardiovascular circuit.

    Regulated by the autonomic nervous system.
- Capillaries
  - Highest total cross-sectional and surface area in the vascular system
  - Thin-walled
  - Sites of nutrient and gas exchange

    Single layer of endothelial cells → facilitates transport
- Veins
  - The vein walls have low muscle content and are highly distensible.
  - Veins and venules have high compliance when pressure is low, whereas arterioles are of low compliance at low pressures.

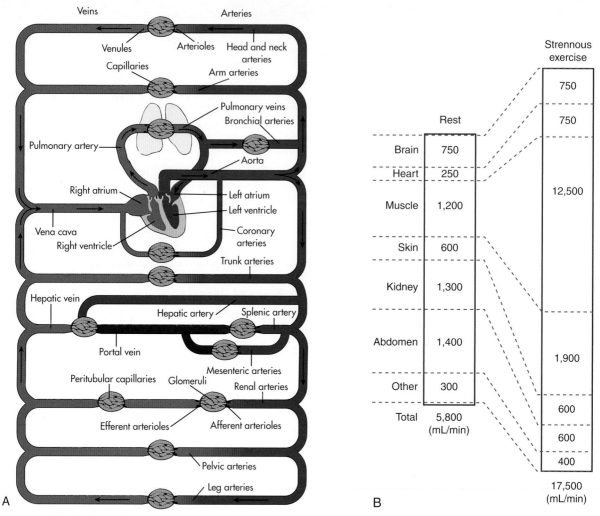

Fig. 9.1 A. The circulatory subsystems of the various organ systems are connected in parallel. B. The distribution of blood to the body's organs and tissues at rest and during strenuous exercise. (A, From Levy M, Koeppen B, Stanton B. *Berne & Levy Principles of Physiology.* 4th Edition. St. Louis, MO: Elsevier; 2005. Fig. 15.1.)

TABLE 9.1 Differences Between Arteries and Veins

	Arteries	Veins
Pressure of transported blood	High-pressure	Low-pressure
Smooth muscle content	+++	+
Blood volume (%)	20	80
Elasticity	+++	−
Compliance	+	+++ (low-pressure) + (high-pressure)

Fast Fact Box 9.1

If the normal blood volume is rapidly expanded (e.g., by blood transfusion) or contracted (e.g., through hemorrhage), most of the volume change is accommodated in the low-pressure portion of the circulation rather than in the arterial high-pressure circulation, whose volume remains relatively constant.

Fast Fact Box 9.2

Compliance is the distensibility of the vessel, or change in volume in the vessel per change in pressure ($C = \Delta V/\Delta P$). Compliance is high when a large volume (ΔV) can be accommodated with small pressure changes (ΔP), and low when small volume changes result in large pressure differences or, stated differently, a large pressure change is required to make a small change in the volume.

This property of veins allows for the accommodation of large volumes of blood in the circulation before development of high venous pressure.
- The high blood volume in the veins is available to return to the heart and lungs when needed, as in the case of exercise or other demand on cardiac output (see Fast Fact Box 9.1 and Fast Fact Box 9.2).

The venous pressure is also a driving force for movement of blood from vein back to heart, a flow known as venous return.
- Normal gravitational forces oppose venous return and need

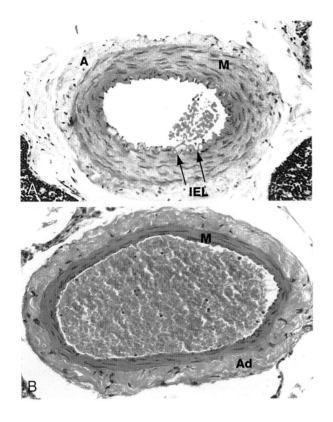

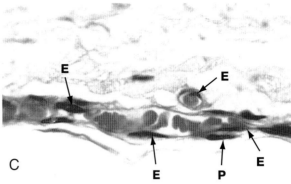

Fig. 9.2 A comparison of the morphology of A) arteries, B) veins, and C) capillaries, demonstrating the higher content of smooth muscle and elastin in the arteries. Artery (axial cross-section): *IEL*, internal elastic lamina; *M*, tunica media, *A*, tunica adventitia. Vein (axial cross-section): *M*, tunica media; *Ad*, tunica adventitia. Capillary (longitudinal cross-section): *E*, endothelial cell; *P*, pericyte. (From Young B, O'Dowd G, Woodford P. *Wheater's Functional Histology: A Text and Colour Atlas*, 6th Edition 2013. Elsevier; Figs. 8.11, 8.14, and 8.22.)

to be overcome by developed venous pressures, particularly in the lower extremities.

- Recalling the relationship between compliance and pressure (C = $\Delta V/\Delta P$), venous pressure may be increased by:
  - Reduced compliance
  - Compression of peripheral veins by muscular contractions of the legs
  - Increased tone of vessels (i.e., by sympathetic nervous system)
  - Increased volume

From the cardiac perspective, venous return is an important component of preload, a topic covered in Chapter 10.

Summary of Arterial Circulation (Fig. 9.3)

- The contraction of the cardiac ventricles, an event called systole, drives blood into the pulmonary arteries and into the aorta. The ventricles then relax, an event called diastole.
- Systole expands the highly elastic aorta, and elastic recoil occurs during diastole.
- This drives the blood out of the aorta and into the smaller arterial branches.
- Because both systole and diastole drive the blood forward, blood never stops moving.
- Flow is very pulsatile in the aorta and becomes less pulsatile as blood moves down the arterial system.
  - Pulsatility is still measured well in small arteries.
- From the aorta, the blood travels through a branching network of vessels of progressively smaller caliber.
- Just before the level of the capillaries are the highly muscular arterioles.
  - The flow of blood into a given capillary bed may be controlled by muscular contraction in structures known as precapillary sphincters.

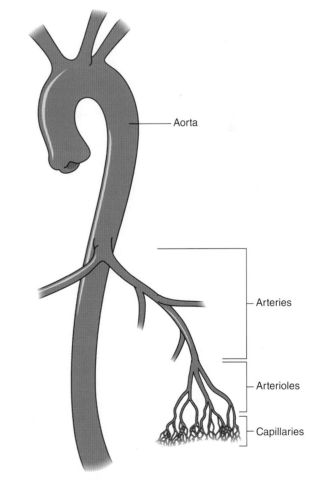

Fig. 9.3 The branches of the vascular tree. The arterioles are noteworthy for their high smooth muscle content, which makes them the main sites of vasoconstriction and vasodilation in the body.

- When constricted, these sphincters result in a diversion through thoroughfare channels directly into the venous sinusoids, bypassing the capillary bed.
- Arterial circulation terminates in the capillaries.
  - Site of nutrient and gas exchange.

SYSTEM FUNCTION

To understand blood pressure, blood flow, and vessel resistance, it is useful to review some basic concepts in physics.

Pressure

Recall from basic gas laws that the pressure, P, of a gas in a container is proportional to the number of moles (n) in the container per volume (V) of the container:

$$P \sim n/V$$

(because $P = nRT/V$, where R is the gas constant and T is temperature in Kelvin).

- This implies that ↓ volume (V) → molecules forced together → more frequent collisions → ↑ force per area → pressure (P). This holds true for fluids in a tube (i.e., vessel).
- Systole: contraction of cardiac muscles → shrinking vessel (ventricle) size → ↑ P
- Diastole: blood emptied into systemic circulation → ↑ V available in aorta → ↓ P

To shrink the ventricle or the aorta, work (W) must be done on the vessel walls (force, F, must be applied over a distance, d):

$$W = F \times d$$

Thus work or energy is necessary to drive the contraction of the vessels.

- In the heart, the energy of muscular contraction is derived from adenosine triphosphate (ATP).
- In the aorta, the kinetic energy of the blood entering from the heart pushes the aortic walls out. That energy is stored as potential energy in the aortic elastin fibers. This is released during vessel contraction during diastole.

Because the work is being done in three dimensions, the work equation can be rewritten for three dimensions:

$$W = P(\Delta V)$$

Note: Because pressure is force per area ($P = F/A$) and volume is equal to distance times area ($\Delta = d \times A$), the equation $W = P(\Delta V)$ can be reduced to $W = (F/A) \times (d \times A)$, which is the same as the more familiar $W = F \times d$.

Pressure Difference

Two types of pressure need be considered in the cardiovascular system (Fig. 9.4):

- Transmural pressure refers to a pressure gradient felt across the vascular wall, at one particular point in the vascular tree.
  - This creates the driving pressure forward through circulation.
  - It requires an opportunity for outflow (i.e., pressure gradient) to move fluid.
- Perfusion pressure or driving pressure, which is the gradient of pressures between two places within the circulation.

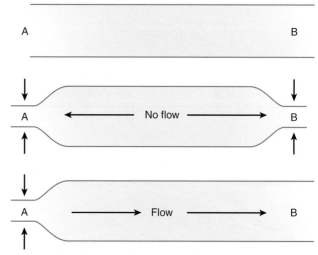

Fig. 9.4 Pressure difference. Flow from point A to point B cannot occur in a vessel without a difference in the transmural pressure at point A versus point B.

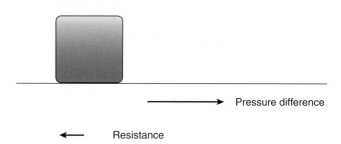

Fig. 9.5 The forces at work on blood flow, depicted as a vector diagram.

The Ohm's law analogy ($I=V/R$, where the current I is analogous to blood flow, voltage V is analogous to the pressure gradient) describes the flow of blood (Q) in liters per minute from point A to point B:

$$Q = \Delta P/R; \text{ or } \Delta P = QR$$

where ΔP is the difference in pressure between point A and point B and R is the resistance (mm Hg/mL/min) to flow along the way from A to B.

From this relationship, we see that blood flow is inversely proportional to blood vessel resistance.

Resistance

- Resistance is related to the amount of friction in the vessel between points A and B.
- The pressure difference is the net force pushing the fluid toward point B, whereas resistance is related to the net force opposing this movement (Fig. 9.5).
- Resistance, like pressure, is a function of the size of the vessel or container.
- Resistance is inversely proportional to vessel radius, as described in Poiseuille's law: $R = 8\eta l/\pi r^4$, where r is the vessel radius, l is the length of the tube, and η is the viscosity of the fluid.
  - The length of the frictional surface and viscosity also contribute to resistance, but they are less important than vessel radius.

- If the blood vessel radius decreases by a factor of 2, then blood flow will decrease by a factor of 16!

It also matters whether resistance is in parallel or series.

Arteries branch from the aorta to supply each organ with blood in a parallel arrangement. The total parallel resistance can be expressed by the following equation:

$$1/R_{Total} = 1/R_1 + 1/R_2 + \cdots + 1/R_n$$

where R_1, R_2, and R_n are the resistances of various arteries in the systemic circulation.

This relationship implies:

- Each artery arranged in parallel receives a fractional amount of the total blood flow
- Total resistance is less than the resistance of any individual artery
- Total resistance decreases when an artery is added in parallel

Blood vessels can also be arranged in series, as is the case within an organ. The total series resistance is the sum of the individual resistances:

$$R_{Total} = R_{artery} + R_{arterioles} + R_{capillaries}$$

This relationship implies:

- Each blood vessel in a series arrangement receives the same total blood flow so that the blood flow through the largest artery supplying the circuit is the same as the total blood flow through all of the subsequent capillaries.
- Total resistance increases when an artery is added in series.

If part of the vascular tree is compressed, an odd phenomenon occurs:

- ↑ P upstream and at site of compression
- ↓ P downstream

This is because of ↑ resistance at the site of obstruction. Consider the diagram in Fig. 9.6.

- Higher R → fewer molecules of fluid to Point B per unit time → ↓ transmural P at point B
- Point A will lose fewer molecules of fluid per unit time → ↑ transmural P at PointA (see Clinical Correlation Box 9.1.)

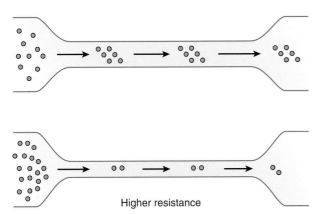

Fig. 9.6 The genesis of a pressure difference as the result of focal increased resistance. The dots represent molecules of fluid in the vessel. Higher resistance, and consequently decreased blood flow, leads to a buildup of fluid molecules upstream of the resistance and a dearth of molecules downstream of the resistance. Fewer molecules means less transmural pressure; more molecules means more transmural pressure.

Clinical Correlation Box 9.1

Neural and humoral factors can increase muscle tone in arterioles to reduce flow and thus pressure to certain downstream areas or to boost upstream pressure. This is the key to cardiovascular regulation of the blood pressure.

The flow of blood within the circulatory system is not only determined by favorable pressure gradients providing the energy for such flow.

- Total energy = potential energy (pressure gradients) + kinetic energy (moving blood)
- As blood moves from larger → smaller vessel, ↑ velocity →↑ kinetic energy, ↓ transmural P
  - Kinetic energy thus drives forward flow (see Clinical Correlation Box 9.2).

Clinical Correlation Box 9.2

Total energy is what counts; if kinetic energy is elevated, the flow could move in a low- to high-pressure direction. This is how blood can continue past a vascular stenosis (narrowed by disease) and how the left ventricle can still eject blood into the aorta in late systole, when aortic pressure >ventricular pressure.

Systemic Pressure, Resistance, and Flow

Let us now consider these concepts relative to the entire cardiovascular circuit.

Mean Arterial Pressure and Systemic Vascular Resistance

What is the pressure difference (ΔP) across the entire systemic arterial system? To answer this question, we must know:

- The aortic pressure at the beginning of the systemic circulation.
  - Weighted average of systolic and diastolic pressure
- The right atrial pressure (RAP) at the end of the systemic circulation.
  - Usually 5 mm Hg or less

The mean arterial pressure (MAP) is calculated from the systolic and diastolic pressure and describes the time-weighted average arterial pressure.

- At low resting heart rates, diastole accounts for approximately two-thirds of the cardiac cycle.
  - MAP = 2/3 [diastolic P] + 1/3 [systolic P]
- At high rates, MAP is more closely approximated by the arithmetic mean of systolic and diastolic pressure.
- Normal MAP ranges from 70 to 110 mm Hg.
  - At MAP below 60 mm Hg, vital organs, such as the brain and kidneys, may be inadequately perfused.

For a MAP of 100 mm Hg and RAP around 5 mm Hg, the driving force for perfusion, ΔP is around 100 mm Hg (see Clinical Correlation Box 9.3).

Clinical Correlation Box 9.3

To estimate the aortic pressures, we use the brachial artery as a substitute for measurement using a blood pressure cuff (sphygmomanometer) and stethoscope. This gives a transmural pressure reading, referred to as the systemic blood pressure (SBP).

The resistance for the entire vascular circuit is called the systemic vascular resistance (SVR), also called the total peripheral resistance (TPR).

$$SVR = (MAP - RAP) / Cardiac\ Output\ (CO) \sim R = \Delta P/Q,$$

- Units are usually converted from mm Hg/L/min to dynes/s/cm^{-5} by multiplying by 80
- Arterioles contribute most resistance to SVR.
  - Downstream pressure drop across arterioles primarily related to:
  Number of parallel vessels
    Diameters (i.e., cross-sectional area)
  - Blood downstream of arterioles has a pressure around 25 mm Hg (see Fast Fact Box 9.3).

Fast Fact Box 9.3

Because the capillaries are the narrowest vessels in the body, one might wonder why they do not create a higher resistance than the arterioles (although they do contribute the next largest component to total resistance). They do not because so many capillaries arise from each arteriole that the total cross-sectional area of a capillary bed is very large, and the resistance is consequently less than at the arteriolar level. The blood downstream of the capillaries (i.e., in the veins) has a pressure of around 10 mm Hg and contributes <10% of the total resistance.

Blood Flow and Cardiac Output

The blood flow through the circulation can be considered as laminar or turbulent.

- Laminar flow is conceptualized streaming or straight-line flow through an ideal tube with the characteristics described in Poiseuille's law.
- Turbulent flow emerges when flow encounters interruption, causing separation of flow velocities.
  - Causes include: narrowed vessel radius (i.e., stenosis), ↑ velocity, ↓ viscosity (i.e., anemia)

The Reynolds number is an index of the factors that determine whether flow will be laminar or turbulent.

- Dimensionless ratio of the inertial forces divided by the viscous forces governing flow.
- Proportional to
  - Velocity of flow (v)
  - Tube diameter (D)
  - Viscosity (μ)
  - Density of liquid (ρ)
- A high Reynolds number implies turbulent flow.
- It is described by:

$$Re = \rho Dv/\mu$$

In laminar flow, the velocity of the stream is greatest at the center of the vessel and slowest at the outermost layer closest to the wall (Fig. 9.7). In turbulent flow, with branching of vessels and eddying currents, the flow is more disorganized and the velocity more variable.

Although blood flow may vary in different portions of the vascular circuit, net blood flow remains relatively constant

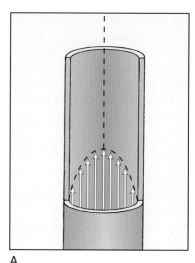

A

Fig. 9.7 Laminar flow with greatest velocity at the center of the vessel and slowest velocity near the vessel wall. (From Levy M, Koeppen B, Stanton B. *Berne & Levy Principles of Physiology*, 4th Edition. St. Louis, MO: Elsevier; 2005. Fig. 20.2A.)

given a steady state of physical and metabolic activity and environmental conditions.

- This is also known as the cardiac output (CO), the volume of blood pumped out of the heart in 1 min.
- Roughly 5 L/min in an adult.
- To standardize CO for individuals of varying size, the cardiac index (CI) is often used and is CO per body surface area in meter^2. The CO may also be expressed as the product of heart rate (HR) and the stroke volume (SV):
- CO = HR × SV
- HR is measured in beats per minute
- SV is the volume of blood ejected into the aorta from the left ventricle with each systolic contraction, is measured in milliliters per beat.
  - SV = end-diastolic volume of the left ventricle (LVEDV) – end-systolic volume of the left ventricle (LVESV)
  - Ejection fraction = EF = SV / LVEDV * 100%
    Normally greater than 60%, may rise up to 90% during exercise.

Capillary Hemodynamics

The capillaries serve as the interface between the circulation and the larger interstitial space.

Please refer to Chapter 8 for a more detailed discussion of the derivation of Starling's law of the capillaries. To review:

$$Q = K [(\Delta P) - \sigma(\Delta \Pi)].$$

- Forces favoring fluid filtration
  - Capillary hydrostatic pressure (P_c)
  - Interstitial oncotic pressure (Π_i)
- Forces opposing filtration
  - Interstitial hydrostatic pressure (P_i)
  - Capillary oncotic pressure (Π_c)
  - K, the filtration coefficient, varies by the surface area, length, thickness, and permeability of the capillary wall
- σ, the reflection coefficient, varies from tissue to tissue depending on permeability to albumin

If L indicates the lymphatic drainage, then the Starling relationship for net flow from the capillary becomes:

$$Q = K_{uf} [(\Delta P) - \sigma (\Delta \Pi)] - L.$$

The Starling forces of the capillary will be addressed in the discussion of heart failure in Chapter 10; gas exchange in the lungs in Chapter 14; renal glomerular filtration in Chapter 17; renal tubular reabsorption in Chapter 18; gastrointestinal fluid absorption in Chapter 24; and cirrhosis of the liver in Chapter 26.

The Regulation of Blood Pressure

Thus by employing Ohm's law, we can find an equation descriptive of the entire vascular tree:

$$MAP = (CO) * (SVR)$$

Of these three variables, blood pressure is monitored and regulated by the brain. Chapter 19 describes the homeostatic system for maintaining a constant blood pressure.
- Baroreceptors are the sensors by which the brain detects changes in blood pressure (Fig. 9.8).
  - Low-pressure baroreceptors exist in the pulmonary vessels and in the cardiac atria.
  - High-pressure baroreceptors exist in the aortic arch, carotid sinus, and in the renal arterioles (Fig. 9.9).
    Baroreceptors in the carotid sinus → CNIX (glossopharyngeal nerve) → medulla
    Baroreceptors in aortic arch → CNX (vagus nerve) → medulla
    Medullary response (Fig. 9.10)
      Efferent signals to systemic arterioles and heart in sympathetic and parasympathetic nerves
      Stimulates adrenal secretion of epinephrine
- The overall response is called the baroreceptor reflex.
  The efferent signals influence the MAP through the modulation of CO and SVR.
- Low BP detected → heart stimulated to pump faster & harder (↑ CO, ↑ SV) → ↑ CO
- ↑ CO → ↑ blood forced from venous to arterial system → ↑ SVR

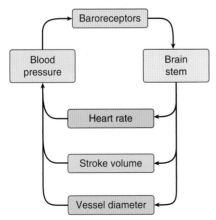

Fig. 9.8 Blood pressure feedback loop. (From Barrett KE, Barman SM, Brooks HL, Yuan JX-J. *Ganongs Review of Medical Physiology*, 23rd Edition. New York: McGraw-Hill; 2010.)

- Low blood pressure may also cause direct arteriolar vasoconstriction in certain vascular beds → ↑ SVR

This ensures adequate blood pressure for perfusion of vascular beds in the brain and heart. However, it necessarily requires shutting down of nonessential vascular beds, that is, skin, intestine (see Clinical Correlation Box 9.4).

Clinical Correlation Box 9.4

The baroreceptor reflex is occasionally used clinically to treat or diagnose tachycardia (rapid heart rate). Massaging the carotid arteries stimulates the baroreceptors there and sends a "high blood pressure" signal to the medulla. Increased parasympathetic output is sent to the heart—intended to decrease heart rate, which would decrease cardiac output and in turn decrease the apparent "high blood pressure." However, in a person who actually has a normal mean arterial pressure, this can lead to a dangerously rapid sinus tachycardia.

As Chapter 19 describes, both the renal and cardiovascular systems play a role in regulating blood pressure.
- The most important renal response to low blood pressure is an increase in salt and water reabsorption in the renal tubules.
- ↑ extracellular fluid volume → ↑ pressure similar to ↑ CO.
  The cardiovascular mechanisms of control are divided into central and local mechanisms.
- The central control mechanism was introduced earlier and will be discussed further.
- Local factors act in paracrine fashion (i.e., near their site of secretion) to influence arteriolar constriction.
- The central and local control systems act in concert to determine vasomotor tone.
  Local control mechanisms dominate in tissues that must preserve perfusion at all costs (i.e., brain, heart) whereas central control mechanisms dominate in "nonessential" tissues (i.e., skin and splanchnic).

Local Control

The various local control mechanisms over vasoconstriction are sometimes called autoregulatory mechanisms because they act independently of the brain. Autoregulatory mechanisms have two primary functions:
1. Maintaining constant blood flow to an organ with a steady metabolic rate in the face of changing blood pressure.
2. Adjusting blood flow to an organ according to local changes in its metabolic activity.
   To maintain constant blood flow, there are multiple safeguards:
- Myogenic response
  - Vascular smooth muscle contracts in response to stretch and relaxes with a reduction in tension.
  - Example: When a person who has been lying down suddenly stands up, blood pools in the lower extremities.
    Vascular stretching leads to arteriolar (precapillary) vasoconstriction, which prevents excess blood flow to the extremities.
    This avoids accumulation of fluid and pressure that would otherwise lead to edema.
  - Presumed mechanism: stretch → activation of Ca^{2+} channels → muscular contraction.

A INNERVATION OF CAROTID SINUS AND BODY

B INNERVATION OF AORTIC ARCH AND BODIES

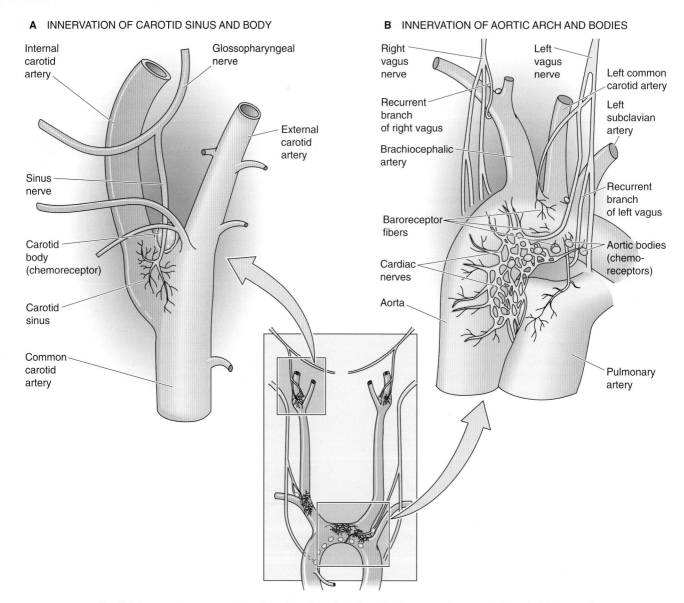

Fig. 9.9 Baroreceptor areas and carotid and aortic bodies. The sits of baroreceptor areas in the carotid sinus and aortic arch. (From Boron W, Boulpaep E. *Medical Physiology*, 3rd Edition. Philadelphia, PA: Elsevier; 2016. Fig. 23.2.)

- The brain and kidney both have relatively constant flow over a given systolic blood pressure range (see Ch. 19)
  Brain: 60 to 160 mm Hg
  Glomerular: 80 to 200 mm Hg
- Chemical response
  - Endothelium produces numerous factors to regulate vascular tone:
    Vasodilators: nitric oxide, prostraglandins, others
    Vasoconstrictors: Endothelin

⚡ **TRAUMA BOX 9.1**

Although the triggers for hereditary angioedema (HAE) attacks are not always clear, traumatic injury is a common one. Patients with an angioedema of the gut wall experience pain that can be misinterpreted as an acute abdomen, as might be seen in acute appendicitis. If such patients are mistakenly taken to surgery, the trauma of the surgical procedure may further exacerbate the angioedema.

🧬 **GENETICS BOX 9.1**

Hereditary angioedema (HAE) is characterized by recurrent bouts of vascular leakage and consequent tissue swelling. Attacks are caused by the accumulation of the vasoactive mediator bradykinin that is produced by the catabolism of high-molecular-weight kininogen by the enzyme kallikrein. Normally, kallikrein's activity is limited by the complement factor C1 Inhibitor (C1INH), but HAE patients have a mutation in the C1INH gene that either abolishes its production or impairs its function.

💊 **PHARMACOLOGY BOX 9.1**

Patients with hereditary angioedema (HAE) have painful swelling typically affecting the face, upper aerodigestive tract, gut, hands, and feet. Laryngeal angioedema can cause fatal airway obstruction. HAE attacks can be treated with infusions of purified C1INH, the use of the kallikrein inhibitor ecallantaide, or antagonism of the bradykinin 2 receptor on endothelial cells by the drug icatibant.

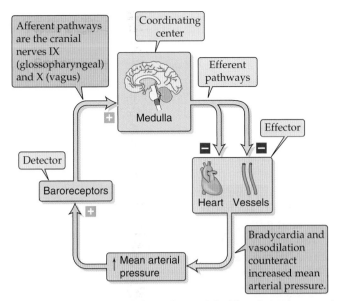

Fig. 9.10 Efferent signaling from the medulla. The glossopharyngeal (*IX*) and vagus (*X*) cranial nerves carry the afferent baroreceptor signaling from nucleus of tractus solitaries of the medulla. (Modified from Boron W, Boulpaep E. *Medical Physiology*, 3rd Edition. Philadelphia, PA: Elsevier; 2016. Fig. 23.1.)

- Increases in the velocity of blood flow through a vessel → reflex secretion of vasodilators

  Presumed mechanism: High flow → increased shear stress → stimulates endothelium to try to reduce BP via vasodilator release (see Trauma Box 9.1, Pharmacology Box 9.1 and Genetics Box 9.1)

The final autoregulatory component is a metabolic mechanism, which adjusts blood flow to a given tissue based on its oxygen needs.

- "Blood goes where blood is needed"
- If ↑ blood flow to one organ system → must ↓ blood flow to another
- ↓ oxygen → accumulation of metabolites serving as vasodilators
  - Including CO_2, H^+ ions, adenosine diphosphate (ADP), adenosine monophosphate (AMP), adenosine, lactic acid, K^+ ions, and inorganic phosphates.
- Decreased $pO2$ can also produce vasodilation that is independent of metabolite accumulation.
  - This occurs through the direct action of hypoxia on smooth muscle mitochondrial energy production.
  - Exceptions: pulmonary vascular bed

    Lungs direct blood flow to regions of greatest O_2 → vasoconstriction of hypoxic areas.

Active or functional hyperemia describes the relationship between tissue metabolism and blood flow.

- Reactive hyperemia → metabolites accumulate → vasodilation
- Example: transient deep red color of a limb following tourniquet release, representing dilated vascular bed

Adrenergic Receptors in Central Control

Let us resume our exploration of the central control of the blood pressure, exploring the role of the nervous system.

- Modulated primarily by the sympathetic nervous system. The parasympathetic nervous system's only serves to decrease the heart rate in response to high blood pressure.

- The main transmitter released from postganglionic sympathetic nerve terminals is norepinephrine (NE).
- NE exerts different effects on vascular smooth muscle depending on the type of receptor expressed in the tissue.
  - Adrenergic receptors are of two main classes with multiple subtypes:
    α
    β
  - Except the heart and brain, arterioles carry α_1 receptors and β_2 receptors.
    Stimulation of α_1 receptors leads to vasoconstriction
    Stimulation of β_2 receptors leads to vasodilatation.
  - Net response depends on number and affinity of each receptor in a given vascular bed.

Table 9.2 summarizes the actions of the sympathetic (adrenergic) receptors on the vasculature. The α_2 adrenoreceptors are also found in blood vessels, particularly in smaller-resistance vessels (see Clinical Correlation Box 9.5).

Clinical Correlation Box 9.5

Oddly, not all catecholamines are made equal. Although both epinephrine and norepinephrine are also produced in the adrenal medulla, catecholamines of adrenal origin have less effect on blood pressure than neural origin. This may be because neurotransmitters in circulation reach vascular smooth muscle in relatively lower concentrations.

Low blood pressure drives sympathetic stimulation and thus vasoconstriction of all vascular beds (except heart and brain), as well as faster, harder cardiac contraction.

- ↑ SVR, CO → ↑ systemic BP → ↑ perfusion of heart and brain

The nervous control of the circulation described in the previous paragraphs is primarily a short-term regulatory mechanism, allowing rapid response to short-term variations in blood pressure.

Humoral Control

More long-term regulation of blood pressure is afforded by the release of vasoactive agents into the bloodstream. These act dually to:

- Increase vascular resistance
- Promote restoration of blood volume, which is ultimately key to resuscitating the hypotensive patient

TABLE 9.2 Adrenergic Receptors

Receptor	Primary Location	Effect of Stimulation
α_1	Blood vessels	Vasoconstriction
α_2	Central nervous system (CNS)	Vasodilation
β_1	Heart	Increase in heart rate (chronotropy) /cardiac contractility (inotropy)
β_2	Blood vessels	Vasodilation

- Included among these agents that act from within the vessel lumen rather than at a nerve terminus are angiotensin, aldosterone, and vasopressin (antidiuretic hormone, or ADH).

The renin-angiotensin-aldosterone axis (RAA) is a key cardiovascular regulatory system that is important not only to normal compensatory responses but also to the pathophysiology of disease states, such as congestive heart failure and hypertension. (The RAA axis will be discussed again in Chapter 19

- Renin is a proteolytic enzyme released from the juxtaglomerular apparatus (JGA) of the kidney into the afferent arteriole of the glomerulus.
  - Responds to apparent low-pressure or low-volume states.
  - May also be stimulated by sympathetic drive.
- Circulating renin cleaves the propeptide angiotensinogen (produced in the liver) to a 10-amino acid peptide, angiotensin I, which has little biological activity.
- Angiotensin I is then rapidly converted to an eight-amino acid peptide angiotensin II (AII) by angiotensin-converting enzyme (ACE), located in the vascular endothelium of the pulmonary vessels.
- AII is a direct, fast acting, potent vasoconstrictor that works primarily by activating the angiotensin II, type 1 (ATI) receptor.

Thus in states of low blood pressure or arterial volume, the signal sensed at the level of the JGA leads to a cascade of events that generate a compensatory AII-mediated increase in peripheral vascular resistance. This serves to complement the baroreceptor reflexes noted earlier to help maintain blood pressure (see Clinical Correlation Box 9.6).

Clinical Correlation Box 9.6

Both angiotensin-converting enzyme and angiotensin II, type 1 receptors are important antihypertensive, pharmacologic targets.

The RAA axis is most active in patients who are salt- or volume-depleted because of:
- Low-salt diet
- Sweating
- Other fluid loss (e.g., hemorrhage).

The vasoconstrictor effect of AII is limited to sensitive vascular beds, such as the renal, cutaneous, and splanchnic circulations. The coronary, cerebral, and pulmonary circulations, as well as the entire venous system, are protected from its effects.

As will be discussed in long-term regulation of blood pressure (see Ch. 19), AII is also an important regulator of blood volume.
- Potent stimulator of the hypothalamic thirst center, promoting oral intake of fluids.
- Acts directly on the renal proximal tubule to enhance the reabsorption of sodium.
- Acts on the adrenal cortex to produce the mineralocorticoid aldosterone, which stimulates reabsorption of sodium from the collecting duct of the nephron.

ADH, or vasopressin, is another key mediator that acts to preserve both volume and osmolality.
- Nine-amino acid peptide hormone
- Synthesized in the hypothalamus and released from the posterior pituitary
- Triggers include
  - Decreased blood volume (as sensed at the level of arterial baroreceptors)
  - Increased plasma osmolality (as sensed by sensitive osmoreceptors in the hypothalamus).
  - Other factors, including physiologic stress (from pain or extreme temperature), may also promote ADH release, whereas alcohol and a variety of medications may inhibit it.
- Two primary functions:
  - ADH binds vasopressin type 2 (V_2) receptor $\rightarrow$ promotes water reabsorption from the distal collecting duct of the nephron. Primary.
  - ADH binds vasopressin type 1 (V_1) receptor $\rightarrow$ promotes vasoconstriction and thereby increase total peripheral resistance. The pressor effect occurs only at higher serum concentrations of vasopressin.

The role of ADH in the regulation of extracellular fluid volume is discussed in detail in Chapters 19 and 29.

Atrial natriuretic peptide (ANP), like ADH, is an important regulator of fluid volume.
- Release triggered by the cardiac stretch receptors.
- Acts to:
  - Antagonize the ADH effect
  - Reduce plasma volume
  - Lower blood pressure
- Mechanism of systemic vasodilation (and subsequent decrease in total peripheral resistance) mediated by cyclic guanosine monophosphate (GMP).
- In volume-expanded states, increases in ANP $\rightarrow$ loss of salt and water in the urine $\rightarrow$ decreased extracellular volume (see Clinical Correlation Box 9.7).

Clinical Correlation Box 9.7

Levels of the related B-type polypeptide (BNP) are used clinically to help characterize states of volume expansion and heart failure. Both conditions are associated with elevated levels because of increased transmural pressures causing atrial and ventricular stretch that results in release of the natriuretic peptide.

PATHOPHYSIOLOGY

There is a broad variety of disease that may affect the vasculature. All have the potential for dire consequences for other organ systems given the role of the vasculature in delivery of oxygen and removal of waste products.

Broadly, we may classify diseases of the vasculature into three main categories:
- Flow obstruction
- Structural integrity
- Autoregulation

Flow Obstruction

Any disease that leads to blockage of a vessel can lead to ischemia or even infarction of vessels downstream because of lack of oxygen delivery.

One of the most common illnesses in the United States, atherosclerosis affects large- and medium-sized muscular arteries, such as the aorta, coronary arteries, and carotid arteries.

- Oxidized low-density lipoprotein (LDL, "bad cholesterol") deposits in vascular wall, causing endothelial cell dysfunction.
- Macrophages adhere to damaged endothelium and release cytokines.
- Macrophages form lipid-filled foam cells within the smooth muscle, causing fatty streaks.
- Smooth muscle hyperplasia and migration to the muscle intima.
- Eventual formation of fibrous plaque, which calcifies and ulcerates.
- Platelets bind and eventually cause vessel thrombosis (clot).

Clots can lead to several pathologies because of obstruction and subsequent limitation in blood flow, including myocardial infarction (MI), stroke, renal artery ischemia or thrombosis, and peripheral vascular disease. Risks for clot may broadly be classified by Virchow's triad:

- Endothelial dysfunction (injury to the vessel, as in atherosclerosis)
- Stasis (blood flow slows or ceases, as in a passenger's legs during a long plane ride)
- Hypercoagulability (dysfunction of the clotting cascade)

Limitation of vessel flow without complete obstruction can still lead to symptoms because of transient ischemia in times of demand. One common example is angina (chest pain) related to myocardial ischemia during exercise, which can be relieved by rest.

Structural Integrity

Several processes can compromise the vessel wall:

- Inflammation
  - May be infectious or autoimmune
  - Diseases causing inflammation of the vessel wall are called *vasculitides*
- Connective tissue disorders
  - May be inherited or autoimmune
  - Many affect collagen, elastin, or other extracellular matrix (ECM) components
- Wall stress

An aneurysm results from weakening of the vessel wall, causing a focal dilation in the vessel wall.

- May occur in any blood vessel.
- Naturally grow in size to minimize pressure
  - Law of Laplace states that T (tension) $\sim$ P (pressure) $\times$ R (radius)
- As size increases, the risk of rupture increases.
  - Rupture occurs when mechanical stress on wall $>$ strength of wall tension

A dissection results when a tear rips down the lumen of the vessel, forming a "false lumen" that rapidly fills with blood.

- Blood influx into the false lumen exerts enough pressure to compromise flow through the vasa vasorum, the vessels feeding the vessel.
- May lead to vessel wall ischemia and necrosis.
- If this occurs in a large vessel, such as the aorta, it may eventually result in a rupture and rapid death from hemorrhage.

Autoregulation

Consider the body's response to acute hemorrhage (bleeding) as a review of blood pressure regulation:

- The initial loss of blood leads to an immediate decrease in the mass of blood contained in the vessels and hence a drop in blood pressure.
- This is sensed at the level of the baroreceptors in the carotid sinus and aortic arch.
  - Decreased stretch → reduced firing to medulla
  - Efferent response → compensatory increase in sympathetic outflow and a decrease in vagal (parasympathetic) tone to the periphery
- Results in massive peripheral vasoconstriction and increased heart rate.
  - Poor blood flow to the periphery results in poor oxygen delivery and the release of vasodilatory metabolites
  - The reflex nervous adjustments compete with the local metabolic and autoregulatory adjustments

However, the ultimate goal is to preserve CO and blood pressure to a level sufficient to maintain perfusion to vital organs, such as the brain and heart.

- Increased sympathetic outflow to the arterioles → constriction of the resistance vessels → increased peripheral vascular resistance → increased blood pressure.
- The decrease in vagal tone and increase in sympathetic discharge increase heart rate.

The kidney and adrenal glands boost this response:

- Sympathetic outflow to the juxtaglomerular apparatus, as well as direct activation of the renal baroreceptors in the afferent arterioles of the nephron.
- Leads to salt and water retention and the expansion of extracellular fluid volume.
- Meanwhile, sympathetic activation of the adrenal gland leads to the generation of circulating catecholamines, which increase vascular resistance and CO.

Ultimately, blood flow is diverted to locations of high priority at the expense of lower-priority places.

- Local vasodilatory effects prevail in the heart and brain, sustaining blood flow to these areas.
- Central vasoconstrictive effects predominate in the muscles, gastrointestinal tract, and skin (and later in the kidneys).

Clinically, this phenomenon manifests as cold, clammy extremities (peripheral vasoconstriction) and decreased urine output (water retention) in the patient who has had a moderate hemorrhage.

SUMMARY

- The vascular circuit from right ventricle to left atrium is the pulmonary circulation. The circuit from left ventricle to right atrium is the systemic circulation.
- The total blood volume is approximately 5 L, and 80% is contained in the low-pressure veins.
- The contraction of the cardiac ventricles is called systole; their relaxation is called diastole. Elastic recoil in the aorta propels blood onward during diastole, ensuring continuous flow.
- The arterial system starts with the aorta and branches into smaller vessels. From large to small, these vessels are called arteries, arterioles, and capillaries. The arterioles are muscular and can be dilated or constricted by neural and hormonal influences.
- Pressure, volume, and mass of fluid are all related at a given point in the vessel: $P \sim n/V$.
- Pressure difference (ΔP) makes a gas or fluid flow from one location to another. High pressure in the vascular circuit relative to downstream cause blood to move forward through the vascular system.
- Resistance (R) is a measure of friction in the vessel, opposing blood flow. It is proportional to the vessel radius (r), a relationship described by Poiseuille's law: $R = 8\eta l/\pi r^4$.
- Ohm's law applied to the entire cardiovascular circuit in the relationship MAP = (CO) × (SVR), where MAP is mean arterial pressure, CO is cardiac output, and SVR is systemic vascular resistance.
- MAP is controlled locally (by factors intrinsic to the vessels themselves), centrally (by reflexes involving the brain) and by the kidneys.
- Local control includes the myogenic response (in which wall stretch leads to vasoconstriction and vice versa), release of nitric oxide, and the release of metabolic vasodilators.
- Central control is through the baroreceptor reflex, where low pressure sensing stimulates the medulla. This leads to increased sympathetic output resulting in increased CO (by increasing heart rate and contractility) and arteriolar constriction in vascular beds other than in the heart and brain.
- Humoral control involves important vasoconstrictors, such as AII and ADH and vasodilators like ANP.

REVIEW QUESTIONS

Directions: Each of the numbered items or incomplete statements in this section is followed by answers or by completions of the statement. Select the one lettered answer or completion that is best in each case.

1. A 22-year-old woman is brought to the emergency room with severe hemorrhaging from open wounds on her lower extremities and a blood pressure of 80/40 mm Hg. The following would best describe her blood vessels:
   A. Vasoconstriction in all vascular beds
   B. Vasoconstriction in central nervous system (CNS) and coronary arteries only
   C. Vasodilation in all vascular beds
   D. Vasoconstriction in all vascular beds except CNS and coronary
   E. Vasodilation in all vascular beds except CNS and coronary

2. During pregnancy, vascular circuits are added in parallel to the systemic circulation as maternal blood vessels grow into the decidua basalis and fill the intervillous spaces with blood. The addition of parallel blood vessels or vascular spaces to the vascular circuit will:
   A. Increase SVR
   B. Decrease SVR
   C. Increase CO
   D. Decrease CO
   E. Not affect SVR or CO

3. Anxiety is known to raise the mean arterial pressure. It may do so by which of the following mechanisms?
   A. Increased stroke volume
   B. Increased parasympathetic output to the sinoatrial node of the heart
   C. Decreased sympathetic output to the arterioles
   D. Increased sympathetic output to the capillaries
   E. Sweat

4. A 61-year-old woman is found to have a 50% narrowing of her right renal artery. What is the expected change in blood flow through the stenotic artery?
   A. Increase to 1/2
   B. Decrease to 1/2
   C. Decrease to 1/4
   D. Increase to 1/16
   E. Decrease to 1/16

5. What is the approximate mean arterial pressure (MAP) of a patient with a systolic pressure of 120 mm Hg and a diastolic pressure of 90 mm Hg?
   A. 80 mm Hg
   B. 90 mm Hg
   C. 100 mm Hg
   D. 110 mm Hg
   E. 120 mm Hg

ANSWERS TO REVIEW QUESTIONS

1. **The answer is D.** She has low blood pressure because of hemorrhage. This would trigger her baroreceptor reflex, causing widespread vasoconstriction of her arterioles with sparing of the coronary arteries in the heart and the arterioles of the brain. The widespread vasoconstriction boosts the SVR and the MAP, and the increased MAP helps sustain perfusion of the heart and brain.

2. **The answer is B.** An additional parallel vascular circuit decreases SVR. This is because adding circuits in parallel is effectively the same as increasing the cross-sectional area (hence radius) of the vascular tree. A larger radius means a lower resistance.

3. **The answer is A.** Anxiety increases sympathetic outflow from the CNS, which boosts the contractility of the heart, leading to larger stroke volumes. CO = heart rate times stroke volume, so increased stroke volume increases CO, elevating the blood pressure. Parasympathetic output slows the heart rate, decreasing CO and MAP. Anxiety can sometimes lead to increases in MAP, followed by parasympathetic reflexes that lower the MAP. This is called the vasovagal reflex (see Ch. 4).

4. **The answer is E.** A 50% decrease in the radius will result in a 16-fold increase in resistance because resistance is inversely related to the fourth power of the radius. Sine blood flow is inversely proportional to the resistance, the expected change in blood flow is a decrease to 1/16 of the original flow.

5. **The answer is C.** Mean arterial pressure (MAP) is approximately the diastolic pressure plus one-third of the pulse pressure (systolic pressure – diastolic pressure), which is mathematically equivalent to [(2 × diastolic pressure) + systolic pressure]/3.

10

The Heart as a Pump

INTRODUCTION

As mentioned in Chapter 9, the heart is the muscular organ that serves as the pump driving the flow of blood through the cardiovascular system.

SYSTEM STRUCTURE

Located in the mediastinum of the chest at the level of thoracic vertebrae T5–T8, the human heart is a four-chambered pump surrounded by a fibrous sac (Fig. 10.1).

- Pericardium
  - Most superficial tissue of the heart.
  - Encases the heart and roots of the great vessels.
  - Two layers.
    The outer fibrous layer of the pericardium functions as a protective shell.
    The inner serous layer secretes pericardial fluid into the potential space created between them.
    This potential space, the pericardial sac, provides a low-friction pocket in which the cardiac muscle can move as it contracts.
- Heart chambers
  - Essentially, heart consists of two pumps.
    The right heart pumps deoxygenated blood into pulmonary circulation.
    The left heart pumps oxygenated blood into systemic circulation.
  - Each pump contains two chambers.
    Atria
    Thin-walled, low-pressure reservoirs.
    Collect venous blood upon return to heart.
    Contract before the ventricles, forcing blood into ventricles for pulmonary or systemic circulation.
    Ventricles
    Thick-walled, high-pressure chambers.
    Each leads outflow tract to arterial root.
    Right ventricle (RV) → pulmonary root.
    Left ventricle (LV) → aortic root.
- Conduction system
  - Extensive branches of tissue specialized for action potential transmission.
    Ensures contraction pattern = optimal pumping of blood.

- Begins in atria and ventricles → terminates in conductive Purkinje fibers → stimulation of cardiac muscle cells.
  Atria: pump blood "down" into the ventricles.
  Ventricle: pump blood "up" into arterial roots.
- Valves (Fig. 10.2)
  - Endothelialized fibrous structures secured to dense, fibrous cardiac skeleton.
  - Atrioventricular (AV) valves separate atria from ventricles.
    Types
    Tricuspid valve (three-leaflet) separates the right heart.
    Mitral valve (bicuspid, or two-leaflet) separates the left heart.
    Function
    Diastole: Remain passively open while blood flows from atria → ventricles.
    Systole: Close because of increasing chamber pressure from ventricular contraction.
    Ventricles contain muscular projections, called papillary muscles, connected to chordae tendineae, fibrous threads attached to free edges of AV valves.
    Ventricular contraction → papillary muscle contraction → chordae tense → AV valve leaflets close.
  - Semilunar valves (all three-leaflet) separate ventricles from arterial roots.
    Types
    Pulmonic valve separates the right ventricle and pulmonary artery.
    Aortic valve separates the left ventricle and aorta.
    Function
    Diastole: Remain closed.
    Systole: Ventricular contraction → rising intraventricular pressure → forces valves open (see Fast Fact Box 10.1 and 10.2).

Fast Fact Box 10.1

Cardiac geography, as is so often the case, is described in precisely the opposite of common sense. The superior-most region of the heart (the top of the atria) is called its base, while the inferior-most region of the heart (the tip of the ventricles) is called its apex.

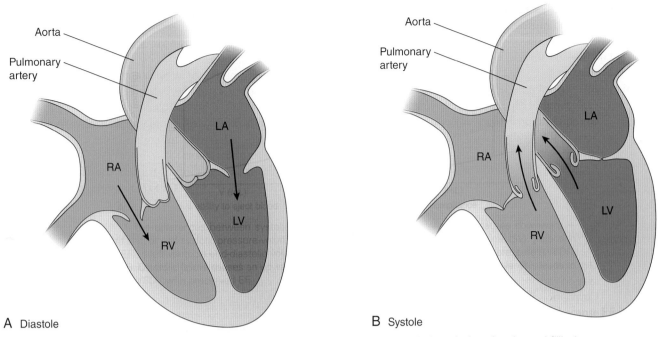

Fig. 10.1 Gross anatomy of the heart. The heart is shown during diastole (ventricular relaxation and filling) and systole (ventricular contraction and ejection). *RA*, right atrium; *LA*, left atrium; *RV*, right ventricle; *LV*, left ventricle.

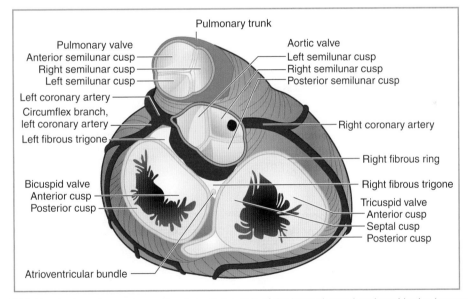

Fig. 10.2 Heart valves. A superior section through the atria of the heart shows the tricuspid valve (separating the right atrium and ventricle) on the right side of the heart, the bicuspid or mitral valve (separating the left atrium and ventricle) on the left side of the heart, the aortic valve (separating the left ventricle and the aorta), and the pulmonary valve (separating the right ventricle and the pulmonary artery). (From Bogart BI, Ort VH. *Elsevier's Integrated Anatomy and Embryology.* Elsevier; 2007. Fig. 4.27)

Fast Fact Box 10.2

The right ventricle (RV) expels its contents into the relatively low-pressure pulmonary arterial tree, and as such its walls are considerably thinner than that of the left ventricle (LV). The RV generates approximately one-seventh of the maximal LV pressure.

Histology

Like the rest of the cardiovascular system, the heart has three layers:

1. Epicardium
   a. Contains fibroelastic connective tissue, blood vessels, lymphatics, and adipose tissue.

2. Myocardium ("cardiac muscle tissue")
   a. Type of striated muscle specialized for rhythmic conduction and contraction.
      i. Like skeletal muscle, contain sarcomeres and sarcolemma.
      ii. Unlike skeletal muscle, contain intercalated discs.
         1. Collections of gap junctions allowing low-resistance communication between adjacent myocytes.
         2. Seen histologically as dark-staining bands between myocytes.
         3. Enable efficient cell-to-cell transmission of action potentials, thus allowing synchronous, ordered, and rapid contraction of myocardium.
      iii. High density of mitochondria (35% of cell volume).
         1. Provide large supply of adenosine triphosphate (ATP) necessary to fulfill cardiac work.
         2. Depends on nearly 1:1 ratio of capillary to myocyte to ensure proper oxygenation (see Clinical Correlation Box 10.1).
3. Endocardium
   a. Layer of endothelium lining the atria and ventricles, and covering the heart valves.

SYSTEM FUNCTION

Excitation-Contraction Coupling

Contraction of an individual myocyte begins with stimulation (i.e., depolarization leading to action potential generation) by the Purkinje fibers or by an adjacent muscle cell. To translate this electrical stimulation into action, the cell must couple this chemical excitation with a mechanical force, a process called excitation-contraction coupling (Fig. 10.3).

- Mediated by $[Ca^{2+}]$, whose intracellular release ultimately converts high-energy chemical bonds into mechanical cross-bridging of actin and myosin filaments.
- Occurs as follows:
  - During phase 2 of depolarization, the sarcolemma and network of T tubules become increasingly permeable to $[Ca^{2+}]$ via L-type Ca^{2+} channels.
    Open by a voltage-dependent mechanism, modulated by cyclic adenosine monophosphate (AMP)-dependent phosphorylation.
  - This small Ca^{2+} influx triggers the larger intracellular release of Ca^{2+} from the sarcoplasmic reticulum.
    $[Ca^{2+}]_{intracellular}$ increases 1 to 2 orders of magnitude from baseline.
  - Ca^{2+} allosterically binds to troponin-c and causes conformational shift.
    At rest, the contractile proteins troponin and tropomyosin are arranged to interfere with the cross-bridging of actin filaments and myosin heads.
    Conformational change in the thin filament that subsequently promotes cross-bridge formation.
  - This leads to contraction.
    Once phase 2 of the action potential ceases, Ca^{2+} release halts, and the intracellular Ca^{2+} is rapidly extruded from the cell and resequestered into the sarcoplasmic reticulum.
  - The resequestration of Ca^{2+} is accomplished by an ATP-driven Ca^{2+} pump stimulated by phosphorylated phospholamban.
  - This leads to relaxation.
    Thus cyclic-AMP-dependent protein kinase has two actions:
  - Accelerates contraction via the phosphorylation of sarcolemmal Ca^{2+} pumps responsible for the initial Ca^{2+} influx during phase 2.

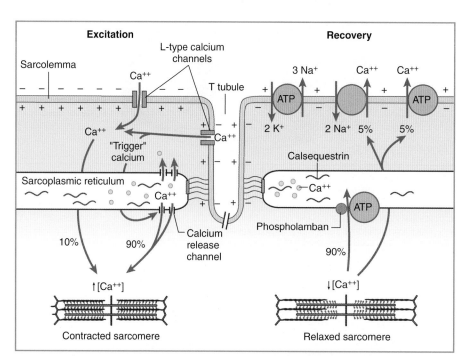

Fig. 10.3 Excitation-contraction coupling. The left side of the diagram shows contraction; the right represents recovery. (From Carroll RG. *Elsevier's Integrated Physiology*. Elsevier; 2006. Fig. 7.7.)

- Accelerates relaxation via the phosphorylation of phospholamban, stimulating resequestration of Ca^{2+} during diastole (see Fast Fact Box 10.3).

Fast Fact Box 10.3

Unlike in skeletal muscle, the Ca^{2+} release from the sarcolemma and T tubule network plays a crucial role in achieving appropriate contraction in the myocyte.

For a more complete description of the various phases of cardiac electrical activity, see Chapter 11.

Three Determinants of Stroke Volume

Three essential determinants of myocardial function are:
- Preload
- Afterload
- Contractility

To use the LV as an example, myocardial function is reflected in the amount of blood the LV ejects during a single contraction, known as the stroke volume (SV).

Clinical Correlation Box 10.1

A common measure of preload is the chamber filling of the left ventricle (LV) just before contraction, or the LV end-diastolic volume.

Preload

The preload is the degree of stretching of the myocardium and its myofibrils before contraction.
- The more blood that has entered a chamber before its contraction, the longer its myofibrils will be before contraction.
- Stretched myofibrils generate more force because stretching results in more actin-myosin cross-bridging (Fig. 10.4).
- Therefore more venous return of blood to the heart → more forceful cardiac contraction.

Experiments show that the tension developed during contraction increases with increasing initial length of the myofibril up to a plateau of maximal tension, beyond which the generated force is inversely related to initial length (Fig. 10.5).

This leads to the principle known as the Frank-Starling relationship.
- Within a certain range, ↑ preload → ↑ SV.

Afterload

The afterload is the force opposing myocardial contraction.
- Reflected by the final length of the myofibrils.
  - Fixed afterload defines the final length of myofibril, regardless of differences in preload.
- If a muscle fiber were attached to a weight on one end, the weight would be the afterload (Fig. 10.6).

In the LV, afterload is determined by the pressure in the aorta.
- The aortic pressure (afterload) hence determines how far the LV can contract during systole and sets the LV end-systolic volume.
  - An LV end-diastolic volume exists because the heart never completely empties itself of blood.

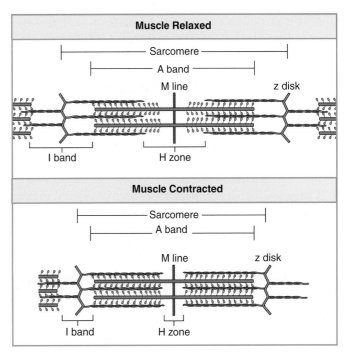

Fig. 10.4 A sarcomere at varying lengths. At greater lengths, there is more actin-myosin cross-bridging, implying a greater force of muscular contraction. This is the basis of the Frank-Starling relationship. (From Carroll RG. *Elsevier's Integrated Physiology*. Elsevier; 2006. Fig. 5.7.)

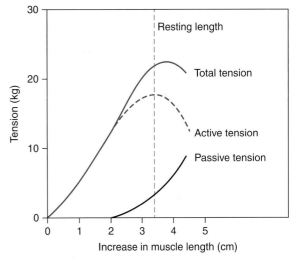

Fig. 10.5 Muscle force versus muscle length. Maximal tension, for myocytes, occurs at a length of 2.0 to 2.4 μm. At shorter lengths (<2.0 μm) the actin filaments actually begin to overlap and interfere with myosin-actin interactions. At lengths greater than 2.4 μm, there is limited actin-myosin interaction at best, producing little active tension.

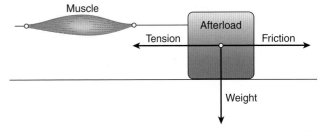

Fig. 10.6 An analogy for afterload. In the analogy, friction is the afterload, which opposes the force of muscle tension.

- The percentage of blood purged from the LV during systole is called the ejection fraction (EF; normal ~60%).
- For a fixed preload, ↑ afterload → ↓ SV and ↓ EF.

Contractility

Contractility, also known as "inotropy," is the force generated by the myocardium under conditions of fixed preload and afterload.
- Directly related to the availability of Ca^{2+} in the cell.
- Measured as maximal force generated in isometric contraction ("same volume," also known as contraction before valve opening) at a fixed preload.
- Changes achieved hormonally via inotropic agents, such as norepinephrine.
- Increased contractility allows the ventricle to contract farther (to a smaller LV end-systolic volume) against a fixed afterload → ↑ SV and ↑ EF (see Clinical Correlation Box 10.2).

Clinical Correlation Box 10.2

Myocardium that is injured and scarred—for example, because of ischemia (poor perfusion from the coronary arteries)—generates a lesser force of contraction than a healthy heart at the same preload and afterload; in other words, injured myocardium possesses less contractility.

The Cardiac Cycle

One cardiac cycle is the period of time from the beginning of one ventricular contraction to the beginning of the next.
- The cardiac cycle consists of two phases: systole and diastole.
- These phases are further subdivided into five divisions:
  - Atrial systole
  - Isovolumetric contraction
  - Ventricular ejection
  - Isovolumetric relaxation
  - Ventricular filling

There are several important physical, electrical, and audible phenomena that repeat during the cardiac cycle (Fig. 10.7). Another way to look at the cardiac cycle is the pressure-volume loop (Fig. 10.8).

Although the cardiac cycle applies to both the left and right hearts, the subsequent discussion focuses on the left heart.

Systole

Systole encompasses the period between the beginnings of the first and second heart sounds, and accounts for about 35% of the cardiac cycle.

Isovolumetric contraction occurs as the ventricles contract against closed valves.
- Quickly achieves a ventricular pressure sufficient to force the atrioventricular valves shut.
- Turbulent flow resulting from the abrupt closure of valves can be auscultated as the first heart sound, known as S1.
- No blood expelled at this time, so ↑ pressure and unchanged volume.

Ventricular ejection occurs when the ventricular pressure exceeds that of the outflow tract, forcing the semilunar valves open to allow flow into the arterial tree.
- First one-third of ejection interval = 70% of the total ejected volume (rapid ejection).

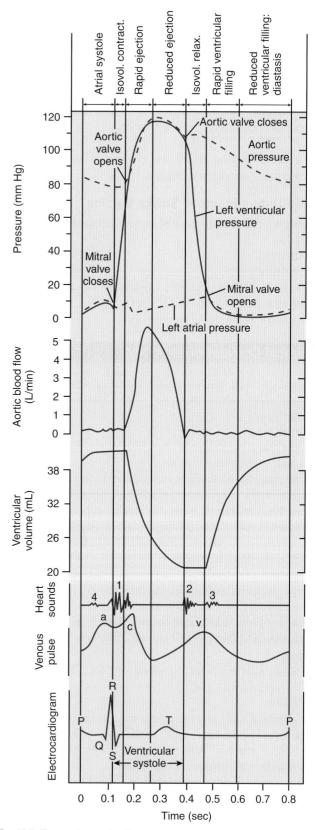

Fig. 10.7 The cardiac cycle. (From Levy M, Koeppen B, Stanton B. *Berne & Levy Principles of Physiology*, 4th Edition. St. Louis, MO: Elsevier; 2005. Fig. 18.8)

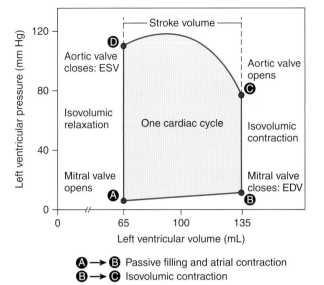

Fig. 10.8 The cardiac cycle depicted as a pressure-volume loop. *EDV*, End-diastolic volume; *ESV*, end-systolic volume.

- During this time, the ventricular pressure continues to rapidly increase, and blood flow is maximal.
- Last two-thirds of ejection interval = 30% of the total ejected volume (slow or reduced ejection).
  - As the displaced volume begins to redistribute further down the arterial system and the force of ventricular contraction decreases, causing ejection to occur at a slower rate.

As the ventricle begins to relax, its pressure eventually falls to a level insufficient to maintain the opening of the semilunar valves. Closure of these valves produces the second heart sound, S2, and marks the end of systole.

Diastole

Diastole, encompassing the period of ventricular relaxation, begins with S2 and encompasses around 65% of the cardiac cycle.

Isometric relaxation occurs with closure of the semilunar valves.

- The ventricular chamber volume remains constant but chamber pressure drops.
- There is a brief positive deflection in the aortic pressure tracing at the start of this phase as the aortic valve closes and the elastic recoil of the aorta begins to squeeze the aortic blood. This is called the dicrotic notch.
- When $P_{ventricle} < P_{atrium}$, the AV valves open.

Ventricular filling occurs as the AV valves open, thereby releasing the pressure buildup in the atria represented by the atrial *v* wave.

- The first third of diastole is the rapid filling phase. It contributes the majority of volume to the ventricular chambers.
- The second third of diastole, known as diastasis, represents effectively free flow from venous conduits to the ventricles; this period contributes minimally to the filling of the ventricles.

Atrial contraction ("kick") takes place during the last third of diastole, where the atria pump and push blood forward.

- Coincides with the P wave electrocardiographically and the *a* wave on the atrial pressure tracing (see Clinical Correlation Box 10.3).

> ### Clinical Correlation Box 10.3
> Atrial kick is incredibly important in a heart in which normal filling of the ventricle is compromised, such as rapid heart rate or severe atrioventricular valve stenoses (conditions that narrow the valve opening).

- Contributes 30% of end-diastolic ventricular volume.

Normal Heart Sounds and Venous Pulsations

The first heart sound, S1, signals the initiation of systole.

- Comprised of two nearly superimposed sounds, the closure of the AV valves.
- Intensity is directly proportional to the distance between the valve leaflets as they begin close.
  - The farther the leaflets must travel to close, the greater the intensity of vibration, and thus sound, that is produced.
- Heard best over the auscultatory zones for each of the valves involved (mitral and tricuspid).

The second heart sound, S2, marks the end of systole.

- Best be heard at the base (top) of the heart.
- The sound of the aortic valve closure, A_2, slightly precedes the pulmonic valve closure, P_2.
  - Because of the greater pressure gradient between the aorta and LV versus the pulmonary trunk and the RV (see Clinical Correlation Box 10.4).

> ### Clinical Correlation Box 10.4
> Physiologic splitting of S2 occurs during inspiration. During inspiration, the negative intrathoracic pressure produces increased venous return to the right heart (from extrathoracic sources via the superior vena cava and inferior vena cava) and also decreases venous return to the left heart (by pooling in the intrathoracic pulmonary venous tree). This change in ventricular volume prolongs ejection from the right heart, thereby delaying P_2, and shortens ejection from the left heart, thereby creating an earlier A_2. These slight changes in the timing of the two components of S2 make them disparate enough to be audible as two distinct sounds by the human ear.

Additional heart sounds include:

- S3
  - Caused by ventricular vibration in early diastole, because of rapid filling.
  - Associated with:
    High output states (normal in children, pregnant women).
    Overfilling (i.e., congestive heart failure).
    Decreased cardiac compliance (i.e., cardiomyopathy).
- S4
  - Caused by ventricular vibration in late diastole, when atrial kick encounters a stiff ventricle → results in turbulent flow.

- Associated with any process that increases stiffness of ventricle (i.e., ventricular hypertrophy).

Clinicians may also observe venous pulsation, which can be seen via the internal jugular (IJ) vein. Because there are no valves intervening between the right atrium and jugular veins, their distention reflects the pressure in the right atrium, and venous pulsation in the IJ reflects the timing of the cardiac cycles.

- Upward deflections.
  - *a* wave (atrial contraction), *c* wave (contraction of the ventricles), and *v* wave (venous collection).
- Downward deflections.
  - *x* wave (atrium relaxes and the tricuspid valve moves downward) and *y* descent (ventricular filling).

If the heart is not pumping adequately (e.g., owing to myocardial ischemia) and too much blood is left behind in the right atrium, the right atrial pressure will be elevated. This in turn will be reflected by the presence of jugular venous distention (JVD).

Oxygen Demand and Supply

The heart has an enormous oxygen demand (8–10 mL O_2/min/100g) because of the necessity of ATP regeneration with each contraction. This demand is represented by the myocardial oxygen consumption (MVO_2), which relates to the work output of the muscle and is determined by:

- Heart rate (↑ contraction cycles / unit time → ↑ ATP use).
- Contractility (↑ actin-myosin cross-bridge cycling → ↑ ATP use).
- Wall tension (↑ afterload, ↑ chamber size, ↓ myocardial thickness → ↑ ATP use).
- Basal energy metabolism (25% of MVO_2).

To match demand, the heart relies on preservation of blood flow via the coronary arteries and stable oxygen content (Eq. 10.1). Note that the heart "feeds itself" first with freshly (and optimally) oxygenated blood via the coronaries, before blood is transported to other organ systems.

$$O_2 \text{ delivery} = \text{coronary blood flow} \times \text{arterial oxygen content}$$
$$= CBF \times CaO_2 \qquad \textbf{(Eq. 10.1)}$$

Coronary artery blood flow relies on the perfusion pressure (driving blood flow from aorta → coronaries) and vascular resistance (see Fast Facts Box 10.4).

Fast Fact Box 10.4

Perfusion pressure = aortic diastolic pressure – left ventricular end-diastolic pressure (LVEDP)

- High pressure differences drive coronary blood flow.
- High resistance (as in coronary atherosclerosis) inhibit coronary blood flow.

Oxygen content is determined primarily by the amount of oxygen bound to hemoglobin in the blood.

- Because of nearly optimal oxygen extraction, oxygen in the coronary capillaries is rapidly consumed and exhausted of its oxygen content.
- This produces a wide arteriovenous difference in oxygen content.

Note that MVO_2 increases with increased AV difference, which represents efficacious oxygen extraction by functional cardiac myocytes (Eq. 10.2)

$$MVO_2 = \text{coronary blood flow} \times$$
$$\text{arteriovenous oxygen content difference}$$
$$= CBF \times [CaO_2 - CvO_2] \qquad \textbf{(Eq. 10.2)}$$

Assuming oxygen content and extraction quality are relatively constant, flow thus becomes the rate-limiting factor for cardiac oxygen consumption. This makes the myocardium particularly vulnerable to ischemia if the coronary blood flow is compromised.

The Regulation of Cardiac Output

The heart must maintain adequate systemic blood flow to meet the metabolic needs of all tissues of the body at all times. To maintain perfusion, the body must:

- Maintain adequate cardiac output (CO).
- Modify systemic vascular resistance as discussed in Chapter 9.

CO, the product of heart rate (HR) and SV, is routinely used as a measure of cardiac performance. Any alterations in SV and HR can influence the CO (Fig. 10.9).

- Extrinsic path: nervous system and reflex arcs → mediate both HR and SV changes.
- Intrinsic path: Frank-Starling mechanism → mediates only SV changes.

Regulation of Stroke Volume

The Frank-Starling mechanism helps to ensure that changes in preload lead to changes in SV and hence CO (Fig. 10.10).

- Changes in preload = changes in LV end-diastolic volume. This may be caused by:
  - Increased cardiac filling (e.g., increased venous return as seen in exercise).
  - Decreased cardiac emptying (e.g., in aortic or mitral regurgitation).
- The greater stretch of the myocardial fibers results in a stronger contraction, leading to the same LV end-systolic volume (LVEDV).
- Thus ↑ preload = ↑ SV = ↑ CO (see Fast Facts Box 10.5).

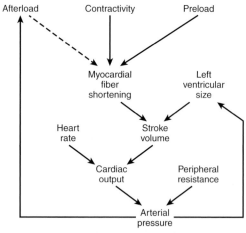

Fig. 10.9 Multiple interactions that influence cardiac output and arterial pressure. The *dashed line* between afterload and myocardial fiber shortening indicates a negative relationship (i.e., high afterload limits myocardial fiber shortening and thus cardiac output).

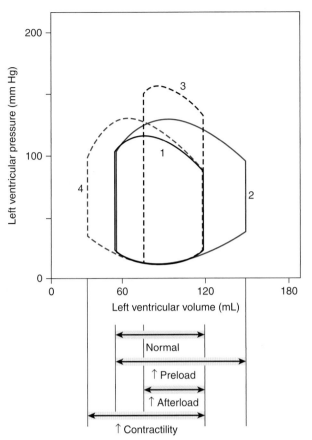

Fig. 10.10 The effect of altered preload, afterload, and contractility on stroke volume (SV). Alterations in these parameters are depicted with pressure-volume loops to illustrate their effects on the entire cardiac cycle. Loop 1 represents the normal cardiac cycle. Loop 2 represents increased preload at the same afterload and contractility as loop 1 (which increases the SV by the Frank-Starling mechanism). Loop 3 represents increased afterload with the same preload and contractility as loop 1. Loop 4 represents increased contractility with the same preload and afterload as loop 1. Stroke volumes are shown below the pressure-volume graph.

Fast Fact Box 10.5

Without the Frank-Starling mechanism, increased venous return to the heart could not be met with increased cardiac output (CO), and the blood would back up in the veins. Inadequate CO with venous backup is what is known as congestive heart failure.

The Frank-Starling mechanism can also indirectly help the heart compensate for increased afterload (i.e., hypertension or aortic stenosis).

- ↑ afterload requires the LV to attain a higher end-diastolic pressure before the aortic valve will open.
  - The heart can only sustain this pressure for a shorter period of time.
  - The valve shuts sooner → ↑ ESV and ↓ SV.
- Importantly, however, this change in SV is rectified on the subsequent contraction.
  - ↓ SV leads to ↑ ESV in the LV, to which the normal volume of blood from the right atrium will be added.
  - This increases LVEDV (preload).

- By Frank-Starling mechanism, this will proportionally increase the force of contraction and thus reestablish the original SV.

The reconstitution of SV, however, comes at the expense of higher end-diastolic filling volumes and pressures. These can have deleterious effects on long-term myocardial performance. Chronic changes in afterload are also compensated physically by structural changes of the heart, which may not be healthy in the long run.

- ↑ afterload → LV must attain higher maximal pressures → ventricle wall is subjected to ↑ transmural pressures.
- Laplace's law dictates that this produces ↑ wall tension and metabolic demand.
- To compensate for the increased wall stress, the heart manipulates other variables in Laplace's law because it cannot modify the transmural pressure.
  - ↑ wall thickness (hypertrophy)
  - ↓ chamber size (concentric hypertrophy)

Contractility is adjusted by baroreceptor regulation and sympathetic tone, as discussed in Chapter 9. Regardless of preload or afterload, ↑ contractility = ↑ SV. T.

In summary:

- ↑ preload and ↑ contractility = ↑ SV and CO
- ↑ afterload = ↓ SV and CO

Regulation of Heart Rate

HR, the second component of CO, is regulated by the sympathetic and parasympathetic nervous systems. The heart is thus richly and strategically innervated by both divisions of the autonomic nervous system (ANS).

- Parasympathetic control is mediated through the vagus nerve.
  - Preganglionic cells arise in the medulla oblongata and synapse with postganglionic cells on or in the surface of the heart.
  - Predominantly innervates the sinoatrial node (containing "pacemaker" cells) and AV node.
  - Primarily affects HR and serves as major determinant of resting HR.
- Sympathetic innervation arises from spinal levels C7 through T6.
  - Preganglionic fibers synapse in the stellate and cervical ganglia with postganglionic fibers, which then directly innervate the heart.
  - Predominantly innervates the ventricular tissue.
  - Primarily affects the contractility of the myocardium, but also necessary to increase HR significantly above 100 beats per minute.

Both divisions of the autonomic nervous system exhibit a tonic and antagonistic stimulation of the heart, allowing for precise manipulation of the HR and contractility.

The medullary baroreceptor reflex is the most important regulatory system governing HR.

- Responds to changes in arterial pressure with changes in HR in parallel with changes in contractility.
- ↓ blood pressure leads to ↑ contractility (↑ sympathetic tone) and ↑ HR (decreased parasympathetic tone).
- ↑ blood pressure leads to ↓ contractility and ↓ HR.

Measuring Cardiac Output

Fick's law allows us to estimate CO by using the law of conservation of mass in oxygen flow.

- O_2 in the pulmonary artery + O_2 added in alveoli = O_2 in pulmonary vein.

Masses can be expressed as mass/time, that is, flow. Flow of O_2 can be calculated as the product of vessel oxygen content $[O_2]$ and arterial blood flow Q.

q_1 = flow of O_2 to alveoli in pulmonary artery (PA) = $[O_2]_{PA} \times Q_{pulmonary}$

q_3 = flow of O_2 from alveoli to pulmonary vein (PV) = $[O_2]_{PV} \times Q_{systemic}$

To calculate the flow of O_2 into the capillary bed from the alveoli (q_2), it is assumed that:

- At equilibrium, this flow equals O_2 consumption of the body
- Blood flow in the pulmonary circulation and systemic circulation is equal and represents CO

Thus, we can calculate CO Q with simple algebraic manipulation:

$$q_1 + q_2 = q_3.$$
$$[O_2]_{pa}\, Q + q_2 = [O_2]_{pv}\, Q$$
$$[O_2]_{pa}\, Q - [O_2]_{pv}\, Q = -q_2$$
$$Q\,([O_2]_{pa} - [O_2]_{pv}) = -q_2$$
$$Q = q_2 / ([O_2]_{pv} - [O_2]_{pa})$$

The O_2 content of the deoxygenated blood ($[O_2]_{pa}$) is measured in catheter-retrieved samples from the pulmonary artery, whereas that of oxygenated blood ($[O_2]_{pv}$) is measured in samples of systemic arterial blood acquired through needle-stick. Finally, O_2 consumption (q_2) is measured by analyzing the volume and O_2 content of expired air.

However, clinicians now commonly use any of a number of alternative, less invasive methods for assessing CO. One of these is the thermodilution method (see Clinical Correlation Box 10.5).

Clinical Correlation Box 10.5

The thermodilution method for measuring cardiac output (CO) uses solid-state circuitry with catheter technology.
- Catheter inserted into venous system.
  - Proximal port → cold saline injected into bloodstream
  - Distal thermistor → Δ resistance with Δ temperature
- Changes in current recorded as function of time as cold saline is injected while voltage held constant (V=IR).
- Temperature curve has exponential decay profile, with parameters as a function of speed at which saline reaches the thermistor.
  - Distance between injection port and thermistor known (catheter length)
  - Δ resistance as a function of time known (thermistor recording)
  - Thus, we can estimate the rate at which saline travels, i.e., CO

PATHOPHYSIOLOGY: HEART FAILURE

Failure of the heart as a pump causes congestive heart failure (CHF), where blood cannot be driven from the low-pressure venous system to the high-pressure arterial system. Blood thus accumulates in the venous system.

For the purposes of discussion, we will focus on left-sided heart failure:
- Blood accumulation in the pulmonary veins causes ↑ hydrostatic pressure of pulmonary vessels and drives fluid into low (atmospheric) pressure in alveoli.
  - This is known as pulmonary edema.
  - Fluid covers the gas exchange membranes, preventing proper oxygenation.
  - Patients experience:
    Dyspnea on exertion (shortness of breath).
    Paroxysmal nocturnal dyspnea (breathless awakening from sleep).
    Orthopnea (shortness of breath while lying supine).
- Blood accumulation in the systemic veins (in more severe CHF) causes ↑ hydrostatic pressure and drives fluid into the interstitial spaces.
  - This is known as peripheral edema.
  - Preferentially affects lower extremities and lower part of lung because gravity causes pooling. These are known as dependent regions.

Physical examination may demonstrate:
- Rales in the lungs (crackles caused by fluid accumulation).
- Jugular venous distention (because of fluid backup in the venous system).
- Pitting edema of the lower extremities.
- S3 or S4 heart sounds.

There are two basic types of cardiac dysfunction that lead to CHF, and they correspond to the two basic phases of cardiac pumping: filling (diastole) and contraction (systole). Fig. 10.11 demonstrates the differences in cardiac function in diastolic and systolic heart failure.

Systolic dysfunction describes any situation in which the heart cannot pump effectively.
- Blood cannot be pushed forward and backs up → ↓ SV and EF and ↑ LVEDV/LV end-diastolic pressure (LVEDP).
- Most common cause is ischemic injury to myocardium because of coronary artery disease (CAD).
- After ischemic injury, the heart gradually enlarges to compensate for lost function (dilated cardiomyopathy).
  - Ischemic injury → ↓ inotropy → ↓ SV/EF.
  - Diastolic filling now begins at a higher ESV and EDV is therefore increased.
  - Over time, the increased filling gradually increases the heart's size. This increases its preload and, by the Frank-Starling mechanism, helps to boost its SV.

Diastolic dysfunction describes any situation in which the heart cannot relax and fill effectively.
- Chamber cannot expand (relax) as usual → ↓ LVEDV, ↑ LVEDP with normal EF.
- Most common cause is chronic hypertension.
  - ↑ afterload → ↑ myocardial thickening + ↓ chamber size to relieve wall stress.
  - ↓ compliance → reduced filling during diastole.
  - This is called hypertrophic cardiomyopathy.
- Other causes include infiltrative disease of the myocardium (as with amyloidosis), causing restrictive cardiomyopathy (see Clinical Correlation Box 10.6).

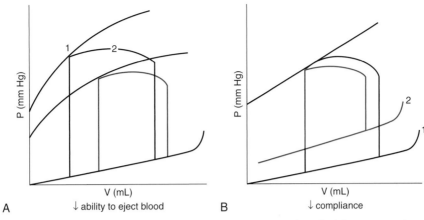

Fig. 10.11 The differences between systolic and Diastolic Failure. A, Systolic failure causes downward + rightward shift of end-systolic pressure-volume relation (ESPVR). This leads to ↓ stroke volume (SV), ↓ ejection fraction (EF), ↑ left ventricle end-diastolic volume (LVEDV), and ↑ left ventricle end-diastolic pressure (LVEDP) (preload). B, Diastolic failure causes an upward shift of passive diastolic pressure-volume curve. This leads to ↑ LVEDP, ↓ LVEDV with preserved EF.

Clinical Correlation Box 10.6

A 57-year-old man with a history of angina and smoking for 40 years presents with severe substernal chest pain, chest pressure, and shortness of breath. Electrocardiogram (ECG) reveals ST-segment elevations consistent with myocardial ischemia. He receives propranolol (a beta-blocker), aspirin, intravenous nitroglycerin, and heparin. An elevated creatine kinase (CK) level confirms myocardial infarction (MI).

MI, or heart attack, refers to the acute event in which blood flow is interrupted to the myocardium.

- Often because of coronary artery disease (CAD), when plaques on the coronary artery endothelium rupture and form thrombi (blood clots) that constrict or completely occlude the artery.
- The three main coronary arteries are the right coronary artery (RCA), left anterior descending artery (LAD), and left circumflex artery (LCx).
- The artery blocked determines the region of injury and the effect on systolic function.

Angina is substernal (midline) chest pain and pressure attributed to cardiac ischemia. Ischemia is a reversible hypoperfusion of the myocardium, which may lead to infarction—actual tissue death—when severe.

- Both manifest in the ECG as ST changes and T wave inversions in the leads corresponding to injured territory.
- The death of myocardial tissue releases intracellular enzymes, such as CK.

Luckily, there are several treatment options available for myocardial ischemia:

- Beta-blockers → ↓ sympathetic tone → ↓ inotropy → ↓ oxygen demand
- Nitroglycerin → vasodilation → ↓ afterload (via arteriodilation), ↓ preload (via venodilation), ↑ heart perfusion (coronary dilation) → ↓ oxygen demand, ↑ oxygen supply
- Aspirin + heparin → ↓ thrombus formation

In chronic systolic CHF, medical management includes medications optimize EF through the following mechanisms:

- Reduce afterload (i.e., antihypertensive [blood pressure-lowering] medications like angiotensin-converting enzyme inhibitors.
- Reduce preload (i.e., diuretics, such as furosemide [Lasix], which relieve the venous system of its congestion by purging fluid in the urine).
- Increase contractility (i.e., digoxin).

Diastolic CHF is more difficult to treat because EF is already normalized.

- Irreversible cardiomyopathies can be treated by heart transplantation.
- Diuresis is typically not used in diastolic dysfunction, the heart already underfills and needs whatever preload it can get.
- β-blocking drugs may help the heart relax and hence to fill in diastolic dysfunction.

Valvular disorders are another group of maladies affecting the heart's ability to act as a pump, which may lead to CHF in the long term.

- Any of the four valves may be affected.
- Stenosis is a narrowing of the valve opening because of valve thickening.
- Regurgitation is a retrograde flow of the blood through the valve because of valvular incompetence (see Genetics Box 10.1, Development Box 10.1, Pharmacology Box 10.1).

GENETICS BOX 10.1

Familial dilated cardiomyopathy is a hereditary disease that results in thinning and weakening of the ventricular tissue and eventually the development of heart failure. Mutations in the TTN gene that encodes the cardiomyocyte sarcomere associated protein titin care the cause in approximately 20% of patients. However, because TTN is a relatively large gene, there are various mutations that are associated with other muscle diseases, including other forms of heart failure and some forms of muscular dystrophy.

DEVELOPMENT BOX 10.1

Although familial dilated cardiomyopathy can manifest at any age, it typically presents in midadulthood with fatigue, dyspnea, arrhythmias, peripheral edema, syncope, and sometime sudden death.

PHARMACOLOGY BOX 10.1

Familial dilated cardiomyopathy is treated like other causes of heart failure with a reduced ejection fraction. Pharmacologic agents include angiotensin converting enzyme inhibitors, angiotensin receptor blockers, beta-blockers, aldosterone antagonists, and hydralazine combined with a nitrate. If pharmacotherapy is insufficient, a device such as a pacemaker or an implantable cardioverter defibrillator is indicated.

SUMMARY

- The cardiac cycle consists of two phases: systole and diastole. These phases are further subdivided into five divisions:
  - Atrial systole
  - Isovolumetric contraction
  - Ventricular ejection
  - Isovolumetric relaxation
  - Ventricular filling
- Oxygen supply depends on coronary blood flow and arterial oxygen content.
- The three determinants of SV are preload, afterload, and contractility.
- SV is the amount of blood expelled from the ventricle during one systolic contraction. The percentage expelled from the ventricle by each stroke is the ejection fraction (normal is >50%).
- Preload is the degree of stretching of the ventricular myofibrils before systolic contraction. It is related to the end-diastolic volume.
- As the LV end-diastolic volume increases, the force generated by the LV will also increase, leading to a proportional increase in the SV. This is known as the Frank-Starling relationship.

- Afterload is the force opposing myocardial contraction. For the LV, this is primarily the aortic pressure.
- Contractility is the force generated by the myocardium under conditions of fixed preload and afterload. It is increased by adrenergic stimulation.
- The Fick principle is a method of calculating cardiac output from the oxygen content of the pulmonary artery and vein and from oxygen consumption:

$$Q = q_2/([O_2]_{pv} - [O_2]_{pa}).$$

- The primary consequence of disordered heart pumping is CHF.
- Two basic types of cardiac dysfunction lead to CHF, corresponding to the two basic phases of cardiac pumping: diastolic dysfunction corresponds to filling, and systolic dysfunction corresponds to contraction.
- The most common cause of systolic dysfunction is ischemia, or injury to the myocardium because of CAD.

REVIEW QUESTIONS

Directions: Each of the numbered items or incomplete statements in this section is followed by answers or by completions of the statement. Select the one lettered answer or completion that is best in each case.

1. A 33-year-old woman reporting exertional chest pain undergoes a Doppler echocardiogram, which shows concentric thickening of the left ventricle, thickened aortic valve leaflets, and a 67-mm Hg pressure gradient from the left ventricle to the aortic root. Which of the following descriptors could best be applied to her cardiac dysfunction?
   A. High preload
   B. Mitral stenosis
   C. Low contractility
   D. Aortic regurgitation
   E. Low ventricular compliance

2. A 70-year-old man with a history of coronary artery disease arrives in the emergency room unresponsive and hypotensive. His respirations are 35 per minute and his heart rate is 140 per minute. If he has had a massive myocardial infraction (MI), the primary cause of his hypotension is:
   A. Dehydration
   B. Peripheral edema with "third-spacing" of fluid

   C. Decreased afterload
   D. Decreased preload
   E. Decreased contractility

3. Total occlusion of the left anterior descending (LAD) artery will have particularly devastating consequences for which part of the heart?
   A. Right ventricle
   B. Left ventricle
   C. Right atrium
   D. Left atrium
   E. Sinoatrial node

4. Echocardiography of a 65-year-old patient with a history of lung cancer and pericarditis is remarkable for a large pericardial effusion. Because of the difference in thickness between the left and right ventricles, pericardial tamponade would most likely first present as:
   A. Pulmonary edema
   B. Shortness of breath
   C. Right ventricular failure
   D. Left ventricular failure
   E. Hypotension

ANSWERS TO REVIEW QUESTIONS

1. **The answer is E.** The patient has aortic stenosis, which has created a chronic obstruction to left ventricular outflow. This in turn has caused hypertrophy of the left ventricle, which decreases its compliance. Low compliance interferes with diastolic filling of the ventricle, leading to low preload, not high.

2. **The answer is E.** Myocardial infarction (MI) lessens the inherent strength (i.e., contractility) of the myocardium. With significantly reduced contractility, the left ventricle cannot sustain the pressure necessary for adequate SV, and the cardiac output falls. In accordance with the analogy to Ohm's law, which says that mean arterial pressure equals cardiac

output times systemic vascular resistance, a drop in cardiac output means a drop in blood pressure (hypotension). Congestive heart failure (CHF) caused by ischemic heart disease does cause peripheral edema and sequestration of fluid in the interstitial tissues does reduce intravascular volume, which in turn reduces preload, which in turn does reduce cardiac output. It is not known in this case whether the patient has CHF, but the primary cause of hypotension is decreased contractility because of MI. If the patient does have CHF with low preload, the original cause of the CHF is still likely to be systolic dysfunction with low contractility because of ischemic heart disease. Finally, low afterload is synonymous with low blood pressure, not the cause of the low blood pressure.

3. **The answer is B.** The LAD provides the main blood supply to the left ventricle.

4. **The answer is C.** The right ventricle is thinner than the left and therefore pericardial tamponade or fluid accumulation in the pericardium would affect the right heart first and cause right-sided ventricular failure. Shortness of breath and pulmonary edema would be expected with left heart failure.

11

Cardiac Electrophysiology

INTRODUCTION

The heart contains specialized tissue for: (1) generating rhythmic action potentials and (2) conducting those action potentials precisely across the heart. This ensures correct timing of atrial and ventricular contraction.

SYSTEM STRUCTURE

Fig. 11.1 depicts the typical pathway of cardiac excitation.
- Action potentials are transmitted from sinoatrial (SA) node to atrioventricular (AV) node.
- Excitation proceeds through atrial muscle and specialized conducting tissues:
  - His bundle
  - Bundle branches
  - Purkinje fibers
- Impulses reach ventricular muscle, initiating muscle contraction.

Coordinated muscular contraction requires the rapid transmission of electrical impulses, which is facilitated by the gap junctions between myocardial cells.
- Gap junctions make the myocardium a functional syncytium (many cells that make the heart function as though it were a single continuous unit of cytoplasm).
- As a result, a stimulus arising at any one point within the ventricle leads to the contraction of both left and right ventricles; likewise, a stimulus arising within the atria leads to the contraction of both left and right atria.

The SA node is normally the functional pacemaker of the heart.
- Under certain pathologic conditions, cells outside the sinus node (within the atria, the AV junction, or the ventricles) may act as independent pacemakers and generate their own intrinsic rhythm for the heart.
- Automaticity is the ability to generate impulses spontaneously, whether innate or acquired as in pathologic states (see Clinical Correlation Box 11.1).

Clinical Correlation Box 11.1

Ectopic automaticity (misplaced automaticity) is important to understanding some of the common cardiac arrhythmias (rhythm disturbances) and electrocardiographic abnormalities seen in clinical practice.

Conduction, the capacity to generate action potentials cell to cell at regular intervals, is another property of myocardial tissue that varies throughout the transmission pathway.
- Speed of conduction varies depending on the location.
  - (Fastest) Purkinje fibers → Atrial muscle → Ventricular muscle → AV node (slowest).
  - Slow conduction at the AV node ensures that the ventricles have adequate time to fill before the signal for ventricular contraction arrives.
  - Differences in conduction vary depending on type of action potentials arising there.

SYSTEM FUNCTION

Cardiac Electrophysiology

Action potentials provide electrical stimulation that is coupled to rhythmic contraction of the heart. Two principal types observed in the heart (Fig. 11.2).
- Fast response seen in conductive cardiac tissue (the myocardial fibers in the atrium, ventricles, His bundle, and Purkinje fiber network).
- Slow response, distinguished by a more prolonged upstroke in electrical potential, seen in the pacemaker fibers of the SA and AV nodes.
  - Only the slow fibers possess automaticity.
  - The slow response is distinguished by smaller amplitude, as well as a slower upstroke (phase 0). This accounts for lower conduction velocity relative to fast-response fibers.

Resting Potential

The sarcolemma of each myocyte is hydrophobic and thus will not permit entry of most charged, hydrophilic ions. Various phases of the cardiac action potential in both slow-response and fast-response fibers can be explained by changes in the permeability of the cell membrane to various ions, primarily:
- Sodium (Na^+)
- Potassium (K^+)
- Calcium (Ca^{2+})

These variations in permeability are accomplished through variations in the configuration and conductance of specialized transmembrane proteins known as ion channels.

Ion channels have two important functional properties:
- Selectivity is the ability of different channels to be selective for specific ions, such as Na^+ or K^+.

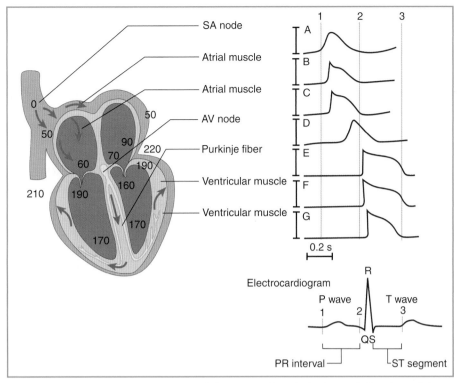

Fig. 11.1 Pacemaker and conductive tissues of the myocardium. Left, Anatomic locations of the various conductive tissues. Right, Action potentials in the various tissues. *AV,* Atrioventricular; *SA,* sinoatrial. (From Carroll R. *Elsevier's Integrated Physiology.* Philadelphia: Mosby Elsevier; 2007. Fig. 7.6.)

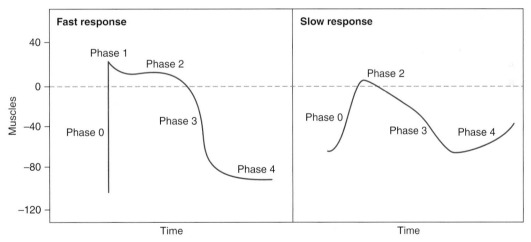

Fig. 11.2 Fast and slow action potentials. Notice the automatic upturn in electrical potential in phase 4 of the slow response.

- Gating is a property that makes ion channels fluctuate between "open" and "closed" states in a voltage-sensitive fashion (i.e., the channel state depends on the electrical potential across the cell membrane at any given time).
  - The total ionic current that flows through the channel is determined by the proportion of time spent in the open versus the closed state.

Myocardial cells, like other cells in the body, are highly permeable to K^+ in their resting state. This permeability to K^+ creates a resting membrane potential, as described in Fig. 11.3.

- The two main driving forces of permeability are electrical forces (as represented by the transmembrane voltage) and chemical forces (as represented by the concentration gradient).
- When electrical forces (accumulation of electronegativity in the intracellular space) equal chemical forces (high intracellular K^+ concentration), equilibrium is achieved.

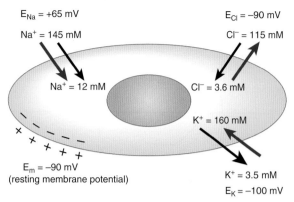

Fig. 11.3 Generation of the potassium (K^+) equilibrium potential. The Na^+,K^+-ATPase drives K^+ into cells, generating high intracellular concentrations and thus creating a favorable chemical gradient for K^+ to diffuse outside the cell. This movement to the extracellular space generates increasing electronegativity on the inside of the cell (K^+ is a positive ion!) and thus decreases the K^+ efflux. Eventually, the electrostatic (K^+ flows in) and chemical forces (K^+ flows out) are equal, producing equilibrium. The *black arrows* indicate the direction of movement favored by the chemical gradient. The *red arrows* indicate the direction of movement favored by the electrical gradient. (From Levy MN, Koeppen BM, Stanton BA. *Berne & Levy Principles of Physiology,* 4th Edition. Elsevier; 2005. Fig. 2.7.)

- The electrical potential inside the cell membrane at this point is known as the equilibrium potential.

Recall that the Nernst equation relates the equilibrium potential for an ion to intracellular and extracellular concentrations:

$$E_K = RT/zF \ln [K^+_o]/[K^+_i]$$

where $[K^+o]$ is the extracellular concentration, $[K^+_i]$ is the intracellular concentration, and E_K is the electrical potential inside the cell. (The other terms of the equation are R, the ideal gas constant, 8.314 J/mol K; T, the absolute temperature in degrees Kelvin; z, the valence of K^+; and F, the Faraday constant, 9.648×10^4 C/mol; ln signifies the natural log function.)

Algebraic manipulation of this equation yields:

$$E_K = 61.5/z \log [K^+_o]/[K^+_i].$$

The Goldman equation is a variation of the Nernst equation that calculates the equilibrium concentration of a membrane with permeabilities to many ions (K^+, Ca^{2+}, Na^+, Cl^-) and that factors in the degree of permeability for each ion.

Table 11.1 shows the distribution of Na^+, K^+, and Ca^{2+} across cardiac cell membranes and the equilibrium potentials that would exist for each if each were the only ion permeability in the membrane.

TABLE 11.1	Ion Distributions and Individual Equilibrium Potentials		
Ion	Extracellular Concentration	Intracellular Concentration	Equilibrium Potential
Na^+	145 mM	10 mM	70 mV
K^+	4 mM	135 mM	−94 mV
Ca^{2+}	2 mM	0.0001 mM	132 mV

- Positive potential indicates a net influx of that ion.
- Negative potential indicates a net efflux of that ion.

The true resting potential of the cardiac cell membrane, reflecting the resting permeability to these three ions, is −90 mV.

- Note that this is close to the Nernst potential for K^+, reflecting that the resting cell membrane is permeable primarily to K^+ ions and not Na^+ or Ca^{2+}.
  - At rest, the cell membrane has a slow inward leak of sodium ions that slightly depolarizes the membrane relative to E_k.
- Hyperpolarization occurs when ion flux renders the cell interior more negative, exaggerating the resting charge difference.
- Depolarization occurs when ion flux renders the cell interior more positive, abolishing the resting charge difference.

The Ionic Basis of the Fast Response

The action potential in myocardial cells is an all-or-nothing response, which requires initiation by a stimulus that raises (depolarizes) the resting membrane potential to a critical value called the threshold potential (roughly −65 mV).

- Stimulation < −65 mV = no response.
- Stimulation ≥ 65 mV = propagation of a normal action potential.

The contour of the fast-response action potential, consisting of five phases, is illustrated in Fig. 11.4.

- Phase 0
- Phase 1
- Phase 2
- Phase 3
- Phase 4 (resting membrane potential)

In these cells, depolarization to threshold potential activates voltage-gated ("fast") sodium channels, causing ↑ Na^+ permeability.

- ↑ Na^+ influx because of favorable concentration and electric gradient.
- This lead to further depolarization of the cell, reflected in the rapid upstroke (phase 0) of the fast action potential.

Sodium channel activation occurs through a dual gating mechanism (Fig. 11.5). The combined position of the two gates (the primary "sliding doors" gate and the secondary "ball-and-chain" gate) determines the state of the sodium channel:

- Closed
- Open
- Inactivated

The positions of the two gates are in turn dependent on the voltage applied across them.

- At resting membrane potential → primary gate closed → no net sodium flux.
- At threshold potential −> both gates open → rapid sodium influx.
- Gradual inactivation through closure of secondary gate → no further sodium flux.

This transition from "open" to "inactivated" accounts for the rapid changes in sodium conductance across the cell membrane and the brief duration of the action potential upstroke. In the inactivated state, the sodium channels are unavailable for

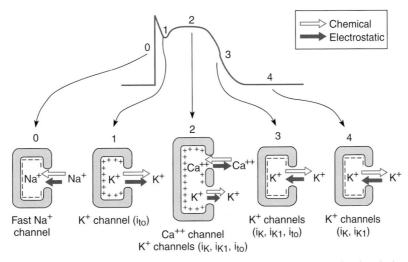

Fig. 11.4 Phases of the fast-response action potential. The *open arrows* represent the chemical gradient and the *filled arrows* represent the electrostatic gradient. i_{to}, i_k, i_{k1} represent currents through various types of K^+ channels. (From Levy MN, Koeppen BM, Stanton BA. *Berne & Levy Principles of Physiology*, 4th Edition. Elsevier; 2005. Fig. 16.5.)

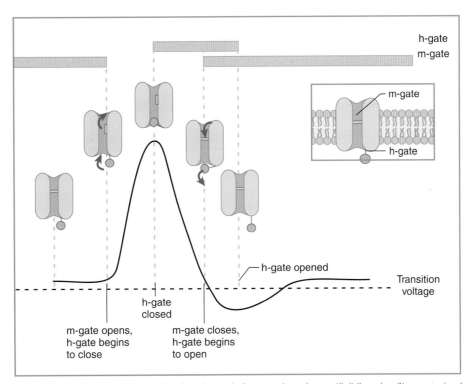

Fig. 11.5 The dual gating of the sodium ion channel. At rest, the primary ("sliding door") m-gate is closed while the secondary ("ball-and-chain") h-gate is closed. While open, both gates are open, allowing flux to occur. While inactivated, the secondary h-gate is closed and prevents further flux, despite the open primary m-gate. (From Carroll R. *Elsevier's Integrated Physiology*. Philadelphia: Mosby Elsevier; 2007. Fig. 4.15.)

recruitment for a second action potential; they are said to be refractory to another threshold-level stimulus.

- The duration of time spent in the inactivated state determines the cellular excitability.
- In nerve and muscle cells, this refractory period is very short—that is, cells recover from the inactivated to the closed (resting) state quickly—whereas in cardiac cells, this period is more prolonged.

- This difference prevents tetany in the myocardium, as discussed later.

In actuality, membrane voltage does not have total control over the sodium channels. They open, close, and inactivate all the time at random (see Genetics Box 11.1, Development Box 11.1 and Pharmacology Box 11.1). The effect of membrane voltage is to skew the probability that a given channel will be in a given state.

GENETICS BOX 11.1

Patients with Brugada syndrome have ventricular arrhythmias that can lead to syncope and cardiac arrest. The disease is a paradigmatic channelopathy. Nearly one-third of patients have a mutation in the SCN5A gene that encodes the alpha subunit of a cardiomyocyte voltage-gated sodium channel. The mutations impair the flow of Na^+ into cardiac cells and dysregulate membrane depolarization and thus action potential generation in cardiomyocytes.

DEVELOPMENT BOX 11.1

The most severe manifestation of Brugada syndrome is sudden death from ventricular fibrillation. Although this can occur at any age, and may be a cause of sudden infant death syndrome (SIDS), the disease typically leads to cardiac arrest in middle aged adults. Because Brugada syndrome can lead to seizures, dyspnea, and ventricular fibrillation when patients are asleep, it is also known as sudden unexplained nocturnal death syndrome (SUNDS).

PHARMACOLOGY BOX 11.1

For patients with Brugada syndrome who have survived a ventricular arrhythmia leading to cardiac arrest, the best treatment appears to be an implantable cardiac defibrillator (ICD). In some situations, either in addition to ICD placement or instead of it, patients can be treated with the antiarrhythmics quinidine and amiodarone. Quinidine, counterintuitively, inhibits Na^+ influx in phase 0 of cardiomyocyte depolarization, as well as K^+ and Ca^{2+} flux across the membrane, leading to slower action potential conduction, myocyte contractility, and thus cell excitability.

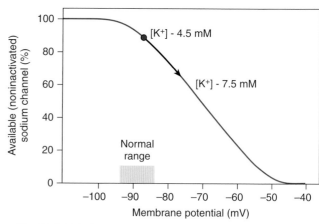

Fig. 11.6 Na^+ channel inactivation versus membrane potential.

TABLE 11.2 Membrane Potential and Effect on Voltage-Gated Sodium Channel Availability

Membrane Potential	Sodium Channel State	Result
< -80 mV	Mostly not inactivated	Available for recruitment
> -65 mV	~75% inactivated	Too few channels available to generate action potential
-65 mV to -80 mV	35%–65% of channels available	Abnormally slow conduction of action potential

It is clear from patch-clamp experiments (techniques that investigate the dynamics of individual ion channels under various electrochemical conditions) that depolarization affects the probability that any given sodium channel will be open or closed (Fig. 11.6 and Table 11.2) (see Clinical Correlation Box 11.2).

Clinical Correlation Box 11.2

If there is poor blood flow to the myocardium, impaired oxygen delivery and glucose prevents adequate generation of adenosine triphosphate (ATP). This prevents proper functioning of the Na^+,K^+-ATPase, which then erodes the normal concentration gradient for K^+ and thus leads to K^+ efflux. This causes mild depolarization that does not reach threshold, and thus causes sodium channel inactivation. This prevents proper action potential generation, leading to slow conduction in ischemic tissue. This can then cause abnormal heart rhythms.

As sodium channels rapidly inactivate, phase 1 begins as transiently activated potassium channels open, leading to gradual efflux of K^+ and repolarization to around 0 mV.

In phase 2, there is a balance between Ca^{2+} influx and K^+ efflux, causing a "plateau" phase.
- L-type calcium channels begin to open at around -40 mV, but both activation and inactivation occur slowly.
- Recall that Ca^{2+} entry is essential to trigger myocyte contraction.

When K^+ efflux exceeds Ca^{2+} influx, phase 3 occurs with return to the resting membrane potential of -90 mV (see Clinical Correlation Box 11.3).

Clinical Correlation Box 11.3

Hyperkalemia, a state of elevated serum potassium, can lead to cardiac rhythm disturbances and sudden death. Why?
- Elevated $[K]_E \rightarrow$ elevated resting membrane potential
  - $[K]_E = 7.5$ mM (normal: 4.0 mM) $\rightarrow E_k = -76.9$ mV (normal: -94 mV)
- Depolarization $\rightarrow$ inactivation of voltage-gated sodium channels $\rightarrow$ cell becomes less excitable $\rightarrow$ smaller amplitude and slower upstroke during phase 0
- AP duration prolonged and ventricular contraction slowed (broad QRS complex on ECG).
- Higher likelihood that aberrant cardiac rhythms can arise because of interruption of normal cardiac conduction.

AP, Action potential; *ECG*, electrocardiogram.

The Ionic Basis of the Slow Response

In cells that exhibit the slow response, such as those in the pacemaker regions of the heart (SA/AV nodes), the action potential consists of only three phases (Fig. 11.7):
- Phase 0
- Phase 3
- Phase 4

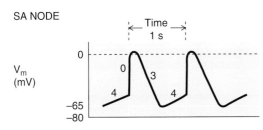

Fig. 11.7 Phases of the slow-response action potential. (From Boron W, Boulpaep E. *Medical Physiology*. 3rd ed. Philadelphia: Saunders Elsevier; 2017. Fig. 21.4a.)

In phase 0, the rapid upstroke is absent because of absence of fast voltage-gated sodium channels.

- Upstroke is instead caused by gradual influx of Ca^{2+} through voltage-gated calcium channels.
- Slow conduction velocity allows for slow transmission from atria→ventricles.

In phase 3, Ca^{2+} channel inactivation leads to predominant K^+ efflux, as in fast response.

The crucial difference between pacemaker cells and fast conduction fibers, however, is in phase 4 of the action potential.

- Pacemaker cells possess a special class of sodium channels allowing for a gradual sodium "leak" inwards during repolarization.
- This produces the I_f, or "funny current" leads to gradual depolarization to threshold value.
- Accounts for automaticity of SA and AV nodes.

Antiarrhythmic Medications

This basic explanation of the action potential is sufficient to understand the mechanism of action of several of the antiarrhythmic drugs, and to explain the genesis of the most common types of cardiac arrhythmias observed in the clinical setting (Table 11.3).

Cardiac Conduction

With the ionic basis of conduction in mind, we can now look at the big picture: myocardial contraction.

Under normal circumstances, the initial impulse for cardiac contraction begins in the SA node, which depolarizes spontaneously in a rhythmic fashion based on the action of the pacemaker sodium currents described earlier.

- The rate of this depolarization is influenced by the balance between adrenergic (sympathetic) and cholinergic (parasympathetic) tone in the body.
  - Stress → ↑ adrenergic tone → ↑ rate of sinus node depolarization → ↑ heart rate (HR).

- Drugs or physiologic maneuvers (carotid massage) → ↑ vagal tone → suppresses sinus rate (see Clinical Correlation Box 11.4).

> **Clinical Correlation Box 11.4**
>
> Because the upstroke of the action potential in pacemaker cells is primarily dependent on the influx of calcium (not sodium) during phase 0, calcium-channel blocking agents (e.g., verapamil and diltiazem) also have the effect of slowing nodal conduction, thereby blocking transmission of impulses to the ventricles and reducing the heart rate.

From the SA node, the cardiac impulse spreads rapidly through the atria (fast-response cells).

- The rate of impulse spread is enhanced by the presence of gap junctions between myocardial cells that connect them into an electrical unit.
- Atrial conduction proceeds in an organized fashion from the SA node → atrial cells → AV node.

Conduction is slowed through the AV node, which possesses slow response (pacemaker) cells similar to the SA node.

- This serves as the final pathway for AV conduction in the normal heart.
- Primary pharmacologic target for management of abnormal rapid heart rhythms originating above the AV node, or supraventricular tachyarrhythmias (SVTs).

Nodal blocking agents all exert their antiarrhythmic effects primarily through their actions at the AV node and are therefore useful agents in the acute management of SVTs:

- Calcium channel blockers
- Beta blockers

Impulses filtered through the AV node proceed down the right side of the interventricular septum through the His bundle. The His bundle divides rapidly into right and left bundle branches, which conduct impulses simultaneously to the right and left ventricles.

These divisions give rise to a complex network of Purkinje fibers that conduct impulses through the remainder of the myocardial syncytium.

- Conduction through the Purkinje fibers is exceptionally fast, allowing rapid, nearly simultaneous activation of the entire endocardial surface of the heart, and thereby allowing coordinated ventricular contraction.
- Ventricular depolarization is not truly simultaneous, however, because of the order of impulse spread.

Class	Medication Examples	Mechanism of Action	Phases Affected	Effect
TABLE 11.3	**Antiarrhythmic Medications and Mechanism of Action**			
I	Quinidine, procainamide, lidocaine	Voltage-gated sodium channel inhibition	0, 3 (fast)	Slow depolarization and raise threshold
II	Metoprolol, propranolol, esmolol	Beta-adrenergic receptor inhibition	4 (slow)	Decrease SA/AV nodal activity and suppress abnormal pacemakers
III	Amiodarone, sotalol	Potassium channel inhibition	3 (fast)	Prolonged AP duration and repolarization
IV	Verapamil, diltiazem	L-type calcium channel inhibition	0, 4 (slow)	Reduced conduction velocity, prolonged repolarization

AP, Action potential; *AV*, atrioventricular; *SA*, sinoatrial.

- The septum depolarizes first, from left to right, simultaneously with the papillary muscles.
- Impulses spread along the epicardial surface through the thickness of the myocardium of both ventricles.
- This causes depolarization of the thinner right ventricle before the left.

Surface Electrocardiography

The pattern of normal impulse spread through the heart can be observed clinically through the use of the scalar electrocardiogram (ECG).

This is possible because electrical current is generated by directional propagation of depolarization and hyperpolarization down a cell (Fig. 11.8).

- When areas of the cell depolarize, the cell surface in that region becomes negatively charged relative to the cell interior.

- When the cell is completely depolarized, the surface is homogenously charged and thus does not generate current.
- When areas of the cell repolarize, the cell surface in that region becomes positively charged relative to the cell interior.

Thus we can measure the electrical current generated by the heart using 10 standard electrodes placed at well-defined points on the body surface (Fig. 11.9).

- From the four limb electrodes, six "leads"—the electrical activity between specific electrodes—can be produced (Table 11.4).
  - Unipolar leads (aVF, aVR, aVF) compare a single electrode to the average of the other limb electrodes.
  - Bipolar leads (I, II, III) compare two electrodes.
- A complete ECG is thus generally referred to as a 12-lead ECG.

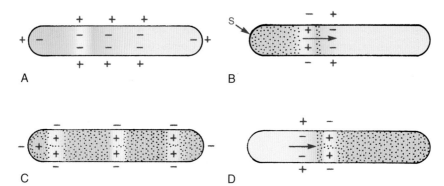

Fig. 11.8 Effect of depolarization and repolarization on electrical current. Recall that electrical current flows from negatively charged to positively charged areas. A, The resting heart muscle cell is polarized; that is, it carries an electrical charge, with the outside of the cell positively charged and the inside negatively charged. B, When the cell is stimulated *(S)*, it begins to depolarize (stippled area). C, The fully depolarized cell is positively charged on the inside and negatively charged on the outside. D, Repolarization occurs when the stimulated cell returns to the resting state. The directions of depolarization and repolarization are represented by *arrows*. Depolarization (stimulation) of the atria produces the P wave on the electrocardiogram, whereas depolarization of the ventricles produces the QRS complex. Repolarization of the ventricles produces the ST-T complex. (From. Goldberger A, Goldberger Z, Shvilkin A. *Goldberger's Clinical Electrocardiography: A Simplified Approach*, 9th Edition. Elsevier; 2018. Fig. 2.1.)

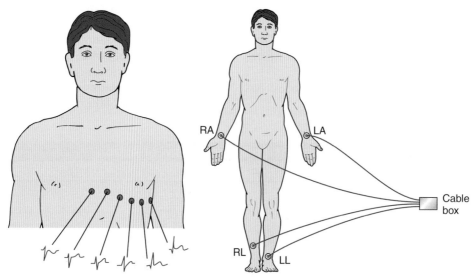

Fig. 11.9 Standard placement of the electrocardiogram (ECG) electrodes. *LA*, Left arm; *LL*, left leg; *RA*, right arm; *RL*, right leg. (From. Goldberger A, Goldberger Z, Shvilkin A. *Goldberger's Clinical Electrocardiography: A Simplified Approach*, 9th Edition. Elsevier; 2018. Figs. 4.1 and 4.3.)

TABLE 11.4 Relationship of Limb Leads to Electrodes

Lead	(+) Electrode	(−) Electrode
aVL	LA	Average of others
aVR	RA	Average of others
aVF	LL	Average of others
I	LA	RA
II	LL	RA
III	LL	LA

LA, Left arm; *LL*, left leg; *RA*, right arm.

Each lead serves as a slightly different vantage point from which to view conduction through the heart. The standard positions of the leads can be divided into two groups:
1. The first group includes the limb leads (I, II, III, aVL, aVR, aVF).
   a. Records myocardial depolarization in the frontal plane—that is, in a coronal plane cutting the body from head to foot.
   b. See Fig. 11.10A.
2. The second group includes the precordial leads (V1–V6).
   a. Records myocardial depolarization in the horizontal (or axial) plane.
   b. See Fig. 11.10B.

In this way, the 12-lead ECG gives the clinician a picture of cardiac conduction that exposes the pattern and timing of depolarization and repolarization of the various portions of the heart.

ECG recording will reveal both direction and magnitude of each electrical impulse:
- When depolarization proceeds in the direction of a given lead, a positive (upward) deflection is recorded on the tracing.
- When depolarization proceeds away from a given lead, a negative (downward) deflection is recorded.
- The more parallel the electrical activity is to the axis of the lead, the greater its magnitude of deflection.
- A perpendicular force to a given lead will not generate any deflection.

Repolarization produces opposite deflections. However, the cell generally repolarizes in the opposite direction as depolarization. Thus for a given area of the heart, depolarization and repolarization tend to produce deflections in the same direction on the ECG tracing.

The standard pattern seen on the ECG tracing during each cardiac cycle takes the form shown in Figs. 11.11 and 11.12. Each deflection from the baseline represents a distinct event in cardiac conduction.

The first hump, or P wave, represents atrial depolarization, which normally proceeds from the SA to the AV node (roughly in a line from the right shoulder to the left foot) in the direction of lead II and opposite that of lead aVR.
- Positive deflection in leads I, II, and aVF.
- Negative deflection in lead aVR.

The PR interval, measured from the onset of the P wave to the beginning of the QRS complex (see later), represents the time it takes for a stimulus initiated in the atrium to proceed through the AV junction to the ventricle. It is isoelectric (see Clinical Correlation Box 11.5).

Clinical Correlation Box 11.5

When conduction through the atrioventricular node is prolonged, the PR interval may also be prolonged, a condition known as first-degree heart block.

The QRS complex signifies ventricular depolarization.
- Q wave
  - As noted previously, impulses arriving from the AV node pass into the ventricles via the His bundle.
  - Because the His bundle travels down the interventricular septum, septal depolarization occurs first, with the left side of the septum being stimulated slightly before the right.
    V6, the lead representing the left side of the heart, shows a small negative deflection (a negative Q wave).
    V1, the lead representing the right side of the heart, will not show this in normal states.
- R wave
  - Conduction proceeds down left and right bundle branches.
  - Simultaneous activation of left and right ventricles.
  - Electrically dominant event is the left-sided depolarization because of thicker, large left ventricle.
    Strong positive deflection (R wave) in left-sided leads (V5/V6).
    R wave becomes progressively larger from leads V1 to V6 (corresponding to placement of the leads relative to the path of left ventricular depolarization).
- S wave
  - Represents final depolarization at the base of the heart. Primarily right ventricle.
  - Negative deflection (S wave) in the left-sided leads (V5/V6) (see Clinical Correlation Box 11.6).

Clinical Correlation Box 11.6

A loss of this progressive R wave transition is seen in myocardial death, and therefore reduced magnitude of ventricular electrical depolarization and contraction. Hence, a loss of *R* wave progression is one cardinal electrocardiogram manifestation of a heart attack in the anterior wall of the left ventricle, clinically termed a myocardial infarction.

Following ventricular contraction and the end of the QRS complex, there is a second isoelectric period known as the ST segment (measured from the end of the QRS complex to the beginning of the T wave).
- Interval between ventricular depolarization and repolarization.
- Deviations in this segment above or below baseline are seen in myocardial ischemia and infarction, and analysis of the ST segment forms the main basis for the ECG diagnosis of those two entities.

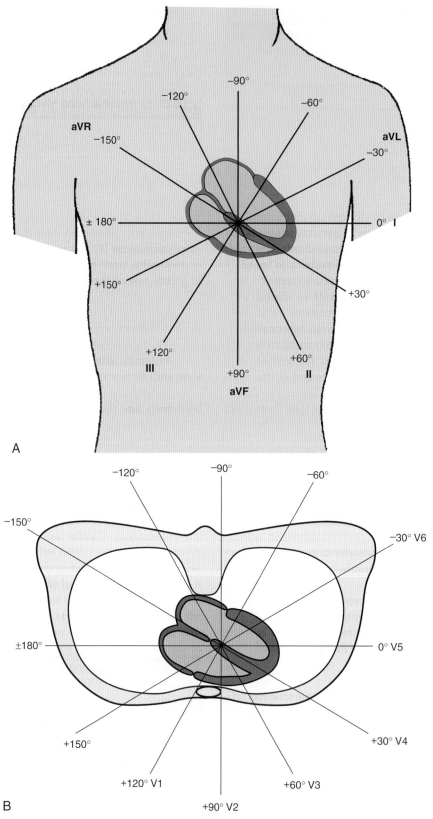

Fig. 11.10 Orientation of electrocardiogram (ECG) leads. A, Each of the six limb leads measures cardiac conduction in the frontal plane. B, Each of the six precordial leads measures cardiac conduction in the horizontal plane. (From Saksena S, Camm JA. *Electrophysiological Disorders of the Heart*, 2nd Ed. Philadelphia: Elsevier; 2011. Figs. 10.2 and 10.4.)

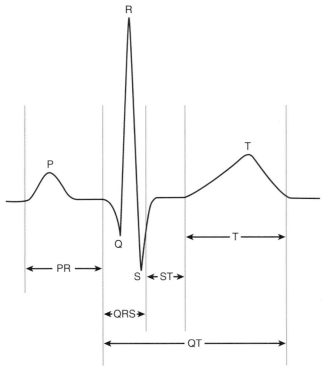

Fig. 11.11 The schematic tracing shows the standard pattern of a cardiac cycle during electrocardiogram (ECG) recording.

The ECG cycle concludes with ventricular repolarization, recorded as the T wave. The duration of the electrical interval from the onset of the QRS complex to the end of the T wave is called the QT interval, a measure of the length of time required for the ventricles to return to their resting state.

The surface ECG reflects the summation of all the action potentials going on simultaneously in individual cells within the myocardium.

- The P wave represents the summation of atrial phase 0 and phase 1 depolarization.
- Atrial repolarization (phases 2 and 3 of the atrial action potential) happens simultaneously with ventricular depolarization and is therefore hidden in the QRS complex.
- For the ventricles, phase 0 and phase 1 of the action potential initiate ventricular contraction and are depicted in the QRS complex.
- The plateau phase (phase 2) of ventricular cells is primarily expressed in the ST segment.
- Repolarization (phase 3) of ventricular cells is reflected in the T wave.

Fig. 11.13 shows an example of a normal surface ECG as recorded in a clinical setting.

PATHOPHYSIOLOGY

As normal cardiac electrophysiology depends on the two functions of automaticity and conduction, arrhythmias arise from either:

- Faulty automaticity
- Faulty conduction

Both of these defects can result from a variety of insults to the myocardium.

Faulty Automaticity

Abnormal automaticity occurs when myocardial tissue outside the nodes begins to drive myocardial contraction. Allows latent pacemaker tissue to escape control. Causes include:

- Slow SA node.
- Ectopic automaticity arises with rate greater than SA node.

One mechanism leading to ectopic beats is after depolarization, in which an increase in Na^+ conductance in myocardial tissue allows depolarization to occur during the refractory period. This leads to extra beats.

Faulty Conduction

Conduction abnormalities include:

- Slowed conduction because of tissue injury.
- Blocked conduction because of tissue injury.
- Bypass tracts, which are alternative conductive pathways, may be present.

A particular type of arrhythmia that can occur in the presence of blocked conduction is a reentrant rhythm. In this situation, unidirectional blocked conduction leads to loops of excitation, mimicking an ectopic pacemaker.

Diagnosing Arrhythmias

The ECG is an important means of diagnosing cardiac arrhythmias.

- Under normal circumstances, as described, a P wave precedes each QRS complex, and a QRS complex follows every P wave.
- This pattern is called normal sinus rhythm.
- This signifies impulses originating in the SA node and proceeding in the familiar fashion to the AV node and then to the ventricles to initiate myocardial contraction.

When conduction begins lower down in the conduction system owing to ectopic or escape rhythms, however, the ECG will likely reflect this aberrant conduction.

- Example: Junctional rhythms
  - Impulses originate below the AV node.
  - Atrial and ventricular depolarization thus occur simultaneously (spreading from this junction).
  - P waves would be hidden within the electrically dominant QRS complex.
  - The ECG would thus display a junctional rhythm, with absent (or perhaps retrograde P waves, because of the reversal of atrial depolarization direction) and regular QRS complexes.

Similarly, the duration of the various intervals on the ECG gives insight into potential defects in the conduction system.

- Prolonged PR signifies slowed conduction through the AV node.
- Widened QRS complex is associated with defects in the ventricular conduction pathways.
- Prolonged QT interval signifies prolonged ventricular repolarization.

The ECG is thus a powerful tool in the clinical analysis of cardiac conduction and a window into the electrical events occurring at the cellular level in the myocardium.

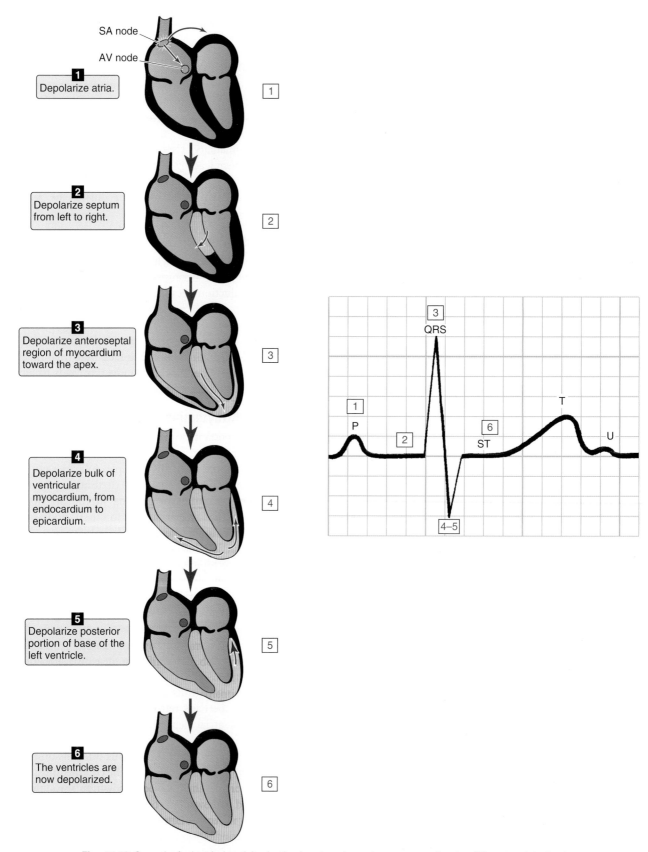

Fig. 11.12 Spread of electrical activity in the heart and events corresponding to different points in the electrocardiogram (ECG). *AV,* Atrioventricular; *SA,* sinoatrial. (Left, from Boron W, Boulpaep E. *Medical Physiology.* 3rd ed. Philadelphia: Saunders Elsevier; 2017. Fig. 21.5. Right, from *Goldberger's Clinical Electrocardiography: A Simplified Approach,* 9th Ed. Philadelphia: Elsevier; 2018. Fig. 2.2.)

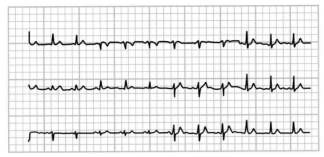

Fig. 11.13 A normal 12-lead electrocardiogram (ECG). This is an actual ECG, recorded in the clinic.

SUMMARY

- The rhythm of electrical discharge underlying cardiac contractions depends on two attributes of the myocardium: automaticity (the capacity to generate action potentials at regular intervals independent of outside influences) and conduction (the capacity to transmit action potentials along prescribed routes).

- The excitatory signal (action potential) for cardiac contraction begins in the SA node, passes to the atrial walls, and then reaches the AV node. The AV node possesses automaticity, but its intrinsic firing rate is slower than that of the SA node, so the SA node sets the pace of AV firing. From the AV node, the excitatory impulse moves into the His bundle in the interventricular septum and then into the Purkinje fibers, and finally into the whole ventricular myocardium.

- The equilibrium resting potential of myocardial cell membranes is –90 mV. The resting potential is determined by the diffusion of K^+ out of the cell, leaving behind negative charge inside the cell. The equilibrium resting potential reflects a balance of chemical and electrostatic forces.

- Conduction is effected by fast-response action potentials. Automaticity is affected by slow-response action potentials. Both types of action potentials proceed in phases.

  Phase 0: Depolarization. In fast action potentials, massive Na^+ influx follows depolarization to threshold. In slow ones, Ca^{2+} influx follows threshold.

  Phase 1: Repolarization begins as K^+ efflux increases.

  Phase 2: Plateau. Na^+ channel inactivation begins and Ca^{2+} influx maintains depolarization.

  Phase 3: Repolarization. K^+ efflux exceeds Ca^{2+} influx as Ca^{2+} channels inactivate.

  Phase 4: In the fast action potential of conduction, this phase represents a return to resting potential. In the slow action potential of pacemaker tissue, phase 4 includes an automatic depolarization, by a Na^+ influx called the pacemaker sodium current, that will lead to threshold and another action potential.

- The ECG measures cardiac conduction through 12 leads. When depolarization proceeds in the direction of a given lead, a positive (upward) deflection is recorded on the tracing, and when it proceeds away from a given lead, a negative (downward) deflection is recorded.

- The P wave is atrial depolarization, which normally initiates atrial contraction.

- The PR interval is transmission through the AV node.

- The QRS complex is ventricular depolarization, which normally initiates ventricular contraction. Atrial repolarization also occurs at this time, hidden in the QRS.

- The ST segment, if abnormally depressed or elevated, may reflect myocardial ischemia or infarction.

- The T wave is ventricular repolarization.

- Abnormal automaticity occurs when latent pacemakers escape from the control of a slowed SA node or when ectopic pacemakers outstrip the SA pace.

- Abnormal conduction may take the form of slowed conduction, blocked conduction, or bypass tracts. Unidirectional block may create a reentrant arrhythmia.

REVIEW QUESTION

1. A 54-year-old woman with renal failure is found to have a serum K^+ level of 8 mM. Her ECG shows wide QRS complexes. Cardiac conduction in this woman's heart is:
   A. Fast, because of bypass tracts
   B. Slow, because of high resting potential
   C. Fast, because of low resting potential
   D. Slow, because of Ca^{2+} channel blockade in the AV node
   E. Slow, because of first-degree AV block

ANSWER TO REVIEW QUESTION

1. **The answer is B.** The woman has hyperkalemia secondary to decreased renal clearance of K^+. Increased plasma K^+ prevents normal K^+ efflux and raises the resting potential of the myocardium. This inactivates Na^+ channels and impairs conduction, reflected in the long (slow) QRS ventricular depolarization. Slow conduction can lead to a variety of serious and unstable arrhythmias.

12

Exercise Physiology

INTRODUCTION

Whether running a marathon or toting a hefty biochemistry book up a staircase, exercising muscle places demand on the body through three mechanisms:

- Increased oxygen and nutrient demand
- Increased waste products of metabolism
- Increased heat generation

The cardiovascular, respiratory, and temperature-regulating systems of the body must adapt to meet the demands of exercising muscles.

SYSTEM FUNCTION

For a discussion of system structure, please refer to Chapters 9 to 11 (cardiovascular system) and Part V (respiratory system).

As previously mentioned, exercise adaptions fall into three main categories:

1. Cardiovascular adaptations
2. Respiratory adaptations
3. Temperature adaptations

Basic Concepts

Isotonic and Isometric Exercise

There are two main types of muscle exercise (Fig. 12.1):

- Isotonic exercise occurs when contracting muscle shortens against a constant load.
- Isometric exercise occurs when contracting muscle increases tension while maintaining its length.

Many common movements and exercises have both an isometric and an isotonic component. The mechanisms described later generally to dynamic exercise (e.g., marathon running) but not to isometric exercise (e.g., weight lifting) (see Fast Fact Box 12.1).

Fast Fact Box 12.1

During sustained forceful isotonic muscle contraction, increased intramuscular pressure can exceed the systolic blood pressure, preventing adequate blood flow from reaching the exercising tissues. Despite the body's other cardiovascular adaptations, this roadblock to oxygen and nutrient delivery to tissues during isometric exercise quickly leads to muscle fatigue.

Performance Measurements

The index of human fitness is maximal oxygen consumption or VO_2 max, expressed in L O_2/min. Its three major determinants include:

- Cardiac output.
- Oxygen carrying capacity of the blood.
- Amount of exercising muscle and ability to use oxygen (i.e., type I fibers) (see Fast Fact Box 12.2).

Fast Fact Box 12.2

Note that only the first determinant, cardiac output, may be changed acutely.

At VO_2 max, there can be no further increase in oxygen uptake despite increases in workload (Fig. 12.2).

- Work can briefly be sustained by anaerobic metabolism.
- This results in lactic acid build-up and prolonged increased oxygen consumption in recovery.

Trained athletes have a significantly higher VO_2 max compared with untrained athletes (Table 12.1).

Cardiovascular Adaptations to Exercise

During exercise, the cardiovascular system undergoes several adaptations to augment its usual function in delivery of oxygen and nutrients and removal of waste products of metabolism. These are summarized in Table 12.2.

Cardiac Output

Recall that, at rest, cardiac output is about 5 L/min. Exercise states are characterized by increased cardiac output, because of increases in both heart rate (HR) and stroke volume (SV). These occur by the following mechanisms:

- Increased HR
  - Diminished parasympathetic outflow to the sinoatrial (SA) node and increased sympathetic activity.
- Increased SV
  - Enhanced sympathetic stimulation of the ventricular myocardium, which boosts the heart's contractility.
  - A modest increase in end-diastolic volume during exercise also contributes, via the Frank-Starling mechanism.

Changes in parasympathetic and sympathetic tone during exercise are mediated by both central and peripheral nervous system (CNS and PNS):

- CNS
  - Anticipation or awareness of exercise.

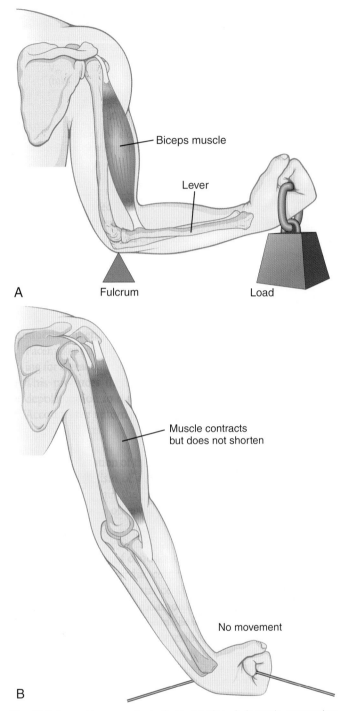

Fig. 12.1 Isometric versus isotonic contraction. A, Isotonic contraction causes muscle to shorten while contracting against a fixed load. B, Isometric contraction increases tension while maintaining muscle length. (A, from Hall JE. *Guyton and Hall Textbook of Medical Physiology*, 13th Ed. Philadelphia: Elsevier; 2015. Fig. 6.16.)

- PNS
  - Mechanoreceptors and chemoreceptors in muscles.
  - Baroreceptors in the carotid sinus and aortic arch. "Reset" to higher baseline pressure during exercise. This means that the body can have increased mean arterial pressure (MAP) relative to baseline without reduction of sympathetic outflow (Fig. 12.3).

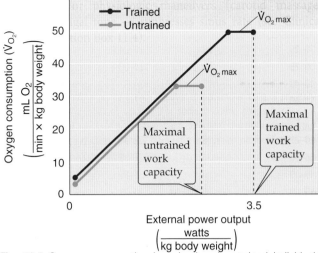

Fig. 12.2 Oxygen consumption in trained and untrained individuals. Note that exercise training increases both maximal work capacity and the corresponding VO₂ max. Muscle work depends on oxygen consumption, but training increases that capacity and thus increases the work that can be accomplished. (From Boron W, Boulpaep E. *Medical Physiology*, 3rd Edition. Elsevier; 2017. Fig. 60.6.)

Increased cardiac output during exercise is primarily a function of HR, which increases with exercise intensity until it reaches a plateau at around 180 beats per minute (see Fast Fact Box 12.3).

Fast Fact Box 12.3

Maximum heart rate = 220 − age (approximately)

Although SV can nearly double in extremely well-trained endurance athletes, in most people it increases only 10% to 35% and reaches its maximal level at a lower intensity of exercise than HR does (Fig. 12.4).

Peripheral Resistance

During exercise, total peripheral resistance decreases, which reduces afterload and contributes to increased SV.

In certain areas, sympathetic activation leads to vasoconstriction and increased resistance, causing decreased blood flow during exercise. These include:
- Splanchnic and renal vasculature
- Vasculature supplying inactive muscles

Meanwhile, resistance in terminal arterioles supplying exercising muscles decreases markedly because of the release of vasoactive substances including:
- Potassium
- Adenosine (a by-product of adenosine triphosphate [ATP] metabolism)
- Lactic acid (a by-product of anaerobic glycolysis)

Blood flow through these vessels can increase up to 25 times over the level at rest. In addition, through the phenomenon of capillary recruitment, blood flows through many muscle capillaries that are not perfused at rest.

Finally, blood flow to the skin initially decreases, owing to sympathetic vasoconstriction, and then increases as body temperature rises (see Fast Fact Box 12.4).

TABLE 12.1 VO₂max Norms Stratified by Age and Gender

Women	Low	Fair	Avg	Good	High	Athletic	Olympic
20–29	<28	29–34	35–43	44–48	49–53	54–59	60+
30–29	<27	28–33	34–41	42–47	48–52	53–58	59+
40–49	<25	26–31	32–40	41–45	46–50	51–56	57+
50–65	<21	22–28	29–36	37–41	42–45	46–49	50+
Men							
20–29	<38	39–43	44–51	52–56	57–62	63–69	70+
30–39	<34	35–39	40–47	48–51	52–57	58–64	65+
40–49	<30	31–35	36–43	44–47	48–53	54–60	61+
50–59	<25	26–31	32–39	40–43	44–48	49–55	56+
60–69	<21	22–26	27–35	36–39	40–44	45–49	50+

Note: VO₂max is expressed in tables as milliliters of oxygen per kilogram of body weight per minute.
(Modified from Astrand I. Aerobic work capacity in men and women with special reference to age, *Acta Physiol Scand Suppl*, 1960;49(169):1-92.)

TABLE 12.2 Summary of Cardiovascular Changes in Exercise

Acute	↑ CO (↑ HR and SV)
	↓ total peripheral resistance
	↑ MAP
	↑ pulse pressure
	↑ venous return
Chronic	Heart chamber enlargement
	Myocardial hypertrophy
	↓ peripheral resistance at rest

CO, Cardiac output; *HR*, heart rate; *MAP*, mean arterial pressure; *SV*, stroke volume.

Fast Fact Box 12.4
Blood flow to the brain does not change during exercise.

Arterial Pressure

Arterial pressure is the product of cardiac output and total peripheral resistance. Recall:
- Total peripheral resistance decreases during exercise.
- Cardiac output increases during exercise.

The cardiac output dominates the response, resulting in an increase of up to 30% in MAP during exercise. Furthermore, because of rapid left-ventricular contraction, systolic pressure increases more than diastolic pressure, resulting in an increased pulse pressure.

Venous Return

To maintain an increased cardiac output during exercise, blood must return more rapidly from the venous circulation to the heart. This increased venous return is caused by four factors:
1. ↑ venous blood pumped toward the heart from compression of veins by muscle contractions.
2. ↑ negative thoracic pressure caused by greater depth and frequency of inspiration, which draws blood back toward the thorax.

3. ↑ sympathetic nervous system tone, resulting in ↑ venoconstriction (i.e., venous tone).
4. ↑ flow of blood from arteries to veins through dilated skeletal muscle arterioles.

A failure to maintain sufficient venous return—in a case of dehydration, for example, when sufficient blood volume is simply lacking—can result in decreased delivery of blood to tissues, and therefore decreased exercise ability (see Genetics Box 12.1, Development Box 12.1, and Pharmacology Box 12.1).

 PHARMACOLOGY BOX 12.1

Pharmacologic treatment of familial hypertrophic cardiomyopathy includes the use of β-adrenergic antagonists (e.g., metoprolol and atenolol), nondihydropyridine calcium channel blockers (such as verapamil) and disopyramide. Their common effects believed to be helpful are reduction of inotropy. In addition, some such drugs may reduce myocardial oxygen demand and increase cardiac blood flow.

 DEVELOPMENT BOX 12.1

Progressive hypertrophy of the interventricular septum can lead to left ventricular outflow obstruction and thus a loss of cardiac output and blood pressure. In addition, patients with familial hypertrophic cardiomyopathy are at an increased risk for arrhythmias. In trained athletes, in whom there is physiologic hypertrophy because of chronic exercise, familial hypertrophic cardiomyopathy may collude to bring about sudden, profound hypotension leading to syncope during exercise with attendant increased inotropy.

GENETICS BOX 12.1

Precisely because exercise has numerous health benefits, we are shocked when we learn that a young person in great shape has died suddenly while exercising. Some such deaths are caused by familial hypertrophic cardiomyopathy, a disease characterized by thickening of myocardial tissue, especially the interventricular septum. Up to one-third of patients have a mutation in the MYH7 gene that encodes the β myosin chain of type II myosin. Thickening of myocardia tissue can lead to diastolic dysfunction and mitral regurgitation manifested as dyspnea.

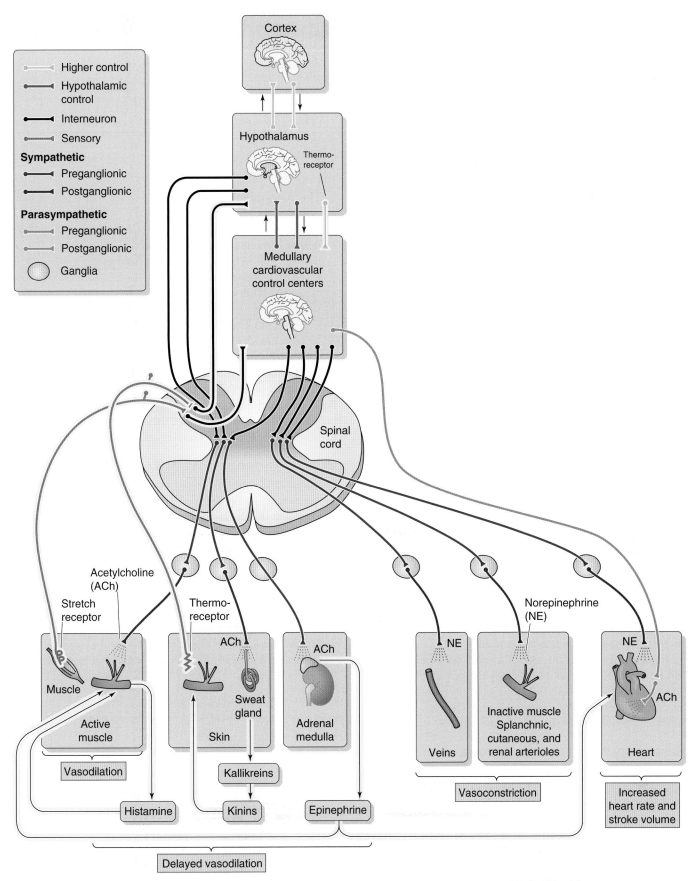

Fig. 12.3 Control of the cardiovascular response to exercise. (From Boron W, Boulpaep E. *Medical Physiology*. 3rd ed. Philadelphia: Saunders Elsevier; 2017. Fig. 25.7.)

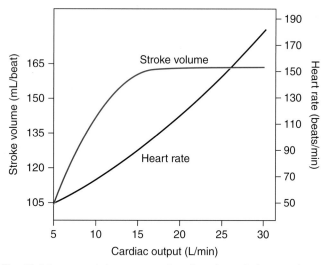

Fig. 12.4 Increases in heart rate and stroke volume during exercise.

The Effects of Chronic Exercise on Cardiovascular Function

Chronic endurance exercise results in:
- Enlargement of the chambers of the heart.
- Hypertrophy of the myocardium.
- Lower total peripheral resistance at rest.

In addition, at rest, the cardiac output of a well-trained endurance athlete equals that of an untrained person. Compared with the untrained person, however, the athlete can achieve this level with a lower HR and a greater SV.

In comparison, chronic isometric exercise results in myocardial hypertrophy but not chamber enlargement. Thus it does not lead to a change in resting HR and SV.

Cardiovascular Limitations on Exercise Capacity

During intense exercise, cardiac output rises to nearly 90% of its maximal level, both HR and SV increasing to nearly 95% of their maximal levels. At the same time, pulmonary ventilation increases to only just over half its maximal level.

It is the cardiovascular system, therefore rather than the pulmonary system, that limits the body's maximal oxygen consumption (VO_2 max) and therefore its ability to exercise. This cardiovascular limitation on exercise ability holds true for both untrained people and trained endurance athlete.

Respiratory Adaptations to Exercise

During exercise, the respiratory system performs the same function—regulating levels of oxygen and carbon dioxide in the blood—as it does when the body is at rest. However, given the changes in blood flow rate and chemical composition of the blood, the respiratory system must make several adaptations. These are summarized in Box 12.1.

Increased Inspiratory Rate and Volume

CNS input leads to increased minute ventilation via:
- ↑ respiratory rate.
- ↑ tidal volume.

This preemptively prevents changes in blood levels of oxygen and carbon dioxide with exercise.

CNS stimulation occurs through several mechanisms (Fig. 12.5):
- Release of epinephrine and potassium
- Central and peripheral receptors sensitive to:
  - Physical movement
  - Temperature changes
  - Blood flow
  - Blood gas concentrations in muscles and the mixed venous blood

As a result, total minute ventilation of the lungs increases abruptly with the onset of exercise and then increases in proportion to its intensity, up to 20 times that of resting level (see Fig. 12.5). Because it is the cardiac output, not the lungs, that ordinarily limits exercise ability, the minute ventilation reaches a plateau as the body achieves VO_2 max.

Increased Pulmonary Blood Flow

Increased cardiac output leads to increased blood flow through the pulmonary vasculature.

Owing to the low resistance and large capacitance of blood vessels in the lung, this increased flow is accomplished with only a modest increase in the pulmonary vascular pressure.

Blood Gases

The oxygen-diffusing capacity (i.e., the rate at which oxygen can cross the alveolar walls into the blood) increases during exercise.
- Occurs as a result of increased pulmonary blood flow.
- This leads to:
  - Increased number of pulmonary capillaries being perfused.

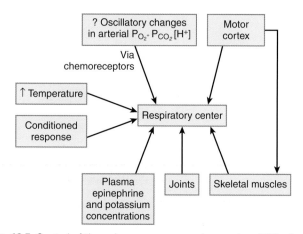

Fig. 12.5 Control of the pulmonary response to exercise. *PCO₂*, Partial pressure of carbon dioxide; *PO₂*, partial pressure of oxygen.

- Diminishing ventilation perfusion (V/Q) mismatches present in the resting lung.

The overall effect of exercise on blood gases is shown in Fig. 12.6.

- Arterial partial pressure of carbon dioxide (PCO_2).
  - Alveolar PCO_2 determines arterial PCO_2.
  - Alveolar PCO_2 is itself a function of the ratio of CO_2 production to alveolar ventilation, which remains constant during moderate exercise.
  - Thus: while venous PCO_2 increases during exercise, alveolar and arterial PCO_2 levels remain relatively constant.
    In fact, during intense exercise—when anaerobic metabolism results in the release of lactic acid into the bloodstream, increasing H^+ and stimulating hyperventilation— alveolar and arterial PCO_2 levels decrease.
- Arterial partial pressure of oxygen (PO_2).
  - Constant during exercise, owing to increased alveolar ventilation, pulmonary blood flow, and oxygen diffusion capacity.
  - In contrast, venous PO_2 decreases.

Because of exercising muscles and other tissues consuming a greater amount of O_2 from the arterial blood to maintain ATP production necessary for continued exertion (i.e., the body approaches VO_2 max).

During intense exercise, the increased production of CO_2 and lactic acid by anaerobic metabolism results in an increase in arterial H^+ (i.e., a lower arterial pH). This surplus of arterial H^+ helps provoke the hyperventilation that accompanies intense exercise.

Temperature Adaptations

Heat is produced during exercise by two mechanisms:

- By-product of metabolic reactions.
- Friction in muscles, joints, and the walls of blood vessels.

All of this heat must be dissipated for the body to maintain thermal homeostasis. To accomplish this, the body uses the following adaptations:

- Sweating
  - Sympathetic-mediated process in which sweat glands actively secrete sweat to the skin surface.
  - Evaporation sweat causes the body to lose heat.
- Recruitment of the skin capillaries.
  - Perfusing them allows heat to escape through the skin.

A failure to dissipate heat adequately can lead to heat stroke, a pathologic condition of increased body temperature that can lead to death if untreated. Such a failure of homeostasis can occur in:

- Extremely hot or humid conditions.
- Too much clothing worn.
- Dehydration
  - Causes the body to vasoconstrict cutaneous blood vessels, leading to a decreased sweat output to preserve fluids.

PATHOPHYSIOLOGY

A number of diseases do not manifest with symptoms until the body is stressed, such as with certain drugs such as nitrates that cause venodilation and thus limit preload, volume depletion, during or following exercise. In nitrate syncope, a patient can lose consciousness after taking a nitrate. In familial hypertrophic cardiomyopathy (see the Genetics, Development, and Pharmacology boxes above), athletes often suffer syncope when they pause or stop exercising. An understanding of exercise is important to clinical practice in three respects:

- Exercise tolerance
  - Patients with diseases, such as congestive heart failure, do not tolerate exercise because they cannot increase cardiac output and ventilation in the way that is necessary to meet muscular demand.
  - Low exercise tolerance predicts worse outcomes.
- Exercise injury
  - Exercise puts stresses on the body that in some circumstances may lead to injury even without underlying chronic disease.
- Primary prevention and treatment implications
  - Exercise limits weight gain, maintains bone strength, lowers the risk of atherosclerosis, and has many other benefits.
  - The importance of physical exercise to cardiovascular and general wellbeing is clear, but there is some controversy surrounding what type of exercise and how much is protective.

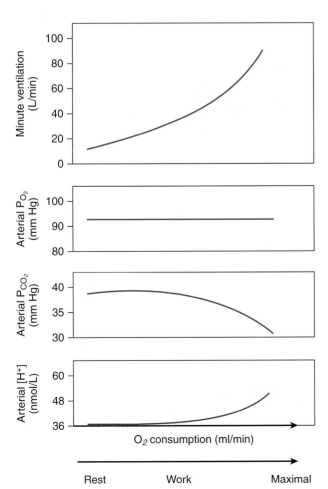

Fig. 12.6 Ventilation, blood gases, and blood acidity during exercise. *PCO₂*, Partial pressure of carbon dioxide; *PO₂*, partial pressure of oxygen.

SUMMARY

The muscles' increased demand for oxygen and nutrients drives the cardiac and respiratory changes seen in exercise.
- Maximal oxygen consumption or VO_2 max is the index of human fitness.
- Isotonic exercise occurs when contracting muscle shortens against a constant load. Isometric exercise occurs when contracting muscle increases tension while maintaining its length.
- Mechanoreceptors and chemoreceptors in muscles detect the increased muscular demand and communicate it to the brain, which increases sympathetic output and decreases parasympathetic output.
- $\uparrow$ HR and SV $\rightarrow$ $\uparrow$ CO during exercise.

- $\downarrow$ vascular resistance in skeletal muscle beds decreases owing to local factors that override the sympathetic activation (i.e., functional sympatholysis) and $\downarrow$ total peripheral resistance.
- $\uparrow$ venous return because of increased venous pressure secondary to muscular flexion, among other causes.
- The cardiovascular system limits muscular oxygen uptake, not the pulmonary system.
- Data from peripheral chemoreceptors and from the cerebral cortex during exercise $\uparrow$ minute ventilation, tidal volume, and respiratory rate.
- Increases in body temperature associated with exercise eventually lead to sweating and vasodilation in the skin.

REVIEW QUESTIONS

Directions: Each of the numbered items or incomplete statements in this section is followed by answers or by completions of the statement. Select the one lettered answer or completion that is best in each case.

1. A 24-year-old woman suffers 3 days of watery diarrhea and then runs a marathon in very hot weather, during which she collapses. If she has collapsed from heat stroke, one reason might be:
   A. She was unable to elevate cardiac stroke volume
   B. She was unable to elevate her heart rate
   C. She was unable to vasodilate the vascular beds in her skin
   D. She was unable to vasodilate the vascular beds in her muscles
   E. She was unable to conduct normal gas exchange
2. Patients with coronary artery disease may suffer angina during exercise because of:
   A. Increased cardiac oxygen supply
   B. Increased cardiac oxygen demand
   C. Increased cardiac production of carbon dioxide
   D. Pulmonary edema
   E. Increased afterload
3. Blood pH may fall during intense exercise from:
   A. Anaerobic metabolism
   B. Aerobic metabolism

   C. Gluconeogenesis
   D. Sweating
   E. Glycogenolysis
4. Which of the following summarizes the effects of exercise on heart rate, stroke volume, and cardiac output, respectively?
   A. $\uparrow, \uparrow, \uparrow$
   B. $\uparrow, \uparrow, \downarrow$
   C. $\uparrow, \downarrow, \downarrow$
   D. $\uparrow, \downarrow, \uparrow$
   E. $\downarrow, \downarrow, \downarrow$
5. Which of the following is not a mechanism for increased venous return during exercise?
   A. Contraction of exercising muscles compresses veins and increases the pumping of venous blood toward the heart
   B. Blood is drawn toward the thorax as a result of increased negative thoracic pressure
   C. An increase in sympathetic nervous system tone results in increased venoconstriction
   D. Dilated skeletal muscle arterioles result in increased flow of blood from arteries to veins
   E. An increase in parasympathetic activity to the sinoatrial node results in venodilation

ANSWERS TO REVIEW QUESTIONS

1. **The answer is C.** Owing to dehydration, the woman was hypotensive. The baroreceptor reflex caused vasoconstriction in the vascular beds in her skin to preserve blood flow to the heart and brain. Vasoconstriction in the skin also had the undesirable effect of preventing cooling of the blood.
2. **The answer is B.** During exercise, increased muscular demand for oxygen leads to increased cardiac output (which in turn increases the flow of oxygenated blood to the muscles). Increased cardiac output requires an increased supply of oxygen to the myocardium. In coronary artery disease, the coronary arteries may not be able to supply the blood and oxygen needed by the myocardium, creating the sensation of angina.

3. **The answer is A.** When muscular demand outstrips the supply of oxygen, the muscles may turn to anaerobic metabolism for energy. Lactic acid is a by-product of anaerobic metabolism. It acidifies the blood, increases the PCO_2, and drives increased respiration by stimulating chemoreceptors.
4. **The answer is A.** Heart rate, stroke volume, and cardiac output will all increase during exercise.
5. **The answer is E.** All of the mechanisms described in choices A, B, C, and D are involved in increasing venous return during exercise. Choice E is incorrect because parasympathetic activity is decreased.

Cardiac Physiology

L.B. is a 68-year-old retired accountant who has noticed worsening shortness of breath while mowing his lawn.

PRESENTATION: HISTORY

L.B. was well until 6 months ago, when he noticed extreme fatigue and lightheadedness when moving from a sitting or lying to a standing position. Initially, he blamed this on lack of sleep because of shortness of breath in bed, relieved by propping his head on two pillows, and frequent trips to the bathroom to urinate during the night. However, he recently found that he could no longer climb a flight of stairs without stopping to rest, and cannot complete chores around the house, such as laundry, mowing the lawn, and gardening. Additionally, when he tried to push himself to finish these tasks, he had episodes of chest "pressure" that were relieved by rest. Additionally, he notes, "It's bizarre, but my boots sure feel tight at the end of the day. Ever heard of anything like that, doc?"

He has no known history of rheumatic fever. Although he has a remote history of smoking less than a pack of cigarettes per week, L.B. is not a current smoker and drinks infrequently. He has no history of hypertension, diabetes, high cholesterol, or heart disease. He admits it has been a few years since his last doctor's appointment, but he thinks his physician might have mentioned a heart murmur before.

DISCUSSION

When taking a history, it is useful to know what level of activity the patient is accustomed to, and if that has changed. In the case of L.B., he experienced a progressive loss of exercise tolerance in the setting of worsening shortness of breath (dyspnea). Dyspnea on exertion is a key symptom of pulmonary edema, which is a common consequence of left-sided congestive heart failure (CHF). When the left ventricle fails to pump enough blood to the aorta, the pulmonary veins become congested with blood. As hydrostatic pressure increases, fluid weeps from the pulmonary vessels into the alveolar spaces, covering part of the gas exchanging surface and impairing oxygenation. This congestion is perceived as shortness of breath, especially during exercise.

Additionally, this patient demonstrates angina-like chest pressure with strenuous exertion, suggesting increased myocardial demand and/or decreased myocardial oxygen delivery. Reduced cardiac output (CO) is also suggested by persistent fatigue and lightheadedness, as well as shortness of breath while lying supine (orthopnea). Lying flat exacerbates pulmonary edema because of increased venous return leading to worsening congestion; however, by propping his head up on two pillows, he reduces venous returns and thus symptoms. Because of failure of the heart to pump, venous congestion tracks back to the systemic circulation. This leads to, among other things, peripheral edema worst in the lower extremities owing to gravity causing venous pooling and subsequent extravasation of fluid into the interstitium. During the night, when the feet are propped up, this pooled fluid may be mobilized back into venous circulation and raise intravascular perfusion pressure, leading to increased urine output.

L.B.'s history does not indicate many risk factors for ischemic disease, besides his gender and his age. To assess the potential cause of his congestive heart failure, we proceed to the physical examination and selected laboratory tests and imaging studies.

PRESENTATION: PHYSICAL EXAMINATION AND LABORATORY VALUES

On examination, L.B. appeared pale. He was afebrile with blood pressure 110/90 mm Hg, heart rate 93 beats/min, and respiratory rate 18 breaths/min. There was jugular venous distension to 10 cm. Cardiac examination was significant for an normal S1 and S2 that splits during expiration, S4 gallop at the apex, and a harsh systolic crescendo-decrescendo murmur at the right upper sternal border radiating to his carotids. Carotid upstrokes seem to be delayed with reduced amplitude. Pulmonary examination demonstrated bibasilar inspiratory crackles on examination. The liver was palpable below the right costal margin. He had 2+ pitting edema in the pretibial and ankle regions, and his nail beds appeared cyanotic. His hands were cool and clammy.

Laboratory tests revealed a low serum sodium of 130 mEq/L and a low normal serum potassium of 3.6 mEq/L. Chloride was 94 mEq/L, and bicarbonate was low at 15 mEq/L. Creatinine was slightly elevated at 1.6 mg/dL (normal <1.3 mg/dL). Blood urea nitrogen (BUN) was high at 45 mg/dL (normal 10–20 mg/dL). A 24-hour urine collection revealed urine output of 500 mL/day (low), urine sodium concentration of 2 mEq/L (low), and urine osmolality of 800 mOsm/kg (toward the concentrated end of the spectrum). Electrocardiogram (ECG) showed mild left ventricular hypertrophy, and chest x-ray (CXR) showed bilateral pulmonary edema in the lower lung fields.

DISCUSSION

Taken altogether, our findings on physical examination confirm our suspicion of congestive heart failure. Pulmonary examination demonstrates inspiratory crackles in the lung bases, indicative of increased congestion typical of pulmonary edema. Venous congestion is evident in distended external jugular veins, engorgement of the liver, and peripheral edema in the lower extremities. Increased systemic vascular resistance (SVR) to support blood pressure is manifested in as peripheral vasoconstriction, with cool and clammy hands, pale skin, and cyanotic nail beds.

The cardiac examination is particularly important in that it suggests a potential cause for L.B.'s congestive heart failure. Aortic stenosis, or pathologic reduction of aortic valve area, produces a characteristic heart murmur caused by turbulent flow during aortic valve opening. Qualities of the murmur include systolic timing (recall the aortic valve opens during systole), crescendo-decrescendo cadence (because of increased turbulence while "cracking" the valve open that decreases with complete valve opening), location at the right upper sternal border (where the aortic valve is located), and radiation to the carotid arteries. As left ventricular pressure increases because of resistance of the stenotic valve, left ventricular hypertrophy and thus diastolic dysfunction results. This is evidenced on physical examination by the S4 gallop (because of a stiffened ventricle) and on ECG. Finally, reduced cardiac output caused by stenotic aortic valve leads to delayed and reduced carotid pulse (pulsus parvus et tardus), as well as narrowed pulse pressure.

L.B.'s laboratory results are also indicative of CHF secondary to aortic stenosis. In CHF, decreased perfusion pressures lead to a number of compensatory changes. The baroreceptor reflex activates the sympathetic nervous system, the renin-angiotensin-aldosterone hormonal axis, and—when hypoperfusion is severe—the secretion of antidiuretic hormone (ADH). Increased sympathetic tone and increased levels of angiotensin II vasoconstrict the arteries to increase the systemic blood pressure (SBP) by increasing the SVR. The baroreceptor reflex also works to increase CO by increasing extracellular fluid (ECF) volume, which occurs because of increased proximal tubular salt (and thus water and urea) reabsorption in the kidney. Increased urea reabsorption under these circumstances is evident in an increased BUN relative to the creatinine level (BUN/Cr >20:1). Finally, increased sympathetic tone raises the HR to boost the CO, and angiotensin II leads to secretion of aldosterone, which increases distal tubular salt reabsorption and potassium secretion in the kidney (reflected in low serum potassium value).

ADH (also known as vasopressin) is also secreted to maintain blood pressure. ADH leads to increased thirst and reabsorption of water without salt, both of which act to dilute the ECF and concentrate the urine (as evidenced by low serum sodium and hyperosmolar urine). Finally, decreased kidney perfusion secondary to third-spacing and low cardiac output may cause a decline in the glomerular filtration rate (GFR) and subsequent elevation of creatinine (Cr).

TREATMENT AND SUBSEQUENT COURSE

After his diagnosis, L.B. received furosemide, a diuretic, to relieve his pulmonary and peripheral edema and oral potassium chloride to preserve his potassium level. However, although these target key symptoms of heart failure, his main issue remained his stenotic aortic valve (likely calcific because of aging). Thus L.B. was also referred to a cardiothoracic surgeon, and he underwent aortic valve replacement with an artificial heart valve. His surgery went well and he recovered without major complications. Six months later, he happily reports that he has been able to resume his daily chores.

DISCUSSION

Diuretics help to minimize pulmonary congestion, but caution must be taken not to lower blood pressure excessively lest the heart lose venous return and subsequently CO. However, management of congestive heart failure centers around treatment of the primary cause, which in this case is the failing aortic valve. Aortic valve replacement requires a median sternotomy (incision through the sternum) and placement on cardiopulmonary bypass (CPB), which recirculates oxygenated systemic blood while the surgeon replaces the heart valve. Full recovery takes up to 3 months and necessitates a period in the intensive care unit (ICU) immediately after surgery. The replacement valve may either be bioprosthetic, which only lasts 10 to 15 years even in elderly patients, or mechanical, which lasts longer but requires chronic anticoagulation with warfarin.

SECTION V

Pulmonary Physiology

13

The Mechanics of Breathing

INTRODUCTION

The use of oxygen for energy extraction is called aerobic respiration. In humans, gas exchange occurs in the air-filled lungs, which exposes the blood of the circulatory system to the air.

- Oxygen in the air of the lungs diffuses into the blood.
- Carbon dioxide brought from the body tissues diffuses out of the blood into the air in the lungs.
- For this exchange to occur effectively, the air rich in carbon dioxide must be expelled and fresh air rich in oxygen must be brought into the lungs. This process is called breathing, or ventilation.

  The important components in the respiratory system are:
- The airways, or conducting zone (trachea and bronchial tree).
- The gas exchange zone.
- The respiratory zone (respiratory bronchioles and alveoli).
- The musculoskeletal apparatus driving breathing (chest wall and diaphragm).
- The control system (central nervous system and chemoreceptors).

  Interactions between these components enable adequate oxygenation and active or passive ventilation.

SYSTEM STRUCTURE: THE THORAX

Air conduction occurs through a system of passages beginning with the trachea and branching continually into smaller and smaller passages (Fig. 13.1). In brief, air follows the following pathway:

1. Upper airways
2. Right and left mainstem bronchi
3. Conducting bronchi (progressively smaller)
   a. Lobar
   b. Segmental
   c. Subsegmental
   d. Bronchioles
   e. Terminal bronchioles
4. Respiratory bronchioles
5. Acini
   a. Contain alveolar ducts and alveolar sacs
   Distal to the terminal bronchioles, gas exchange begins to occur.

Histology

The overall histologic architecture of the bronchial tree is relatively consistent from the trachea to the bronchioles, with a sharp transition at the respiratory portion.

- Trachea
  - Fibroelastic connective tissue lined by two cell types
    Ciliated columnar epithelial cells
    Mucus producing goblet cells
  - C-shaped rings of hyaline cartilage provide support along anterior and lateral surfaces (Fig. 13.2).
  - Semirigid support with high elastin content resists collapse but also accommodates changes in size:
    Expansion during inspiration
    Recoil during expiration

Clinical Correlation Box 13.1

The mucociliary elevator represents a joint effort of the ciliated epithelial cells and mucus-secreting goblet cells to move mucus and trapped debris to the pharynx. Toxins from cigarette smoking damage the ciliated epithelial cells. This results in accumulation of secretions and debris from the lungs.

- Distal conducting airways
  - Cartilage rings less frequent, disappearing completely in bronchioles.
  - Cilia shorten with fewer goblet cells. See Clinical Correlation Box 13.1
  - Smooth muscle layer increases (more control of diameter).
- Alveoli
  - Type I pneumocytes.
    Thin, flat cells that form gas-diffusion barrier.
  - Type II pneumocytes.
    Rounded, infrequent.
    Produce surfactant which lowers surface tension in alveoli, which prevents alveolar collapse (see Fast Fact Box 13.1).

Fast Fact Box 13.1

There are over 300 million alveoli in the adult lung, covering a total surface area approximately equal to the size of a tennis court.

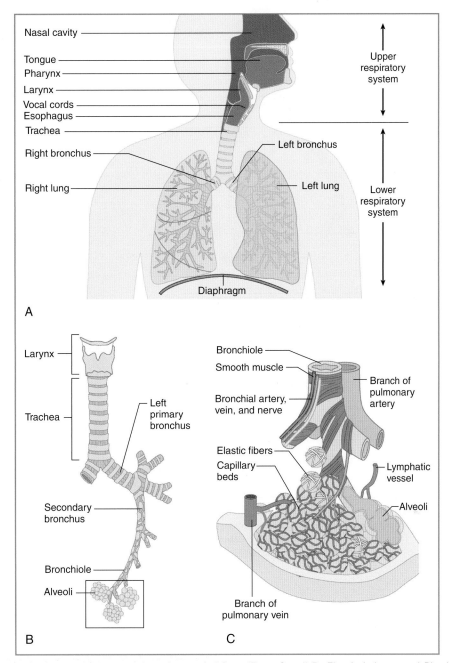

Fig. 13.1 Overview of the anatomic pathway of airflow. (From Carroll R. *Elsevier's Integrated Physiology.* Philadelphia: Mosby Elsevier; 2007. Fig. 10.2.)

Gross Anatomy

The lung may be divided into lobes, which are not symmetrical because of the need to accommodate the heart on the left side (Fig. 13.3A).

- Right
  - Upper
  - Middle
  - Lower
- Left
  - Upper
    Lingula, a small portion of this lobe, corresponds to the "middle" lobe.
  - Lower

The lobes are further subdivided into bronchopulmonary segments, which are shaped like pyramids with apices pointing toward the hilum of the lung (Fig. 13.3B). Each is supplied by:
- Segmental bronchus. See Clinical Correlation Box 13.2

Clinical Correlation Box 13.2

A state known as atelectasis results when one or more bronchopulmonary segments collapse. This might happen when a mucus plug obstructs a segmental bronchus, blocking the movement of air into that segment. Atelectasis can occur after surgery or another cause of limited mobility. Such patients often spontaneously sigh in an unconscious manner to expand the collapsed alveoli. Collapse of entire lung, however, cannot be corrected by this strategy, however, and requires an invasive procedure such as placement of a chest tube.

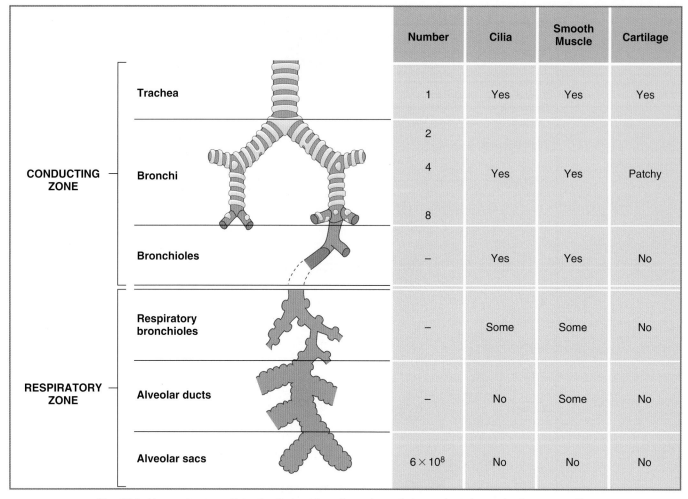

	Number	Cilia	Smooth Muscle	Cartilage
CONDUCTING ZONE Trachea	1	Yes	Yes	Yes
Bronchi	2 4 8	Yes	Yes	Patchy
Bronchioles	–	Yes	Yes	No
RESPIRATORY ZONE Respiratory bronchioles	–	Some	Some	No
Alveolar ducts	–	No	Some	No
Alveolar sacs	6×10^8	No	No	No

Fig. 13.2 Airway structure. Note the C-shaped cartilage rings of the trachea that maintain patency. The fractal-like branching of the respiratory "tree" is reflected in the geometric progression of airway numbers and allows for the accommodation of a relatively massive surface for gas exchange within the limited volume of the thoracic cavity. (From Costanzo L. *Physiology*, 6th Ed. Philadelphia: Elsevier; 2017. Fig. 5.1.)

- Segmental artery (branch of pulmonary artery).
- Segmental vein (branch of pulmonary vein).

There are no attachments between the lungs and the chest wall except at the hilum, where the lungs are suspended by the mediastinum, primary bronchi, pulmonary arteries, and pulmonary veins.

The pleura, which has two layers, surrounds the lungs (Fig. 13.4).

- The visceral pleura adheres to the lung.
- The parietal pleura adheres to the chest wall and diaphragm, the principal muscle of breathing.
- The potential space between them is called the pleural space.
  - This contains only a small amount of pleural fluid, secreted by the superficial mesothelium of the pleura, which lubricates the movement of the lungs inside the chest wall.
  - Lymph ducts continually drain the fluid from the pleural space into the hilar lymph nodes and from there conveys it to the thoracic duct.

- This drainage keeps the pleural space a potential space; a near vacuum. See Clinical Correlation Box 13.3

Clinical Correlation Box 13.3

Note that if the pleural space is punctured and air is introduced into the pleural space (pneumothorax) this space will no longer have a negative pressure, but will be equal to atmospheric pressure. Thus the lung collapses on that side. If the pneumothorax is a tension pneumothorax (i.e., air can enter but not escape from the puncture wound), air progressively accumulates in the pleural space and pushes the mediastinum to the opposite hemithorax. This can block venous return to the heart with devastating effects. Please see the pathophysiology section at the end of this chapter for a more complete discussion.

As a result, during inhalation, when the diaphragm pulls down on the parietal pleura, the parietal pleura cannot be pulled away from the visceral pleura. The diaphragm contracts and pulls the parietal pleura, which is vacuum-suctioned to the visceral pleura, and the lung is pulled open (see Clinical Correlation Box 13.4).

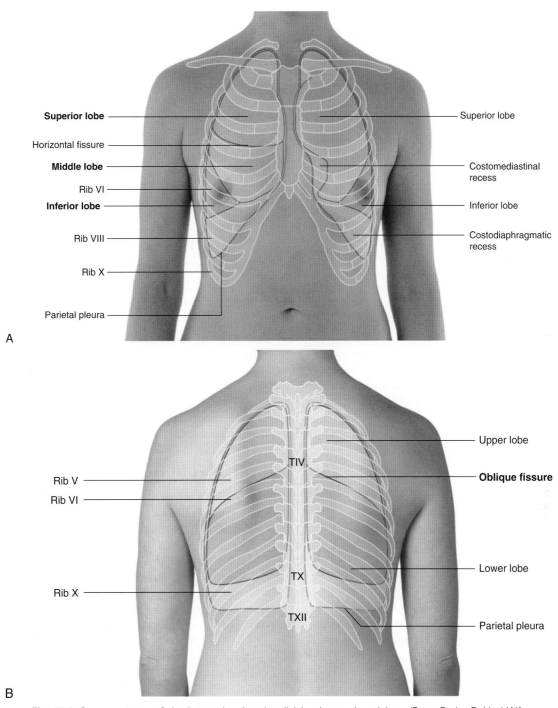

Fig. 13.3 Gross anatomy of the lungs showing the division into various lobes. (From Drake R, Vogl WA, Mitchell A. *Gray's Anatomy for Students*, 4th Ed. Philadelphia: Elsevier; 2019. Fig. 3.39.)

Clinical Correlation Box 13.4

When patients cannot breathe for themselves and require a machine for ventilation, the positive transpulmonary pressure is generated by increasing P_{alv} with respect to P_{pl} and P_{bs}. Because mechanical ventilation relies on positive P_{alv}, it is sometimes referred to as positive-pressure ventilation.

P_{alv}, Alveolar pressure; P_{bs}, body surface pressure; P_{pl}, pleural space pressure.

The chest wall is the semirigid musculoskeletal apparatus (ribs, sternum, spine, respiratory musculature) that serves to:
- Protect and support the heart and lungs
- Modify the volume of the thoracic cavity during breathing.

The most important muscle in this system is the dome-shaped diaphragm, which forms the floor of the thoracic cavity.

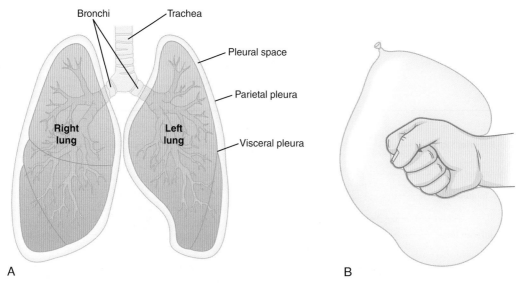

Fig. 13.4 A, The pleural surfaces. The visceral pleura is the outermost cell layer covering the lungs, while the parietal pleura lines the inside of the thoracic cavity. Normally, a small volume of pleural fluid is trapped between these two surfaces, allowing them to slide over one another easily, but keeping them in close contact with respiration. B, The pleural surfaces are formed when the lungs "grow into" an anlage of developing tissue. The fist represents the lung tissue, while the balloon represents the pleural tissue. The balloon surface in direct contact with the fist is analogous to the visceral pleural, while the "opposite side" of the balloon represents the parietal pleural that adheres to the inner aspect of the chest wall (not shown). The volume in the balloon represents the pleural space.

- The diaphragm contracts in a downward direction during inspiration, generating negative intrathoracic pressure to expand the lungs.
- The diaphragm relaxes during expiration, moving upwards and thus increasing intrathoracic pressure to empty the lungs.
- The diaphragm is innervated by the phrenic nerves, which originate at cervical roots C3, C4, and C5 (see Fast Fact Box 13.2).

Fast Fact Box 13.2   "C3, C4, C5, keep the diaphragm alive"

Any injury at or above C3 can result in paralysis of the diaphragm, respiratory failure, and death.

Accessory breathing muscles may assist the diaphragm during exercise or in disease states that compromise breathing function.
- Intercostal muscles
  - Divisions
    External intercostal muscles
    Internal intercostal muscles
    Innermost intercostal muscles
    Transversus thoracis muscles
  - Function
    Manipulate the ribs to increase or decrease the dimensions of the thoracic cavity.
    Recruited during forced or active inspiration.
- Scalenes
- Sternocleidomastoids
  - Elevates the sternum and is only activated at increased respiratory volumes.
- Anterior serrati

- Alae nasi
  - Flare the nostrils.
  Under respiratory stress, such as in the case of an asthma attack, these accessory muscles of inspiration can become overworked.

SYSTEM FUNCTION: THE BELLOWS

It is useful to imagine the lungs as a bellows, the tool used to force air into a fireplace.
- Inspiration: Bellows open → pressure inside plummets → air rushes in to fill expanded volume.
- Expiration: Bellows compressed → pressure inside skyrockets → air forcefully expelled.
  Inspiration involves the contraction of the muscles of inspiration (primarily the diaphragm) and is thus considered an active process. In contract, expiration occurs when these muscles relax.
- The recoil forces in the elastic lung tissue naturally contract the lung again when unopposed by the diaphragm, driving air back out of the lungs.
- Expiration is therefore a passive process with twice the duration of inspiration.
- During exercise or in disease states, the accessory breathing muscles may assist in expiration, actively supplementing the passive process (see Clinical Correlation Box 13.5).

Clinical Correlation Box 13.5

A substantial amount of damage to the smallest airways is necessary to change flow or resistance. Consequently, diseases, such as bronchiolitis obliterans, chronic obstructive pulmonary disease, and asthma can progress fairly far in the small airways before the patient notices symptoms and before changes in the lungs are detectable.

Pulmonary Pressures and Compliance

Transmural Pressure and Elastic Recoil Pressure

A transmural pressure is defined as the difference between the pressure inside and outside of the container.

$$P_{transmural} = P_{in} - P_{out}$$

A positive transmural pressure ($P_{in} > P_{out}$) works to expand a container. A negative transmural pressure ($P_{in} < P_{out}$) works to collapse a container.

There are three transmural pressures that determine the dynamics of ventilation:

- Pressure across the lungs and airways, or transpulmonary pressure (P_L)
- Pressure across the chest wall (P_{CW})
- Pressure across the respiratory system (P_{RS})

The transpulmonary pressure (also known as P_{lung} or P_L) is the transmural pressure across the lungs (Fig. 13.5). It determines the degree of inflation of the lungs.

$$P_{transpulmonary} = P_{alveoli} - P_{pleural\ space} = P_{alv} - P_{pl} = P_L$$

- P_{pl} is generally negative.
- In static conditions (i.e., before a breath is inhaled or exhaled), $P_{alv} = P_{mouth}$.
- If $P_{alv} < 0$, the lung tends to contract and leads to expiration. If $P_{alv} > 0$, the lung tends to expand and leads to inspiration (see Genetics Box 13.1, Development Box 13.1 and Pharmacology Box 13.1).

🧬 GENETICS BOX 13.1

Some of patients with early onset emphysema have α1 antitrypsin deficiency because of a mutation in SERPINA1. This gene encodes the protein that antagonizes the enzyme neutrophil elastase. There are multiple alleles of this gene, the normal version being designated M, whereas others like the Z and S alleles have point mutations that impair the protein's function. Patients with the MM genotype (homozygous for the normal gene) have no disease, whereas those with an ZZ, SS, or SZ have the disease.

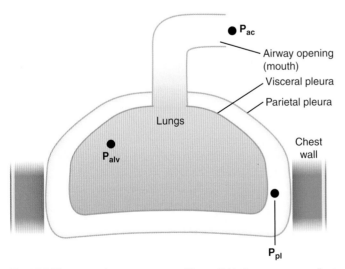

Fig. 13.5 The transpulmonary pressure (P_{lung} or P_L) is the pressure gradient across the lungs, and is defined and calculated as the difference between the alveolar pressure (P_{alv}) and the pressure of the pleural space (P_{pl}).

🧬 DEVELOPMENT BOX 13.1

Although chronic obstructive pulmonary disease affects middle age to older adults who often have a history of smoking more than 10 to 15 years, patients with alpha 1 antitrypsin deficiency tend to be younger (age 20–50 years) and often are nonsmokers. They progressively lose elastic recoil of lung tissue because of the unopposed action of neutrophil elastase. This disrupts the balance of forces that help keep the airways open, resulting in air trapping in their overly compliant lungs. Symptoms include dyspnea, cough, wheezing, and sputum.

💊 PHARMACOLOGY BOX 13.1

Like other patients with chronic obstructive pulmonary disease, patients with symptomatic α1 antitrypsin deficiency respond to inhaled bronchodilators, such as albuterol and ipratropium with decreased airflow obstruction. But the intravenous administration of α1 antitrypsin pooled from human donors, a form of replacement therapy called "intravenous augmentation" directly addresses the pathobiology of the disease and helps preserve the elastic recoil of lung tissue and potentially slowing disease progression.

In static conditions, P_L is equivalent to the elastic recoil pressure (P_{el}) of the lung.

- The lung has an innate tendency to collapse that is counterbalanced by the tendency of the elastic chest wall to "spring out."
- This pressure difference creates a "vacuum" in the pleural space (see Clinical Correlation Box 13.6).

Clinical Correlation Box 13.6

Coughing, or exhalation at high velocity, is initiated by irritant receptors in the large airways and mediated by the medulla.

- Initiates tremendous inspiration
- Seals the epiglottis and vocal cords
- Abdominal muscles contract to generate high intrathoracic pressure
- Seal is abruptly released, driving air out at high velocity

The trachea can add resistance through contraction of the smooth muscle connecting its cartilage rings, resulting in a smaller diameter.

- Recall that $A_1V_1 = A_2V_2$ (A = cross sectional area, V = fluid velocity)
- Thus smaller diameter → higher velocity
- High intrathoracic pressures generated by abdominal musculature overcome the tendency of increased resistance to limit flow ($Q = P/R$)

Thus this high speed mobilizes debris and helps to clear phlegm and mucus.

- The force with which the lungs tend to collapse is the elastic recoil pressure, which is defined as the difference between the pressure outside of the lung (P_{pl}) and inside the lung wall (P_{alv}):

$$P_{el} = P_{alv} - P_{pl}$$

The pressure of expansion or contraction (P expansion or contraction, or $P_{E/C}$) for the lungs is defined as the net result of recoil pressure and transmural pressure across the lungs.

$$P_{E/C} = P_L + P_{el}$$

- When the lungs are neither expanding nor contracting, P_L and P_{el} are equal and opposite and $P_{E/C} = 0$.
- In general, the positive transpulmonary pressure opposes the lungs' recoil pressure because of connective tissues in the lung parenchyma, such as elastin and collagen. However,

it is the recoil pressure of the lung that drives contraction and exhalation.

The tendency for the chest wall to "spring out," increasing the intrathoracic volume, is the P_{CW} may be represented as:

$$P_{CW} = \text{Ppleural space} - \text{Pbody surface} = P_{pl} - P_{bs}$$

Thus the transmural pressure across the entire respiratory system is represented as a balance between elastic recoil and chest wall expansion:

$$P_{RS} = P_{alv} - P_{atm} = (P_{alv} - P_{pl}) + (P_{pl} - P_{bs}) = P_{alv} - P_{bs}$$

Compliance

The shape of transmural pressure-volume (PV) curves for elastic containers like the lung is determined by the elastic recoil properties of the container walls.
- When recoil pressure is constant overall volume, the transmural PV has a linear relationship.
  - ↑ Transmural pressure against a constant recoil pressure → ↑ container volume in a direct proportion to change in transmural pressure.
  - Higher recoil force = decreased slope (more pressure required to achieve same change in volume).
  - Lower recoil force = increased slope (less pressure required to achieve same change in volume) (Fig. 13.6).

Compliance (C) is defined as the slope of this curve, or the change in volume in the lung (ΔV) that occurs for a given change in transmural pressure (ΔP) (Fig. 13.7). Compliance is thus inversely proportional to elastic recoil.

$$C = \Delta V / \Delta P$$

Recall that the linear relation between transmural pressure and volume implies a recoil force that is uniform over all volumes. However, the transmural PV curves are not linear in the lung and chest wall (Fig. 13.8).
- Like a rubber band being stretched, greater ΔV leads to greater recoil force (and thus greater difficulty in expanding the lungs).
- This tends to progressively flatten the transmural PV curve.

The Lung/Chest Wall Counterbalance and the Breathing Cycle

The transmural PV curves for the lungs and chest wall in isolation differ due their differences in recoil properties.
- Lungs (Fig. 13.9)
  - If transmural P is ≤ 0, the recoil force of the lung acts unopposed and the lung collapses (atelectasis).
  - At larger lung volumes, ↓ C because of ↑ recoil force.
  - Eventually, volume expansion cannot occur and further ↑ in pressure leads to alveolar rupture (barotrauma).
- Chest wall (Fig. 13.10).
  - As transmural P becomes increasingly negative, C approaches zero/
  - If transmural P = 0, the chest wall tends to maintain 60% of thoracic capacity volume because of inherent recoil outwards.
  - As transmural P becomes more positive, the chest cavity will continue to expand.
  - However, at a certain point, the chest wall's recoil forces direct inward (similar to the lung) and resist further expansion.

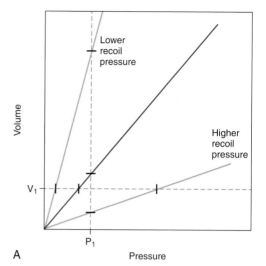

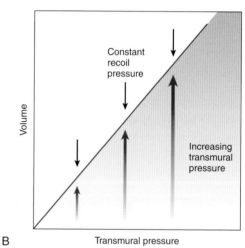

Fig. 13.6 The pressure-volume (PV) curve for a container with a collapsing elastic recoil pressure that remains uniform at all volumes. A, A container with a lower recoil pressure requires a lower transmural pressure to sustain a given volume, V1. A container with a higher recoil pressure requires a higher transmural pressure to sustain the same volume V1. At a given transmural pressure P1, a container with a lower recoil pressure has a higher volume compared with a container with a higher recoil pressure. B, Transmural and recoil pressures oppose one another, and changes in their difference (the net pressure gradient) determine the container volume.

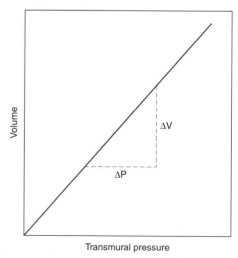

Fig. 13.7 Compliance is the slope of the transmural pressure-volume curve ($\Delta V / \Delta P$).

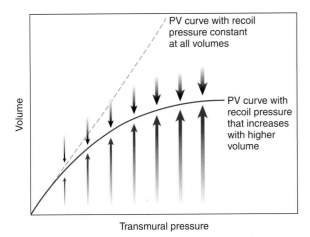

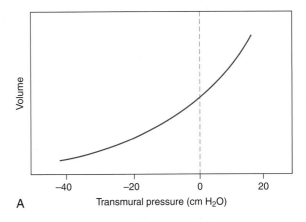

Fig. 13.8 The pressure-volume (PV) curve for a container with a collapsing elastic recoil pressure that increases as volume increases. This increased elastic recoil pressure at higher volumes limits volume expansion and flattens the PV curve. The lower slope at higher volumes is decreased compliance.

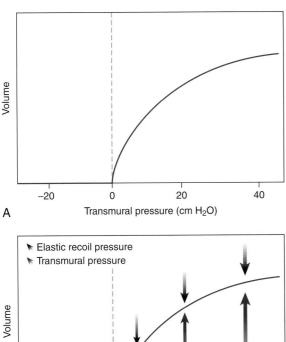

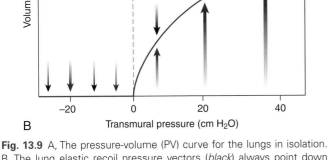

Fig. 13.9 A, The pressure-volume (PV) curve for the lungs in isolation. B, The lung elastic recoil pressure vectors (*black*) always point down because that pressure always favors volume contraction. The transmural pressure vectors (*red*) point down (left side) when the transmural pressure is negative, which also favors volume contraction. But they point up (right side) when the transmural pressure is positive, which favors volume expansion. In situ, the lungs cannot achieve zero volume (i.e., complete deflation) because they adhere to the chest wall by means of the pleural fluid that keeps the visceral and parietal pleural surfaces connected. If this connection is broken, as can occur with a pneumothorax, the lungs can completely collapse. (Modified from Thibodeau GA, Patton KT. *Anatomy & Physiology*, 10th Ed. Philadelphia: Elsevier; 2019. Figure 36-5.)

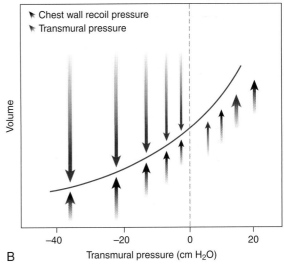

Fig. 13.10 A, The pressure-volume (PV) curve for the chest wall in isolation. B, The chest wall elastic recoil pressure vectors (*black*) always point up because that pressure always favors volume expansion. The transmural pressure vectors (*red*) point down (left side) when the transmural pressure is negative, which favors volume contraction. But they point up (right side) when the transmural pressure is positive, which favors volume expansion. The figure does not show that at higher volumes this curve levels off because beyond a certain volume the chest wall resists further expansion. Above that critical volume, the chest wall has a collapsing recoil force like that of the lungs, which would be illustrated by *black arrows* pointing down.

However, in a living person, the lung and chest wall work in unison as a single container (the chest wall/lung system) with its own elastic recoil properties.

The Counterbalance

When the lungs are in the body, the collapsing force exerted by the lungs is countered by the force exerted by the chest wall to try to expand.

- The lungs maintain a small volume even at negative transmural pressures because of the recoil of the chest wall.
- The chest wall does not expand as much at higher transmural pressures because of the recoil of the lungs.
- At volumes greater than 60% of capacity, the chest wall's recoil force changes direction to become a collapsing force like lung recoil. The combined system has a lower compliance than either system in isolation.
- $1/C_T = 1/C_L + 1/C_{CW}$

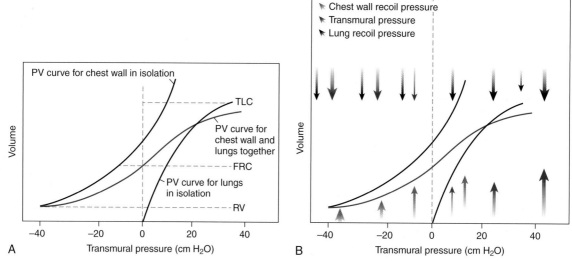

Fig. 13.11 A, The pressure-volume (*PV*) curve for the lungs and chest wall together, connected by the pleural space. The curve reflects PV relationships over artificially induced changes in transmural pressure in the absence of physiologic contraction of respiratory muscles such as the diaphragm. B, In this system, the chest wall recoil pressure vectors (*gray arrows*) generally favor volume expansion, the lung recoil pressure vectors (*black arrows*) always favor volume contraction, and the transmural pressure vectors (*red arrows*) favor volume contraction when the transmural pressure is negative (left side) and volume expansion when the transmural pressure is positive (right side). Note that near TLC, the chest wall recoil pressure points down, indicating that beyond a critical volume it too favors volume contraction. This reflects the decreased compliance of the lung and chest wall combined system compared with the isolated lungs at high volumes. *FRC*, Functional residual capacity; *RV*, residual volume, *TLC*, total lung capacity.

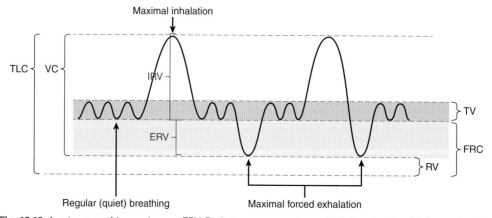

Fig. 13.12 A spirogram of lung volumes. *ERV*, Expiratory reserve volume; *FRC*, Functional residual capacity; *IRV*, inspiratory reserve volume; *RV*, residual volume, the lung volume left over after maximum exhalation of the entire VC; RV cannot reach 0 except in the case of total bilateral lung collapse; *TLC*, total lung capacity, the maximum lung volume attainable by forceful inhalation; *TV*, tidal volume, the volume inhaled and exhaled during relaxed breathing; *VC*, vital capacity, the maximum volume change that can be achieved by forceful inhalation and exhalation.

Fig. 13.11 depicts the PV relationships of the chest wall/lung system in the absence of muscular exertion with the pressure gradients adjusted by artificial means to obtain specific lung volumes and to measure system compliance.

- With no muscular exertion and epiglottis open (keeping alveoli and external atmosphere in equilibrium), there is no pressure gradient between the outside and inside of the chest wall/lung system (transmural pressure = 0).
- Thus the opposing recoil forces of the lung and chest wall are balanced.
- The system settles into a resting state at a lung volume referred to as functional residual capacity (FRC). This is equivalently

the volume of air remaining in the lungs after expiring a tidal volume (TV), or a normal breath.

Fig. 13.12 depicts the spirogram, with lung volumes generated during different ventilatory states. The lung spaces are divided between air in the conducting airways and air in the alveolar spaces. Note that capacities represent the sum of two or more volumes.

- Total lung capacity (TLC) = inspiratory reserve volume (IRV) + tidal volume (TV) + expiratory reserve volume (ERV) + residual volume (RV).
- Functional residual capacity (FRC) = ERV + RV.
- Vital capacity (VC) = IRV + TV + ERV = TLC − RV.

Inspiration

A cycle of breathing entails changes in the counterbalance of forces that dictate thoracic volume.

- In a living person, the breathing cycle begins at FRC.
  - With the glottis open, the transmural pressure is 0.
- The contraction of the diaphragm or accessory muscles results in chest wall expansion by creating a bellows effect and drawing air into the lungs.
- As the lungs fill with air, the force of the muscular action on the chest wall overcomes the recoil force of the lungs and shifts the balance of the combined system toward expansion of the lungs to a larger volume.
- As the lung volume increases, lung compliance decreases and the lungs' recoil force increases, thereby progressively opposing further increases in lung volume.
- The maximum volume the lungs can achieve during inspiration is the TLC.

Expiration

- After inspiration, the respiratory muscles can relax, shifting the balance of forces in favor of lung recoil.
- The chest wall/lung system will passively return to its resting state at FRC as air flows out of the lungs.
- Although expiration is a passive process at rest, abdominal contraction can force air out of the lungs, driving lung volume down below FRC.
- However, the chest wall recoil force opposes this contraction of the chest wall/lung system below the system's resting state at FRC. Once the abdominal muscles relax, the system passively reexpands to FRC.
- The minimum volume the lungs can achieve is the residual volume (RV). Beyond this point, the abdominal muscles and lung recoil forces cannot overcome the recoil forces of the chest wall.

Transmural Pressures During the Breathing Cycle

We can more closely analyze this cycle by considering the transmural pressures at each phase (Fig. 13.13, Table 13.1).

At Functional Residual Capacity

- Transmural pressure of the chest wall/lung system is 0.
- Transpulmonary pressure is positive to keep the lung open.
  - The chest wall and lung pulling away from each other creates a "vacuum" in the pleural space relative to P_{bs} and P_{alv}.
  - Thus decreasing Pout (P_{pl}) increases P_L.
- Pressure across the chest wall is negative to keep the chest wall slightly compressed.
  - This occurs because Pin (P_{pl}) is negative and Pout (P_{bs}) is 0 (see Clinical Correlation Box 13.7).

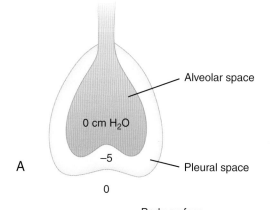

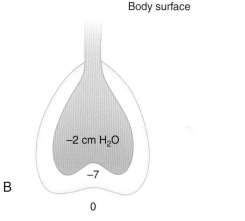

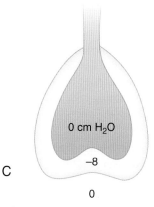

Fig. 13.13 Pressures in the alveolar space, the pleural space, and at the body surface, (A) at functional residual capacity, (B) during inspiration, and (C) at end-inspiration.

TABLE 13.1 Transmural Pressures During the Breathing Cycle

Phase	PRS ($P_{alv} - P_{bs}$)	PL ($P_{alv} - P_{pl}$)	P_{CW} ($P_{pl} - P_{bs}$)	Overall Effect
FRC	0	+	-	No movement
Inspiration	+	++	−	Lungs expand
Expiration	-	+	—	Lungs collapse

FRC, Functional residual capacity; P_{alv}, alveolar pressure; P_{bs}, body surface pressure; P_L, transpulmonary pressure; P_{pl}, pleural space pressure; *PRS*, pressure across the respiratory system.

Clinical Correlation Box 13.7

If the pleural space fills with air (pneumothorax), blood (hemothorax), or excess fluid (pleural effusion), then the "vacuum" effect of the pleural space is lost. As a result, the movement of the parietal and visceral pleura is uncoupled, and a restrictive ventilatory defect (inability of the lungs to expand properly) will occur.

During Inspiration

During inspiration, the respiratory muscles supplement the chest wall's tendency to expand the thoracic cavity (see Fig. 13.11).

- P_{pl} drops even lower, which causes P_{CW} to become more negative and P_L to become more positive.
  - Expanding forces of muscles with expanding recoil force of the chest wall overcomes the collapsing P_{CW}.
  - P_L overcomes the lungs collapsing recoil force.
  - Thus the entire chest wall/lung system expands.
- P_{alv} drops because of the increase in alveolar volume, causing air to rush into the lungs.

At End-Inspiration

At end-inspiration, the rush of air into the lungs has raised the P_{alv} back up to the atmospheric pressure of zero cmH_2O.

- The transmural pressure across the chest wall is more negative than at FRC (but the muscles resist this collapsing force).
- The transpulmonary pressure is more positive than at FRC, holding the lungs open.
- Muscles cease to contract.

During Expiration

Without the force of the muscles acting to expand the chest wall, the negative P_{pl} is now enough to cause the collapse of the chest wall, and the recoil force of the lungs now overcomes the reduced positive transpulmonary pressure.

- The contracting lungs squeeze the alveolar air and raise alveolar pressure, and the air rushes out of the mouth and nose.
- As the alveolar pressure drops back to zero, the lungs contract down to FRC.
- The breathing muscles no longer pull at the pleural space and the recoil force of the lung on the pleural space is less because the lung is no longer as stretched and is more compliant.
- The pleural space pressure assumes the less negative value with which it began the breathing cycle at FRC.

Alveolar Stability

Surface tension depends on the strong adherence of water molecules to one another via hydrogen bonding (Fig. 13.14). These water molecules line the alveoli.

- Major determinant of the recoil force of the lungs.
- Particularly strong at the air/water interface.
  - Because of lack of upward attractive forces and thus stronger hydrogen bonding creating a more strongly adherent layer of molecules at the surface.

The contractile surface forces tend to collapse the alveoli (and hence the lung). Recall Laplace's law describes the transmural pressure (P) needed to keep the alveoli open with a given surface tension (T) and radius (r):

$$P = 2T/r.$$

- P is directly proportional to surface tension (T) and inversely proportional to radius (r).
- P is equal and opposite to the recoil force of the alveoli.
- Small or collapsed alveoli ($\downarrow r$) require a higher transmural pressure to open.
  - Residual volume $\downarrow$ P required for inflation and thus reduces muscular work.

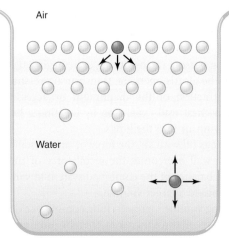

Fig. 13.14 Surface tension. The *circles* represent water molecules. The *arrows* represent the forces acting on the highlighted molecules because of hydrogen bonds with other water molecules.

- Surface tension (T) may be reduced through the use of surfactant, pro.
  - Surfactant consists primarily of the hydrophobic lipid dipalmitoyl phosphatidylcholine, which interferes with water–water hydrogen bonding that accounts for surface tension.
  - Surfactant therefore $\downarrow$ T and thus $\downarrow$ recoil force of the lungs, and makes inflation easier (see Clinical Correlation Box 13.8).

Clinical Correlation Box 13.8

Neonatal respiratory distress syndrome (RDS) is a disease affecting premature infants (especially before 28–32 weeks of gestation) characterized by insufficient surfactant production in the immature lungs. This increases alveolar surface tension and thus recoil force, causing alveoli to collapse (atelectasis) and making inflation extremely difficult. Recall that elastic recoil is inversely related to compliance (C = 1/E), such that these babies have extremely low lung compliance. The high compliance of the infant chest wall because of lack of rib cage ossification or costal cartilage calcification also tends to distort the rib cage during respiratory distress and wastes further energy. Together, this disorder can lead to severe hypoxemia and even death. However, aerosolized surfactant can improve their symptoms dramatically.

Several other forces help stabilize the alveoli and prevent them from collapsing. The two most important of these are:

- Interdependence
  - Alveoli, alveolar ducts, and other air spaces are adjacent to one another and mechanically dependent on each other.
  - The collapsing force in one alveolus thus stents open adjacent alveoli.
- Airway closure
  - During late expiration, transmural pressures of the airways tend to collapse the airways.
  - This traps some air distal to the area of collapse (i.e., in the alveoli) and helps keep the alveoli open at low lung volumes.

Airway Flow and Resistance

Expansion and contraction of the thoracic cavity lead to pressure gradients (ΔP) that drive air flow (Q) from the body surface (i.e., mouth and nose) to the alveoli and back out again.

- Flow of air is directly proportional to ΔP and inversely proportional to resistance (R).
- This is analogous to Ohm's law in electricity: $Q = \Delta P/R$.

If flow through the conducting airways is assumed to be laminar—nonturbulent and parallel to the walls of the airways—the airflow can be described by Poiseuille's law:

$$Q = \Delta P \pi r^4 / 8 \eta l$$

where r is the radius of the tube, η is fluid viscosity, and l is the length of the tube. Plugging in Ohm's law, we find:

$$R = 8 \eta l / \pi r^4$$

- Resistance is directly proportional to the viscosity of the air and the length of the tube, and inversely proportional to the radius of the tube to the fourth power.
  - Small changes in the radii of the airways have a dramatic effect on the resistance and thus on the flow of air into and out of the lungs.
  - The greatest point of resistance is the medium-sized bronchi.
    The bronchioles, the smallest airways, branch in parallel and thus have greater cross-sectional area with reduced resistance compared with the medium-sized airways (see Clinical Correlation Box 13.9).

There are two main determinants of airway resistance:
- Bronchial smooth muscle tone
  - Bronchioles are surrounded spirally oriented smooth muscles.
  - Contraction ↓ radius and ↑ resistance, resulting in partial obstruction of the airways.
  - Triggers include:
    Parasympathetic stimulation
    Irritants
    Leukotrienes
    Low carbon dioxide levels
    Histamine (see Clinical Correlation Box 13.10)

Clinical Application Box 13.10

Asthma is an obstructive lung disease in which patients have abnormally increased tone of bronchial smooth muscle following exposure to irritants, causing constricted air flow. Asthma exacerbations can be triggered by inflammation (i.e., upper respiratory infection) or exposure to environmental irritants (i.e., allergens or cold air). Treatment often features inhaled B2 agonists, such as albuterol, which provide sympathetic stimulation, cause bronchial dilation and lower airway resistance.

- Lung volume
  - Radial traction of the bronchi from surrounding lung tissue stents the bronchi open.
  - ↑ lung volume → ↑ recoil force → ↑ radial traction → ↑ bronchial diameter → ↓ resistance.
Airway resistance is particularly important in two phenomena:
- Forced expiration
  - At end-inspiration: P_{pl} is negative, P_{alv} is 0, and positive transmural pressure stents the airways open.
  - Contraction of abdominal muscles causes P_{pl} and P_{alv} to rise sharply, pushing air of lungs ($P_{alv} > P_{AW} > P_{mouth} = 0$).
  - High alveolar pressure creates a negative transmural pressure ($P_{AW} - P_{alv}$) across the airways, constricting them (Fig. 13.15).
  - This imposes limits on the flow velocity achievable by forced exhalation (see Fast Fact Box 13.3).

Clinical Correlation Box 13.9

During exercise and certain disease states, normal "quiet breathing" cannot move the necessary volume of air in and out of the lungs to provide adequate oxygenation to the body. In this scenario, *accessary muscles* of breathing supplement the usual mechanisms.
- Accessory muscles of inspiration include external intercostal, sternocleidomastoid, scalenes, and anterior serrati m.
  - Contract in synchrony with the diaphragm, elevating the ribs and allowing them to pivot on the spine and sternum in addition to raising the sternum.
  - This serves to increase the: (1) lateral and (2) anteroposterior diameter of the thorax, increasing total intrathoracic volume.
- Accessory muscles of expiration include rectus abdominus and internal intercostal m.
  - Rectus pushes the diaphragm up → decreased intrathoracic volume.
  - Internal intercostals pull the ribs down → decreased intrathoracic volume.
  - This assists the lung's natural recoil mechanism.
The effect of each group of intercostals is generally characterized as the "bucket handle" effect, as depicted.

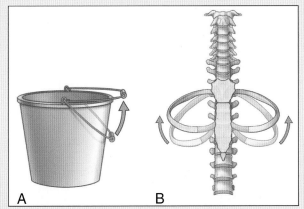

A   B

(Modified from Thibodeau GA, Patton KT. *Anatomy & Physiology*, 10th Ed. Philadelphia: Elsevier; 2019. Figure 36.5)

Fast Fact Box 13.3

The equal pressure point theory suggests that this flow velocity limitation occurs at a particular point. The theory posits that airway pressures decrease from the alveoli to the mouth, and defines the equal pressure point (EPP) as that point where the pressure surrounding the airway (P_{alv}) is equal to the pressure inside the airway.
- Beyond EPP: $P_{alv} > P_{AW}$ → airway is compressed with resistance to flow
- Before EPP: $P_{alv} < P_{AW}$ → airway remains open to flow
  If the EPP occurs in the cartilaginous conducting airways, the structure will remain open because of the structural integrity imposed by cartilage. If the EPP occurs in the non-cartilaginous bronchioles and smaller airways, the structure may transiently collapse.

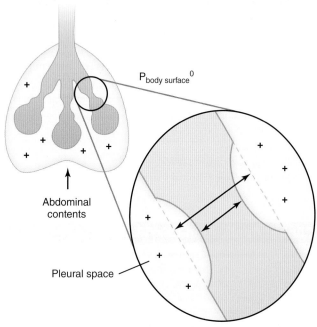

Fig. 13.15 Airway constriction during forced expiration. Airway constriction decreases airway radius and thus resistance to airflow.

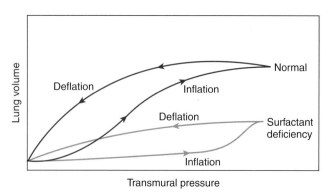

Fig. 13.16 Hysteresis. Even under normal physiologic conditions, on inflation, the lung demonstrates decreased compliance at low volumes. On deflation, the lung demonstrates decreased compliance at high volumes. The lower pair of curves illustrates the additional loss of compliance on both inflation and deflation in the setting of surfactant deficiency. P_L, Transmural pressure.

- Hysteresis (Fig. 13.16)
  - Defined as the change in lung compliance during inflation versus deflation, reflected in distinct transmural PV curves.
    Low lung volumes → $C_{inflation} < C_{deflation}$
    High lung volumes → $C_{inflation} > C_{deflation}$
  - Difference in compliance is thought to be mediated by two factors:
    The presence of surfactant, which interrupts hydrogen bonding during inhalation and creates more uniform alveolar recruitment during exhalation.
    Airway resistance because of initial turbulence during inhalation (as air movement begins), because the coefficient of static friction > coefficient of kinetic friction.

PATHOPHYSIOLOGY: DISORDERS OF PULMONARY MECHANICS

Pulmonary pathology may emerge from any component of the respiratory system, including the chest wall and lung. Suspected disorders may be assessed using pulmonary function tests, or "PFTs."
- Patient inhales maximally and exhales forcefully into spirometer.
- This allows us to record specific lung volumes and compare them to predicted values for each patient:
  - TLC
  - RV
  - VC
  - FRC
  - Forced expiratory volume in 1 second (FEV_1) and forced vital capacity (FVC).
    Patient blows down from TLC to RV as hard and fast as possible.
    Normal FEV1:FVC is around 80% to 110% predicted.
  Using the results of PFTs, one can distinguish two broad varieties of respiratory dysfunction (Fig. 13.17):
- Restrictive
- Obstructive

Restrictive Lung Disease

In restrictive lung disease, the main cause of pathology is reduced lung volume. PFTs in restrictive lung disease typically demonstrate:
- ↓ TLC (<80% predicted), VC, RV.
- FEV1/FVC normal (no increased resistance to outflow).
  Broadly, the pathophysiology of restrictive lung disease lies in either:
- Decreased lung compliance (equivalently, increased elastic recoil); or
- Decreased thoracic expanding forces.

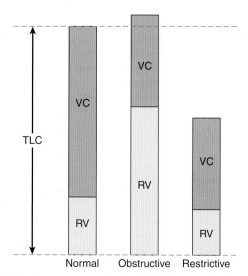

Fig. 13.17 Physiologic and pathophysiologic lung volumes. In obstructive lung diseases, total lung capacity (TLC) and residual volume (RV) are increased, and vital capacity (VC) may be decreased because of the increased RV.

Causes of restrictive lung disease can be remembered with the acronym "PAINT":

- Pleural disease (e.g., effusion, tumor)
- Alveolar disease (e.g., edema, pneumonia, hemorrhage)
- Interstitial disease (e.g., a stiffened lung through collagen reorganization and fibrosis)
- Neuromuscular disease (i.e., amyotrophic lateral sclerosis [ALS])
- Thoracic cage disease (i.e., obesity or kyphoscoliosis)

Lung volumes are low and can result in decreased alveolar ventilation, which can lead to hypoxia. Parenchymal abnormalities associated with some of these conditions can also contribute to hypoxia through $\dot{V}/\dot{Q}$ mismatch (see Ch. 14).

Obstructive Lung Disease

In obstructive lung disease, the main cause of pathology is impaired outflow. PFTs in obstructive lung disease typically demonstrate:

- ↑ TLC, RV
- ↓ FEV1/FVC (<0.75 predicted)

Broadly, the pathophysiology of obstructive lung disease lies in either:

- Increased lung compliance (equivalently, decreased recoil); or
- Increased airway resistance.
  - To produce flow into the lung across elevated resistance, the intrathoracic pressure must be lower than outside atmospheric pressure. A good inspiratory effort can usually accomplish this.
  - To produce flow out of the lungs against increased resistance, however, abdominal musculature must be recruited.
  - Intrathoracic pressure must rise very high to combat higher transpulmonary pressure and push air out of the lung. Unfortunately, high intrathoracic pressures can lead to airway collapse and further increase airway resistance.
  - This difficulty of expiration thus causes air trapping, leading to increased RV and eventual dynamic hyperinflation.

The most common cause of obstructive lung disease is cigarette smoking. Specific manifestations of obstructive lung disease include:

- Emphysema
  - Inflammation destroys elastin and alveolar walls → ↑ TLC/RV and lung compliance.
  - Because of high lung volumes and the prolonged duration of forced expiration, alveolar ventilation is decreased and can result in hypoxia.
- Chronic bronchitis
  - Hyperplasia and hypersecretion of mucus glands in response to irritants (i.e., tobacco smoke).
- Bronchiectasis
  - Dilation and scarring of the airways because of persistent severe infections.
- Asthma
  - Abnormally increased bronchial smooth muscle tone in response to irritants or inflammation.

Gross Structural Disruptions of the Thoracic Bellows

Airway Obstruction

Airway obstruction is one of the most common causes of death in trauma victims. Thus the airway is the first and most important component in the initial evaluation of a trauma patient (or any unconscious patient).

- The most common cause of airway obstruction in an unconscious patient is the tongue.
  - When a person becomes unconscious, the tongue may relax back into the pharynx and obstruct the airway.
  - A simple maneuver like a head tilt/chin lift or a jaw thrust will draw the tongue up out of the airway.

Partial airway obstruction may also occur through separate mechanisms including (Fig. 13.18)

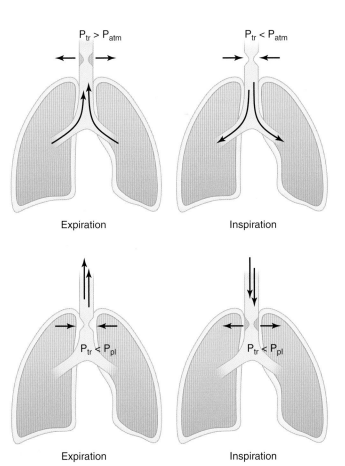

Fig. 13.18 Expiration and inspiration with partial airway obstruction. The transmural pressures across the trachea inside the thoracic cavity are opposite those outside the thoracic cavity. P_{atm}, Atmospheric pressure; P_{tr}, transmural pressure; P_{pl}, pleural space pressure.

- Swallowing a foreign object.
- Tumors infiltrating the airway.
- Infection leading to extreme swelling (i.e., in epiglottitis).

Importantly, partial airway obstruction presents with different symptoms depending on whether the obstruction occurs in the upper or lower respiratory tract.

- Upper airway: Obstruction exaggerates normal tracheal narrowing during inspiration, causing inspiratory stridor (prolonged high-pitched gasping sound). During expiration, the positive pressure in the airway forces the airway open, and air is exhaled easily.
- Lower airway: Obstruction exerts positive pressure leading to airway collapse on exhalation, producing an audible expiratory wheeze.

Both will lead to respiratory distress evidenced by increased rate of breathing (tachypnea) and sensation of shortness of breath.

Pneumothorax

There are two varieties of pneumothorax:

- Open pneumothorax (Fig. 13.19)
  - Occurs when a hole in the chest wall connects the pleural space and the atmosphere.
  - P_{pl} "vacuums" air into the pleural space, expanding the chest wall and collapsing the lung. This tends to compromise ventilation and oxygenation.
  - On each subsequent breath, air is drawn in via the pleural space because it has less resistance than the actual airways.
  - Emergency treatment consists of covering the hole in the chest wall with an occlusive dressing (air-tight and water-tight). Eventually, the wound must be surgically closed and a chest tube placed in the pleural space to withdraw the air.
- Tension pneumothorax (Fig. 13.20)
  - Disruption in the visceral pleura connects the airways with the pleural space. This may occur if there is an anatomic abnormality such as a bronchopulmonary fistula or if a structurally relatively weak area of lung tissue ruptures when an individual is exposed to decreased atmospheric pressure such as decompression at high altitude.
  - P_{pl} "vacuums" air into the pleural space during inspiration, but air cannot escape during expiration because the lung tissue acts like a one-way valve. This may occur if there is an anatomic abnormality such as a bronchopulmonary

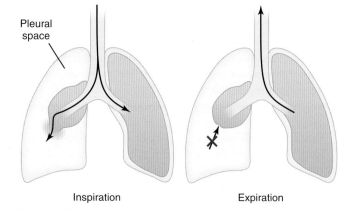

Fig. 13.20 A tension pneumothorax during inspiration and expiration. The one-way valve effect leads to progressive inflation of the pleural space.

fistula or if a structurally relatively weak area of lung tissue ruptures when an individual is exposed to decreased atmospheric pressure such as decompression at high altitude.

- On each subsequent breath, more air is trapped and leads to lung collapse on that side.
- As pressure continues to increase, the heart and the opposite lung are also compressed; an imminently life-threatening situation.

Signs include decreased breath sounds (because of lung collapse), massive jugular distension (because blood cannot return to the compressed heart), deviation of the trachea to the side opposite the injury, and shock (high heart rate, low blood pressure).

- Treatment entails decompression of the tension pneumothorax by inserting a chest tube through the chest wall into the pleural space and removing the air. Emergency decompression for a tension pneumothorax is also possible by inserting a needle into the second intercostal space in the mid-clavicular line on the side of injury.

Flail Chest

Occurs when two or more adjacent ribs are broken in two places. This leads to a disruption in the integrity of the chest wall (Fig. 13.21).

- During inspiration, the negative intrathoracic pressure will cause this disconnected section of the chest wall to be drawn inward.

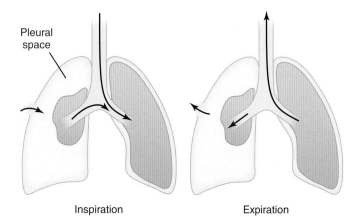

Fig. 13.19 An open pneumothorax during inspiration and expiration.

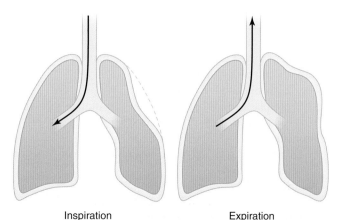

Fig. 13.21 Flail chest during inspiration and expiration.

- During expiration, the positive intrathoracic pressure will push this section of the chest wall out.
- Because these motions are the opposite of what normally occurs during breathing, they are termed paradoxical chest wall motion.

AGING: ALTERED LUNG MECHANICS

Alterations in lung function also occur as part of the normal aging process. Overall, oxygenation and exercise tolerance decline with age.
- ↑ lung compliance, ↓ recoil force

- Decreased radial traction on airways → earlier closure → air-trapping at end-expiration.
- ↑ FRC, RV, TLC
- ↓ VC, FEV$_1$
- ↓ Diffusion capacity and chemoreceptor function.

SUMMARY

- Respiration entails the airways, gas exchange zone, respiratory zone, musculoskeletal apparatus, and control (central nervous system) system.
- Inspiration is active, while expiration is normally passive because of the recoil forces in the lung.
- Transmural pressures across the respiratory system determine its behavior at different points of ventilation.
    - Elastic recoil pressure of the lung: $P_{el} = P_{alv} - P_{pl}$
    - Elastic recoil pressure of the chest wall: $P_{CW} = P_{pl} - P_{bs}$
    - Elastic recoil pressure of the system: $P_{RS} = P_{alv} - P_{bs}$
- Compliance is a measure of the recoil properties of the container and is inversely proportional to elastic recoil.

$$C = \Delta V / \Delta P$$

- The elastic recoil pressures of the lung and the chest wall are equal and opposite at FRC.

- Surface tension tends to collapse the alveoli, and accounts for the majority of elastic recoil within the lung. These effects are mitigated by surfactant.
- Airway flow is described by Ohm's law and is most prominently affected by airway radius. The two most determinants for radius are bronchial smooth muscle tone and lung volume.
- The two broad categories of ventilatory defects are restrictive disease and obstructive disease, which can be distinguished by PFTs.
    - Restrictive: ↓ Lung volumes because of ↓ respiratory compliance or muscle weakness.
    - Obstructive: ↓ Outflow and increased lung volumes and are because of increased compliance or increased airway resistance.

REVIEW QUESTIONS

Directions: Each of the numbered items or incomplete statements in this section is followed by answers or by completions of the statement. Select the one lettered answer or completion that is best in each case.

1. A 68-year-old woman with pulmonary fibrosis presents with worsening exertional dyspnea. The mechanism of her pulmonary disease is consistent with which of the following pulmonary function test results?
   A. FEV1/FVC high, low VC, low TLC, low RV
   B. FEV1/FVC normal, low VC, low TLC, low RV
   C. FEV1/FVC normal, high VC, high TLC, high RV
   D. FEV1/FVC low, low VC, low TLC, low RV
   E. FEV1/FVC low, high VC, high TLC, high RV

2. A 3-year-old boy with dyspnea and wheezing is brought to the pediatric emergency room shortly after he swallowed a coin. His chest x-ray would be consistent with a partial airway obstruction at which of the following locations?
   A. Alveolus
   B. Bronchiole
   C. Larynx
   D. Oropharynx
   E. Trachea

3. A 28-year-old man presents with Guillain-Barré syndrome, an ascending polyneuropathy that may occur after a viral prodrome. He will need ventilatory assistance if his disease weakens muscles innervated by which of the following nerve root levels?
   A. C3, C4, C5
   B. C6, C7, C8
   C. T1, T2, T3
   D. T3, T4, T5
   E. L1, L2, L3

4. A thin 70-year-old man with a barrel-shaped chest who smoked two packs of cigarettes/day since he was 18 years presents with worsening exertional dyspnea. On physical exam, no breath sounds were heard. His pulmonary function test results were as follows: FEV1 40% predicted before and after albuterol administration, TLC 170% predicted, FEV1/FVC .6, RV 320% predicted. His likely diagnosis is:
   A. Asthma
   B. Chronic bronchitis
   C. Chest wall weakness
   D. Emphysema
   E. Interstitial lung disease

ANSWERS TO REVIEW QUESTIONS

1. **The answer is B.** Pulmonary fibrosis is a restrictive lung disease, in which decreased compliance of the respiratory system leads to decreased lung volumes. In the case of pulmonary fibrosis, this decreased compliance results from increased lung recoil force, whereas in a patient with neuromuscular weakness, it results from a decreased capability to expand the thoracic cavity. A patient with a restrictive lung disease will have no difficulty with the expiration of air, and consequently the FEV1/FVC ratio should be normal. A pattern of high lung volumes and low FEV1/FVC ratios would be more consistent with an obstructive pulmonary disease, such as asthma or emphysema, with their characteristic difficulties with outflow of air.

2. **The answer is E.** Audible expiratory wheezes result from intrathoracic airway obstruction, such as in the trachea or a bronchus. The negative intrathoracic pressure of inspiration allows airways within the thorax to open, but the positive pressure against the airways during expiration will result in their collapse if an obstruction is present, resulting in a wheeze. An object the size of a coin is too large to pass through the branching bronchi to lodge in the small-diameter bronchioles. Alveoli lie distal to the bronchioles and are the sites of gas exchange. If an object were lodged in the larynx, inspiratory flow might be hindered, resulting in the high-pitched inspiratory gasps of stridor.

3. **The answer is A.** The most important muscle in the respiratory system is the diaphragm, which is innervated by the phrenic nerves from cervical roots C3, C4, C5. During inhalation, the diaphragm contracts, pulling down the floor of the thoracic cavity and allowing the lungs to expand. The accessory breathing muscles can assist the diaphragm in its work during exercise or some disease states, but none of them can fully substitute for the diaphragm. Involvement of the entire diaphragm by a disease process necessitates mechanical ventilation to help the patient breathe.

4. **The answer is D.** The patient's FEV1 is low, his TLC is elevated, his FEV1/FVC ratio is less than 0.75 (a clinical indicator for obstructive disease), and RV is greatly elevated. The TLC is not less than 80% predicted, therefore this is likely not a restrictive process (so it is not chest wall weakness or interstitial lung disease). Because FEV1 does not improve at all with albuterol administration, and because this is not an acute attack, this is likely not asthma. As mentioned before, he has the clinical indicator for an obstructive disease (FEV1/FVC < 0.75), such as chronic bronchitis or emphysema. These two disease processes typically can both be caused by smoking, but classically have very different presentations. Patients with chronic bronchitis can be remembered as "blue bloaters" whereas emphysema patients can be remembered as "pink puffers". Chronic bronchitis is accompanied by chronic cough and sputum, leading to a fixed airway obstruction which leads to dyspnea after work and at rest. A characteristic finding on auscultation is rhonchi, which this patient does not have. Because emphysema is caused by destruction of lung parenchyma with decreased elastic recoil, TLC and RV are usually greatly increased, as is FRC, because of dynamic hyper-inflation, which also causes the barrel-like appearance of the chest. Cough is rare in these patients.

Gas Exchange in the Lung

INTRODUCTION

Why do we breathe? The vital importance of breathing was clear even in ancient times, when people believed that the air we breathe, or *pneumo*, gives rise to the spirit. Oxygen in the air enables active cellular metabolism, enabling optimal function at the cellular level and ultimately proper functioning of all of the body's organ systems.

Ultimately, the lungs bear two important responsibilities:
- To provide oxygen to cells to enable energy release via oxidative phosphorylation;
- To maintain physiologically optimal pH (alongside the kidneys) through control of carbon dioxide, a waste product of cellular metabolism, in the blood.

The lungs perform these tasks through passive gas exchange between the atmosphere and the blood, absorbing oxygen from air and releasing carbon dioxide into air. Breathing or ventilation—the mechanical function of the lung—makes effective gas exchange possible.

SYSTEM STRUCTURE: THE DISTAL RESPIRATORY TREE AND PULMONARY CIRCULATION

Please refer to Chapter 13 for a more in-depth discussion of lung structure. However, it is useful to review and expand upon some of these basic tenets with attention to pulmonary gas exchange.

Recall that the trachea gives rise to large airways that progressively branch during descent into the lungs, ultimately leading to the respiratory bronchioles and alveoli that participate in gas exchange (Fig. 14.1).
- The large airways allow passage of air but do not perform gas exchange (i.e., they are conducting airways).
- The volume occupied by the conducting airways, where gas exchange does not occur, is also known as anatomic dead space.
The walls of the alveolar compartments, across which gas exchange occurs, are only about two cells thick (Fig. 14.2).
- The alveolar lumen is lined by type I pneumocytes, flat, thin cells that lie adjacent to the basement membrane.
- Alveoli are enmeshed in extensive plexus of capillaries, whose walls are composed of flat, thin endothelial cells.
- Other cells appear intermittently in the alveolar wall do not constitute the gas exchange surface, but still serve vital functions.
  - Type II pneumocytes (secretion of surfactant)
  - Fibroblasts (lay down basement membrane, which is composed of collagen and elastin)
  - Macrophages
  - Clara cells (main secretory cell type in distal conducting airways, defend against pollutants and aid in repair)

From one alveoli to the next, we would encounter the following cell types:
- First alveolar space → type I pneumocyte → basement membrane → capillary endothelial cell wall → blood → opposite capillary wall → basement membrane → type I pneumocyte → second alveolar space

Pulmonary circulation, consisting of the pulmonary arteries, capillaries, and veins, is supplied by the right ventricle pumping deoxygenated blood into the pulmonary trunk.
- The pulmonary trunk feeds into dual pulmonary arteries.
- These each contribute to capillaries surrounding the alveoli, which participate in gas exchange.
- Oxygenated blood is then carried into the pulmonary vein, which supplies the left ventricle for propulsion of oxygenated blood to the rest of the body.

However, the lungs also contain bronchial arteries, which carry oxygenated blood from systemic circulation to feed the lungs.
- These primarily feed the walls of large airways, which (unlike alveoli) cannot rely on direct oxygen absorption.
- Bronchial arteries arise from the thoracic aorta and posterior intercostal arteries.
- However, deoxygenated bronchial blood ultimately feeds back into the pulmonary veins (see Fast Fact Box 14.1).

Fast Fact Box 14.1
Because of dual blood supply from the bronchial and pulmonary arteries, the lungs are more resistant to infarction.

Fig. 14.3 shows the functional units of the lung, including the two pulmonary arterial supplies.

SYSTEM FUNCTION: OXYGENATION AND THE CLEARANCE OF CARBON DIOXIDE

Our first consideration in understanding gas exchange is the behavior of gases in general. For this, we will briefly review the principles of gases from introductory chemistry in the context of clinical medicine.

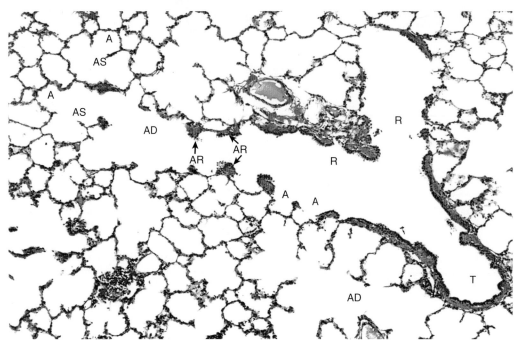

Fig. 14.1 The respiratory bronchioles and alveoli. *A,* Alveolus; *AD,* alveolar duct; *AR,* alveolar ring; *AS,* alveolar sac; *R,* respiratory bronchiole; *T,* terminal bronchiole. (From Young B, Woodford P, O'Dowd G. *Wheater's Functional Histology*, 6th Ed. Philadelphia: Elsevier; 2014. Fig. 12.12.)

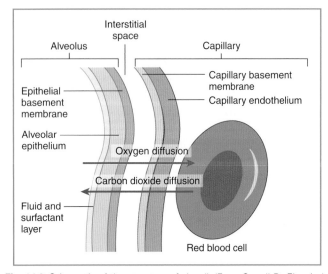

Fig. 14.2 Schematic of the structure of alveoli. (From Carroll R. *Elsevier's Integrated Physiology.* Philadelphia: Mosby Elsevier; 2007. Fig. 10.11.)

Gases

For both a single gaseous species and a mixed gas (such as that in atmospheric air and the alveoli), the relationships among different parameters of this gas are expressed within the ideal gas law:

$$PV = nRT \qquad \textbf{(Eq. 14.1)}$$

where P = pressure exerted by gas, V = volume occupied by gas, n = number of moles of gas, R = empirically determined constant, and T = temperature of the gas.

In a mixture of gases, one can express the amount of a particular species of gas as the partial pressure. This same term can also be used to describe the amount of a particular species of gas that has been dissolved in the blood. The partial pressure of a given gas is related to the total pressure of the gas mixture in proportion to the mol fraction of the given gas.

$$P_1/P_T = n_1/n_T \qquad \textbf{(Eq. 14.2)}$$

where P_1 = partial pressure of gas 1, P_T = total pressure, n_1 = moles of gas 1, and n_T = total moles in gaseous mixture.

Given that n_T in a gaseous mixture is the sum of its components, this relationship implies Dalton's law of partial pressures, or:

$$P_T = P_1 + P_2 + P_3 \ldots P_n \qquad \textbf{(Eq. 14.3)}$$

Using these relationships, we can better understand the movement of gas from blood to alveoli (Fig. 14.4).

- Molecules in atmospheric gas dissolve into blood *in proportion* to the quantity of each gas in the mixture.
- The greater the partial pressure, the more molecules that will dissolve into blood. (see Fig. 14.4A)
  - High P_1 = high efflux into blood = high blood concentration
  - Low P_1 = low efflux into blood = low blood concentration
- Net dissolution of a given gas continues until equilibrium is achieved between influx and efflux (see Fig. 14.4B) (see Clinical Correlation Box 14.1).

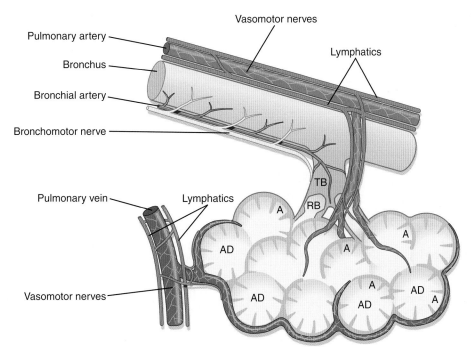

Fig. 14.3 The functional units of the lung. *A*, Alveoli; *AD*, alveolar ducts; *RB*, respiratory bronchioles; *TB*, terminal bronchioles. (From Koeppen BM, Stanton BA, *Berne and Levy Physiology*, 7th Ed. Philadelphia: Elsevier; Fig. 20.7.)

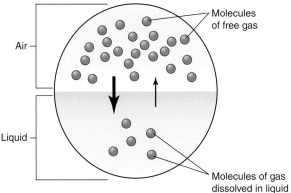

A Before equilibrium is achieved

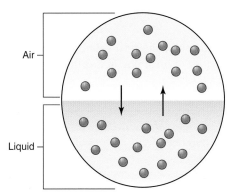

B At equilibrium

Fig. 14.4 Equilibrium vapor pressure. A, The large amount of free gas and small amount of dissolved gas means more molecules randomly move into solution than come out. The amount of dissolved gas increases, which in turn increases the number of molecules coming out of solution. B, The amount of free gas depletes and the amount of dissolved gas increases until the rates of gas-liquid crossover become the same in both directions.

> ## Clinical Correlation Box 14.1
>
> What happens when you submit an arterial blood gas (ABG)?
>
> The sensors in blood gas analyzers yield readings in partial pressure, yet they do not measure partial pressure directly. Instead, the sample is exposed to O_2 and pH-sensitive electrodes covered in a permeable membrane. These electrodes then read out the number of millivolts in proportion to the quantity of O_2 and CO_2 in solution. This millivolt reading is then converted to an equilibrium partial pressure using a reference measurement.
>
> The reference measurements are derived from electrode sampling of blood from a tonometer with a known equilibrium partial pressure of O_2 or CO_2.
> - Acquire millivolt reading for known PCO_2 and PCO_2
> - Correlation forms basis for linear conversion from millivolts → equilibrium partial pressure for a patient sample
> - Recalibration must occur with sufficient frequency (i.e., every personnel shift) to ensure accuracy

By using this convention to describe the amount of blood gas, we can readily predict the direction of change of blood oxygen content when systemic venous blood (the same as pulmonary arterial blood), for example, is exposed to alveolar air.

- The venous blood would be at equilibrium at 40 mm Hg partial pressure of oxygen (PO_2).
- On exposure, a higher alveolar PO_2 (P_AO_2) will drive more oxygen into solution until a new equilibrium is reached (e.g., 100 mm Hg), with the blood and the alveolar air at the same PO_2.
- The equilibrium PO_2 is higher than blood's initial PO_2 and lower than alveolar air's initial PO_2 (Fig. 14.5).

For a list of the most physiologically significant partial pressures, please refer to Table 14.1.

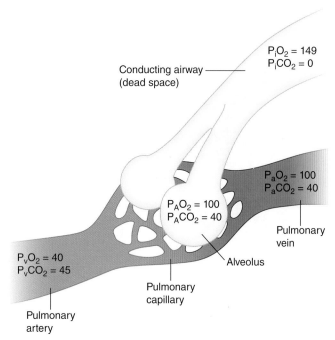

P₁O₂ = 149
P₁CO₂ = 0

Conducting airway
(dead space)

P_aO₂ = 100
P_aCO₂ = 40

P_AO₂ = 100
P_ACO₂ = 40

Pulmonary
vein

P_vO₂ = 40
P_vCO₂ = 45

Alveolus

Pulmonary
capillary

Pulmonary
artery

Fig. 14.5 Equilibration of partial pressures between the alveolus and the blood. The partial pressures shown in the alveolus are those after inspired air has mixed with the end expiratory alveolar air and after this mixture has equilibrated with blood. Subscripts: i refers to inhaled air, A refers to the alveolus, a refers to arterial blood, v refers to venous blood.

Ventilation

During periods of rest (i.e., in between breaths or while holding one's breath), the composition of air within the gas-exchanging portion of the lung (the alveolar gas) will remain dynamic.

- Peripheral tissues continuously absorb O_2 from systemic blood and offload CO_2.
- Blood returning to the lung from the body tissues is thus O_2-poor and CO_2-rich.
- If ventilation is not occurring, this blood continuously absorbs O_2 from the alveolar gas and deposits CO_2 in return via simple diffusion.
- Therefore O_2 levels in alveolar gas are continuously going down while CO_2 levels are going up.

Ventilation can thus be seen as an effort to keep alveolar gas O_2-rich and CO_2-poor by blowing off gas low in O_2 and high in CO_2 and replacing it with atmospheric gas, which has the opposite proportions. This maintains the alveolar gas to blood gas gradients necessary to promote continued clearance of CO_2 and absorption of O_2.

Before inhalation, the lung volume is at functional residency capacity (FRC) as described in Chapter 13. Inspiration adds the tidal volume (V_T) to the preexisting volume at FRC (Fig. 14.6)

- The tidal volume is composed of two components, V_A and V_D.
  - 2/3 of V_T is added to the expanded alveoli, and is called V_A.
  - 1/3 of V_T is added to the expanded dead space, and is called V_D.
  - $V_A + V_D = V_T$
- V_A mixes with the preexisting FRC volume.
  - PO_2 rises above FRC levels but drops below that of atmospheric air.
  - PCO_2 drops below FRC levels but rises above that of atmospheric air (~0).

With expiration, the same tidal volume is blown off and the new V_A (with higher CO_2, lower O_2 composition) leaves the alveoli. Now, there is a better gradient for O_2 absorption and CO_2 clearance in the alveoli (Fig. 14.7).

This paradigm leads to two important tenets:
- With decreasing respiratory rate, alveolar gas at FRC will have more time to accumulate CO_2 and lose $O_2 \rightarrow \uparrow P_ACO_2$ and $\downarrow P_AO_2$.
- With decreasing tidal volume, less V_A will be added to FRC with constant CO_2 production $\rightarrow \uparrow P_ACO_2$ and $\downarrow P_AO_2$.

Stated another way, V_A and f (the frequency of breathing in breaths per minute) have an inverse relationship with the amount of alveolar CO_2 (P_ACO_2), and a direct relationship with the amount of alveolar O_2 (P_AO_2). Thus the partial pressures of O_2 and CO_2 in alveolar gas are a function of the net size of the addition of V_A to alveolar gas per unit time, $\dot{V}_A$. Note the dot notation that stands for the first derivative. It indicates that this is a flow rate—a change in volume over time. V_A is the alveolar volume (units in mL) while dot V_A is the alveolar ventilation flow rate (units in mL/min). This ventilation rate can be expressed as the magnitude of V_A multiplied by the frequency of V_A's addition to alveolar gas. In other words,

$$\dot{V}_A = V_A f$$

where V_A = the portion of the tidal volume added to alveolar gas, f = the frequency of breathing in breaths per minute, and $\dot{V}_A$ is the alveolar ventilation.

TABLE 14.1 **Important Partial Pressures With Typical Values**		
Partial Pressure	**Symbol**	**Normal Value (mm Hg)**
Alveolar partial pressure of oxygen	P_AO_2	100–105
Alveolar partial pressure of carbon dioxide	P_ACO_2	40
Arterial partial pressure of oxygen = PO_2 in pulmonary vein	P_aO_2	95–100
Arterial partial pressure of carbon dioxide = PCO_2 in pulmonary vein	P_aCO_2	40
Inspired partial pressure of oxygen	P_iO_2	149[a]
Inspired partial pressure of carbon dioxide	P_iCO_2	0.3 (negligible)
Venous partial pressure of oxygen = PO_2 in pulmonary artery	P_vO_2	40
Venous partial pressure of carbon dioxide = PO_2 in pulmonary artery	P_vCO_2	45

[a]Assuming (BT)PS, that is, saturated pressure because it is inside the body.

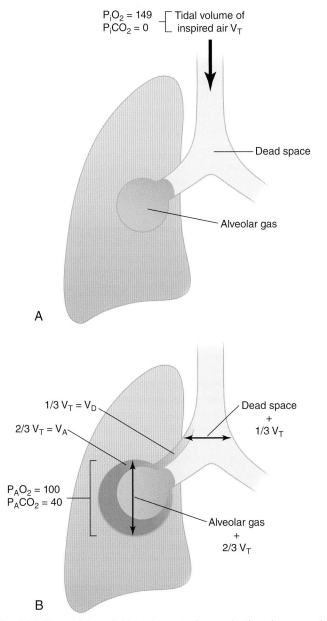

A

$P_IO_2 = 149$
$P_ICO_2 = 0$ — Tidal volume of inspired air V_T

— Dead space

— Alveolar gas

B

$1/3 V_T = V_D$

$2/3 V_T = V_A$

$P_AO_2 = 100$
$P_ACO_2 = 40$

Dead space + $1/3 V_T$

Alveolar gas + $2/3 V_T$

Fig. 14.6 The addition of tidal volume to the conducting airways and alveoli. Two-thirds of the tidal volume is added to the gas-exchanging alveolar space and one-third to the anatomic dead space, assuming all alveoli are open and participating in gas exchange. For simplicity, the alveolar space is represented by one large schematic alveolus in one lung. A, At functional residual capacity (FRC): before the addition of a tidal volume V_T. B, At FRC + V_T after the addition of a tidal volume V_T. All partial pressures are measured in mm Hg.

From the above relationships come the definitions of hyperventilation and hypoventilation.

- Hyperventilation ($P_ACO_2 < 38$ mm Hg) refers to elimination of CO_2 exceeding its rate of production, leading to a decreased P_aCO_2 in the blood (hypocapnia; $P_aCO_2 < 38$ mm Hg).
  - An increased breathing frequency is known as tachypnea, and is not synonymous with hyperventilation.
- Hypoventilation ($P_ACO_2 > 42$ mm Hg), similarly, is not simply a decreased rate of breathing but a decrease in alveolar ventilation relative to CO_2 production. When the

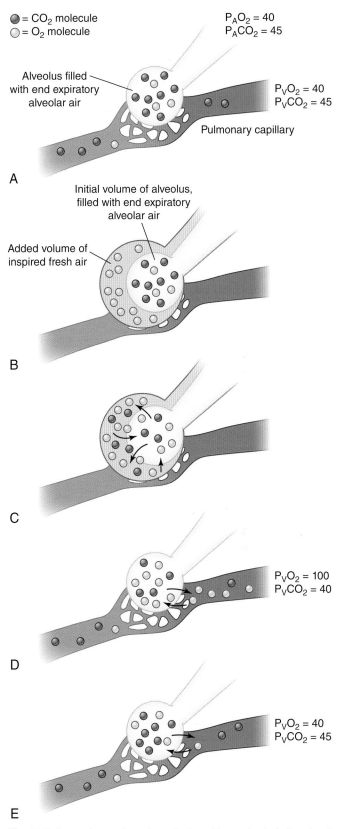

= CO_2 molecule
= O_2 molecule

$P_AO_2 = 40$
$P_ACO_2 = 45$

Alveolus filled with end expiratory alveolar air

$P_VO_2 = 40$
$P_VCO_2 = 45$

Pulmonary capillary

A

Initial volume of alveolus, filled with end expiratory alveolar air

Added volume of inspired fresh air

B

C

$P_VO_2 = 100$
$P_VCO_2 = 40$

D

$P_VO_2 = 40$
$P_VCO_2 = 45$

E

Fig. 14.7 Gas exchange throughout the breathing cycle. A, At functional residual capacity (FRC), preinspiration, the alveolus filled with end expiratory alveolar air. B, At FRC + tidal volume (V_T), after inspiration, the added volume of inspired, fresh atmospheric air. C, At FRC + V_T, end expiratory alveolar air mixing with inspired fresh air. D, Back to FRC, after expiration. E, At FRC, after gas exchange has again created end expiratory alveolar air. All partial pressures are measured in mm Hg.

elimination of CO_2 is less than its production rate, the consequence is an increased P_aCO_2 (hypercapnia; $P_aCO_2 >$ 42 mm Hg).

The Alveolar Ventilation Equation

The relationship between alveolar ventilation and P_ACO_2, described earlier, can be stated mathematically in the alveolar ventilation equation:

$$\dot{V}_A = \left(\dot{V}_{CO_2} / P_ACO_2\right)(K) \qquad \textbf{(Eq. 14.4)}$$

where $\dot{V}_{CO_2}$ is the rate of CO_2 production and K is a constant that includes conversion from standard temperature (22° C) to body temperature (37° C).

$\dot{V}_{CO_2}$ represents the mass of CO_2 being produced in the peripheral tissues in accordance with the cells' production and its diffusion into the blood.

Unless the metabolic rate in the tissues changes, $\dot{V}_{CO_2}$ remains constant.

- Instead of representing an anatomic lung volume, $\dot{V}_{CO_2}$ is the volume per time that would be occupied by the mass of CO_2 produced if this CO_2 were at standard temperature (295.15K) and pressure (760 mm Hg) in dry ($PH_2O = 0$ mm Hg) air.

As $\dot{V}_A$ goes up and dilutes this constant amount of CO_2 production in the alveolar gas, the alveolar partial pressure of CO_2 (P_ACO_2) goes down.

One might at first think that the same sort of equation could be written for the relationship between $\dot{V}_A$ and P_AO_2, but it cannot because the relationship between $\dot{V}_A$ and P_ACO_2 is linear, but the relationship between $\dot{V}_A$ and P_AO_2 is not linear over the entire physiologic range. Although increased $\dot{V}_A$ will increase P_AO_2, it does not do so in a linear relationship because unlike CO_2, there is a significant amount of O_2 in the inspired air.

Diffusion

The average distance between blood and alveolar air in the lung is less than 1.5 μm, which ensures that simple diffusion is possible. In the healthy lung, blood equilibrates with respect to O_2 and CO_2 after traveling about one-third of the length of the pulmonary capillary. The equation that describes the determining factors for diffusion rate is Fick's law:

$$\dot{V}_G = (P_A - P_C)(A)(S) / (T)(MW) \qquad \textbf{(Eq. 14.5)}$$

where $\dot{V}_G$ = volume of gas transferred across the membrane per unit time, P_A = partial pressure of the gas in the alveolus, P_C = partial pressure of the gas in the capillary, A = area of membrane of transfer, S = solubility of the gas in blood, T = thickness of membrane, and MW = molecular weight of the gas.

Because O_2 and CO_2 both have a rapid diffusion rate and equilibrate early in the capillary, they display perfusion-limited gas exchange, wherein the amount of O_2 and CO_2 gas exchange is limited by alveolar perfusion.

- No matter how fast the diffusion time, if less blood is delivered per time to the alveolar capillary, less CO_2 will cross over into alveolar air and less O_2 will cross over into blood.

- This is because only a certain amount of these gases can be dissolved into the blood plasma, or bound to hemoglobin (or buffered by HCO_3^-, as in the case of CO_2).
- Thus increasing perfusion rate ensures that new blood is present that can undergo immediate gas exchange (see Fast Fact Box 14.2. Also Genetics Box 14.1, Pharmacology Box 14.1, and Development Box 14.1).

Fast Fact Box 14.2

The fact that O_2 exchange is perfusion-limited means increases in heart rate will increase oxygenation.

 GENETICS BOX 14.1

Patients with cystic fibrosis (CF) have mutations in the CFTR gene that encodes a transmembrane Cl^- channel. The movement of Cl^- helps regulate the water content of respiratory tract mucus. Without normal Cl^- transport, patients produce tenacious, abnormally viscous mucus. In the lungs, this mucus impairs gas exchange and obstructs airways, causing respiratory distress with dyspnea, coughing, and wheezing. It is hoped that the CRISPR gene editing technology will allow for the safe correction of mutated CFTR genes and cure of CF.

 PHARMACOLOGY BOX 14.1

Antibiotics (particularly inhaled antibiotics that combat alveolar bacteria while limiting systemic effects) are useful in treating respiratory bacterial infections in patients with cystic fibrosis (CF). Inhaled β-2-adrenergic agonists, such as albuterol, can help acute symptoms. Airway mucus can be made less viscous with inhaled DNAse I (dornase α), an endonuclease that digests neutrophil DNA. Depending on the specific CF transmembrane conductance regulator (CFTR) mutation, CF patients can benefit from Ivacaftor, a small molecule that augments the function of the Cl^- channel in patients with selected "gating" mutations. It can be combined with Lumacaftor or Tezacaftor, agents that improve mutant CFTR protein folding.

 DEVELOPMENT BOX 14.1

With chronic mucus hypersecretion, airflow obstruction, and repeated respiratory infections, cystic fibrosis (CF) patients progressively develop airway damage with scarring and distortion of the normal architecture called "bronchiectasis." This impairs clearance of mucus and fluid from the airways, and leads to chronic cough and mucus hypersecretion. Patients also produce hyperviscous mucus in the gastrointestinal tract, and patients frequently have mucus obstructing their pancreatic ducts, leading to damage to this endocrine and exocrine organ and leading to diabetes and malabsorption. In affected males, accumulation of mucus in the vas deferens leads to infertility.

The exchange of other more slowly diffusing molecules, like carbon monoxide (CO), is known as diffusion-limited gas exchange.

- Blood may need to travel the whole length of the capillary before equilibrating.
- Thus higher rate of blood flow will actually decrease gas exchange for these substances as blood would spend less time in the capillary before being swept downstream (see Clinical Correlation Box 14.2).

Alveolar and Arterial Partial Pressures

The rapidity with which alveolar gas equilibrates with blood has fundamental implications for pulmonary physiology.

- Partial pressures of O_2 and CO_2 in the alveolus (P_AO_2 and P_ACO_2) exactly match the partial pressures of O_2 and CO_2 in the blood leaving the alveolus (P_aO_2 and P_aCO_2).
- In other words: $P_AO_2 = P_aO_2$ and $P_ACO_2 = P_aCO_2$.

If all alveolar partial pressures of O_2 and CO_2 were the same in every alveolus, the arterial partial pressure would match that one number. However, as the following discussion will show, the alveolar partial pressures are not perfectly uniform across the entire lung.

Ventilation-Perfusion Relationships: $\dot{V}_A/\dot{Q}$ Mismatch

In the normal lung, as well in pathologic states, the alveolar ventilation $\dot{V}_A$ varies in different parts of the lung. In addition, the blood flow $\dot{Q}$ varies from one part of the lung to another.

Consequently, different parts of the lungs have a different ventilation-perfusion ($\dot{V}_A/\dot{Q}$) ratio.

An imbalance in this ratio is termed a $\dot{V}_A/\dot{Q}$ mismatch.

Varying the regional $\dot{V}_A$ with respect to blood flow introduces regional variations in the alveolar partial pressures of O_2 and CO_2.

↑ regional $\dot{V}_A$ ~ regional hyperventilation → ↑ regional P_AO_2 and P_aO_2, ↓ regional P_ACO_2 and P_aCO_2.

↓ regional $\dot{V}_A$ ~ regional hypoventilation → ↓ regional P_AO_2 and P_aO_2, ↑ regional P_ACO_2 and P_aCO_2.

Varying the regional $\dot{Q}$ with respect to alveolar minute ventilation also introduces regional variations in the alveolar partial pressures of O_2 and CO_2.

↓ regional $\dot{Q}$ with respect to $\dot{V}_A$ ~ ↑ regional $\dot{V}_A$ because of reduced CO_2 delivery and O_2 absorption → ↑ regional P_AO_2 and P_aO_2, ↓ regional P_ACO_2 and P_aCO_2.

↑ regional $\dot{Q}$ with respect to $\dot{V}_A$ ~ ↓ regional $\dot{V}_A$ ~ regional hypoventilation → ↓ regional P_AO_2 and P_aO_2, ↑ regional P_ACO_2 and P_aCO_2.

The alveolar ventilation equation predicts this. With a lower $\dot{V}_{CO_2}$ in the alveolar ventilation equation and the same $\dot{V}_A$, P_ACO_2 would be lower and hence local P_aCO_2 would be lower as well.

Given the effect of changes in $\dot{V}_A$ and $\dot{Q}$ described earlier, it is the $\dot{V}_A/\dot{Q}$ ratio that determines regional partial pressures.

High $\dot{V}_A/\dot{Q}$ increases partial pressures of O_2 but decreases partial pressures of CO_2

Low $\dot{V}_A/\dot{Q}$ decreases partial pressures of O_2 but increases partial pressures of CO_2

When extreme, $\dot{V}_A/\dot{Q}$ mismatches have specific names.

When $\dot{V}_A$ is zero and hence $\dot{V}_A/\dot{Q} = 0$, it is called a shunt.

- Collapse of part of the lung (atelectasis).
- Filling of alveoli with inflammatory debris (consolidation), as in pneumonia.

When $\dot{Q}$ is zero and hence $\dot{V}_A/\dot{Q} = \infty$ it is called physiologic dead space.

- Large airways with lack of blood supply to participate in gas exchange.
- Pulmonary embolism (blockage of arterial supply with clot).

Because $\dot{V}_A/\dot{Q}$ mismatches are regional, what effect do they have on the overall P_aO_2 and P_aCO_2?

Shunt (low $\dot{V}_A/\dot{Q}$) impairs gas exchange.

- This causes pulmonary capillary blood to approach P_vO_2 and P_vCO_2, that is, decreasing P_aO_2 and increasing P_aCO_2 in the blood from these mismatched regions.
- This poorly ventilated blood will mix with a larger amount of better-ventilated blood in the pulmonary vein.
- Overall effect: ↓ systemic P_aO_2 (mild, not significant in the healthy lung), and ↑ systemic P_aCO_2 (mild).

Dead space makes no contribution per se to blood gas composition because by definition no blood ever sees this part of the lung.

- In this region of poor gas exchange, the P_AO_2 and P_ACO_2 will approach the partial pressure values of the gases in inspired air.

The higher P_aO_2 and lower P_aCO_2 blood from these high $\dot{V}_A/\dot{Q}$ areas mixes with all the blood in the pulmonary vein.

- Overall effect: ↓ P_aCO_2 (mild), no change in P_aO_2 (because of saturation of oxygen-carrying molecules in the blood under normal conditions).

The nature of the oxyhemoglobin dissociation curve (Fig. 14.8) accounts for the way that regional changes affect overall values of PO_2 (see Ch. 15).

- The dissolved O_2 and CO_2 are not the only pools of O_2 and CO_2 in the blood.
- O_2 and CO_2 are also bound to the protein hemoglobin.

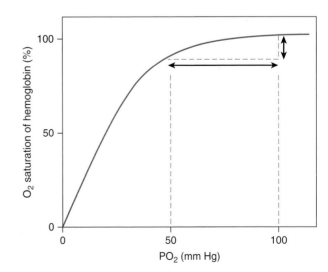

Fig. 14.8 The oxyhemoglobin dissociation curve. A significant increase in PO_2 yields a much less significant increase in total O_2 content. Note that even though this curve is highly nonlinear, a portion of it can be approximated as linear, using the "40-50-60, 70-80-90" rule: when partial pressure of oxygen (PO_2) = 40 mm Hg, oxygen saturation (SaO_2) = 70%, when PO_2 = 50 mm Hg, SaO_2 = 80%, and when PO_2 = 60 mm Hg, SaO_2 = 90%.

- ↑ blood PO_2 or PCO_2 will drive greater amounts of these gases into association with hemoglobin.
- The vast majority of the total blood O_2 content is accounted for not by the dissolved O_2, measured in partial pressure, but in hemoglobin-associated O_2 (Table 14.2).

For a clearer picture of blood oxygen content, imagine that blood were a building with a small foyer and a large interior, and O_2 molecules were people crowding into the building.

- At high P_AO_2, O_2 would pass through the foyer as dissolved O_2 and crowd into the large interior as hemoglobin-associated molecules until the interior were full, at which time the door to the interior would be sealed shut.
- With continued high P_AO_2, the O_2 would crowd into the foyer as high P_AO_2-dissolved O_2, but could not get into the interior.
- Thus even though the foyer would get more and more tightly packed, the overall number of people in the building would not be affected significantly.

In other words, at P_aO_2 values greater than 50 mm Hg (where hemoglobin is already nearly saturated with oxygen), increases in P_aO_2 do not produce significantly increased hemoglobin association and hence do not significantly elevate the total O_2 content.

Therefore the high P_aO_2 blood from the high $\dot{V}_A/\dot{Q}$ areas contributes little total O_2 content to the blood of the pulmonary vein.

- This does not raise the overall P_aO_2 significantly.

On the other hand, at P_aO_2 values less than 50 mm Hg (where hemoglobin is not near saturation), decreases in P_aO_2 do significantly reduce total oxygen content.

Consequently, when blood from low $\dot{V}_A/\dot{Q}$ areas mixes with an equal amount of blood from high $\dot{V}_A/\dot{Q}$ areas, the blood from the regionally low $\dot{V}_A/\dot{Q}$ area does significantly reduce overall oxygen content.

- This reduces the overall P_aO_2.

CO_2's hemoglobin dissociation curve is more linear; variations in P_aCO_2 are truer reflections of variations in total blood CO_2 content (Fig. 14.9).

For this reason, when low $\dot{V}_A/\dot{Q}$ blood and high $\dot{V}_A/\dot{Q}$ blood mix, the $PaCO_2$ normalizes.

In summary (Fig. 14.10):

Low $\dot{V}_A/\dot{Q}$ lowers P_aO_2 and high $\dot{V}_A/\dot{Q}$ has a negligible effect on P_aO_2

High $\dot{V}_A/\dot{Q}$ can compensate for low $\dot{V}_A/\dot{Q}$ in the case of P_aCO_2 but not in the case of P_aO_2.

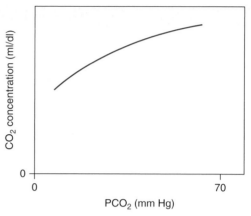

Fig. 14.9 The CO_2 dissociation curve.

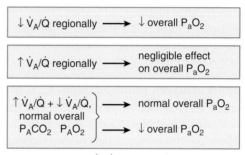

Fig. 14.10 The effect of the $\dot{V}_A/\dot{Q}$ ratio on the overall partial pressures of O_2 and CO_2. Even if the overall P_aO_2 is normal, low $\dot{V}_A/\dot{Q}$ can decrease overall P_aO_2, creating an A-a gradient.

The Alveolar Gas Equation

What is the importance of low P_aO_2, and how may it be caused? The answer to this question is useful in the differential diagnosis because certain disease states lower P_aO_2 by low $\dot{V}_A/\dot{Q}$, while other disease states lower P_aO_2 by different means.

The alveolar gas equation, or alveolar air equation, can be used by a physician at the bedside to determine whether a patient's low P_aO_2 is because of low $\dot{V}_A/\dot{Q}$.

- The alveolar gas equation enables physicians to calculate P_AO_2.

Because average P_AO_2 is sometimes higher than P_aO_2 owing to low $\dot{V}_A/\dot{Q}$, as described earlier, we can compare our P_AO_2 value from the alveolar gas equation with measured P_aO_2.

If there is a difference, which we term an A-a gradient, we know that low $\dot{V}_A/\dot{Q}$ exists.

TABLE 14.2 Amount of Oxygen and Carbon Dioxide Carried by Various Transporters in the Blood (Typical Values)

Transporter Mechanism	% O_2 by Volume		% CO_2 by Volume	
	Artery	Vein	Artery	Vein
Dissolved	1.4%	0.9%	4.9%	5.3%
Hemoglobin-bound	98.6%	99.1%	90.2%	87.4%
HCO_3^- bound	0%	0%	4.9%	7.3%

Assumes $P_AO_2 = 100$ mm Hg, $P_ACO_2 = 40$ mm Hg. $P_vO_2 = 40$ mm Hg, $P_vCO_2 = 45$ mm Hg.

The alveolar gas equation is as follows:

$$P_AO_2 = P_IO_2 - (P_ACO_2/R) + F \qquad \textbf{(Eq. 14.6)}$$

where P_IO_2 is the partial pressure of O_2 in inspired air, R is the respiratory exchange ratio equal to 0.8, and F is a correction factor (equal to $(1-R)/R*F_IO_2*P_ACO_2$) that can be discounted at an F_IO_2, or O_2 mol fraction, less than 50%, such as the atmospheric F_IO_2 of 21%.

- P_IO_2 is calculated for water-saturated air (i.e., P_B-P_{H2O}; barometric pressure minus the partial pressure because of water).
  - PO_2 for dry air is (21%) * (atmospheric pressure or 760 mm Hg) = 159 mm Hg.
  - At normal body temperature of 37° C, water vapor pressure at saturation = 47 mm Hg.
  - Thus PO_2 for air saturated with water vapor, as it is in the lung airways, is (21%) * (760 – 47 mm Hg) = 149 mm Hg. R represents the ratio of the amount of CO_2 produced out of blood into alveolar air per amount of O_2 extracted from the alveolar air ($\dot{V}CO_2/\dot{V}O_2$.)
  - R is approximately equal to 0.8 on a "normal" protein diet, but is equal to 1 on a high-carbohydrate diet, and 0.7 on a high-fat diet.
    This is because the oxidation of fat, for example, produces less CO_2 than that of carbohydrates per unit of oxygen.
    What does the alveolar gas equation mean?
- Imagine a theoretical "first breath" that filled the entire space of the lungs with atmospheric air at P_IO_2 of 149 mm Hg. Now the alveolar gas is depleting in O_2 content and accumulating CO_2 content.
- According to R, we know that alveolar gas loses 1.2, or 1/0.8, mol O_2 for every 1 mol CO_2 produced, when R = 0.8.
- Therefore we know the amount that P_AO_2 has dropped from its initial P_IO_2 of 149 mm Hg is equal to the amount that P_ACO_2 has increased from its P_ICO_2 of 0 mm Hg multiplied by 1.2 mol of O_2 decrease per mol of CO_2 increase. Restated:

$$\Delta P_AO_2 = (\Delta P_ACO_2) \qquad \textbf{(Eq. 14.7)}$$
$$*(1.2 \text{ mol } O_2 \text{ consumed / mol } CO_2 \text{ produced})$$

This may be rephrased as:

P_IO_2 [initial P_AO_2] $- P_AO_2$ [P_AO_2 after exchange]
$= (P_ACO_2$ [P_ACO_2 after exchange]
$- P_ICO_2$ [initial P_ACO_2]$)(1.2)$; with $P_ICO_2 = $ to 0 mm Hg

such that:

$$P_AO_2 = P_IO_2 - P_ACO_2/R$$

and therefore $P_AO_2 = P_IO_2 - P_ACO_2/0.8$ **(Eq. 14.8)**

Because P_ACO_2 is not particularly sensitive to $\dot{V}_A/\dot{Q}$ mismatch, the average P_ACO_2 is considered always to be equal to P_aCO_2. Therefore with an arterial blood gas (ABG) test that gives us P_aO_2 and P_aCO_2, and with P_IO_2 known to be 149 mm Hg, we can calculate P_AO_2 and compare it to P_aO_2 to obtain our A-a gradient (see Clinical Correlation Box 14.3).

The Physiologic A-a Gradient

Even under normal physiologic conditions, there is a small A-a gradient of 5 or 10 mm Hg. In fact, the normal A-a gradient is equivalent to approximately 10 + 3 (age 30 years)/10 for people who are over 30 years old.

Several normal anatomic features account for this finding:
1. Areas of high and low $\dot{V}_A/\dot{Q}$ are naturally present in the lung (Fig. 14.11).
   - Blood flow and ventilation both increase from the apex (top) to base (bottom) of the lungs. However, blood flow increases out of proportion to ventilation.
   - This results in:
     Lower $\dot{V}_A/\dot{Q}$ at the base
     Higher $\dot{V}_A/\dot{Q}$ at the apex
   - These regional differences in ventilation and blood flow in the healthy lung are in part determined by gravity.
   - Ventilation
     The dependent area of the lung (i.e., the inferior area when lying supine or lung base when standing) bears the weight of the lung tissues above it and compresses the pleural space, making pleural pressure at the lung base less negative and reducing the transpulmonary pressure at the lung base.

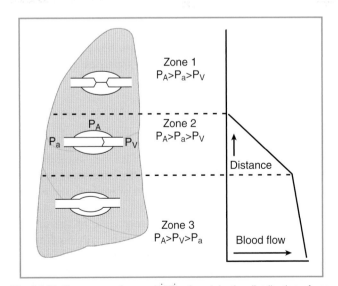

Fig. 14.11 One cause of normal $\dot{V}_A/\dot{Q}$ mismatch: the distribution of ventilation and blood flow across the lung. Ventilation is higher at the apex of the lung, blood flow higher at the base. Gravity draws more blood flow to the bottom of the lung (and dependent lung), and the weight of the superior lung tissue compresses the inferior lung tissue slightly, shrinking the alveolar spaces. P_a, Arterial partial pressure; P_A, alveolar partial pressure; P_V, venous partial pressure. (From Carroll R. *Elsevier's Integrated Physiology*. Philadelphia: Mosby Elsevier; 2007. Fig. 10.13.)

Recall that transpulmonary pressure is what causes the lung to open; lower transpulmonary pressures should mean reduced opening of the lung and a smaller alveolar ventilation volume per breath. However, compliance of the lung is actually greater at the base at FRC.

Thus alveolar ventilation at this level will in fact be greater than at the apex of the lungs.

- Blood flow

  Gravity increases blood flow to the bases.

  The pulmonary vessels' smooth muscle tone is much lower than in the systemic vessels, and therefore the vessels accommodate this downward flow in a way that systemic vessels would not.

  Pulmonary vessels in the dependent lung are thus more distended than those at the lung apex.

2. The bronchial arteries naturally form an anatomic shunt.
   - Recall that the bronchial arteries supply non–gas-exchanging tissues in the lung with oxygenated blood from the left heart.
   - This blood then returns to the left heart via the pulmonary vein, dumping its deoxygenated blood into the systemic arterial system without having first been ventilated.
   - This constitutes an anatomic shunt, that is, blood flowing through the lung returning to the left heart unventilated and deoxygenated.

3. The thebesian veins also create an anatomic shunt.
   - They return used, deoxygenated blood from the coronary arteries directly into the left ventricle.

The normal anatomic shunts account for approximately 5% of the circulating blood volume at a given time.

Pulmonary Blood Flow

The pulmonary arteries carry deoxygenated blood and the systemic arteries carry oxygenated blood. The lung vessels carry blood from right heart ventricle to left heart atrium, whereas the systemic vessels carry blood from left heart ventricle to right heart atrium. There are, however, two other major differences between pulmonary arteries and systemic arteries:

- Blood pressure
- Regulation of blood flow

Pulmonary Blood Pressure

The pulmonary arterial blood pressure is much lower than the systemic blood pressure (Fig. 14.12). To understand why this must be so, consider the Starling forces at work on the pulmonary blood vessel (see Ch. 9).

- The pulmonary capillaries run very close to the outside atmosphere, and therefore the pressure surrounding the pulmonary capillaries is much lower than the pressure surrounding the systemic capillaries. Consequently, the pulmonary arterial system maintains a lower pressure than systemic blood pressure.
- If the pressure in the pulmonary capillaries were the same as the pressure inside systemic capillaries, there would be a large hydrostatic pressure gradient for fluid extravasation across the pulmonary capillary walls.

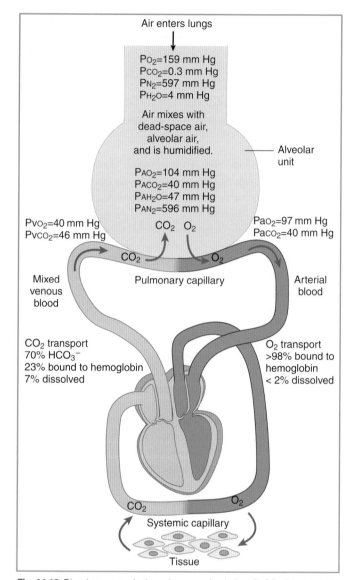

Fig. 14.12 Blood pressures in the pulmonary circulation. $PaCO_2$, Arterial partial pressure of carbon dioxide; PaO_2, arterial partial pressure of oxygen; P_VCO_2, venous partial pressure of carbon dioxide; P_VO_2, venous partial pressure of oxygen. (From Carroll R. *Elsevier's Integrated Physiology*. Philadelphia: Mosby Elsevier; 2007. Fig. 10.9.)

- This would cause fluid to flow into the thin lung interstitium, which then reflects into the alveolar spaces and covers the gas-exchanging surfaces.
- This would impair subsequent gas exchange.

The body keeps pulmonary arterial pressure low by maintaining low muscle tone in the smooth muscles of the pulmonary arteries. However, in times of stress (i.e., cardiac output during exercise bringing increased blood flow), recruitment and distention maintains low intravascular pressure.

- Small, low-pressure pulmonary vessels that remain closed most of the time passively open during high blood flow.
- These recruited vessels increase the pulmonary vascular volume to accommodate the increased blood volume, which reduces vascular resistance and thereby keeping the pressure down (in accordance with Ohm's law, $\Delta P = Q \times R$) (see Clinical Correlation Box 14.4).

Clinical Correlation Box 14.4

The differential diagnosis of hypoxemia revolves around the presence or absence of an elevated A-a gradient, which serves as a marker for pathologic $\dot{V}/\dot{Q}$ mismatch.

- Hypoxemia with a normal A-a gradient may indicate:
  - Hypoventilation
  - Low fraction of inspired oxygen (FiO_2; which may be iatrogenic, or because of low O_2 in atmosphere as in high-altitude conditions)

- Hypoxemia with an elevated A-a gradient may indicate:
  - Shunt (i.e., pneumonia, acute respiratory distress syndrome or ARDS)
  - Increased dead space (i.e., pulmonary embolism)

Note that if hypoxemia presents with an elevated A-a gradient but is correctable with administered oxygen, this suggests that increased dead space ($\dot{V}/\dot{Q} = \infty$) is the cause of the hypoxemia. Administering O_2 will not reduce hypoxemia in a patient with a shunt.

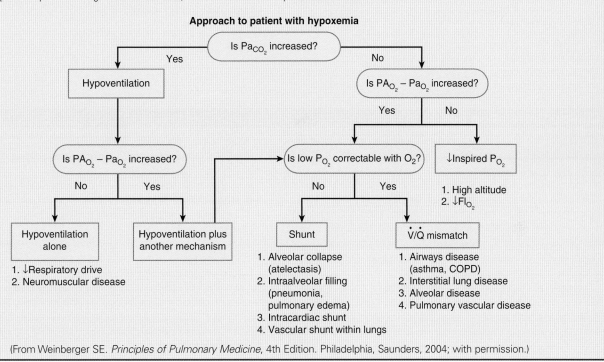

Approach to patient with hypoxemia

(From Weinberger SE. *Principles of Pulmonary Medicine*, 4th Edition. Philadelphia, Saunders, 2004; with permission.)

The Regulation of Pulmonary Blood Flow

The regulation of pulmonary blood flow is also much different from the regulation of systemic blood flow. Whereas hormones and the autonomic nerves predominantly govern the systemic arteries' tone, locally acting nonneurohumoral factors alone govern pulmonary vascular tone.

- The main factor is the P_AO_2.
- Low P_AO_2 causes constriction in the pulmonary arterioles neighboring those alveoli.

  This makes teleologic sense given the anatomy of the lung.
- A small pulmonary artery is surrounded by the alveoli it supplies.
- Under this anatomic set up, the lung automatically reduces the blood flow to any alveoli that are not well ventilated and hence have a low P_AO_2.

  This regulatory process, known as pulmonary hypoxic vasoconstriction, combats $\dot{V}_A/\dot{Q}$ mismatching.
- When hypoxia affects all alveoli uniformly (i.e., global hypoxia, which takes place during hypoventilation or at high altitude) global hypoxic vasoconstriction ensues.
- This increase in vascular resistance across all pulmonary vascular beds results in pulmonary hypertension, which can lead to right-sided heart failure.

PATHOPHYSIOLOGY

Disorders of gas exchange encompass dysfunction of:
- Ventilation
- Diffusion

  Pathologic $\dot{V}_A/\dot{Q}$ mismatching

  All of these disorders can result in low PaO_2, or hypoxia in the blood, which is called hypoxemia, and is defined as P_aO_2 under 80 mm Hg.

Disorders of Ventilation

Recall that hypoventilation means a decreased $\dot{V}_A$ owing to decreased frequency of breathing and/or shallow breathing (small tidal volumes). Hypoventilation can be caused by:
- Primary respiratory depression, a neurologic lack of respiratory drive.
  - Causes include:

    Narcotics

    Other derangements of the respiratory center in the medulla.
- Restrictive ventilatory defects, which limit the expansion of the lungs and hence reduce V_T and $\dot{V}_A$.
  - Causes include:

    Dysfunction of respiratory musculature, as in neurodegenerative diseases, such as amyotrophic lateral sclerosis.

Decreased lung compliance, as in pulmonary fibrosis.

- Obstructive ventilatory defects, which impede the expiration of air, cause the lung to overfill and make it difficult to inspire a good tidal volume for exchange.
    - Causes include:
    Asthma
    Chronic obstructive pulmonary disease (COPD)
        Upper airway obstruction decreases the volume of $\dot{V}_A$ with each breath.
    - Causes include:
    Tumors
    Airway edema (i.e., in anaphylaxis)
    Laryngospasm
    Foreign bodies

Hypoxemia

The globally decreased $\dot{V}_A$ leads to a global decrease in P_AO_2 and hence a decrease in P_aO_2, or hypoxemia. As we will see later, hypoventilation also increases P_aCO_2 which can lead to hypercapnia ($P_aCO_2 > 42$ mm Hg), which has important pathophysiologic consequences.

Low atmospheric PO_2 at high altitudes has the same effect on P_aO_2 as does hypoventilation. It creates hypoxemia by a global, as opposed to regional, decrease in P_AO_2 (see Clinical Correlation Box 14.5).

Respiratory Acidosis and Alkalosis

Hypoventilation can cause not only hypoxemia, but also high P_aCO_2, which is called hypercarbia, or hypercapnia. Remember that CO_2 levels affect the bicarbonate buffer system in the blood through this relationship:

$$CO_2 + H_2O \leftrightarrow H_2CO_3 \leftrightarrow H^+ + HCO_3^- \quad \textbf{(Eq. 14.9)}$$

Therefore increased P_aCO_2 increases the concentration of H^+ in the blood and thus decreases blood pH.

- Hypoventilation and hypercarbia can therefore create primary respiratory acidosis.
- Conversely, disease that leads to proton wasting and metabolic alkalosis, such as vomiting or hyperaldosteronism, can cause a physiologic compensatory hypoventilation in the lungs to preserve blood CO_2 and hence reduce blood pH.

Hyperventilation, which is less common clinically as a primary cause of illness, yields increased P_aO_2 and decreased P_aCO_2.

- Decreased P_aCO_2 in turn creates alkalosis, or lowers blood pH.

- The body consequently uses hyperventilation to combat nonrespiratory disease states that cause acidosis.

Disorders of Diffusion

Any thickening of the gas-exchanging membrane, as in pulmonary edema or fibrosis, can cause a diffusion defect.

- Recall that diffusion defects make O_2 transfer diffusion-limited rather than perfusion-limited, which impedes oxygenation when the heart rate increases.
- Conditions that cause diffusion defects therefore result in poor exercise tolerance.

Pathologic $\dot{V}_A/\dot{Q}$ Mismatch

We have already touched on the physiologic A-a gradient because of low $\dot{V}_A/\dot{Q}$. Pathophysiology, however, can create larger A-a gradients whose associated hypoxemia may be life-threatening. Certain disease processes lead to the formation of shunts ($\dot{V}/\dot{Q} \to 0$), which include:

- Pneumonia, an infection of the distal lung tissues, will fill the alveoli with exudate and inflammatory debris, which will block local alveolar ventilation → shunt (see Clinical Correlation Box 14.5).

- Pulmonary edema will fill the alveoli with fluid from transudate and thus prevent adequate ventilation from reaching the blood → shunt.

- Acute respiratory distress syndrome (ARDS) will fill alveoli with inflammatory debris and exudate → shunt.

Other disease processes lead to the formation of excessive dead space ($\dot{V}/\dot{Q}$ approaches infinity), which include:

- Pulmonary embolism, when an object (such as a blood clot) that clogs a pulmonary artery and prevents alveolar perfusion.

- Recall that dead space was not supposed to lower PaO_2. Why does the patient become hypoxemic?
  Pulmonary embolism blocks the perfusion of a (presumably) well-ventilated area of the lung.
  Because there is a finite reserve of well-ventilated lung areas (Zone 3), blood is then diverted to the more poorly-ventilated lung region (Zones 1 or 2).
  This ultimately leads to low $\dot{V}/\dot{Q}$ in these regions.

SUMMARY

- The partial pressure of a gas is proportional to its mol fraction in the gas mixture:

$$P_1 / P_T = n_1 / n_T = X_1$$

- Increases in the partial pressure of oxygen in the alveolus shift the equilibrium toward increased oxygen into blood. Decreases in the partial pressure of carbon dioxide in the alveolus shift the equilibrium toward release of carbon dioxide out of blood and into alveolar air.

- Inspiration adds a tidal volume, V_T, to the lung spaces. One-third of V_T is added to the anatomic dead space in the conducting airways (V_D). Two-thirds of V_T are added to the gas-exchanging alveolar space (V_A):

$$V_A + V_D = V_T$$
$$(1/3)(V_T) = (V_D)$$
$$(2/3)(V_T) = (V_A)$$

Alveolar minute ventilation, $\dot{V}_A$, is defined as V_A times f, where f is the frequency of breathing in breaths per minute.

$$\dot{V}_A = (V_A)(f)$$

The larger the V_A added to the alveolar space per unit time, $\dot{V}_A$, the higher the P_AO_2 of alveolar air and the lower the P_ACO_2 of alveolar air.

The alveolar ventilation equation describes the relationship between $\dot{V}_A$ and P_ACO_2:

$$\dot{V}_A = (\dot{V}CO_2 / P_ACO_2)(K)$$

- Fick's law describes diffusion of gases between blood and air:

$$\dot{V}_G = (P_A - P_C)(A)(S)/(T)(\sqrt{MW})$$

- Rapid diffusion of O_2 and CO_2 makes the gas exchange of these molecules perfusion-limited. CO is a slow-diffusing molecule whose gas exchange is diffusion-limited.

- Rapid diffusion of O_2 and CO_2 means that the arterial blood leaving the alveoli shares the PO_2 and PCO_2 of alveolar air; that is, regionally:

$$P_AO_2 = P_aO_2 \text{ and } P_ACO_2 = P_aCO_2$$

The ratio of $\dot{V}_A/\dot{Q}$ an area (the ventilation-perfusion relationship of that area) determines the regional alveolar and arterial partial pressures of O_2 and CO_2.

When the $\dot{V}_A/\dot{Q}$ relationship is imbalanced, this is called $\dot{V}_A/\dot{Q}$ mismatch. Low regional $\dot{V}/\dot{Q}$ (~0) is referred to as a *shunt*, whereas high $\dot{V}/\dot{Q}$ (approaching infinity) is referred to as dead space.

The difference between P_aO_2 and P_AO_2 is an A-a gradient. An A-a gradient greater than 5 to 10 mm Hg for patients under 30 years old is indicative of a pathologic $\dot{V}_A/\dot{Q}$ mismatch.

- The alveolar gas equation is used to calculate P_AO_2 from P_IO_2 and P_ACO_2, which are always known or measured. At sea level, P_IO_2 = 149 mm Hg. $P_ACO_2 = P_aCO_2$, which is determined by drawing an ABG. R = 0.8 for a normal protein diet.

$$P_AO_2 = P_IO_2 - (P_ACO_2/R)$$

Imbalanced $\dot{V}_A/\dot{Q}$ ratios in normal lungs create a physiologic A-a gradient. These imbalances are caused by gravitational effects on blood flow and ventilation and to the anatomy of the bronchial and coronary vasculatures.

- Pulmonary blood pressures are lower than systemic blood pressures to prevent fluid extravasation into the alveoli. Pulmonary blood pressure is kept low through the mechanisms of recruitment and distention.

Pulmonary blood pressure is regulated locally by pulmonary hypoxic vasoconstriction, which combats $\dot{V}_A/\dot{Q}$ mismatching. Chronic global hypoxia can lead to pulmonary hypertension.

Diseases that affect gas exchange can lead to low P_aO_2, or hypoxemia. These diseases are divided into disorders of ventilation, disorders of diffusion, and disorders of low $\dot{V}_A/\dot{Q}$.

REVIEW QUESTIONS

Directions: Each of the numbered items or incomplete statements in this section is followed by answers or by completions of the statement. Select the one lettered answer or completion that is best in each case.

1. A 49-year-old man with pulmonary edema reports new-onset shortness of breath when walking upstairs. Thickening of the gas exchange membranes by his disease has resulted in which of the following?
   A. Carbon monoxide exchange is now diffusion-limited.
   B. Oxygen exchange is now diffusion-limited.
   C. Carbon dioxide exchange is now perfusion-limited.
   D. Carbon monoxide exchange is now perfusion-limited.
   E. Oxygen exchange is now perfusion-limited.

2. A 72-year-old woman who recently underwent hip replacement surgery develops a large left lower lobe pulmonary embolus. The ventilation and perfusion status in the alveoli of her affected lobe could best be described by which of the following?
   A. $\dot{V}_A$ is 0, $\dot{Q}$ is normal.
   B. $\dot{V}_A$ is 0, $\dot{Q}$ is low.
   C. $\dot{V}_A$ is normal, $\dot{Q}$ is high.
   D. $\dot{V}_A$ is normal, $\dot{Q}$ is normal.
   E. $\dot{V}_A$ is normal, $\dot{Q}$ is 0.

3. A 65-year-old woman has right middle lobe pneumonia. Her blood gas on room air indicates a P_aO_2 of 57 mm Hg and a P_aCO_2 of 32 mm Hg. If P_1O_2 on room air is 149 mm Hg, what is her A-a gradient?
   A. 25 mm Hg
   B. 52 mm Hg
   C. 60 mm Hg
   D. 92 mm Hg
   E. 109 mm Hg

ANSWERS TO REVIEW QUESTIONS

1. **The answer is B.** In healthy lungs, the diffusion of carbon dioxide and oxygen across the alveolar membrane is rapid. In a healthy person, the degree of carbon dioxide and oxygen exchange is determined instead by the amount of blood flow to the capillary, which is perfusion-limited exchange. In diseased lungs where the alveolar membranes are thickened, the diffusion of oxygen is slower, and oxygen exchange becomes perfusion-limited. During states of increased blood flow, such as exercise, there is decreased oxygen exchange in the lung with thickened membranes, which can result in symptoms of exercise intolerance. Carbon monoxide has a slower diffusion rate, even in the healthy lung, and is consequently diffusion-limited in both normal and abnormal conditions.

2. **The answer is E.** In a pulmonary embolus, a blood clot blocks the flow of blood to a part of the lung, resulting in no perfusion to the affected area ($\dot{Q}$ = 0). The alveoli in the affected region are still exposed to air by ventilation, but there is no blood supply for gas exchange. The affected region becomes physiologic dead space. In situations where there is adequate blood flow but no ventilation ($\dot{V}_A$ = 0), this is called a shunt. A shunt exists both in pneumonia, where the alveoli are filled with inflammatory cells and exudate, and in the case of atelectasis, where the alveoli have collapsed.

3. **The answer is B.** The simplified, clinically useful form of the alveolar gas equation is as follows:

$$P_AO_2 = P_1O_2 - P_ACO_2 / 0.8$$

The average P_ACO_2 is considered to be equal to P_aCO_2. With a P_aCO_2 of 32 mm Hg and a P_1O_2 of 149 mm Hg on room air (where F_1O_2 = 0.21), P_AO_2 will be 109 mm Hg. The P_aO_2 from the blood gas is 57 mm Hg. The difference between P_AO_2 and P_aO_2 yields an A-a gradient of 52. An A-a gradient of more than 5 to 10 mm Hg is abnormal. The acute inflammation and exudate of pneumonia typically causes both an A-a gradient and a shunt.

15

Gas Transport

INTRODUCTION

For successful cell respiration to occur, multiple systems must work in unison for the transport of oxygen (O_2) and carbon dioxide (CO_2):

- Respiratory system
- Hematologic system
- Cardiovascular system

Both O_2 and CO_2 traverse these systems (blood, alveoli, and tissues) via simple diffusion.

- O_2 : air $\rightarrow$ alveoli $\rightarrow$ pulmonary capillaries $\rightarrow$ systemic circulation $\rightarrow$ tissue
- CO_2: tissue $\rightarrow$ systemic veins $\rightarrow$ pulmonary arteries $\rightarrow$ alveoli $\rightarrow$ air

SYSTEM STRUCTURE: OXYGEN RESERVOIRS AND HEMOGLOBIN

To begin, we first ask: How much oxygen demand does the body actually have?

- Each 100 mL of arterial blood contains a mass of oxygen equivalent to about 20 mL.
- With a cardiac output of 6 L/min, we can calculate that approximately 1200 mL of oxygen is delivered to the body per minute.
- Of the 1200 mL of O_2/min, the body tissues consume 300 mL/min and the remaining 900 mL flows back to the heart each minute in the venous blood.

To keep up with this level of oxygen demand, a majority of blood oxygen content must be bound to hemoglobin (Hb) inside red blood cells, with only a small remainder dissolved in the plasma in free solution (see Genetics Box 15.1, Development Box 15.1, Environmental Box 15.1, Pharmacology Box 15.1 and Fast Fact Box 15.1).

GENETICS BOX 15.1

Patients with mutations in the CYB5R3 gene have autosomal recessive methemoglobinemia, a condition in which there is impaired conversion of methemoglobin (hemoglobin in the ferric Fe^{+++} state) to ferrohemoglobin (the ferrous Fe^{++} state). The Fe^{+++} ions cannot reversibly bind oxygen, and the affinity of any remaining Fe^{++} ions is increased, consequently left shifting the O_2 dissociation curve, limiting tissue delivery of O_2. Type I disease affects only erythrocytes, while type II affects all cells.

DEVELOPMENT BOX 15.1

Patients affected by type I methemoglobinemia have cyanosis, dyspnea on exertion, and may have headaches and fatigue. Patients with type II disease have failure to thrive, developmental delay, and cognitive impairment.

ENVIRONMENTAL BOX 15.1

In addition to hereditary methemoglobinemia, there are acquired versions because of drugs (e.g., dapsone, benzocaine, and inhaled nitric oxide). Chemicals, such as aniline and other dyes, pesticides, the naphthalene chemical in moth balls, benzene-derived solvents, and hydrogen peroxide, are among the numerous agents that may be used in work settings and can cause methemoglobinemia.

PHARMACOLOGY BOX 15.1

The cyanosis of type I hereditary methemoglobinemia can be treated with methylene blue, riboflavin, and ascorbic acid. Unfortunately, these treatments have not proved effective in preventing the cognitive impairment and developmental delay of type II disease. For acquired methemoglobinemia, removal of the causative agent is of primary import, although methylene blue and ascorbic acid are often used as well. In the specific case of dapsone-induced disease, cimetidine is effective in the long term for patients who must remain on that drug.

Fast Fact Box 15.1

Oxygen extraction varies from organ to organ. A 25% oxygen extraction rate is an average of the body; the heart extracts almost all oxygen it receives, while the kidneys only extract a small percentage.

Oxygen Reservoirs

What if oxygen were only carried in free solution?

- Henry's law states that amount of gas dissolved in any liquid is proportional to its partial pressure.
- There is only 0.003 mL of dissolved O_2 per 100 mL of blood for each mmHg of PO_2.
- If PO_2 around 100 mm Hg (normal), 100 mL of blood only contains 0.3 mL of dissolved O_2 (not nearly enough!)

To load the blood with the O_2 we need, the blood must contain an O_2 reservoir, Hb, which binds dissolved O_2 molecules and removes them from free solution.

- This prevents the plasma from reaching its saturation point (0.3 mL O_2/100 mL blood).

- Thus more O_2 can diffuse out of alveolar gas into solution.
- This tends to increase the O_2-carrying capacity of blood by over 60-fold (1.39 mL O_2 per g of saturated Hb).

To calculate the total O_2 content in the blood, or CaO_2 (measured in mL O_2 per 100 mL blood), we can rearrange Henry's law to yield:

$$CaO_2 = 1.39 \text{ mL } O_2/\text{g sat-Hb} * SpO_2$$
$$*15 \text{ g Hb}/100 \text{ mL blood} + P_aO_2$$
$$*0.0034 \text{ mL } O_2/100 \text{ mL blood}/\text{mmHg } P_aO_2$$

where SpO_2 is the O_2 saturation in the arterial blood, and P_aO_2 is the partial pressure of O_2 in the arterial blood.

Hemoglobin Structure and Cooperativity

Recall from Chapter 7 that Hb possesses a unique structure that facilitates its interaction with O_2 (Fig. 15.1).
- Two α and two β polypeptide chains.
- Each subunit contains a heme group, a porphyrin ring with a central iron atom that can reversibly bind oxygen.

Hb switches between two major conformational states: tense (T) and relaxed (R) (Fig. 15.2).
- T form (also known as, reduced Hb or deoxyhemoglobin)
  - In the absence of oxygen, the four subunits are tightly bound to each other with electrostatic interactions.
  - Relatively low affinity for oxygen.
- R form
  - O_2 noncovalently binds to the central iron atom of the porphyrin ring of one subunit, producing a conformational shift.
  - Because the subunits are in close apposition, the change in one subunit to the R conformation induces all of the other subunits to change to the R form via mechanical and electrostatic interactions.

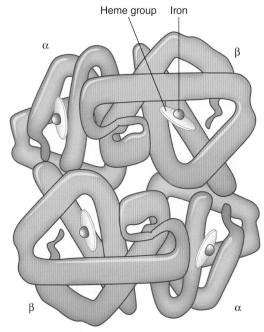

Fig. 15.1 Hemoglobin is composed of four subunits. Each subunit contains a heme group.

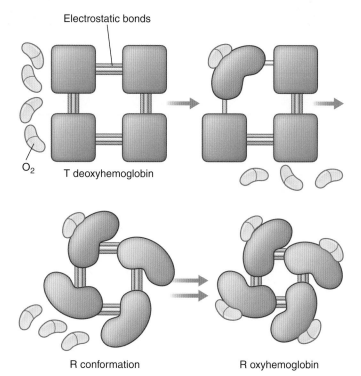

Fig. 15.2 Changes in hemoglobin conformation and oxygen affinity. The T conformation has a low affinity for oxygen, and the R conformation has a high affinity for it. Oxygen binding promotes the R conformation and therefore more oxygen binding.

- The R form has 500 times higher affinity for oxygen than the T form and displays cooperativity (i.e., binding of O_2 to one subunit makes it easier for the other three to bind O_2).

This sequence essentially occurs in reverse when O_2 is unloaded into peripheral tissues after being carried through the arterial system.

SYSTEM FUNCTION: OXYGEN AND CARBON DIOXIDE TRANSPORT

The presence of two oxygen reservoirs and the structure of hemoglobin facilitates:
- The loading of O_2 in the pulmonary capillaries.
- The unloading of O_2 at the tissues.
- The adaptation of Hb to meet changing metabolic demands.

The O_2-Hemoglobin Equilibrium Curve

The interaction between Hb and O_2 at the molecular level is described by the O_2-Hb equilibrium curve, a graph of PO_2 versus O_2 content of Hb (expressed as % of maximum O_2 saturation) (Fig. 15.3).
- Sigmoidal relationship owed to the allosteric properties of Hb.
  - Initial flat curve represents low PO_2 state, with largely T form Hb with low affinity for O_2.
  - Thus the rapidly rising slope represents the progressively increased O_2 affinity of the R form.
  - As Hb becomes saturated and cannot accommodate additional O_2 molecules, the curve flattens.

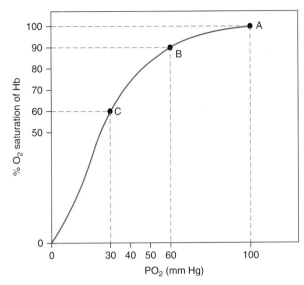

Fig. 15.3 The O_2-hemoglobin equilibrium curve. From point A to point B, PO_2 drops by 40 mm Hg but O_2 saturation drops by only 10%. From point B to point C, O_2 saturation drops by about 30% and PO_2 drops by only 30 mm Hg. A narrow range of this oxyhemoglobin dissociation curve can be approximately as linear; PO_2s of 40, 50, and 60 mm Hg correspond roughly to O_2 saturations of 70%, 80%, and 90%.

Past this point, large increases in PO_2 produce only small increases in the amount of O_2 loaded onto Hb (see Clinical Correlation Box 15.1 and Box 15.2).

Clinical Correlation Box 15.1

A simple rule for remembering the O_2-hemoglobin equilibrium relationship is:

"40-50-60 for 70-80-90"

A PO_2 of 40, 50, and 60 mmHg corresponds to O_2 saturation of 70%, 80%, and 90%, respectively.

Clinical Correlation Box 15.2

Pulse oximetry measures O_2 saturation via a probe connected to the patient's fingernail. This transmits two wavelengths of red light that are absorbed differently by oxy- and deoxyhemoglobin. A photodetector then measures the amount of each wavelength transmitted to determine a ratio of oxy:deoxyhemoglobin, whereby the O_2 saturation can be calculated. However, for the A-a gradient and information about alveolar ventilation, an arterial blood gas must be measured.

- This relationship creates certain physiologic advantages in the loading of O_2 in the lungs and unloading in the periphery.
  - What happens when PO_2 drops from 100 mg to 60 mm Hg? (Fig. 15.3 A→B)
    O_2 saturation drops only to 90% ("flat" part of the curve). Thus oxygen loading is not compromised even if PO_2 drops significantly.
    O_2 partial pressure difference between alveoli and arterial blood (100–60 mmHg) drives continued O_2 diffusion even after Hb is 90% saturated.

- What happens when peripheral tissues remove a large amount of O_2 from Hb? (Fig. 15.3 B→C)
  The steep slope of the curve ensures that a large amount of O_2 may be removed with only a small drop in capillary PO_2.
  This produces a favorable PO_2 gradient from capillaries→tissue, driving oxygenation of downstream tissues. Ultimately, Hb buffers O_2 content such that PO_2 and oxygen diffusion remain relatively constant.
- The P_{50} (PO_2 corresponding to 50% Hb saturation) serves as an index of the position of the O_2-Hb curve.

Hb's Adaptation to Changing Oxygen Requirements

In times of increased oxygen demand, Hb can respond by decreasing its affinity for oxygen and thus increasing oxygen unloading at the tissues. This triggered by four markers of increased metabolic activity affecting the interaction of O_2 with Hb.

- Heat
  - Laws of chemical equilibrium dictate that $\uparrow T \rightarrow \uparrow$ dissociation.
- PCO_2
  - CO_2 covalently binds Hb subunits to form carbaminohemoglobin (Fig. 15.4), which favors the T conformation.
- H^+ concentration
  - Binds specific Hb sites to favor the T conformation.
- 2, 3-bisphosphoglycerate (2,3-BPG) concentration.
  - Normal intermediate in the glycolysis pathway.
  - Binds specific Hb sites to favor the T conformation.

Therefore when the markers of oxygen demand are increased, Hb will have a lower affinity for O_2. This manifests as a "right shift" on the O_2-Hb equilibrium curve, wherein O_2 saturation is lower for a given PO_2 (Fig. 15.5).

- The effect of PCO_2 and H^+ is specifically referred to as the Bohr effect, whereas its foil is known as the Haldane effect (Table 15.1).
- In states of low PO_2, this produces increased tissue oxygenation because of decreased affinity of Hb for O_2, which is then unloaded into tissues (O_2 saturation is lower for the same PO_2) (see Fast Fact Box 15.2 and 15.3).

Fast Fact Box 15.2

To remember the factors promoting rightward shift, recall the phrase:

"CADET, face RIGHT"

[CO_2, Acid, 2,3-DPG, Exercise, Temperature]

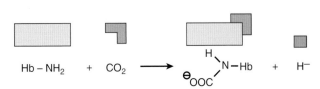

Fig. 15.4 The formation of carbaminohemoglobin from CO_2 and hemoglobin.

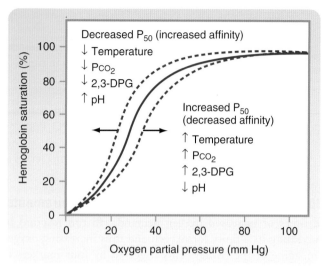

Fig. 15.5 The Bohr effect. When the markers of increased metabolic demand are increased, decreases in hemoglobin's oxygen affinity lead to increased oxygen extraction from hemoglobin. (From Koeppen BM, Stanton BA, *Berne & Levy Physiology*, 7th Ed. Philadelphia: Elsevier; Fig. 24.5.)

TABLE 15.1	**The Basics of the Bohr and Haldane Effects**	
Bohr Effect	**Haldane Effect**
CO_2 and H^+ binding to Hb→decreased Hb affinity for O_2	Deoxygenation of Hb →increased Hb affinity for CO_2
Shifts O_2-hemoglobin curve RIGHT	Shifts CO_2-blood curve LEFT

CO_2, Carbon dioxide; *H^+*, hydrogen ion; *Hb*, hemoglobin; *O_2*, oxygen.

Fast Fact Box 15.3

Hemoglobin may also respond to physiologic oxygenation needs by promoting release of nitric oxide (NO), a potent vasodilator. This is because oxyhemoglobin binds NO tightly but deoxyhemoglobin does not, thus allowing hemoglobin to serve as an NO "sink" to be released in hypoxic tissues.

If metabolic activity is decreased, as reflected in low amounts of these metabolic markers, the curve can shift left and cause increased affinity of Hb for O_2. Two other states can produce this effect are:
- Increased fetal hemoglobin (Hbf) (see Clinical Correlation Box 15.3).

Clinical Correlation Box 15.3

Fetal hemoglobin (Hbf), most often found in the fetal circulation during pregnancy, allows the fetus to extract O_2 from the mother's blood with a greater affinity. This is important because the fetus does not yet have a functioning respiratory system, and thus depends on the oxygen in its mother's blood while in the womb. The main functional difference between Hbf and adult Hb is that Hbf does not bind 2,3-DPG as strongly as adult Hb, resulting in an increased affinity of Hbf for O_2 that tends to shift the curve to the *left*.

- Increased carbon monoxide (CO) (see Clinical Correlation Box 15.4).

Clinical Correlation Box 15.4

Carbon monoxide (CO) is a colorless, odorless gas formed by the incomplete combustion of any carbon material that can be highly toxic to humans. It interferes with tissue oxygenation through two mechanisms.
- Binds hemoglobin with affinity 250× that of oxygen, thus serving as a competitive inhibitor for oxygen loading.
- Inhibits unloading of oxygen because of carboxyhemoglobin (CO+hemoglobin) favoring the R conformation, thus producing a leftward shift in the curve.
  It is treated through administration of 100% O_2, sometimes via hyperbaric oxygen treatment, which can overcome the competitive inhibition.

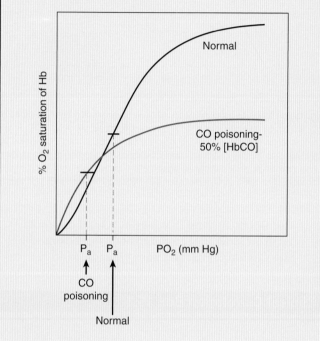

Patients with CO poisoning appear "cherry red" instead of blue-purple as in

CO_2 Transport

How much CO_2 does the body actually generate at rest?
- Cellular metabolism in the tissues of a resting adult produces a mass of CO_2 equivalent to 200 mL/min of CO_2.
- Each 100 mL of venous blood contains about 50 mL of carbon dioxide.
- Therefore 3 L of CO_2 is delivered to the lungs per minute (cardiac output of 6 L/min times 500 mL/L).
- However, only 200 mL is extracted by the pulmonary alveoli for excretion to maintain a steady state. This occurs for two reasons:
  - Kidneys share the burden of handling CO_2 produced by cellular metabolism.
  - Brain and kidneys regulate CO_2 excretion such that some amount remains in the blood at all times as part of the bicarbonate buffer system.

CO_2 exists in blood in three forms:
- Around 5% dissolved in plasma.
  - CO_2 is 20× more soluble in plasma than O_2, with a solubility constant of 0.06 mL CO_2/100 mL blood/mm Hg $PaCO_2$.

- Therefore dissolved CO_2 contributes to a significant proportion of the exhaled CO_2.
- Around 5% covalently bound to Hb as carbaminohemoglobin.
- Around 90% bicarbonate.

Bicarbonate, the major form of CO_2, is carried mostly in plasma, but it is formed in the red blood cell (RBC) and plays a major role in the chloride shift (Fig. 15.6).

$$CO_2 \leftrightarrow H_2CO_3 \leftrightarrow H^+ + HCO_3^-$$

- CO_2 from tissues enters the RBC and is converted to carbonic acid, which undergoes spontaneous dissociation into H^+ and HCO_3^-.
- In the peripheral blood, HCO_3^- is exchanged for Cl^- ions in the plasma. H^+ ions are scavenged by Hb to prevent excessive acidemia.
- In the lungs, Cl^- is exchanged for HCO_3^- in the plasma and the reverse reaction occurs, allowing CO_2 release.

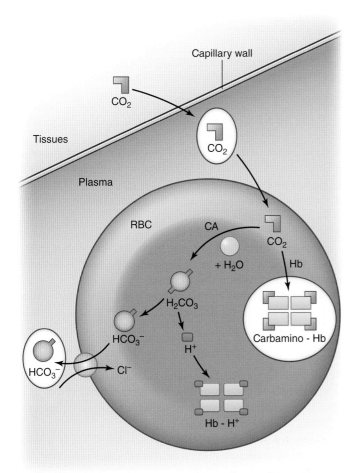

Fig. 15.6 Transport of CO_2 from tissues to venous plasma to red blood cells (*RBCs*). In the RBCs, the reaction between CO_2 and H_2O is catalyzed by carbonic anhydrase to form H_2CO_3, which dissociates into H^+ and HCO_3^-. HCO_3^- exchanges with a Cl^- to leave the RBC (chloride shift). This buffering process occurs in deoxyhemoglobin. The HCO_3^- is then transported to the lung to deliver CO_2 via the aforementioned reactions in reverse.

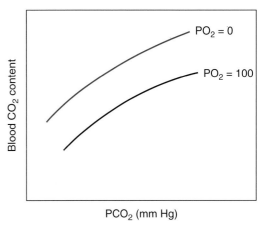

Fig. 15.7 The CO_2-blood equilibrium curve. The two lines show the curve in oxygenated versus deoxygenated blood, illustrating the Haldane effect.

The CO_2-Blood Equilibrium Curve

The CO_2-blood equilibrium curve relates total CO_2 content to PCO_2. In contrast to the O_2 Hb curve, however, the relationship is essentially linear (Fig. 15.7). This occurs because of:

- Lack of molecular cooperativity in CO_2 loading.
- Lack of saturation point for CO_2 at PCO_2 values compatible with human life, that would otherwise lead to a flattened upper curve.

If Hb is less saturated with oxygen, the CO_2-blood equilibrium shifts leftward.

- Deoxyhemoglobin has greater affinity for CO_2 and is a better scavenger for H^+ ions.
  - Removal of H^+ tends to drive the equation toward formation of more carbaminohemoglobin, by Le Chatelier's principle.
- In deoxygenated states, the blood can thus transport more CO_2 for a given PCO_2.
- This is known as the Haldane effect (see Table 15.1) and tends to enhance removal of CO_2 from oxygen-consuming tissues.

Coupled CO_2 and O_2 Transport

The mechanisms involved in the transport of O_2 from the lungs to the periphery and CO_2 from the periphery to the lungs are coupled and facilitate each other (Fig. 15.8). To summarize:

- Periphery
  - Bohr effect (Fig. 15.9).
    Uptake of CO_2 into RBCs $\rightarrow \uparrow$ carbonic acid $\rightarrow \uparrow [H^+]$ in RBCs $\rightarrow$ *right shift* of O_2-Hb curve $\rightarrow$ higher PO_2 for given O_2 saturation $\rightarrow$ greater PO_2 gradient between capillaries and tissues $\rightarrow$ facilitates O_2 unloading.
  - Haldane effect
    Low oxygen $\rightarrow$ deoxyhemoglobin formation $\rightarrow$ increased affinity for CO_2 & $H^+ \rightarrow \uparrow [HCO_3^-]$, carbaminohemoglobin $\rightarrow$ lower PCO_2 for given CO_2 content $\rightarrow$ greater PCO_2 gradient between capillaries and tissues $\rightarrow$ facilitates CO_2 loading,
- Lungs
  - O_2 loading $\rightarrow$ oxyhemoglobin $\rightarrow \uparrow [CO_2] \rightarrow$ higher PCO_2 for given CO_2 content $\rightarrow$ increased PCO_2 gradient for CO_2 diffusion into alveolar gas $\rightarrow$ facilitates CO_2 unloading.

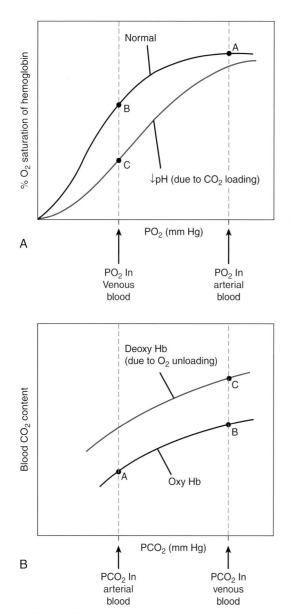

Fig. 15.8 The coupling of O_2 and CO_2 transport. A, The effect of CO_2 loading on O_2 unloading. Without the Bohr effect, there would be less unloading of oxygen in the tissues (point A → point B). With the Bohr effect from CO_2 loading there is more unloading of oxygen in the tissues (point A → point C). B, The effect of O_2 unloading on CO_2 loading. Without the Haldane effect, there would be less CO_2 loading (A → B). With the Haldane effect from O_2 unloading, there is more CO_2 loading (A → C).

- CO_2 unloading → R conformation of Hb → O_2 loading increased → lower PO_2 for given O_2 content → greater PO_2 gradient for O_2 diffusion to the blood → facilitates O_2 loading.

PATHOPHYSIOLOGY

Disorders of oxygen transport result in inadequate oxygen delivery to tissues. This may result in hypoxia, defined as low PO_2, and/or hypoxemia, defined as decreased PO_2 specifically in arterial blood (P_aO_2 <80 mm Hg).

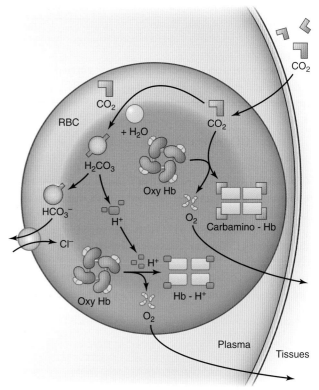

Fig. 15.9 The effect of CO_2 on hemoglobin. By two distinct pathways, CO_2 promotes the T conformation of hemoglobin and thereby promotes unloading of O_2 into the tissues. *Hb*, Hemoglobin; *RBC*, red blood cell.

Recall from Chapter 14 that hypoxemia has three important causes:

1. Low atmospheric or inspired PO_2 (i.e., because of high altitude, room air dilution, or iatrogenic if ventilation fails to deliver properly).
2. Hypoventilation (i.e., because of muscle weakness or drugs causing respiratory dysfunction.
3. $\dot{V}/\dot{Q}$ mismatch (i.e., shunt or dead space).

Hypoxemia may lead to tissue hypoxia. However, tissue hypoxia may occur in absence of hypoxemia because of disorders in gas transport. Why is this the case?

A clinical example, anemia, will help illustrate this point, as well as help explain the difference between PO_2, O_2 saturation, and O_2 content.

Anemia

Recall from Chapter 7 that anemia is defined as a reduction in the concentration of Hb in blood. Several entities lead to anemia; however, they fall into three major categories:

- Acute or chronic blood loss.
- Decreased production of RBCs (i.e., B12 or folate deficiency, decreased erythropoietin production because of kidney dysfunction).
- Increased destruction (i.e., immune-mediated lysis).

Anemia leads to hypoxia by reducing the oxygen-carrying capacity of blood.

- The normal Hb concentration of blood is about 15 g/100 mL. Because 1 g of Hb can carry 1.39 mL of O_2, the O_2

capacity of normal blood will be approximately 21 mL O_2/100 mL blood.

- In contrast, an anemic patient with a Hb concentration of 7.5 g/100 mL will have an O_2 capacity of 10.5 mL/100 mL. In this case, the patient displays:
- Normal gas exchange.
- Normal PO_2 (i.e., not hypoxemic).
- Normal O_2 saturation (amount of oxyhemoglobin expressed as a percentage of total Hb).
- Normal O_2-Hb dissociation curve.

However, if O_2 content, expressed as total mL O_2/100 mL blood, is plotted against PO_2, the curve of the anemic individual is very different (Fig. 15.10).

- Less O_2 will be delivered to the tissues per 100 mL of blood.
- Cardiac output is increased to compensate, since recall: O_2 delivery = cardiac output * O_2 content of blood.

Owing to this increased work and tissue hypoxia, patients develop fatigue and headaches. They also develop skin pallor because Hb imparts the red color to their blood (see Clinical Correlation Box 15.5).

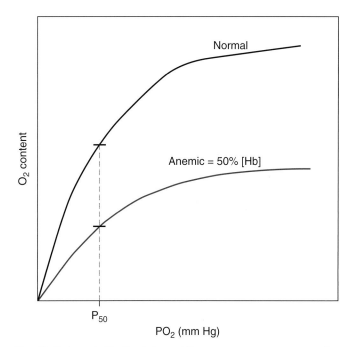

Fig. 15.10 Anemia. The Y axis is total O_2 content, not percent saturation of hemoglobin as on the O_2-hemoglobin equilibrium curve. Note that the P_{50} of the patient with anemia remains the same.

Anemia can be treated acutely with blood transfusions if severe. Otherwise, treatment is dictated by the primary cause.

Clinical Correlation Box 15.5

Interestingly, an anemic patient with respiratory compromise will be less cyanotic (bluish tinge to the skin) compared with other patients in respiratory disease. This is because oxyhemoglobin is bright red while deoxyhemoglobin is purple, and given a normal O_2 saturation, an anemic patient will have a less-than-normal absolute amount of purple deoxyhemoglobin and will therefore be less cyanotic. Accordingly, a person with an abnormally high hematocrit (polycythemia) will be more cyanotic at the same O_2 saturation.

SUMMARY

- The blood carries two O_2 reservoirs: (1) 4% dissolved O_2 in solution and (2) 96% O_2 bound to the protein hemoglobin (Hb) inside red blood cells.
- The PO_2 is directly proportional to the quantity of O_2 dissolved in blood. There is 0.0034 mL of dissolved O_2 per 100 mL of blood for each mm Hg of PO_2.
- Total oxygen content in the blood relies on both sources of oxygen:

$$CaO_2 = 1.39 \text{ mL } O_2 / \text{g sat-Hb} * SpO_2$$
$$* 15 \text{ g Hb} / 100 \text{ mL blood} + P_aO_2$$
$$* 0.0034 \text{ mL } O_2 / 100 \text{ mL blood} / \text{mm Hg } P_aO_2$$

- Hb is composed of four subunits, each containing an iron-based heme group. Each heme group can bind one O_2 molecule.
- Hb's subunits can be arranged in T conformation (tense) or R conformation (relaxed). The T conformation has a low affinity for O_2 and the R conformation has a high affinity for O_2.
- O_2 binding of one subunit to O_2 in the T conformation shifts the other three subunits into R conformation. This property of Hb, called cooperativity, means that O_2 binding promotes further O_2 binding. Conversely, dissociation of O_2 from Hb promotes more dissociation of O_2 from Hb.

- As PO_2 increases, more O_2 molecules associate with Hb. The O_2-Hb equilibrium curve precisely defines this relationship between PO_2 and Hb saturation. Hb is 90% saturated at a PO_2 of roughly 60 mm Hg.
- CO_2 exists in blood in three forms: (1) 5% dissolved in plasma; (2) 5% covalently bound to Hb as carbamino-hemoglobin; and (3) 90% bicarbonate.
- The CO_2-blood equilibrium curve describes the relationship between total CO_2 content and PCO_2. Because there is no physiologic saturation point for CO_2 content, this curve is more linear than the O_2-Hb equilibrium curve.
- The Bohr effect occurs because CO_2 and H^+ interacts with Hb to shift it into T conformation and reduce its affinity for O_2. It manifests as a rightward shift of the O_2-Hb equilibrium curve.
- The Haldane effect occurs because of the fact that deoxyhemoglobin has a higher affinity for CO_2 and manifests a leftward shift in the CO_2-blood equilibrium curve.
- The Bohr and Haldane effects account for the coupling of O_2 and CO_2 transport (in the lungs O_2 loading and CO_2 unloading promote each other; in the tissues O_2 unloading and CO_2 loading promote each other) and for increased O_2 delivery in the presence of high metabolic demand.
- In anemia, total oxygen content is reduced without reducing PO_2 or Hb saturation.

REVIEW QUESTIONS

Directions: Each of the numbered items or incomplete statements in this section is followed by answers or by completions of the statement. Select the one lettered answer or completion that is best in each case.

1. A 9-year-old boy with a family history of a hemoglobinopathy is analyzed for hemoglobin mutations. He is found to have a mutation that decreases the oxygen affinity of his hemoglobin. The mechanism by which this happens might be which of the following?
   A. The mutation enhances the binding of carbon monoxide to hemoglobin
   B. The mutation increases cooperativity between hemoglobin molecules
   C. The mutation decreases the binding of carbon dioxide to hemoglobin
   D. The mutation inhibits the association of the subunits of hemoglobin
   E. The mutation decreases the binding of hydrogen ions to hemoglobin

2. A 15-year-old girl with hemolytic anemia (increased destruction of red blood cells) reports fatigue and headaches. Her total oxygen content is reduced by which of the following mechanisms?
   A. Decreased PO_2
   B. Increased hemoglobin oxygen saturation
   C. Increased amount of hemoglobin
   D. Decreased amount of hemoglobin
   E. Decreased hemoglobin oxygen saturation

3. A 37-year-old man is running the Marine Corps Marathon. The increased oxygen demand of his body is met by which of the following mechanisms?
   A. Increased oxygen affinity of hemoglobin
   B. Decreased oxygen affinity of hemoglobin
   C. Acute increase in hemoglobin production
   D. Increased oxygen loading in lungs
   E. Decreased levels of carbon dioxide in blood

ANSWERS TO REVIEW QUESTIONS

1. **The answer is D.** The cooperativity of hemoglobin results from the association of its subunits. If one subunit binds oxygen and shifts to the higher-oxygen–affinity R conformation, it triggers shifts to the R conformation in the three other subunits. Mutations that prevent the close association of hemoglobin's subunits will result in the loss of this cooperativity and a decrease in oxygen affinity. The binding of carbon dioxide and hydrogen ions to hemoglobin stabilizes the low-oxygen–affinity T conformation of hemoglobin. The binding of carbon monoxide results in the formation of carboxyhemoglobin, which increases the oxygen affinity of hemoglobin by shifting it into the R conformation.

2. **The answer is D.** In anemia, the number of red blood cells is decreased, which results in a decreased amount of hemoglobin available to bind oxygen. A patient with anemia will have normal gas exchange in the lungs and will have a normal PO_2. Hemoglobin oxygen saturation is the amount of oxyhemoglobin expressed as a percentage of total hemoglobin. While this patient's total hemoglobin is decreased, her amount of oxyhemoglobin is decreased by a similar degree. Therefore her oxygen saturation will be normal.

3. **The answer is B.** Increased metabolic activity results in elevated levels of heat, carbon dioxide, hydrogen ions, and 2,3-bisphosphoglycerate, all of which stabilize the low-oxygen–affinity T conformation of hemoglobin. During exercise, oxygen loading of hemoglobin in the lungs is relatively unchanged by these factors because of the high PO_2. However, in the tissues where PO_2 is low, the stabilization of hemoglobin's lower oxygen affinity by these factors results in increased unloading of oxygen to the tissues.

16

The Regulation of Breathing

CORE CONCEPTS (FIGS. 16.1 AND 16.2)

- To function properly, the human respiratory system must:
  - Respond to oxygen demands.
  - Maintain a constant range of oxygen and carbon dioxide in blood.
- Respiration is governed by both voluntary and involuntary neural pathways.
  - Voluntary control allows talking, eating, and drinking.
  - Involuntary control allows respiration through wakefulness and periods of unconsciousness (i.e., sleep).
- Neural pathways mediating respiration are sensitive to changes in O_2, CO_2, and H^+ content in the peripheral blood.

SYSTEM STRUCTURE AND FUNCTION

The Role of the Central Nervous System

The respiratory cycle uses specific neurologic circuits and muscular groups (Table 16.1):
- Stimulation of respiratory centers → efferent nerves → activation of motor neurons in cervical, thoracic, and lumbar spinal cord → innervation of diaphragm, intercostal muscle (m.), and abdominal m. (respectively) → inspiration (see Clinical Correlation Box 16.1).

Clinical Correlation Box 16.1

Efferents from cervical motor neurons C3–C5 form the phrenic nerves, which drive relaxed tidal breathing. The phrenic nerves provide the only motor supply the diaphragm, which upon contraction expands the volume of the thoracic cavity and draws air into the lungs. Damage to the phrenic nerve or its cervical roots, as with traumatic head and neck injury, may lead to diaphragmatic paralysis and mechanical ventilation dependence.

Mnemonic: "C3, 4, 5, keeps the diaphragm alive!"

- Cessation of stimulation → inspiratory muscles relax → lung recoils because of elasticity of lungs → passive expiration.
- Activation of additional expiratory muscles (abdominal recti & internal intercostal m.) → active expiration.

Voluntary and involuntary impulses are transmitted through different pathways in the spinal cord (Fig. 16.3):
- Voluntary nerve fibers are located within the dorsolateral corticospinal tracts.
- Involuntary nerve fibers are located within the medial portion of anterior horn.

There are three main respiratory control centers in the central nervous system (CNS): the medulla, the pons, and the cerebral cortex.

1. Medulla (reticular formation) (Fig. 16.4)
   - Dorsal respiratory group (DRG)
   - Maintains inspiratory rhythm during tidal breathing
   - Located in the nucleus tractus solitarii
   - Modulated by chemoreception (PCO_2, PO_2, pH), mechanoreception (lung stretch), and nociception.
   - Receives input from the vagus (CNX) and glossopharyngeal (CNIX) nerves (n.)
   - Produces a "ramp signal" to phrenic n. to regulate respiratory rate and tidal volume (Fig. 16.5).
   - Ventral respiratory group (VRG)
   - Augments active respiration (i.e., during exercise)
   - Composed of:
     Nucleus paraambiguus (active during inspiration)
     Caudal nucleus retroambiguus (active during exhalation)
     Rostral nucleus retrofacialis (active during exhalation)
     Pre-Bötzinger complex (central rhythm generation)
   - Receives stimulation from the DRG
   - Increases DRG ramp signal and recruits expiratory m. of respiration (i.e., abdominal recti).
2. Pons (see Fig. 16.4)
   - Pneumotaxic center
   - Coordinates speed of inhalation and exhalation.
   - Located in the upper pons (nucleus parabrachialis)
   - Inhibits DRG and thus lowers the threshold for ramp signal cessation
     ↑ pneumotaxic signal → ↓ ramp signal duration → ↓ duration of inspiration, ↓ tidal volume, ↑ respiratory rate (RR)
     ↓ pneumotaxic signal → ↑ ramp signal duration → ↑ duration of inspiration, ↑ tidal volume, ↓ RR
   - Apneustic center
   - Coordinates speed of inhalation and exhalation
   - Located in the caudal pons adjacent to the DRG and VRG
   - Receives inhibitory input from the pneumotaxic center
   - Stimulates DRG and thus raises the threshold for ramp signal cessation
     ↑ apneustic signal → ↑ ramp signal duration → ↑ duration of inspiration, ↑ tidal volume, ↓ RR
     ↓ apneustic signal → ↓ ramp signal duration → ↓ duration of inspiration, ↓ tidal volume, ↑ RR
3. Cerebral Cortex
   - Function: Voluntary hypo- or hyperventilation (see Genetics Box 16.1, Pharmacology Box 16.1, Fast Fact Box 16.1, and Fast Fact Box 16.2).

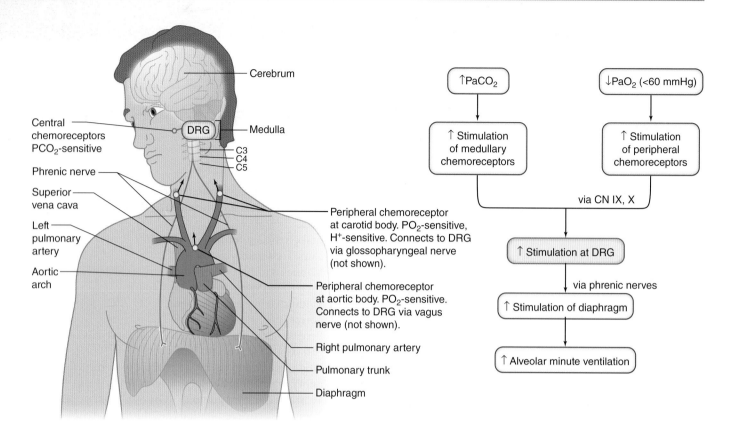

Fig. 16.1 Regulation of the respiratory cycle is accomplished through several essential components. Peripheral and central receptors communicate with respiratory control systems located in the brainstem to alter parameters of the respiratory cycle, such as rate and tidal volume. Furthermore, the cerebral cortex can exert a degree of voluntary control over breathing through communication with the same centers. *DRG*, Dorsal respiratory group.

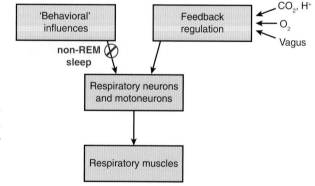

Fig. 16.2 Conceptual model showing that efferent output from respiratory neurons and motoneurons is controlled by behavioral influences and feedback regulation. (© Richard L. Horner, PhD, University of Toronto. From *Murray and Nadel's Textbook of Respiratory Medicine.* pp. 1511-1526.e1. © 2016. Fig. 85.5.)

TABLE 16.1	**Summary of the Phases and Anatomic Changes Within the Respiratory Cycle**	
Phase	**Muscles Activated**	**Lung Action**
Inspiration	Diaphragm (C3–C5), external intercostal muscle, abdominal muscle	Active expansion
Passive expiration	None	Passive recoil
Active expiration	Internal intercostal muscle, abdominal recti	Augmented recoil

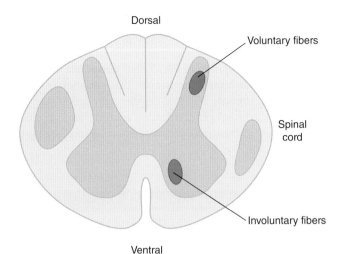

Fig. 16.3 The location of voluntary and involuntary nerve fibers in a cross-sectional view of the spinal cord.

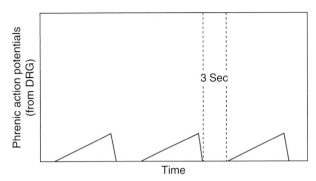

Fig. 16.5 The inspiratory ramp signal. Neurons within the dorsal respiratory group (*DRG*) initiate inspiration with a weak burst of action potentials that gradually increases in amplitude over the next few seconds and then ceases for approximately 3 seconds until the cycle begins anew.

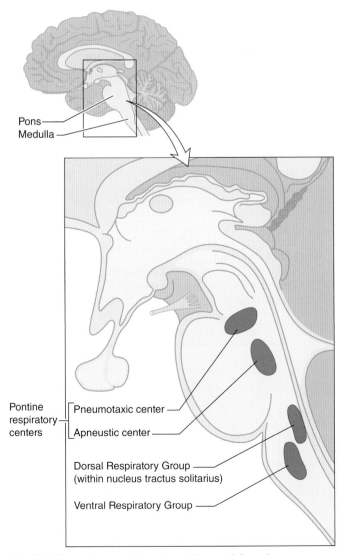

Fig. 16.4 Respiratory control centers in the medulla and pons.

🧬 GENETICS BOX 16.1

Congenital central hypoventilation syndrome is a rare disease that underscores the critical importance of involuntary control of breathing. Affected children hypoventilate (especially when sleeping), retain carbon dioxide, and do not reflexively increase ventilation in response to higher CO_2 levels. This disease is caused by a mutation in the PHOX2B gene that encodes a protein important in the development of central nervous system (CNS) chemoreceptor areas. The mutation alters a single amino acid and results in this potentially life-threatening disease.

💊 PHARMACOLOGY BOX 16.1

Central sleep apnea is a disease in which the involuntary respiratory drive is abnormal. It can be treated with acetazolamide, a medication that induces a mild metabolic acidosis (see Ch. 22 on acid base balance) and thereby stimulates respiration. Theophylline antagonizes phosphodiesterase, increasing concentrations of cyclic adenine monophosphate (cAMP) leading to catecholamine stimulation of various tissues including central respiratory centers.

Fast Fact Box 16.1

The advantages of a "ramp signal" are 2-fold:
1. Gradual increase in lung volume (rather than a gulp of air)
2. Subtle control of ventilatory rhythm
   - Δ rate of AP firing → Δ ramp slope
   - Δ threshold for ramp signal cessation → Δ ramp height

Fast Fact Box 16.2

"Apneusis" refers to a deep, prolonged inspiratory gasp (↑TV, ↓RR).

RR, Respiratory rate; *TV*, tidal volume.

The Role of Central Chemoreceptors

Under normal conditions, central chemoreceptors just below the ventrolateral surface of the medulla supply the most important sensory inputs to the medullary respiratory centers.

Instead of relaying input peripheral chemoreceptors, they detect chemical changes in their immediate environment and transmit this information to the respiratory centers in the medulla and pons.

The central chemoreceptors react to the arterial partial pressure of carbon dioxide ($PaCO_2$). $PaCO_2$ affects the central chemoreceptors indirectly by increasing the cerebrospinal fluid (CSF) H^+ concentration, which stimulates the central chemoreceptive neurons (Fig. 16.6). $PaCO_2$ and H^+ are related to one another by the blood buffer equation (see Ch. 22):

$$PaCO_2 \leftrightarrow H_2CO_3 \leftrightarrow H^+ + HCO_3^-$$

Given that the central chemoreceptors respond directly only to H^+, one might conclude that low arterial pH (high H^+ concentration) would stimulate the chemoreceptors. However, this is not the case: cationic H+ ions cannot cross the blood-brain barrier. Instead, increasing $PaCO_2$ drives dissolved CO_2 across the blood-brain barrier, which increases the CO_2 content of CSF. CO_2 is then readily hydrated to carbonic acid, which then dissociates to produce bicarbonate and H^+. These H^+ ions then bind the central chemoreceptors, which stimulates an increase in respiratory drive (Fig. 16.7).

In other words:

$\downarrow$ ventilation $\rightarrow \uparrow PaCO_2 \rightarrow \downarrow$ CSF pH $\rightarrow$ central chemoreception activation $\rightarrow \uparrow$ ventilation

This serves two main purposes:
1. Maintenance of respiratory drive to provide sufficient tissue oxygenation.
2. Homeostatic regulation of $PaCO_2$ and thus stable blood pH.

Although it has been demonstrated that peripheral chemoreceptors are primarily involved in the acute respiratory response to acidic blood pH (acidemia), central chemoreceptors may play a role in the chronic response to acidemia (see Physiology Integration Box 16.1).

Physiology Integration Box 16.1

In the carotid bodies, decreased oxygen arterial partial pressure (PaO_2) appears to cause a decrease in K^+ influx through oxygen-sensitive K^+ channels in the glomus cells. The drop in PaO_2 also stimulates adenylate cyclase, leading to an increase in cyclic adenosine monophosphate (AMP) that further inhibits the K^+ channels. The resultant change in the membrane potential causes an influx of calcium ions through calcium channels, leading to increased cell excitability and transmission of the signal to the dorsal respiratory group (DRG) through the pathways noted earlier.

The Role of Peripheral Chemoreceptors

Under normal conditions, $PaCO_2$ is the primary stimulus for respiratory drive in the periphery. This is because $PaCO_2$ is a direct, near-linear reflection of blood CO_2 content, whereas oxygen saturation of hemoglobin is stable for a wide range of arterial partial pressure of oxygen (PaO_2) values under physiologic conditions. However, pathologically low PaO_2 values will trigger peripheral chemoreceptors to increase ventilation (see Fast Fact Box 16.3).

Fast Fact Box 16.3

Recall that arterial oxygen partial pressure (PaO_2) varies from 60 to 100 mm Hg while oxygen saturation remains within the 90% to 100% range.

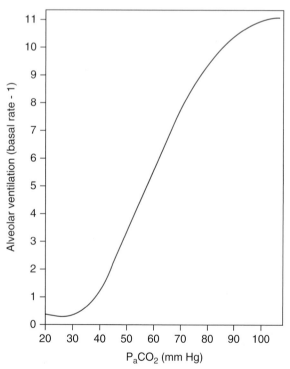

Fig. 16.6 The effects of increased arterial partial pressure of carbon dioxide (*PaCO₂*) on respiration. Increased $PaCO_2$ drives dissolved CO_2 across the blood-brain barrier, leading to decreased pH; hydrogen ions then stimulate the medullary center to increase respiratory rate. This, in turn, allows more CO_2 to be "blown off" and aids in correction of hypercapnia/acidemia. Note that minute ventilation increases when the $PaCO_2$ rises above 40 mm Hg.

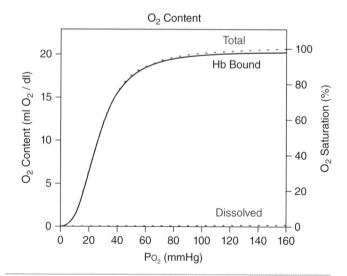

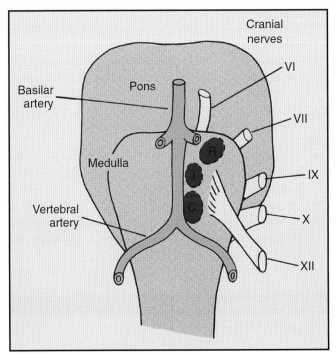

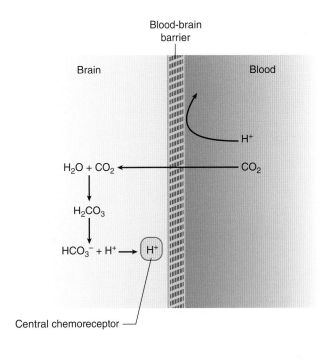

Fig. 16.7 A, The medullary respiratory control centers. B, The stimulation of central chemoreceptors. Although chemoreceptors ventral to the medulla respond primarily to H^+, these charged molecules cannot cross the blood-brain barrier. Instead, carbon dioxide, which readily crosses this barrier, is hydrated in the central nervous system to H_2CO_3 that releases H^+ ions, which then stimulate the central chemoreceptors. (A. from Levy MN, Koeppen BM, Stanton BA. *Berne & Levy Principles of Physiology,* 4th Edition. Elsevier; 2005. Fig. 31.8.)

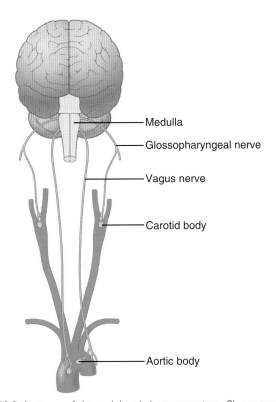

Fig. 16.8 Anatomy of the peripheral chemoreceptors. Chemoreceptors located in the carotid bodies (at the bifurcation of the common carotids) and in the aortic bodies (along the arch of the aorta) play an integral role in stimulating an increase in ventilation in response to hypoxemia. (From Guyton AC, Hall JE. *Guyton and Hall Textbook of Medical Physiology,* 13th Edition. Elsevier; 2015. Fig. 42.4.)

In humans, there are two types of peripheral chemoreceptors:
- Carotid bodies
  - Located at the bifurcation of the common carotid arteries bilaterally (Fig. 16.8).
  - Afferent impulses → glossopharyngeal nerves (CN IX) → stimulation of DRG → regulation of respiratory cycle.
- Aortic bodies
  - Located above and below the arch of the aorta (see Fig. 16.8).
  - Afferent impulses → vagus nerves (CN X) → stimulation of DRG → regulation of respiratory cycle.

The anatomy of the carotid and aortic bodies is designed to maximize the ability of the peripheral chemoreceptors to respond to changes in the PaO_2. Because of their location at areas of high arterial blood flow, each receives more than 2000 mL/100 g of tissue per minute. This means that only a negligible amount of oxygen is removed for chemoreception, and thus they can respond to true changes in PaO_2.

The peripheral chemoreceptors in the carotid and aortic bodies have an important role in the response to hypoxemia because they alone can increase ventilation when arterial hypoxemia occurs. This allows them to override the normal $PaCO_2$-mediated regulation of respiration (Fig. 16.9):
- Threshold for neuronal activity: PaO_2 below 100 mm Hg
- Threshold for increased ventilation: PaO_2 below 55 to 60 mm Hg

PaO_2 levels below 50 mm Hg correspond to an oxygen saturation of hemoglobin below 90%—and the point at which oxygen delivery to the tissues is threatened. Any further decrease in PaO_2 has a very potent stimulatory effect on the peripheral chemoreceptors (see Clinical Correlation Box 16.2).

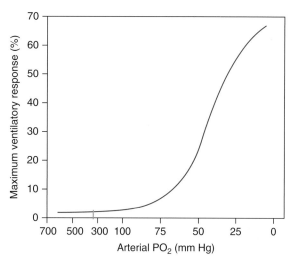

Fig. 16.9 The response of peripheral chemoreceptors to hypoxemia. The peripheral chemoreceptors are designed to sense drops in oxygen arterial partial pressure (PaO$_2$) to below 50 mm Hg, the point at which the hemoglobin buffer system begins to fail to adequately oxygenate peripheral tissues. Below this critical set point, the activity of these receptors increases at a rapid rate to stimulate an increase in ventilation.

Clinical Correlation Box 16.2

Because the peripheral chemoreceptors are designed to respond to changes in dissolved O$_2$ in the arterial supply, low oxygen content resulting from insufficient functional hemoglobin will not trigger the chemoreceptors. Thus disorders, such as anemia, carbon monoxide poisoning, and methemoglobinemia, will not trigger increased ventilation despite low oxygen levels.

Like the central chemoreceptors, the peripheral chemoreceptors respond to elevated PaCO$_2$ by stimulating an increase in ventilation from the DRG in the medulla. The effect on ventilation is less potent than that mediated through the central chemoreceptors, but occurs 5 times faster. This allows the body to react quickly to changes in PaCO$_2$, such as during exercise. Acidic blood pH will also prompt increased ventilation by the same mechanism, to "blow off" CO$_2$ and correctively raise pH to physiologic levels.

Other Sensors

Even though respiration is primarily regulated by the CNS response to changes in PaCO$_2$, other mechanical and physical stimuli may modulate the rate and pattern of breathing via the stimulation of peripheral receptors.

- The Hering-Breuer reflex
  - Mediated by stretch receptors found within the smooth muscles of the small airways.
  - Stimulated by an increase in transmural pressure during lung overinflation.
  - Mechanoreception → stimulation of vagus nerve (CN X) → inhibition of medullary and pontine respiratory centers → contraction of the expiratory muscles & period of *apnea* (termination of breathing after end-expiration).
  - Prominent in newborns, lesser role in regulation of respiration in adults.

- J receptors
  - Named for their location in juxtaposition with capillaries in the alveolar walls.
  - Stimulated by toxins in the pulmonary circulation and by the distention of the pulmonary vessels, as can occur in pulmonary edema secondary to left heart failure.
  - Mediate tachypnea (rapid breathing) and the sensation of dyspnea (shortness of breath).
- Irritant receptors
  - Irritant and C-fiber receptor neurons are located in the epithelium of the large airways (trachea, bronchi, and bronchioles).
  - Stimulated by various noxious agents.
  - Mediate diverse reflexive responses, including coughing, sneezing, mucus secretion, and bronchoconstriction (see Clinical Correlation Box 16.3).

Clinical Correlation Box 16.3

The cough reflex is an example of how irritant receptors function to clear the airways of debris. When irritant receptors are exposed to noxious stimuli, vagal afferent nerves signal the central nervous system (CNS) respiratory centers to direct the inspiration of a large volume of air. The epiglottis and vocal cords are then closed to seal this inspired volume within the lungs. The muscles of expiration contract against this seal to generate extraordinarily high intrapulmonary pressures. When the seal is broken as the epiglottis and vocal cords are reopened, this pressure expels the air and ideally the source of the initial noxious stimulus from the lungs. This reflex is inhibited by alcohol, which may account in part for the prevalence of aspiration pneumonia in alcoholics.

- Chest wall receptors
  - Recall: inspiratory m. contain receptors that relay information pertaining to preload (stretch before contraction) and afterload (force opposing contraction) to the CNS (see Ch. 10).
  - Promote reduced change in ventilation over a range of preload and afterload through reflexes occurring at the level of the spinal cord.
  - Excessive afterload (i.e., restrictive lung disease or increased airway resistance) stimulates spindle receptors and relays to CNS, resulting in the sensation of *dyspnea*.

Sleep

Sleep, defined as the state of unconsciousness during which an individual can be aroused by stimuli, is marked by alterations in respiratory drive with resultant changes in the patterns of respiration.

Sleep is generally divided into two major stages:

1. Slow-wave sleep, named for the brain waves that predominate during this stage.
2. Rapid-eye-movement (REM) sleep, a type of sleep marked by prominent brain activity.

Disturbances in breathing that can occur during these stages may have long-term deleterious effects on several organ systems (see Clinical Correlation Box 16.4).

Clinical Correlation Box 16.4

Case Study

A 55-year-old obese man is admitted to the internal medicine service complaining of swollen legs and shortness of breath worsening over several months. He also notes a long history of daytime sleepiness. Electrocardiogram (ECG) demonstrates sinus tachycardia and findings consistent with an enlarged right atrium. Chest x-ray reveals enlarged heart with prominent pulmonary vasculature. After ruling out imminently life-threatening conditions, what is your next step?

Sleep apnea comes in two forms:

1. Central sleep apnea
   - Abnormality in respiratory drive.
   - Intermittent cessation of rhythmic activity of central respiratory centers → loss of inspiratory muscle activity.
   - Hundreds of apneic periods overnight lead to low arterial O_2 saturation and microarousals.
   - Associated with obesity, central nervous system (CNS) malformations, and pseudotumor cerebri.
2. Obstructive sleep apnea
   - Abnormality in body mechanics ("bull neck" in obese individuals).
   - Weight of excess tissue on upper airways (which normally relax during sleep) leads to obstruction of pharynx.
   - Hundreds of microarousals to reinitiate ventilation throughout night.

Consequences of untreated sleep apnea include:

   - Hypersomnolence (sleepiness interfering with daily life).
   - Pulmonary hypertension and edema because of chronic pulmonary vasoconstriction in response to hypoxemia.

Diagnosis is made via polysomnography, which tracks respiratory patterns and blood oxygen levels during sleep. If diagnosed, patients benefit from supplemental night-time oxygen and/or continuous positive airway pressure (CPAP) to stent the airway open and maintain oxygenation.

Normal Mechanisms of Breathing During Sleep

A significant difference between the waking and the sleeping individual is the tone of skeletal muscles.

- In the waking individual, the muscles of the upper airway (nasopharynx, oropharynx, and larynx) are tonically active and maintain the patency of the upper airway.
- As the diaphragm contracts and the intrapleural and alveolar pressures drop below that of the atmosphere to initiate inspiration, pressure in the upper and lower airways also decreases relative to subatmospheric levels.
- Thus without the contribution of the upper airway muscles, tissues of the upper airway tend to collapse, increasing airway resistance and the work of respiration. In the case of obstructive sleep apnea (Fig. 16.10), occlusion of the airway occurs with relaxation of the upper airway musculature. Arousal is necessitated to increase upper airway tone and allow the passage of air.

The regulation of breathing by the respiratory centers in the CNS also differs in the sleep state. Respiratory drive is suppressed in sleep by a decrease in neural activity within the respiratory centers in the medulla. This results primarily from a loss of excitatory influences from other brain centers, such as the reticular activating system (RAS), which are inhibited during sleep.

In slow-wave sleep, $PaCO_2$ increases in proportion to the decrease in alveolar ventilation. In addition, the drive for respiration in response to increased $PaCO_2$ is blunted, permitting this rise in $PaCO_2$ to occur without a subsequent increase in ventilation.

In REM sleep, the $PaCO_2$-mediated drive for respiration is further attenuated. Thus the hypoxemia-stimulated increase in respiratory drive via peripheral chemoreceptors becomes important in maintaining the oxygen saturation of arterial blood. During REM sleep, irregular patterns of breathing are observed, resulting from the influence of increased brain activity on the normal rhythmic pattern of respiration originating in the medullary and pontine respiratory centers.

Responses to High Altitude

Recall that atmospheric pressure at a given height is simply a function of how much gas "bears down" from above. At sea level, there is considerably more air mass pushing down from above (>14 pounds per square inch) than in the Himalayas. Although the fractional concentration (or mol fraction) of oxygen remains constant at around 21% at all altitudes, the partial pressure of oxygen, PO_2, declines with higher altitudes. PO_2 at sea level is 21% of 760 mm Hg, or 160 mm Hg, whereas PO_2 on Mt. Everest might be 21% of 250 mm Hg, or 53 mm Hg (!) (Fig. 16.11).

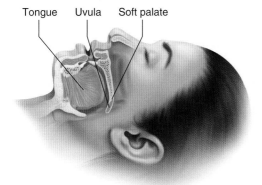
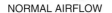

Tongue   Uvula   Soft palate

NORMAL AIRFLOW

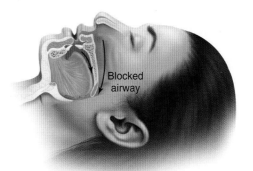

Blocked airway

OBSTRUCTIVE SLEEP APNEA

Fig. 16.10 Anatomic basis of obstructive sleep apnea. (From Yoost BL, Crawford LR. *Fundamentals of Nursing: Active Learning for Collaborative Practice*, 2nd Edition. Elsevier; 2020. Fig. 33.2.)

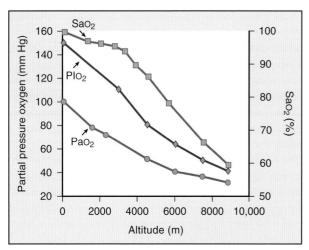

Fig. 16.11 Reduction in oxygen arterial partial pressure (PaO_2) (mm Hg) and oxygen saturation (SaO_2) (%) with increasing altitude. (From Lawley JS, Roach RC, Hacket PH. High-altitude physiology. In: Cushing TA, Harris NS, Auerbach PS (eds). *Auerbach's Wilderness Medicine*, Seventh Edition. Elsevier; 2017. Fig. 1.1.)

$\downarrow$ atmospheric pressure $\rightarrow$ $\downarrow$ partial pressure of inspired oxygen (P_IO_2 $\rightarrow$ $\downarrow$ partial pressure of oxygen in the alveolus (P_AO_2) and in arterial blood (P_aO_2) $\rightarrow$ potential hypoxemia.

The responses of the lungs to high altitude may be acute or chronic.

Acutely, the lungs respond to hypoxemia as described later:

1. Hypoxemia drives hyperventilation through stimulation of the peripheral chemoreceptors. This partially reverses the low alveolar P_AO_2 to maintain favorable gradients for the diffusion of O_2 into the blood. The central chemoreceptors do not contribute to increased ventilation because the $PaCO_2$ is low at high altitude; the hypoxia-driven hyperventilation eliminates more CO_2 than usual, dropping $PaCO_2$ in the blood and creating a respiratory alkalosis (see Ch. 22). This can be treated with acetazolamide.

2. Hypoxemia triggers increased cardiac output to increase total oxygen delivery to the tissues at lower PaO_2.

3. Hypoxic pulmonary vasoconstriction increases pulmonary arterial pressure. However this increases the work of the right side of the heart as it pumps against increased resistance, leading to hypertrophy of the right ventricle long-term.

Beyond a certain altitude, even very high alveolar minute ventilation cannot produce adequate oxygenation, and respiratory failure ensues. This is why mountain climbers wear oxygen masks and airplanes are equipped with supplemental oxygen in the event of cabin depressurization.

At a habitable high altitude, however, these acute responses attenuate over a period of days as the body makes adjustments to life at a slightly lower PaO_2:

1. Hypoxia stimulates erythropoietin production in the kidneys. Erythropoietin causes the bone marrow to produce more red blood cells, increasing the hematocrit and raising the oxygen-carrying capacity of the blood. Thus even though PaO_2 is lower and hemoglobin is less saturated with oxygen, there is more total hemoglobin available, ensuring adequate delivery of oxygen to the tissues.

2. The concentration of 2,3-bisphosphoglyceric acid (DPG) increases in response to hypoxemia, right-shifting the oxyhemoglobin dissociation curve to decrease affinity of hemoglobin for O_2 to facilitate O_2 unloading into the tissues (see Box 16.1 and Clinical Correlation Box 16.5).

BOX 16.1 Collaboration Between the Lungs and Kidneys in the Regulation of $PaCO_2$ and pH

Although the central chemoreceptors are primarily responsible for governing the arterial carbon dioxide partial pressure ($PaCO_2$) level, what happens when a disease state impairs the lungs' capacity to ventilate? In such a case, the $PaCO_2$ climbs because of hypoventilation and, despite increased ventilatory drive, ventilation obviously cannot be increased. The increased $PaCO_2$ lowers the blood pH through the blood buffer equation.

Fortunately, the kidney tubular cells also respond to pH. Acid pH prompts the kidney to excrete H^+ ions and to generate more bicarbonate, thus reversing the acidity through bicarbonate buffering. The kidney thereby compensates for one of the sequelae of a pathologic deficiency in ventilation (respiratory acidosis). The kidney cannot, however, compensate for decreased oxygenation as a result of hypoventilation. The kidneys' response to hypoxemia includes decreased renal perfusion, leading to decreased glomerular filtration (GFR). The decreased GFR leads to increased sodium reabsorption, which increases circulatory volume. Under these conditions, supplemental oxygen given to a hypoxemic patient can reverse these changes, and as the kidneys (no longer suffering from hypoxia) decrease their reabsorption of filtered sodium, sodium and water leave the body in the urine. Thus, under these conditions, oxygen can act as a diuretic.

An increased $PaCO_2$ also leads to increased sodium bicarbonate reabsorption, again with a consequent increase in circulating volume. This can lead to a condition known as cor pulmonale. Thus, the compensatory mechanism of the kidneys to opposed respiratory acidosis can have negative consequences on cardiac function.

Conversely, if a disease state (or a drug) impairs the kidneys' ability to regulate blood pH (metabolic acidosis), assuming normal respiratory centers and mechanical ventilation, the chemoreceptors can sense the change in $[H^+]$.

Clinical Correlation Box 16.5

Case Study

A 30-year-old man who was skiing in the Rocky Mountains at 3500 m collapses on a trail and the local physician is called. On examination, he exhibits dyspnea (shortness of breath), cough, headache, and extreme fatigue. Arterial blood gas (ABG) reveals a pH of 7.6, a carbon dioxide arterial partial pressure ($PaCO_2$) of 19 mm Hg, and an oxygen arterial partial pressure (PaO_2) of 38 mm Hg. Oxygen is administered at 6 L/min via nasal cannulation and a helicopter is called for evacuation. What is the diagnosis?

High-altitude pulmonary edema can occur in otherwise healthy individuals who rapidly ascend to high altitudes. Recall that the pulmonary arteries constrict in the poorly-ventilated areas of the lung to divert blood flow to better-ventilated areas (hypoxic vasoconstriction). However, at high altitude, reduced PaO_2 leads to reduced alveolar oxygen pressure (PAO_2) across the entire lung. This results in uniform vasoconstriction across all pulmonary vascular beds, leading to pulmonary hypertension. High microvascular pressure eventually leads to stress failure of the pulmonary capillary walls, resulting in alveolar fluid exudation and pulmonary edema.

This patient displays hypoxemia (PaO_2 of 38 mm Hg) because of the loss of functional alveoli from edema. Furthermore, his hypoxemia drives hyperventilation via peripheral chemoreceptors, leading to reduced $PaCO_2$ and increased pH (alkalosis) relative to baseline.

Patients are treated with oxygen administration, descent to lower altitude, and, if possible, a hyperbaric chamber to raise PaO_2 and alleviate pulmonary hypoxic vasoconstriction.

Responses to Exercise

Many physiologic changes occur during increased activity, including increased consumption of O_2 and an increased production of CO_2. The excess CO_2 produced by the highly active muscles is carried through the venous circulation to the lungs, thus increasing venous PCO_2. To match these changes in gas concentrations in the body, respiratory rate is increased. As described earlier, joint and muscle receptors activated by movement also increase breathing rate at the beginning of exercise.

Although the mean PO_2 and PCO_2 values are stable during exercise, arterial pH may decrease during strenuous exercise because of lactic acidosis. This triggers the central chemoreceptor relay to the medulla as described earlier.

The cardiovascular effect of increased pulmonary blood flow caused by increased cardiac output during exercise also has an effect on respiration. The increased blood flow increases perfusion, thus making the distribution of V/Q ratios more even throughout the lung, resulting in decreased physiologic dead space and increased gas exchange during exercise.

PATHOPHYSIOLOGY: ABNORMAL PATTERNS OF BREATHING

A myriad of respiratory patterns are observed in the context of dysfunction in respiratory control. These pathophysiologic states may result from structural changes in the CNS, respiratory abnormalities, behavioral disorders, or cardiovascular disease.

Cheyne-Stokes Breathing

Cheyne-Stokes breathing is characterized by cyclic waxing and waning of tidal volume separated by periods of apnea (Fig. 16.12). This periodic pattern of respiration represents an instability of respiratory control that may be observed in association with hypoxia, CNS disease, congestive heart failure, drug overdose, and occasionally sleep. In some cases, Cheyne-Stokes breathing is thought to be caused by a delay in feedback to central and peripheral chemoreceptors secondary to an increase in circulatory transit time.

In conditions, such as congestive heart failure, in which circulatory time is markedly delayed, changes in respiratory drive from the respiratory centers in the CNS lag behind changes in arterial blood gases originating from the lungs. This can lead to periodic Cheyne-Stokes breathing. On the other hand, CNS injury occurring at the level of the brain stem can also cause a "block" in information relay between the peripheral and central chemoreceptors, producing Cheyne-Stokes respirations.

Biot's Breathing

The pattern of respiration in Biot's breathing is characterized by prolonged periods of apnea interrupting normal respiratory cycles. Although the mechanism of Biot's breathing has not been elucidated, it is thought to represent a form of Cheyne-Stokes breathing, resulting from CNS disease.

Kussmaul Breathing

An increase in the rate of ventilation along with an increase in tidal volumes is observed in Kussmaul breathing. Seen most commonly in the setting of diabetic ketoacidosis, it represents an attempt to compensate for metabolic acidosis by blowing off carbon dioxide, thereby raising the pH of the blood. However, with prolonged metabolic acidosis, tissues become depleted of bicarbonate and the inspiratory muscles become fatigued. This results in severe acidosis and death.

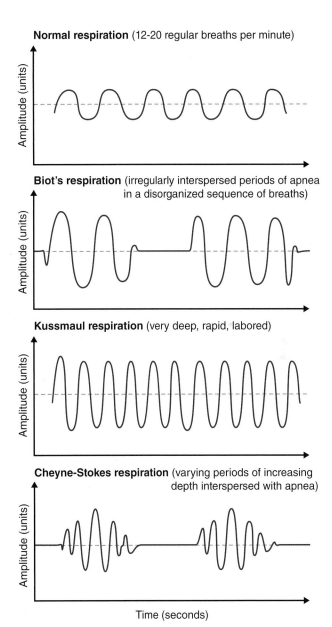

Fig. 16.12 Cheyne-Stokes breathing. Note the episodic periods of hyperventilation and apnea. The periods of apnea are associated with a decrease in arterial O_2 saturation.

SUMMARY

- The major respiratory control centers lie in the medulla, pons, and cerebral cortex.
- The DRG, located in the medulla, is the primary control center in the regulation of respiration, especially inspiration. It generates rhythmic ramp signals that connect to the diaphragm via the phrenic nerves. The signals lead to rhythmic diaphragmatic contraction and relaxation, the basis of breathing.
- The VRG augments active respiration.
- The pneumotaxic and apneustic centers, located in the pons, influence inspiratory volume and respiratory rate.
- The central chemoreceptors in the ventral medulla prompt the DRG to increase ventilation in response to elevated $PaCO_2$. The CO_2 level is the primary driver of respiration under normal circumstances.
- The peripheral chemoreceptors in the carotid bodies and the aortic bodies prompt the DRG to increase ventilation in response to decreased PaO_2. Peripheral respiratory drive becomes especially significant when PaO_2 falls to below 60 mm Hg. They also prompt the DRG to increase ventilation in response to decreased pH (increased H^+ concentration).
- Other receptors influence breathing through reflex arcs. These include stretch receptors in the smooth muscles of small airways, J receptors in the pulmonary interstitium, and irritant receptors in the epithelium of the large airways.
- During sleep, respiratory drive decreases and pharyngeal muscle tone decreases. Sleep apnea may occur if pharyngeal occlusion occurs, requiring arousal for recovery of muscle tone and successful inspiration.
- High altitude can cause hypoxemia and hyperventilation because of maladaptive physiologic responses. Adaptation to chronic habitation at high altitude leads to increased hemoglobin production and enhances oxygen-carrying capacity of the blood.
- Exercise increases O_2 consumption and CO_2 production, but does not change arterial PO_2 or PCO_2. Arterial pH may decrease during strenuous exercise. Changes include increased ventilation rate, increased cardiac output, increased pulmonary blood flow, decreased physiologic dead space, and increased gas exchange.
- Disease states may lead to abnormal breathing patterns. Examples are Cheyne-Stokes breathing, seen in CNS injury and congestive heart failure, and Kussmaul breathing, seen in diabetic ketoacidosis.

REVIEW QUESTIONS

Directions: Each of the numbered items or incomplete statements in this section is followed by answers or by completions of the statement. Select the one lettered answer or completion that is best in each case.

1. A 25-year-old man with a history of polysubstance abuse presents to an emergency department after being found unresponsive at an inner-city nightclub. On arrival, the patient was cyanotic with small pupils (miosis), and responded only to deep, painful stimuli. Needle tracks were observed along the upper extremities. His heart rate was 56 beats per minute, blood pressure, 95/60 mm Hg, and temperature, 35.4° C (95.8° F). Strikingly, his respiration rate was abnormally low at only 6 breaths per minute, and he would occasionally stop breathing entirely, prompting frequent checks by his nurse. What is the most likely cause of his hypoventilation?
   A. Central sleep apnea
   B. Respiratory depression secondary to opioid use
   C. Profound metabolic alkalosis secondary to vomiting
   D. Alcohol intoxication
   E. Benzodiazepine intoxication

2. A 26-year-old man who lives at sea level travels to Colorado for a ski trip. Upon arrival at high altitude, however, he experiences severe dyspnea. The mechanism by which he adjusts acutely to high altitude includes which of the following?
   A. Hyperventilation via hypercarbia-driven stimulation of J receptors
   B. Hyperventilation via stimulation of peripheral chemoreceptors by low arterial pH
   C. Increased hematocrit via hypoxia-driven stimulation of erythropoietin production
   D. Hyperventilation via hypercarbia-driven stimulation by central chemoreceptors
   E. Hyperventilation via hypoxia-driven stimulation by peripheral chemoreceptors

3. A 42-year-old man with severe hypertension has a cerebrovascular accident localized to his medulla and requires mechanical ventilation. The nuclei of the tractus solitarius, the home of the dorsal respiratory group (DRG), appear to be involved. Involvement of the DRG is most likely to obliterate which function of respiratory control?
   A. Stimulation of expiratory muscles
   B. Regulation of rate of respiration
   C. Management of depth of lung inflation
   D. Stimulation of inspiration via a ramp signal
   E. Regulation of inspiratory lung volume

ANSWERS TO REVIEW QUESTIONS

1. **The answer is B.** In the postoperative period, opioids are a critical but preventable cause of respiratory depression. Opioids mainly affect central rhythm generation via inhibition of the pre-Botzinger complex, the "pacemaker" within the VRG. Patients experience reduced respiratory drive and exhibit hypoventilation with both reduced tidal volumes and respiratory rate. Patients thus may require frequent arousals from caretakers after opioid overdose (or, even in the postoperative care unit!). Furthermore, patients exhibit additional vital sign abnormalities, such as relative bradycardia, hypotension, and hypothermia that are not generally seen in abuse of alcohol or benzodiazepines. Bolus doses of naloxone, an opioid reversal agent, can relieve both coma and respiratory depression in opioid overdose.

2. **The answer is E.** At high altitude relative to sea level, the decreased atmospheric pressure results in lower PaO_2 and lower $PaCO_2$. Peripheral chemoreceptors in the carotid and aortic bodies are stimulated by low PaO_2, triggering hyperventilation. Peripheral chemoreceptors are also activated by low arterial pH (high H^+ concentration). At high altitude, a respiratory alkalosis (high arterial pH) exists because more CO_2 than usual is eliminated by hypoxia-induced hyperventilation. Central chemoreceptors are activated by increased levels of $PaCO_2$ and thus are not involved in the acute adjustment to high altitude. Stimulation of erythropoietin production by hypoxia is part of the chronic response to high altitude. J receptors are thought to mediate tachypnea in certain pathophysiologic states, but by either toxins or distention of pulmonary vessels, not by hypercarbia.

3. **The answer is D.** The DRG acts to generate the rhythm of respiration, which it does via initiation of a series of weak action potentials that gradually increase in amplitude, known as a ramp signal. The ventral respiratory group (VRG) in the medulla helps stimulate the muscles involved in expiration under conditions of labored respiration. The pneumotaxic center in the pons regulates both inspiratory volume and respiratory rate. The apneustic center of the pons is thought to manage the depth of lung inflation in inspiration.

Pulmonary Physiology

A.Y. is a 33-year-old woman with a history of severe asthma requiring multiple admissions and intubations, who initially presented to the emergency room with shortness of breath, wheezing, and chest pain.

PRESENTATION: HISTORY

A.Y. had been in her usual state of health until this morning, when she had a sudden sensation of "tightness" in her chest accompanied by wheezing and shortness of breath. She cannot name a precipitant, but noted that a newscaster this morning reported that this was the coldest day so far of the year. She went to a local emergency department. On initial evaluation, she was found to be tachypneic, tachycardic, hypoxic with oxygen saturation (SaO_2) 80%, and sitting in a "tripod" position (see Fig. 16.1.1). On arrival, she received albuterol by nebulizer, intravenous solumedrol (a steroid), and supplemental oxygen by nasal cannula.

She denied sick contacts, fevers, congestion, increased cough, myalgias, chills, sputum production, nausea/vomiting, and recent illness. She also reported no leg swelling or change in number of pillows upon which she slept at night. She has taken all medications as prescribed, including daily leukotriene inhibitor, inhaled corticosteroid, and long-acting β2-agonist therapy in addition to "as-needed" short-acting acting β2-agonists. She reported that cold weather, upper respiratory infections, and ragweed pollen have triggered her symptoms in the past.

DISCUSSION

Based on her symptomatology, as well as an extensive history of asthma complications, this is most likely an acute asthma exacerbation. Exposure to a variety of stimuli (such as allergens, irritants, and cold weather) causes mast cell activation, leading to release of factors including histamine, leukotrienes, and prostaglandins that promote airway smooth muscle contraction. Bronchial constriction and subsequent airflow limitation lead to the sensation of dyspnea (shortness of breath), chest tightness, and wheeze characteristic of this disease.

Vocal cord dysfunction is another possible diagnosis, but tends to have stridor or wheezing that is predominantly inspiratory rather than expiratory and prominent over the neck. Pulmonary embolism is plausible given the acute onset of her symptoms, but less likely given her prominent wheezing and known asthma history. Respiratory infection is unlikely as she is afebrile with no sputum production, cough, chills, or myalgias. COPD (chronic obstructive pulmonary disease) is unlikely given

she has no history of smoking, cough, or sputum production. Finally, the absence of leg edema (swelling) and orthopnea (dyspnea exacerbated by lying flat) suggest against pulmonary edema secondary to congestive heart failure.

PRESENTATION: PHYSICAL EXAMINATION AND LABORATORY VALUES

On initial examination, A.Y. was afebrile with a blood pressure of 133/77 mm Hg. She was somnolent and unable to speak in full sentences. Pulmonary examination revealed tachypnea at 26 breaths per minute, scattered inspiratory and expiratory wheezes in bilateral lung fields, and use of accessory respiratory muscles. Her oxygen saturation was 80% while breathing room air and 95% on 2 L/min of supplemental oxygen by nasal cannula. Her cardiovascular examination was unremarkable except for tachycardia at 111 beats per minute. A.Y.'s abdominal and neurologic examinations were unremarkable. She had no lower extremity edema.

Arterial blood gas was notable for a pH of 7.19, arterial partial pressure of oxygen (PaO_2) of 61 mm Hg, arterial partial pressure of carbon dioxide ($PaCO_2$) of 66 mm Hg, and bicarbonate of 27 mEq/L. Her chest radiograph was unremarkable. Her peak expiratory flow rate were less than 25% of her personal best.

DISCUSSION

Her physical examination reveals diffuse wheezing resulting from difficulty in expiration likely caused by bronchoconstriction. The use of accessory muscles of respiration at rest is also abnormal. Often, contraction of the scalene muscles during inspiration is the first sign of impending respiratory failure, with contraction of the trapezius and sternocleidomastoid only occurring late in the process. Her somnolence and inability to speak in full sentences further signal a possible life-threatening asthma exacerbation. Her examination is not suggestive of respiratory infection or cardiac disease.

Her bloodwork demonstrates a severe acute respiratory acidosis with elevated $PaCO_2$ at 61 mm Hg and markedly decreased pH at 7.19, with appropriate bicarbonate compensation at 27 mmol/L. Her low pH triggers central respiratory centers leading to hyperventilation, consistent with the tachypnea noted on examination. She is hypoxemic, but her PaO_2 has not yet fallen below 60 mm Hg, which would trigger her peripheral chemoreceptors to drive hyperventilation. Finally, her peak expiratory flow rates were markedly reduced from her baseline values, consistent with limited expiration. Ultimately, her lab results are

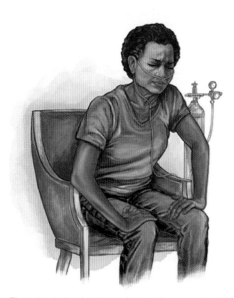

Fig. 16.1.1 The tripod sign in this patient with an acute asthma exacerbation. This patient, like many with acute dyspnea (shortness of breath) caused by conditions, such as chronic obstructive pulmonary disease, is leaning forward sitting with her hands on her distal anterior thighs/knees. This position helps recruit accessory muscles of respiration, such as the scalene, sternocleidomastoid, and pectoralis major muscles. (Netter illustration used with permission of Elsevier Inc. All rights reserved. www.netterimages.com)

suggestive of hypercapnic respiratory failure, characterized by a $PaCO_2$ above 50 mm Hg.

Key fact: Recall that we can assess for adequate bicarbonate compensation by assuming that the $[HCO_3^-]$ rises by 1 mmol/L from its reference value of 24 mmol/L for every 10 mm Hg increase in pCO_2 above its reference value of 40 mm Hg.

TREATMENT AND SUBSEQUENT COURSE

Given her alarming arterial blood gas results, A.Y. was immediately treated with several doses of a combined inhalation solution containing a short-acting β-2 agonist and an anticholinergic medication (ipratropium bromide). After 30 minutes, she was alert and able to speak in full sentences. Her oxygen saturation recovered to 99% on room air. A repeat arterial blood gas demonstrated resolved acidemia with a pH of 7.41.

Overnight, she had no complications and reported complete resolution of her symptoms. Her physical examination revealed only trace wheezes in bilateral lung fields. Once arrangements were made for discharge, she was given an additional oral corticosteroid to taper (reduce dose) over the next 5 days. She was given strict instructions to return to the emergency room if any of her symptoms recurred.

DISCUSSION

A.Y.'s diagnosis upon admission was acute exacerbation of her known asthma complicated by hypercapnic respiratory failure. Thankfully, she responded rapidly to several pharmacologic interventions in addition to supplementary oxygen support. Asthma is now considered a syndrome, not a single disease. Various molecular and cellular processes can lead to episodic bronchoconstriction that manifests clinically as asthma. These are sometimes referred to as asthma "endotypes". Examples include allergic asthma, in which allergen specific IgE sensitizes mast cells, and exercise induced asthma in which exertion (often in cold, dry air) precipitates exacerbations.

β-2-agonists relax the smooth muscle of the airways, alleviating bronchoconstriction. Anticholinergic agents, such as ipratropium bromide, further act as bronchodilators. Corticosteroids inhibit the synthesis of numerous proinflammatory mediators and promote the apoptosis of inflammatory cells such as eosinophils. Leukotriene inhibitors act at the late stage of the inflammatory response, antagonizing the effects of cysteinyl leukotrienes (among the most potent bronchoconstricting molecules known) at their receptor. Additional agents not used in this patient include theophylline, a phosphodiesterase and adenosine inhibitor, and omalizumab, a monoclonal antiimmunoglobin E antibody. Other biologic agents include: 1) dupilumab, which binds to the alpha chain shared by the receptor for interleukins-4 and -13, thereby inhibiting the skewing of immune responses to a Th2, generally "allergic" phenotype; 2) Benralizumab, which binds to the interlukin-5 receptor critical to the survival of eosinophils; and 3) mepolizumab, which likewise deprives eosinophils of interleukin-5 by binding to the cytokine itself and stearically hindering it from finding its receptor. Avoidance of potential triggers is, of course, always the ideal!

SECTION VI

Renal Physiology

17

Renal Structure and Function

INTRODUCTION

The kidney is the principal organ of homeostasis. The kidney's filtration of blood, and modification of that filtrate by epithelial transport, produces urine to accomplish the following functions:
- Control of the composition of body fluids, the concentration of electrolytes, and the excretion of metabolic waste products and foreign substances.
- Control of body fluid volume and osmolality.
- Regulation of the acidity of the blood.

The kidney also performs hormonal and metabolic functions, including:
- Production and secretion of erythropoietin (EPO)
- Activation of vitamin D
- Gluconeogenesis (the synthesis of glucose from amino acids and other noncarbohydrate precursors, which also occurs in liver and muscle tissue)

In this chapter, we focus on the initial step in urine formation, the production of a plasma ultrafiltrate by the process of glomerular filtration.

SYSTEM STRUCTURE: THE KIDNEY

The kidneys are retroperitoneal organs, lying alongside the vertebral column at the level of the T12-L3 vertebrae (see Fast Fact Box 17.1).

Fast Fact Box 17.1

Each adult kidney weighs between 115 and 170 g, and is approximately the size of the human fist.

Fig. 17.1 shows the gross anatomic features of the human kidney and urinary system.
- The medial side of the kidney has an indentation, the hilum, where the renal artery and nerves enter the kidney and the renal veins exit.
- The funnel-shaped renal pelvis also exits at the hilum.
- The ureter, forming a contractile conduit that pushes the urine from the kidney to the bladder.

The kidney can be divided into two regions:
1. Outer region called the cortex
2. Inner region called the medulla

The medulla forms 10 to 18 cone-shaped structures, the renal pyramids.
- The apex of each pyramid, called the papilla, projects into the urinary collection space.

- Urine expressed from each papilla is collected by a minor calyx, the smallest branch of the urinary collection system → coalesce to form major calyces → form the renal pelvis.
- In between the renal pyramids are renal columns, also called columns of Bertin, that are considered to be extensions of renal cortical tissue.

The Vasculature

The kidney is one of the most well-perfused tissues in the human body, receiving 20% of 25% of total cardiac output (~1.25 L/min). The disproportionately large amount of blood flow the kidney receives allows it to excrete large quantities of nitrogenous waste products (see Clinical correlation Box 17.1).

Clinical Correlation Box 17.1

It is important that the kidney has the ability to regulate renal blood flow and glomerular filtration rate independently. In some disorders of reduced blood volume or increased osmolarity, the kidney has the ability to compensate through mechanisms that reduce renal blood flow.

The renal vascular system is illustrated in Fig. 17.2.

The renal artery enters the kidney at the hilum → interlobar arteries → arcuate arteries → interlobular arteries → afferent arterioles → glomerular capillaries → coalesce to form the efferent arterioles → peritubular capillaries, a capillary network surrounding the renal tubules.
- Each glomerulus is a discrete functioning unit connected to its own afferent and efferent arteriole.
- A subset of the peritubular capillaries called the vasa recta supplies the tubules in the medulla.
- As blood exits the peritubular capillaries, it enters the venous system, which follows approximately the same course as the arteries (see Fast Fact Box 17.2).

Fast Fact Box 17.2

The renal circulation has two sets of capillary beds in sequence: glomerular and peritubular. Blood exiting the glomerular capillaries remains in the arterial system and passes through the peritubular capillaries before entering the venous system. The kidney is one of a few organs with this unusual circulatory anatomy (another is the pituitary gland).

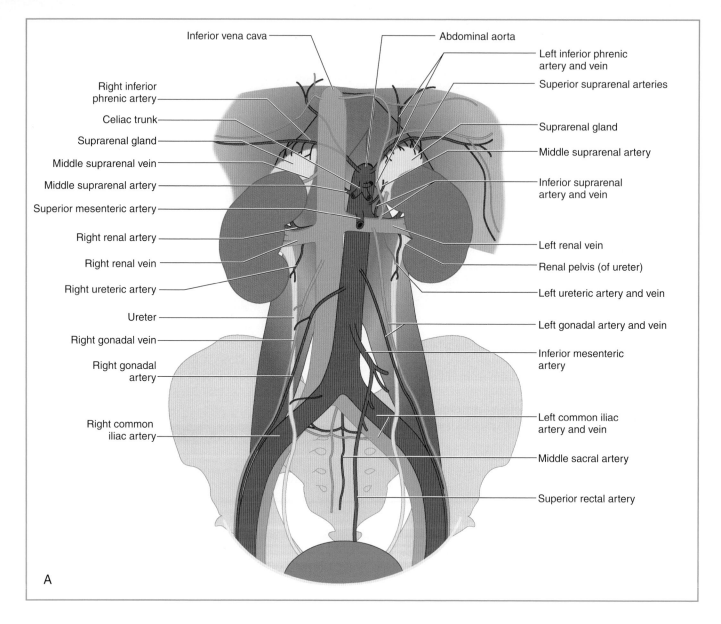

Inferior vena cava

Abdominal aorta

Left inferior phrenic artery and vein

Superior suprarenal arteries

Right inferior phrenic artery

Celiac trunk

Suprarenal gland

Middle suprarenal vein

Middle suprarenal artery

Superior mesenteric artery

Right renal artery

Right renal vein

Right ureteric artery

Ureter

Right gonadal vein

Right gonadal artery

Right common iliac artery

Suprarenal gland

Middle suprarenal artery

Inferior suprarenal artery and vein

Left renal vein

Renal pelvis (of ureter)

Left ureteric artery and vein

Left gonadal artery and vein

Inferior mesenteric artery

Left common iliac artery and vein

Middle sacral artery

Superior rectal artery

A

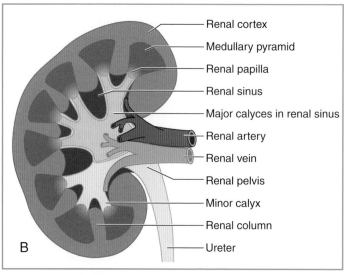

Renal cortex

Medullary pyramid

Renal papilla

Renal sinus

Major calyces in renal sinus

Renal artery

Renal vein

Renal pelvis

Minor calyx

Renal column

Ureter

B

Fig. 17.1 Gross anatomy of the kidney. A, The urinary system. B, The kidney. (From Bogart BI, Ort VH. *Elsevier's Integrated Anatomy*. Philadelphia: Mosby Elsevier; 2007. Figs. 6.2 and 6.6.)

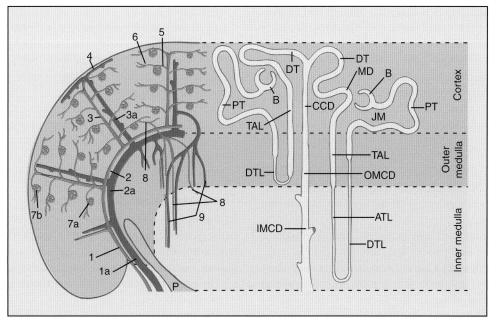

Fig. 17.2 Organization of the vascular system of the human kidney: 1, interlobar arteries; 1a, interlobar veins; 2, arcuate arteries; 2a, arcuate veins; 3, interlobular arteries; 3a, interlobular veins; 4, stellate vein; 5, afferent arterioles; 6, efferent arterioles; 7a, 7b, glomerular capillary networks; 8, descending vasa recta; 9, ascending vasa recta. Right, Organization of the human nephron. A superficial nephron is illustrated on the left, and a juxtamedullary (*JM*) nephron is illustrated on the right. The loop of Henle includes the straight portion of the proximal tubule (*PT*), descending thin limb (*DTL*), ascending thin limb (*ATL*), and thick ascending limb (*TAL*). B, Bowman's capsule; *CCD*, cortical collecting duct; *DT*, distal tubule; *IMCD*, inner medullary collecting duct; *MD*, macula densa; *OMCD*, outer medullary collecting duct; *P*, pelvis. (From Levy MN, Koeppen BM, Stanton BA. *Berne and Levy Principles of Physiology*, 4th Edition. Elsevier; 2005. Fig. 36.2.)

Why does the renal circulation have such an unusual design? Each of the kidney's two capillary beds has a specialized function:

- The glomerular capillaries = filter large volumes
- The peritubular capillaries = reabsorb fluid and solute

Flow regulation through each of these capillary beds is critical to kidney function.

The Nephron

The functional unit of urine formation in the kidney is the nephron (Fig. 17.3). Each kidney contains approximately 1 million nephrons (range of approximately 600,000–1.2 million) (see Clinical Correlation Box 17.2).

Clinical Correlation Box 17.2

The kidney cannot regenerate nephrons. When nephrons are lost from disease or by normal aging, the kidneys compensate with adaptive changes in the remaining nephrons. This is the basis for living donor kidney transplants, as the donor can survive with only one kidney.

The glomerulus, the initial part of the nephron, filters plasma into the urinary space of a surrounding pouch called Bowman's capsule (the parietal epithelium of the glomerulus and its basement membrane) → The filtrate then flows into the proximal convoluted tubule → medullary proximal straight tubule (Pars recta) and the loop of Henle, a hairpin-shaped structure divided into the → thin descending limb, the thin ascending limb, and the thick ascending limb → continues to the distal tubule. A specialized segment of the distal tubule, at a

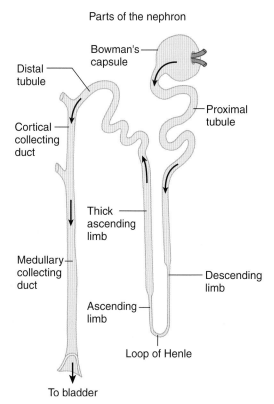

Parts of the nephron

Fig. 17.3 Basic components of the nephron. (From Carroll R. *Elsevier's Integrated Physiology*. Philadelphia: Mosby Elsevier; 2007. Fig. 11.1.)

point where the tubule passes between the afferent and efferent arterioles, makes up the macula densa → distal tubules from several nephrons empty into a cortical collecting duct → then become medullary collecting ducts in the outer medulla. The medullary collecting duct descends to the tip of the renal papilla (inner medulla), emptying into the collecting system.

Nephrons can be broadly divided into two groups:

1. Superficial cortical nephrons have glomeruli in the outer regions of the cortex and short loops of Henle, which lack a thin ascending limb and barely dip into the medulla.
   - Their peritubular capillaries form extensive networks surrounding the tubules, allowing for an efficient exchange of substances and water between the tubules and the circulation.
2. Juxtamedullary nephrons have glomeruli near the medulla, and their loops of Henle travel deep into the medulla.
   - Note that all glomeruli are in the cortex. Juxtamedullary nephrons have vasa recta. These long, thin peritubular capillaries travel alongside the loops of Henle into the medulla and then loop back toward the cortex.
   - The vasa recta play an important role in the concentration of urine and in nature, mammals that must excrete concentrated urine have the longest nephron loops.

The Glomerulus

During development, the glomerular capillaries push into the closed end of the proximal tubule, like a fist pressing into a balloon (Fig. 17.4).

- This invagination forms Bowman's capsule (the punched-in "balloon"), made up of two epithelial layers: the inner visceral layer tightly enveloping the "fist" of glomerular capillaries, and the outer parietal layer.
- The space between these two, which remains connected to the lumen of the proximal tubule, forms the urinary space, or Bowman's space. The visceral epithelial cells, or podocytes, tightly envelope the capillaries, adhering to them with foot processes. The histology of the glomerulus is illustrated in Fig. 17.5.

Fig. 17.6 is a closer view of the layers that substances must cross in traveling from the blood into Bowman's space. These layers make up the filtration barrier.

- The first layer is the capillary endothelium. The endothelium has many holes, or fenestrations, that make it highly permeable to water and also allow small molecules, including many plasma proteins, to pass freely.
- The second layer is basement membrane containing collagen type IV and negatively charged proteoglycans. The basement membrane provides a charge barrier for the negatively charged plasma proteins.
- The third layer is the visceral epithelium. In the visceral epithelium, small spaces between the podocytes, called filtration slits, are bridged by a thin diaphragm. The filtrate passes through the filtration slits and flows around the foot processes into Bowman's space.

The Juxtaglomerular Apparatus

As shown in Fig. 17.5, the region where the distal tubule passes between the afferent and efferent arterioles contains a set of structures, the macula densa and the juxtaglomerular cells, known together as the juxtaglomerular apparatus.

- The epithelial cells of the distal tubule in this region form the macula densa.
- The juxtaglomerular cells are modified smooth muscle cells in the arteriolar walls adjacent to the macula densa. They secrete the enzyme renin, stored in intracytoplasmic granules.

The important role these structures play in the autoregulation of renal blood flow (RBF) will be discussed later in this chapter.

SYSTEM FUNCTION: THE KIDNEY

Three distinct processes determine the amount of a substance excreted in the urine (Fig. 17.7).

1. Glomerular filtration generates a cell-free and protein-free ultrafiltrate by glomerular filtration which continues through Bowman's space
2. Tubular reabsorption from the tubule lumen back into the peritubular capillaries
3. Tubular secretion from the peritubular capillaries into the tubule lumen

The processes are related in the following mass balance equation:

$$\text{Amount of substance excreted} = \text{amount filtered} + \text{amount secreted} - \text{amount reabsorbed}$$

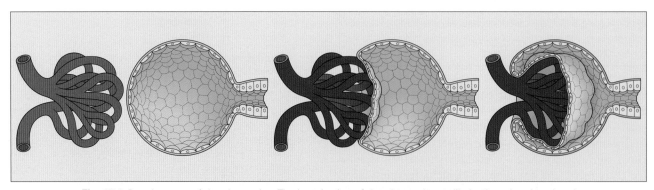

Fig. 17.4 Development of the glomerulus. The invagination of the glomerular capillaries into the closed end of the proximal tubule forms Bowman's capsule. (From Lowe JS, Anderson PG. *Stevens & Lowe's Human Histology*, 4th Ed. Philadelphia: Mosby Elsevier; 2014. Fig. 15.6.)

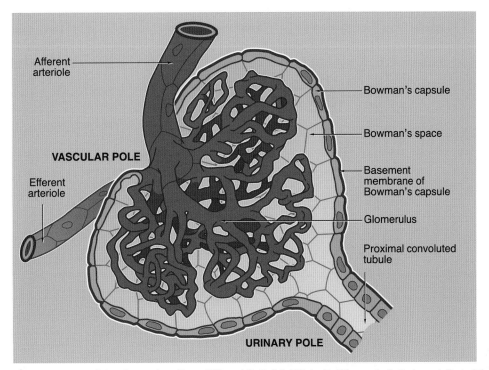

Fig. 17.5 Histology of the glomerulus. (From O'Dowd G, Bell S, Wright S. *Wheater's Pathology: A Text, Atlas and Review of Histopathology*, 6th Ed. Philadelphia: Elsevier; 2019. Fig. 15.2a.)

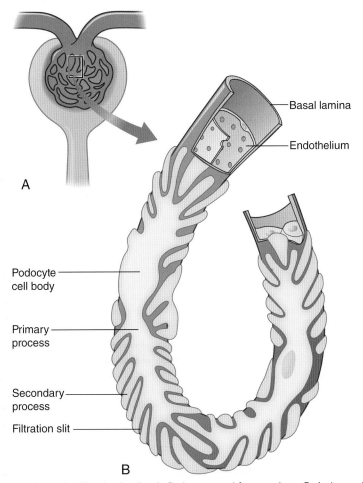

Fig. 17.6 The glomerular filtration barrier. A, Podocytes and fenestrations. B, A closer view of the same.

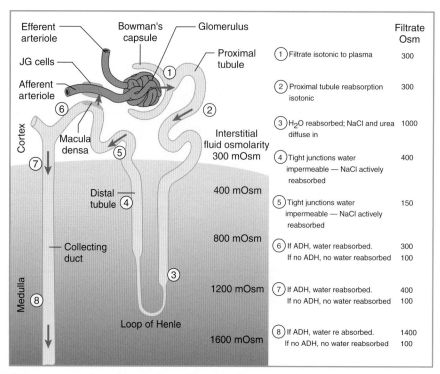

Fig. 17.7 Three essential renal mechanisms. The general processes in the nephron that determine urine composition are glomerular filtration, reabsorption, and secretion. (From Carroll R. *Elsevier's Integrated Physiology.* Philadelphia: Mosby Elsevier; 2007. Fig. 11.18.)

Glomerular Filtration

Glomerular filtration requires substances traveling from the glomerular capillaries into the urinary space to traverse the filtration barrier, composed (sequentially) of a fenestrated capillary endothelium, the negatively charged basement membrane, and the filtration slits between podocytes (Fig. 17.8). The driving force for filtration is the mechanical energy from contraction of the heart. This force is greatest during systole, and there is a pressure wave in the afferent and efferent arterioles. All the energy expended by the kidney after filtration is due to electrochemical gradients for specific solutes, flow along the peritubular capillaries and the tubular lumen, with the contribution of metabolic energy in the form of ATP.

- Freely filtered into ultrafiltrate:
  - Water
  - Small molecular-weight solutes, whether positively or negatively charged (e.g., sodium, chloride, bicarbonate, and small peptides and proteins) are freely filtered (Fig 17.9).
- Excluded from ultrafiltrate:
  - Small molecules bound to proteins in plasma (e.g., calcium bound to albumin)
  - Large negatively charged macromolecules (e.g., albumin)
  - Large positively charged macromolecules (e.g., immunoglobulins) (see Clinical Correlation Box 17.3).

Measuring Glomerular Filtration Rate

Glomerular filtration rate (GFR) is the volume of plasma that is filtered in the glomeruli per unit time. It represents only a fraction of blood flow through the glomerular capillaries (~20%)

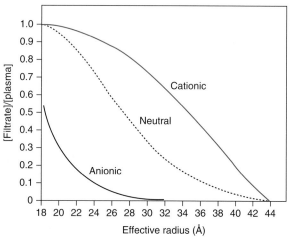

Fig. 17.8 Filtration rates of dextrans. Larger molecules and negatively charged molecules are less freely filtered. A filterability value of 1 indicates that the molecules are filtered as freely as water; a value of 0 implies that they are not filtered at all.

Clinical Correlation Box 17.3

In some renal diseases, the glomerular basement membrane is damaged and loses its negative charge. The consequences of this injury and loss of surface area are predictable. The filtration barrier becomes more permeable to the negatively charged plasma proteins, and large amounts of protein (mostly albumin) are lost in the urine where it can be measured clinically, a condition called *proteinuria*. Extreme losses of albumin from the plasma can lead to a shift in fluid from the blood vessels to the extracellular spaces because of decreased oncotic pressure, leading to edema. Severely low albumin resulting from heavy proteinuria is one of the causes of edema in the condition called nephrotic syndrome (see Ch. 19).

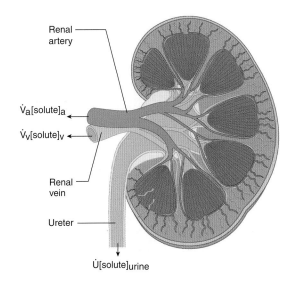

$$\dot{V}_a[solute]_a = \dot{V}_V \times [solute]_V + \dot{U} \times [solute]_{urine}$$

Fig. 17.9 The excretion of a substance S into the urine. We can write a mass balance of the earlier equation when two conditions are met: (1) substance S is freely filtered, (2) the tubule does not absorb or secrete substance S. (From Carroll R. *Elsevier's Integrated Physiology.* Philadelphia: Mosby Elsevier; 2007. Fig. 11.1.)

as the majority of substances are not filtered. A normal value is 125 mL/min, or 180 L/day. It is interesting to note by analogy that 20-25% of cardiac output goes to the kidney. Just as only a fraction of blood from the heart goes to the kidneys, so only a fraction of blood flow to the kidney gets filtered.

Note that because renal arterial flow and venous flow are so much greater than the urine flow rate, we presume that the arterial and venous flow rates are equal. The renal artery plasma flow rate is ~800 mL/min, and the urine flow rate is ~1 mL/min, so the renal venous flow rate will be ~799 mL/min. We presume that 800 mL/min = 799 mL/min for ease of calculation.

- At 125 mL/min this tremendous filtration rate is the first step in a process that allows the kidneys to regulate the composition and volume of body fluids in the subsequent segments of the renal tubule.

GFR acts as an indicator of kidney function as a whole in clinical settings. Estimating a patient's GFR has several important clinical applications, from assessing the degree of damage to the kidneys to determining appropriate doses of medications (because many medications are excreted in the urine).

We can measure GFR by using substances that are freely filtered in the glomerulus but are neither secreted nor reabsorbed in the tubules. "Freely filtered" means that filtered plasma holds the same concentration of a substance as unfiltered plasma. Inulin (different from insulin) is one such substance, which is found in dahlia roots and the Jerusalem artichoke. Not all solutes are freely filtered. Factors that may affect the filtration rate of a solute include the molecular weight, the charge, and whether the solute binds to other macromolecules in the plasma.

- Because inulin is neither secreted nor reabsorbed, all the inulin that is filtered by the glomerulus is excreted in the urine (Fig. 17.10). Broadly, filtered solute is equal to GFR multiplied by the plasma solute concentration. This is known

as the filtration rate of the solute, in units of mg/min. Likewise, the excreted solute is equal to the urine flow rate ($\dot{V}$) multiplied by the urine solute concentration. This is known as the excretion or elimination rate of the solute in the urine, in units of mg/min. Note that the filtration rate of a solute is different than GFR, which is the filtration rate of water. We can state this concept as a mass balance equation:

Filtered inulin = Excreted inulin

Recall that the mass of a solute equals the concentration of the solute times the volume of the solution. Thus the amount of inulin filtered per minute equals the volume of plasma filtered per minute—the GFR—times the plasma inulin concentration, $[inulin]_P$. Similarly, the amount of excreted inulin equals the urine flow volume per minute ($\dot{V}$) times the concentration of inulin in the urine, $[inulin]_U$. It is critical to be consistent with units. Choose the units and do a dimensional analysis of all calculations.

- We can then rewrite the mass balance equation as:

$$GFR \times [inulin]_P = \dot{V} \times [inulin]_U$$
$$GFR = \dot{V} \times [inulin]_U / [inulin]_P$$

- Thus if we infuse inulin into a patient so that it reaches a steady-state plasma concentration, we can measure the volume of urine and the inulin concentrations in the plasma and urine to obtain an estimate of the patient's GFR (see Clinical Correlation Box 17.4). We can measure the inulin concentration in peripheral venous blood and use that value for renal arterial concentration because none of the structures that the venous blood will pass through on its way to the kidney has any appreciable ability to eliminate water or solutes from the plasma.

Clinical Correlation Box 17.4

When physicians want to estimate glomerular filtration rate (GFR), they use a common clinical technique for estimating GFR which entails measuring levels of creatinine, a product of creatine phosphate hydrolysis in skeletal muscle. It enters the plasma from muscle at a relatively fixed rate determined by the muscle mass of the individual. In the kidney, creatinine is filtered by the glomerulus and is secreted to a small extent but not reabsorbed. Thus measuring plasma and urine creatinine levels and urine volume per time (a standard is 24 hours) allows us to estimate GFR.

The filtration faction, or the fraction of renal plasma flow (RPF) filtered through the glomerulus, can be calculated using the GFR and RPF, the volume of plasma that enters the kidney per minute. This is different from GFR, the number of milliliters per minute that is filtered.

Filtration fraction = GFR/RPF

Normally, this fraction is approximately 20%. In other words, of the plasma entering the kidney, 20% is filtered through the glomerular capillaries and the other 80% exits the glomeruli via the efferent arterioles and continues on to the peritubular capillaries.

Measuring RPF requires a substance that is completely eliminated from the plasma entering the kidney, and thus is

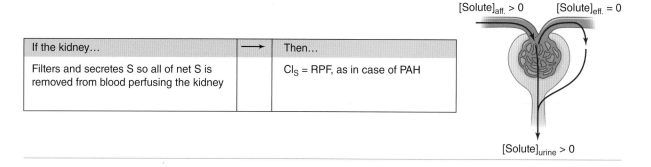

If the kidney...	→	Then...
Filters and secretes S so all of net S is removed from blood perfusing the kidney		$Cl_S = RPF$, as in case of PAH

If the kidney...	→	Then...
Filters and secretes S so some but not all of net S is removed from blood perfusing the kidney		$Cl_S < RPF$ and $Cl_S > GFR$

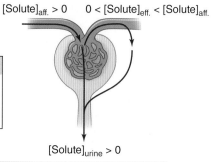

If the kidney...	→	Then...
Filters but neither secretes nor resorbs S		$Cl_S = GFR$, as in case of insulin

If the kidney...	→	Then...
Filters and resorbs all filtered S so none of net S is removed from blood perfusing the kidney		$Cl_S = 0$, as in case of glucose, amino acids, etc. (in normal physiology)

If the kidney...	→	Then...
Filters and resorbs some of filtered S		$Cl_S < GFR$

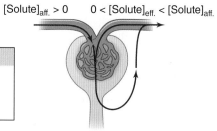

Fig. 17.10 The clearance of S under different types of renal handling. *Cls*, Clearance of S; *GFR*, glomerular filtration rate; *PAH*, paraaminohippurate; *RPF*, renal plasma flow.

completely excreted in the urine. Because no substance is completely filtered (as not all plasma water is filtered) a substance that is completely eliminated must require a secretory mechanism to eliminate in excess of filtration. Thus even if a solute has a small molecular weight, no inhibition of filtration due to charge, and no appreciable binding to other plasma macromolecules, in other words it is freely filtered, that filtration rate will still not equal RPF. You never filter all of your plasma.

- A commonly used substance that approximates these characteristics at low concentrations is paraaminohippurate (PAH). Thus, for low concentrations of PAH (<<Km), the clearance is equal to RPF, as the venous concentration of PAH will be 0.

Using a similar calculation as that to determine GFR by inulin, the mass of PAH entering the kidney per minute equals the plasma volume entering the kidney per minute (the RPF) times the concentration of PAH in the plasma, $[PAH]_P$. The mass of PAH excreted in the urine per minute equals the urine flow rate (V in units such as mL/min) times the concentration of PAH in the urine, $[PAH]_U$. Thus:

$$RPF \times [PAH]_P = \dot{V} \times [PAH]_U$$
$$RPF = \dot{V} \times [PAH]_U / [PAH]_P$$

This equation lets us estimate RPF by using an infusion of PAH and measuring the urine output and the concentrations of PAH in the plasma and urine. Other methods that do not require complete elimination of the solute into the urine can be used to measure RPF, (see Genetics Box 17.1, Development Box 17.1 and Pharmacology Box 17.1).

GENETICS BOX 17.1

A dramatic alteration in renal structure occurs in patients with autosomal dominant polycystic kidney disease, with the progressive formation of numerous fluid filled cysts in both kidneys. Most such patients have a mutation in either the PKD1 gene or the PKD2 gene. How the products of these genes (polycystin-1 and -2, respectively) lead to cyst formation is incompletely understood.

DEVELOPMENT BOX 17.1

In autosomal dominant polycystic kidney disease, as multiple cysts deriving from various nephron segments grow and coalesce, renal function progressively declines. Affected patients can manifest with hematuria, flank pain from renal hemorrhage or kidney stone formation, or proteinuria. As the glomerular filtration rate declines, generally around age 50 years in PKD1-driven disease and in patients in their 70s in PKD2-driven disease, hypertension and other manifestations of renal failure ensue. Some patients also develop cysts in other organs (thyroid, liver, spleen.)

PHARMACOLOGY BOX 17.1

Treatment of autosomal dominant polycystic kidney disease is largely symptomatic and supportive. In addition to counseling patients to adopt a low sodium diet, hypertension can be treated with angiotensin converting enzyme inhibitors and angiotensin receptor blockers. Tolvaptan, a vasopressin receptor antagonist, decreases the rate of loss of glomerular filtration rate. Octreotide, a long acting version of somatostatin may decrease the rate of fluid accumulation in cysts.

RBF (RBF) can be derived from RPF.

- Recall that hematocrit (HCT) equals the percentage of blood volume occupied by red blood cells (e.g., an HCT of 40% indicates that a fraction of 0.4 of total blood volume is made up of red blood cell mass).
- Everything else is the plasma; thus, (1 – HCT) represents the fraction of blood volume occupied by plasma. In the example of a HCT of 40%, the fraction of blood that is plasma is 0.6. Consequently,

$$RPF = (RBF)(\text{fraction of blood that is plasma})$$
$$RPF = (RBF)(1 - HCT)$$
$$RBF = RPF / (1 - HCT)$$

If we measure the RPF, we calculate RBF. By determining the RBF and with knowledge of the cardiac output, we can assess what percentage of the cardiac output is directed into the kidneys.

Renal Clearance

Clearance refers to the volume of incoming plasma from which all substance is removed and excreted into the urine per minute.

- A solute that is neither secreted nor reabsorbed, such as inulin, has a clearance that actually corresponds to a real value of plasma volume filtered.
- A solute that is secreted extensively, such as PAH, never actually reaches the renal vein. Although the solute is fully cleared from plasma, the total renal plasma volume never left the circulation.

Note that the value for the clearance of any specific substance S is a calculated number used to describe the way the kidney handles substance S. The kidney may leave some of S in the blood, but we still say there was clearance of S. The clearance of S is a calculated theoretical number answering this question:

Given the amount of S excreted by the kidney (amount filtered + amount secreted – amount reabsorbed), what volume of incoming plasma per minute would have to be totally cleared of S to surrender that amount of excreted S?

It may help to imagine that the plasma flowing through the kidney comes in two volume compartments (Fig. 17.11):

- The first compartment contains the S that will not be excreted after filtration, secretion, and reabsorption
- The second compartment contains the S that will be excreted after filtration, secretion, and reabsorption. This imagined volume containing the S that is destined for excretion is the volume that is "cleared" of S.

Then imagine that the two compartments coalesce upon leaving the kidney in the veins, after being worked on by filtration, secretion, and reabsorption. Imagine that the S from the nonexcreted compartment diffuses into the cleared compartment. That is how we can have a clearance for S without removing all of S from the RPF.

We can derive a general formula for clearance by beginning with a mass balance equation for hypothetical substance S.

As before, $[S]_P$ and $[S]_U$ represent the concentrations of S in the plasma and urine, and V represents the volume of urine produced per minute.

- Now, we will denote the clearance of S as Cl_S, the volume of plasma per minute from which S has been removed and excreted into the urine. Using the concept of mass balance, we write:

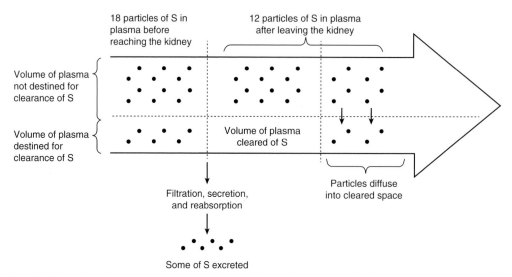

18 particles of S in plasma before reaching the kidney

12 particles of S in plasma after leaving the kidney

Volume of plasma not destined for clearance of S

Volume of plasma destined for clearance of S

Volume of plasma cleared of S

Particles diffuse into cleared space

Filtration, secretion, and reabsorption

Some of S excreted

Fig. 17.11 Two imaginary compartments of plasma laden with substance S. Each dot represents a particle of substance S. One compartment is destined for renal clearance of S and one is not.

Mass cleared from the plasma/time = Mass found in the urine/time

Because mass/time equals concentration times volume/time, we find that:

$$[S]_P \times Cl_S = [S]_U \times V$$

$$Cl_S = [S]_U \times V / [S]_P$$

Looking back to our earlier equations, we verify that the clearance of inulin equals the GFR and the clearance of PAH equals the RPF. We can also verify that the units of clearance are mL/min (the units for concentration cancel out and V, the urine flow rate or volume of urine per minute, can be measured in mL/min). These units are in accordance with our definition of clearance as the volume of plasma being cleared of a substance per minute.

Determinants of Glomerular Filtration Rate and Renal Blood Flow

As in other capillary beds, the rate of fluid filtered by the glomerulus is determined by the balance of oncotic and hydrostatic forces. These forces are illustrated in Fig. 17.12.

The balance of forces is summarized in the Starling relationship, wherein flow is proportional to an ultrafiltration coefficient and the driving forces that apply:

$$GFR = K_f \left[(P_{GC} - P_{BS}) - \sigma(\Pi_{GC} - \Pi_{BS}) \right]$$

The ultrafiltration coefficient (K_f) is proportional to the hydraulic conductivity (L_p) of the glomerular capillary and the surface area available for filtration.
- The hydraulic conductivity, in turn, represents the flux of water per unit time for a defined pressure gradient and surface area.
- The physical properties of the glomerular filtration barrier, particularly the fenestrations in the endothelium, make it highly permeable. Consequently, in the kidney, the hydraulic permeability is more than 50 to 100 times greater than many other peripheral capillary beds, accounting in large part for the high filtration rate in the glomeruli.

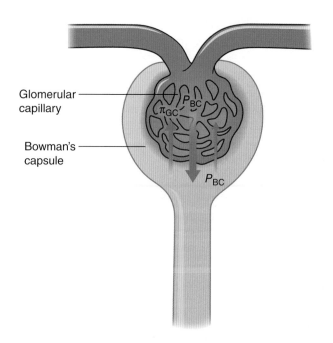

Glomerular capillary

Bowman's capsule

Fig. 17.12 Starling forces in the glomerulus. Π_{GC}, Oncotic pressure in the glomerulus; P_{BS}, hydrostatic pressure in Bowman's capsule; P_{GC}, hydrostatic pressure in glomerulus. (The oncotic pressure in Bowman's capsule, Π_{BC}, is close to zero.)

The hydrostatic pressure in the glomerular capillary (P_{GC}) favors filtration, whereas the hydrostatic pressure in Bowman's space (P_{BS}) opposes it.
- Normally, the glomerular capillary pressure is significantly greater than the pressure in Bowman's space.
- Thus the net hydrostatic force, $P_{GC} - P_{BS}$, favors filtration.

The oncotic pressure in the glomerular capillaries (Π_{GC}) opposes filtration.
- Because the glomerular ultrafiltrate is nearly protein-free, the oncotic pressure in Bowman's space, Π_{BS}, is close to zero.
- Therefore the net oncotic pressure favors absorption into the glomerular capillaries (see Clinical Correlation Box 17.5).

Clinical Correlation Box 17.5

Dialysis

When the kidneys fail to regulate the composition of the blood, whether acutely or chronically, it is sometimes necessary to restore the blood composition to desired levels by machine. This process is called dialysis, and there are two forms: hemodialysis and peritoneal dialysis. In hemodialysis, the patient's blood is circulated through an extracorporeal circuit, where it is pumped through selectively permeable synthetic capillary tubing (the dialysis membrane) bathed in an electrolyte solution similar in osmotic concentration to that of normal plasma, but devoid of urea and creatinine and with desired concentrations of solutes, such as potassium and bicarbonate (the dialysate). Because the dialysate is low in substances that accumulate in the blood during kidney failure, the dialysate provides a favorable gradient to remove unwanted solutes from the blood by passive diffusion into the dialysis solution. The mechanism responsible for the movement of fluid from the blood to the dialysate is similar to the Starling factors that govern glomerular filtration. The membrane has intrinsic parameters of surface area and hydraulic conductivity, and pressure gradients favoring ultrafiltration are achieved through the use of blood and dialysate pumps.

In peritoneal dialysis, dialysate fluid is infused by catheter into the patient's abdominal cavity where the peritoneal membrane provides the surface for unwanted solute removal (by diffusion) and ultrafiltration. The peritoneum provides a large surface area, and the pressure gradients that drive ultrafiltration from body fluids to intraperitoneal space are osmotic gradients achieved by infusing concentrated glucose solutions into the abdomen. In a diabetic, this could result in hyperglycemia. Unwanted substances diffuse into the fluid, which is withdrawn through the catheter. In many cases, chronic kidney disease leads to dialysis. Renal transplantation is also used to treat advanced renal failure. Usually, kidney function declines to nearly 10% of normal before dialysis is indicated.

The reflection coefficient (σ) corrects for the effect of oncotic pressure gradient on ultrafiltration.

- It can range from 0 to 1, depending on the effectiveness of proteins in retaining water across the capillary wall.
- The glomerular capillaries are relatively impermeable to proteins, therefore σ is close to 1, and oncotic pressure becomes an important driving force.
- For capillaries that are permeable to all solutes, ($\sigma = 0$), ultrafiltration would only depend on hydraulic pressure gradients.

Fig. 17.12 shows the dynamics of the Starling forces along the length of the glomerular capillary.

- Net hydrostatic pressure across the wall of the capillary ($P_{GC} - P_{BS}$) is relatively constant along the length of the capillary because of low resistance to flow.
- In the initial portions of the glomerular capillaries, the glomerular oncotic pressure (opposing filtration) is significantly lower than the net hydrostatic pressure (favoring filtration), so the balance of forces favors filtration.
- As the blood travels along the capillary, protein-free fluid is filtered into the urinary space, making the proteins remaining in the capillaries more and more concentrated, thereby raising the glomerular oncotic pressure. The oncotic pressure continues to increase until it may become as strong as the net hydrostatic pressure.
- At this point, the forces for and against filtration balance out, and filtration ceases (filtration pressure equilibrium). Filtration pressure equilibrium, however, is not inevitable. At high plasma flow rates, a balance of pressures favoring and opposing filtration will not be achieved, because there will be

less of an increase in plasma oncotic pressure, despite high filtration. In the situation of very high plasma flow rates, GFR will reach a maximum value.

Fig. 17.13 graphs the hydrostatic pressures within the lumen of the blood vessel along the renal arterial system.

- Observe that the greatest drops in pressure occur along the afferent and efferent arterioles, segments with highly regulated resistance.
- As in any hydrostatic system, when fluids encounter segments of high resistance (R) in a tube, kinetic energy is lost to overcome the resistance and maintain constant flow (Q). The loss of kinetic energy is reflected in the drop in pressure (ΔP) as fluid travels along the tube. This is the fundamental principle behind the Ohm's law analogy.

$$Q = \Delta P / R \text{ or } \Delta P = Q \times R$$

It is important to distinguish this ΔP from ($P_{GC} - P_{BS}$). Although both reflect the conversion of potential energy to kinetic energy as fluid move from area of high pressure to area of low pressure, the ΔP in Ohm's law refers to the pressure difference within different segments of the vessel, ($P_{GC} - P_{BS}$) refers to pressure difference across the wall of the vessel.

- Note also that in the peritubular capillaries, the hydrostatic pressure is much lower than in the glomerular capillaries. In the peritubular capillaries, consequently, the oncotic forces

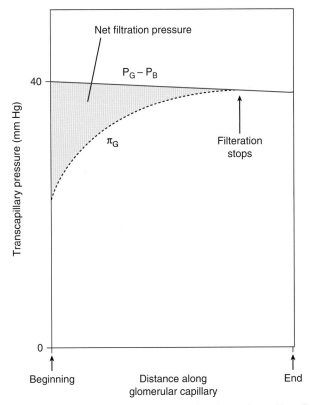

Fig. 17.13 Changes in Starling forces along the glomerular capillary. The *solid line* is net hydrostatic pressure and the *dotted line* is net oncotic pressure. The net hydrostatic pressure remains fairly constant, whereas the net oncotic pressure increases as the proteins in the glomerular capillary become increasingly concentrated.

favoring reabsorption are greater than hydrostatic forces favoring filtration, and net reabsorption takes place.

- On the whole, efferent arteriolar resistance plays a particularly important role in determining the Starling relationships in the glomerulus and the peritubular capillary. It maintains P_{GC}, and therefore GFR, with consequent increase in Π_{GC}.
- In addition, downstream from the efferent arteriole, the peritubular capillary hydrostatic pressure will be decreased by the efferent arteriolar resistance. Thus we see an important role of efferent resistance on both glomerular filtration and tubular reabsorption.

RBF is determined by systemic blood pressure, as with that of other organs. Unlike with other organs, however, the kidney has precise mechanisms for autoregulation of flow, changing its vascular resistance mainly in the afferent and efferent arterioles, in response to changes in systemic blood pressure. These mechanisms maintain relatively constant RBF and GFR when the systemic blood pressure ranges from approximately 80 to 170 mm Hg (Fig. 17.14).

The Effects of Changes in the Starling Relationship on G Glomerular Filtration Rate

The determinants of GFR are the:
- Filtration coefficient (K_f)
- Starling driving forces

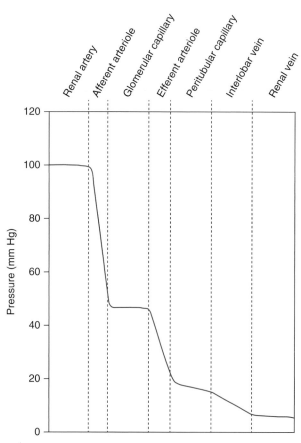

Fig. 17.14 Changes in renal blood flow (RBF) and glomerular filtration rate (GFR) as systemic blood pressure changes. Note that RBF and GFR remain relatively constant at systemic blood pressures between 80 and 170 mm Hg.

These variables can be affected by physiologic and pathologic processes. From the principles of capillary flow we have outlined, we can predict how these changes would affect GFR. It is important to think of GFR as a continuous function of its determinants.

Changes in K_f

The filtration coefficient, K_f, depends on both the permeability of the filtration barrier and the total surface area available for filtration.
- Various disease processes can affect these parameters.
- K_f can also be decreased by constriction of mesangial cells within the glomerular tuft, which can be mediated by hormones, such as angiotensin-II (Clinical Correlation Box 17.6).

Clinical Correlation Box 17.6

In glomerulonephritis, the glomerular capillary basement membrane can become thickened or damaged, reducing its permeability. These chronic changes eventually lead to a decreased K_f, and (from the Starling equation) to a decreased glomerular filtration rate.

Changes in P_{BS}

Normally, the hydrostatic pressure in Bowman's space is low. When the flow of urine is completely blocked downstream, however, such as with a kidney stone lodged in the ureter, the urine backs up and the pressure in Bowman's space builds. This increase in P_{BS} opposes glomerular filtration, so the GFR decreases.

Changes in Π_{GC}

We noted earlier that as protein-free plasma filters out of the glomerular capillaries, the remaining proteins become more concentrated, increasing glomerular oncotic pressure.
- As the RBF increases, the amount of plasma filtering out represents a smaller fraction of the total amount of plasma passing through the capillaries.
- Consequently, the oncotic pressure in the capillaries increases less rapidly.
- By this mechanism, increases in RPF decrease the average glomerular oncotic pressure.
- Decreased glomerular oncotic pressure favors increased filtration, thereby increasing the GFR.
- Thus increasing RPF tends to increase GFR.

Changes in P_{GC}

The glomerular hydrostatic pressure depends on the arterial pressure and the resistance of the afferent and efferent arterioles.
- Greater arterial pressure increases the glomerular hydrostatic pressure, thus increasing the GFR.
- Increased afferent arteriolar resistance decreases the hydrostatic pressure and the GFR, whereas increased efferent arteriolar resistance increases the GFR (see Fast Fact Box 17.3 and Clinical Correlationgz Box 17.7).

Fast Fact Box 17.3

To visualize these effects, we can think of glomerular filtration as water leaking through a hole in a hose. If we increase the pressure in the hose by opening up the faucet, more water will leak. If we squeeze the hose before the hole (i.e., if we increase the resistance in the afferent vessel), less water will leak out. Conversely, if we squeeze the hose past the hole (increasing the resistance of the efferent vessel), the flow through the hole will increase.

Clinical Correlation Box 17.7

The net effect on glomerular filtration rate (GFR) of efferent arteriolar constriction depends on the balance of changes in renal blood flow and glomerular hydrostatic pressure. In hypotension or when the major renal arteries narrow because of atherosclerosis (renal artery stenosis), renal plasma flow is decreased, hydrostatic pressure in glomerulus (P_{GC}) is also decreased, and GFR is reduced. This reduction in P_{GC} and GFR can be minimized by an increase in efferent arteriolar resistance, because of angiotensin-II vasoconstriction.

The Regulation of Renal Blood Flow and Glomerular Filtration Rate

In our analysis of the effects of Starling force changes on GFR, we ignored the kidney's ability to compensate for such changes. In fact, the kidney actively regulates RBF and GFR. Furthermore, long-term compensatory mechanisms exist that alter overall renal function (see Clinical Correlation Box 17.8).

Clinical Correlation Box 17.8

We would predict that a loss of nephrons would lead to decreased surface area for filtration and thus to decreased glomerular filtration rate (GFR). In reality, however, the kidney has a tremendous ability to compensate for nephron loss, with the remaining nephrons adjusting their perfusion, function, and size. For example, if a healthy adult donates a kidney to a sibling with kidney failure, overall GFR in the donor may fall only by 20% instead of 50% (a value predicted by a loss of one-half the renal mass). It is not until the kidney's compensatory abilities are exceeded that we notice larger decreases in GFR. This is a common theme in many organ systems, known as physiologic reserve.

Autoregulation

We have already observed that the kidney maintains relatively constant flow despite wide fluctuations in systemic blood pressure from approximately 80 to 170 mm Hg.

Two mechanisms play a role in this autoregulation of flow:
1. Myogenic autoregulation involves the constriction of afferent arterioles in response to wall stretch.
   - The stretching of smooth muscle cells in the walls of arterioles is thought to open calcium channels in their membranes, increasing the influx of calcium ions and thereby triggering contraction.
   - Accordingly, when a rise in arterial pressure stretches the afferent arteriole, the arteriole contracts.

- The increase in afferent arteriolar resistance offsets the pressure increase, maintaining constant RBF and GFR.
2. Tubuloglomerular feedback involves structures in the juxtaglomerular apparatus, which sits between the distal tubule and vascular supply.
   - An increase in arterial blood pressure increases RBF and GFR, which leads to a greater amount of fluid delivered to the distal tubule.
   - In the setting of high flow, there will be maximum solute transport out of the tubule lumen.
   - As filtered fluid reaches the distal tubule, elevated chloride remains in the tubule. Evidence indicates that the macula densa cells sense this increase in the chloride concentration and activate an effector mechanism that increases resistance in the afferent arteriole.

Increased afferent arteriolar resistance decreases RBF and GFR, returning them to their initial levels.

Synthetic Functions

Although most of the energy consumed by the kidney is directed toward solute transport by specialized epithelial cells, renal cells perform some very important synthetic functions.

Erythropoietin

EPO is the hematopoietic growth factor that is produced primarily in renal tissue (and to a lesser degree, in the liver).
- EPO acts in the bone marrow to stimulate the production of new red blood cells, and its production in the kidney is increased when oxygen levels in the blood are chronically depressed.
- It is not surprising that cells in the interstitium of the kidney, situated largely at the cortical-medullary border, contain a heme-like protein that acts as an oxygen sensor.
   - In hypoxic conditions, this sensor leads to an increase in a hypoxia-inducible transcription factor, which induces the EPO gene to produce more hormone.

Gluconeogenesis

The cells of the renal proximal tubule are the only renal cells that are gluconeogenic, and during a fast, they contribute significant amounts of glucose to the circulation.
- Renal gluconeogenesis is under hormonal control (by glucagon, corticosteroids, epinephrine) and is also increased in metabolic acidosis in concert with the production of alpha ketoglutarate and $2NH_3$ from glutamine (metabolic acidosis will be discussed in Ch. 22).
- The proximal tubule cells are specialized not only for gluconeogenesis, but also to donate the newly made glucose to the circulation. The activity of hexokinase (the enzyme catalyzing the first step in glycolysis) is lowest in proximal tubule cells and highest in the distal nephron where energy is derived from glycolysis.
- As a result, glucose reabsorbed by proximal tubule cells (approximately 900 mmol/day) or made by gluconeogenesis does not undergo glycolysis, but rather is available for transport back to the circulation.

Vitamin D

The mitochondria of the proximal tubule are the site of activation of 25-OH D3 to the active form, 1,25-OH D3. Vitamin D metabolism will be discussed in Chapter 33.

PATHOPHYSIOLOGY

Renal dysfunction, or renal failure, is typically classified according to the duration of the pathologic process.

- Acute renal failure describes a rapid and frequently reversible deterioration of renal function, marked by a drop in GFR.
- Chronic renal failure, in contrast, is a more sustained, often progressive and irreversible decrease in renal function.

Both can result from a wide variety of causes. The list of the kidney's functions (with which we began this chapter) gives us an idea of the kinds of clinical consequences of either acute or chronic renal failure.

For instance, we might predict that renal failure will cause derangements in electrolyte concentrations, accumulations of metabolic toxins, volume overload, or acid-base imbalances. As we acquire a more sophisticated understanding of the various functions of the kidney in the following chapters, we can make more detailed predictions regarding the precise consequences of renal dysfunction. Because of the kidneys' great ability to compensate, a disease process generally has to affect both kidneys before any clinical findings arise.

Types of Acute Kidney Injury

For now, we will focus on acute kidney injury to illustrate the physiologic principles we have discussed in this chapter.

A useful framework for categorizing the many causes of acute renal failure divides them according to the location of the primary disease process. In this classification, the causes of acute renal failure fall into the following three categories:

- Prerenal: Decreased GFR owing to compromise in the blood flow to the kidney.
- Intrinsic: Disease involving any of the various components of the kidney—the glomerulus, the tubules, the interstitium, or the microvasculature—leading to decreased GFR.
- Postrenal: Obstructions of the urinary tract, anywhere from the renal pelvis to the urethra, resulting in kidney dysfunction by increasing hydrostatic pressure in Bowman's space, impeding glomerular filtration.

Prerenal

Normal fluctuations in fluid intake, heart rate and contractility, and vascular tone produce daily changes in blood flow to the kidney.

- It is only when pathologic decreases in RBF exceed the kidney's ability to compensate that GFR falls far enough to be classified as prerenal failure.
- Anything that causes a drop in cardiac output can cause acute prerenal failure, from myocardial infarction to hemorrhage to vomiting and diarrhea.

- Some conditions and clinical scenarios can also selectively decrease RBF relative to overall cardiac output. If prerenal causes are repaired, the kidney returns to normal function (see Clinical Correlation Box 17.9).

Intrinsic

Glomerulonephritis refers to a group of autoimmune disorders that involve inflammation in the glomerular capillaries.

- Inflammatory cells or proliferating glomerular cells interfere with the passage of filtrate out of the glomerular capillary, and these cells may therefore acutely reduce the GFR. They reduce the K_f by decreasing the surface area of filtration. Other glomerular conditions, such as diabetic nephropathy, may result in chronic reductions in GFR (chronic renal failure).
- Tubular and renal interstitial disease can also reduce GFR and cause acute renal failure. The most common variety of tubulointerstitial disease is acute tubular necrosis. Acute tubular necrosis may result from drug toxicity (e.g., because of the administration of certain antibiotics) or severe renal ischemia.
- Tubular pathology decreases GFR independently of glomerular pathology through two mechanisms:
  - The first is through dysfunction of tubuloglomerular feedback. With tubular pathology and impaired proximal reabsorption, heavier flow may reach the distal tubule. As occurs in tubuloglomerular feedback under normal conditions, the macula densa then senses the increased flow and triggers vasoconstriction of the afferent arteriole, lowering blood flow to the glomerulus and decreasing GFR.
  - The second mechanism is increased pressure in the tubule, similar to postrenal failure. Poor absorption of fluid and cellular debris associated with tubular disease may block tubular outflow and, in turn, create an unfavorable hydrostatic gradient for glomerular filtration. There may also be a backleak of tubular fluid, a mechanism not seen in the normal tubule (see Clinical Correlation Box 17.10).

Clinical Correlation Box 17.10

An Example of Glomerulonephritis

Goodpasture disease is an autoimmune condition in which the body forms antibodies against collagen type IV, a major component of the glomerular basement membrane. The deposition of antibodies in the basement membrane begins an inflammatory process that destroys the integrity of the filtration barrier. Red and white blood cells can thus penetrate the glomerulus. The inflammatory cells can also block the glomerular capillary lumens, decreasing the total area available for filtration and thereby reducing the glomerular filtration rate (GFR). As discussed in later chapters, one of the consequences of reduced GFR is hypertension. The clinical findings of red blood cells in the urine and hypertension are features of the nephritic syndrome.

Postrenal

We noted earlier that blockage of a ureter by a renal stone can increase the pressure in Bowman's space and decrease the GFR in the kidney.

- If only one ureter is blocked, the other kidney is able to compensate, and the overall GFR is generally unaffected.

- When urine flow from both kidneys is blocked, however, renal failure can ensue. This condition of urinary "backup" is known as obstructive nephropathy see Fast Fact Box 17.4 and Clinical Correlation Box 17.11).

Fast Fact Box 17.4

Hydronephrosis is the anatomic appearance of a dilated collecting system, the consequence of obstruction.

Clinical Correlation Box 17.11

One common cause of bilateral urinary flow obstruction in men is benign prostatic hyperplasia, a condition in which the prostate enlarges, compressing the urethra as the urethra passes through the prostate. In addition to reducing the glomerular filtration rate, the increased pressure in the urinary space can eventually damage the kidneys, resulting in permanent injury.

SUMMARY

- The initial step in urine formation by the kidneys is the generation of a plasma ultrafiltrate by glomerular filtration.
- The glomerular filtration barrier filters substances by size and charge, eliminating large, negatively charged molecules, and generating a largely protein-free ultrafiltrate.
- The glomerular ultrafiltrate is further modified by exchange between the tubules and the peritubular capillaries; that is, by reabsorption and secretion.
- The amount of substance excreted = the amount of substance filtered + the amount secreted – the amount reabsorbed
- Knowledge of how particular substances (e.g., inulin, creatinine, and PAH) are handled by the kidney allows us to measure GFR, RPF, and RBF, and to understand clearance.

- GFR is determined by the balance of oncotic and hydrostatic forces.
- GFR and RBF are actively regulated by autoregulatory mechanisms that seek to maintain constant flow and by neural and hormonal mechanisms that respond to changing physiologic demands.
- The kidney has various synthetic functions, including production of EPO in response to hypoxia, gluconeogenesis, and activation of vitamin D.
- Renal failure means a drop in GFR. The three categories of acute renal failure are prerenal, intrinsic, and postrenal.

REVIEW QUESTIONS

Directions: Each of the numbered items or incomplete statements in this section is followed by answers or by completions of the statement. Select the one lettered answer or completion that is best in each case.

1. A 39-year-old man with insulin-dependent diabetes mellitus demonstrates thickened glomerular capillary basement membranes on renal biopsy. The decreased GFR resulting from his diabetic nephropathy is caused by which of the following?
   A. Increased hydrostatic pressure in Bowman's space (Fig. 17.15)
   B. Decreased glomerular oncotic pressure
   C. Increased total filtration area of kidney
   D. Decreased permeability of filtration barrier
   E. Decreased oncotic pressure in Bowman's space

2. A 63-year-old man with a history of urinary hesitancy is found to have a large asymmetric mass in his prostate gland. Upon biopsy, he is diagnosed with prostate cancer. His disease

places him at risk for which of the following mechanisms of renal failure?
   A. Prerenal failure secondary to hemorrhage
   B. Prerenal failure because of tubular damage
   C. Intrinsic renal failure because of glomerular damage
   D. Postrenal failure because of renal artery stenosis
   E. Postrenal failure because of increased pressure in the urinary space

3. A 3-year-old male child has a condition that leads to an absence of charge on the proteoglycans in his glomerular basement membrane. An investigation of his urine might reveal which of the following?
   A. Increased amounts of negatively charged small molecules
   B. Increased amounts of negatively charged large molecules
   C. Increased amounts of positively charged small molecules
   D. Increased amounts of positively charged large molecules
   E. No discernible difference from a normal child's urine

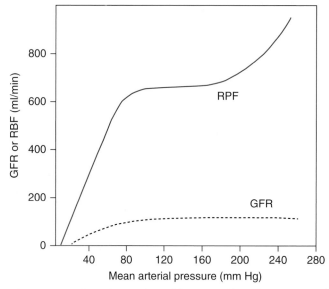

Fig. 17.15 Hydrostatic pressures along the renal arterial system. Note the pronounced drops in pressure along the efferent and afferent arterioles and the difference in pressures in the glomerular and peritubular capillaries.

ANSWERS TO REVIEW QUESTIONS

1. **The answer is D.** By the Starling equation $\{GFR = K_f\,[(P_G - P_B) - \sigma(\Pi_{GC} - \Pi_{BS})]$ we can predict that the GFR is decreased by decreases in the filtration coefficient, K_f. The thickened glomerular capillary membranes characteristic of diabetic nephropathy have two effects on K_f. The thickening of the membrane itself reduces its permeability. Once the disease progresses far enough, entire glomeruli can become nonfunctional, which would reduce the total surface area available for filtration. Either of these effects can reduce K_f. The pressure in Bowman's space (P_B) is typically low, except in situations when the outflow of urine is obstructed, such as by a urinary calculus. Decreased glomerular oncotic pressure would actually increase GFR. The oncotic pressure in Bowman's space is usually close to zero in a healthy individual with protein-free urine.

2. **The answer is E.** In this patient, the prostate tumor is likely placing increased pressure on his urethra, making it more difficult for him to void his bladder. This can result in bilateral urinary flow obstruction and hydronephrosis with a subsequent decrease in GFR because of the increased pressure in Bowman's space. The patient has no history of hemorrhage, making that an unlikely cause of prerenal failure. Intrinsic renal failure is a term used to describe disease processes that affect the kidneys directly, such as autoimmune disorders or drugs that damage the glomeruli or tubules themselves. Renal artery stenosis is a cause of prerenal failure.

3. **The answer is B.** The loss of negative charge will not result in increased amounts of negatively charged small molecules in the urine because in all situations, small molecules are freely filtered. Negatively charged large molecules, such as albumin, will be more likely to traverse the filtration meshwork of the glomerular basement membrane. Each 10 g/L of plasma albumin has approximately 2.5 mEq/L negative charge. A neutral charge to the basement membrane instead of a negative charge might decrease the filtration of positively charged macromolecules.

18

Tubular Transport

INTRODUCTION

The body faces multiple challenges met by the kidneys, including acid base balance, regulation of the concentrations of electrolytes such as potassium, and control of blood pressure. Two of the most critical are (1) the management of extracellular fluid volume by the handling of sodium and water and (2) the removal of metabolites and dietary components that are useful at low concentrations but toxic at high concentrations. Evolutionarily, animal species did not have a mechanism to concentrate urine until the arrival of mammals.

As we saw in chapter 17, the glomerular filtration rate (GFR) in mL/min is normally approximately 20% of renal plasma flow (RPF). That means that ingested toxins or metabolic waste products cannot be removed completely from the body by the kidney by filtration alone. Since their accumulation would be lethal to the organism, a necessary component of normal renal function is the secretory mechanisms involving membrane transport in the tubular structures of the nephron. Operating on low concentrations of toxic substances in the renal plasma, the transporters can secrete close to 100% of these solutes if they are working at the unsaturated portion of their transport kinetic relationships. Such is the case with para-amino hippurate (PAH, see Ch. 17).

These renal tubular transporters, however, are not limited to the secretion of ingested toxins, and therefore have other functions – namely, to secrete similar but normal endogenous metabolites that are useful within a physiologic range. For these molecules, removing them entirely would cause disease, but allowing them to accumulate above a certain concentration would also cause disease. The kidney must therefore regulate the serum concentrations of these molecules by a combination of filtration, secretion, and reabsorption. These same mechanisms allow the kidney to control the movement of water, saving it when extracellular fluid volume (and thus blood pressure) is too low or when the concentration of electrolytes like sodium is too high by concentrating the urine, and removing it when extracellular fluid volume (and thus blood pressure) is too high or when the concentration of electrolytes like sodium is too low by diluting the urine. The reason for high filtration rates in most mammals is that reabsorption of solutes in excess of water allows the kidney to produce dilute urine in the late distal nephron under appropriate circumstances.

In general, the control of osmolality is achieved by the handling of free water. The control of extracellular fluid volume is achieved by the handling of sodium.

The body faces a major dilemma concerning ingested nitrogen containing substances. On the one hand, molecules such as ammonia are toxic at sufficiently high concentrations. On the other hand, nitrogen containing substances also perform critical metabolic functions. The turnover of proteins requires a critical mass of protein precursors, so some organic nitrogen must be available to form amino acids. Ammonia, a waste product produced by protein catabolism, is converted by the urea cycle to urea, mostly in the liver. Urea is also critical to the concentrating mechanism of the kidney. Glomerular filtration allows for large amounts of filtered nitrogen products to be excreted into the urine while some (but not complete) reabsorption of urea occurs by the renal tubules. A large portion of the filtered urea is not eliminated – it is saved to maintain the ability of the kidney to concentrate the urine – and the amount that is eliminated must match the amount ingested to maintain nitrogen balance. Since most protein is approximately ⅙th nitrogen by weight, the mass of urea nitrogen (there are two nitrogen atoms per molecule of urea) excreted daily must equal ⅙th of the mass of protein ingested. Thus, for example, if 10 gm of nitrogen appear in the urine in a 24 hour period, that means that the patient is consuming 60 gm of protein daily. This is known as the protein catabolic rate, which in a healthy person is equivalent to the daily protein intake and requires that the concentration of urea in the blood be constant. *Azotemia* results when too much urea is retained. *Uremia* ensues when this increased urea concentration causes toxicity.

The processes of glomerular filtration, tubular reabsorption, and tubular secretion determine the composition of the urine and the blood leaving the kidney. This enables the kidney to maintain blood volume and solute levels within the body regardless of external conditions.

Homeostasis is achieved through regulated tubular transport of solutes in both directions (reabsorption and secretion), as well as reabsorption of water. This chapter will describe:
- Mechanisms of reabsorption and secretion
- Specialization of different parts of the tubule for transporting various substances
- Cellular transporters that convey substances across the tubule walls

SYSTEM STRUCTURE: FUNCTIONAL ANATOMY OF THE KIDNEY TUBULE

Recall that the nephron is the functional unit of the kidney, composed of (Fig. 18.1):
- Glomerulus, where the initial filtration of blood occurs

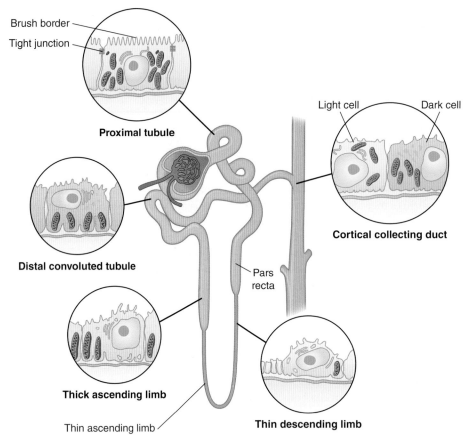

Fig. 18.1 The nephron. Although only depicted on the proximal tubule cell, tight junctions and the lateral intercellular space are present in the epithelium in all parts of the tubule. The pars recta is the straight portion of the proximal tubule.

- Tubule, where reabsorption and secretion occur
  The tubule is further broken down into:
- Proximal tubule
- Loop of Henle
- Distal tubule
- Collecting duct
- Juxtaglomerular apparatus (regulatory structure)
  Transport takes place in every part of the tubule. The epithelial cells are connected to each other along the entire tubule by tight junctions, which separate the cell surface into (Fig. 18.2):
- An apical-luminal side facing the tubule lumen
- A basolateral side facing the interstitium and the peritubular capillaries
- Between the cells is an area known as the lateral intercellular space.
  The proximal tubule is located in the cortex of the kidney along with the glomerulus:
- Ultrafiltrate from the glomerulus flows directly into the proximal tubule
- The initial convoluted portion, the proximal convoluted tubule, has more surface area for transport than the straight portion
- The following straight portion—the pars recta—conducts less transport

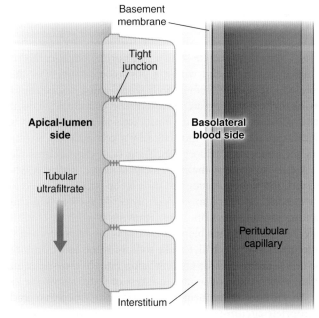

Fig. 18.2 Two distinct surfaces of tubular cells. The apical-luminal side refers to the inside of the tubule, where the ultrafiltrate flows. The basolateral side constitutes the outside of the tubule and faces the peritubular capillaries. The tight junctions in between the epithelial cells separate the tubule lumen from the outside.

The loop of Henle is a U-shaped structure that dips into the medulla of the kidney. The filtrate in the lumen encounters the three sections of the loop of Henle in the following order:

- The thin descending limb is permeable to water but impermeable to salt.
- The thin ascending limb is impermeable to water, but the passive permeability to salt is high.
- The thick ascending limb actively, rather than passively, transports salt out of the lumen into the interstitium. As the filtrate passes through the thick ascending limb, sodium is pumped out, the fluid becomes hypotonic, and it eventually passes into the distal tubule.

The distal convoluted tubule is located in the cortex of the kidney.

- Cells located in the distal tubule are cuboidal and have extensive infoldings of the basolateral membranes and numerous mitochondria.
- Multiple neighboring distal convoluted tubules empty into a common collecting duct.

Collecting ducts receive fluid from distal convoluted tubules in the cortex and transport the fluid through the medulla. The portion of the duct that receives fluid from the distal tubule is known as the cortical collecting duct, which becomes the medullary collecting duct as it passes into the medulla.

- The cortical collecting duct has a large lumen and is composed of two main cell types (with distinct roles that will be discussed later in the chapter):
  - Principal cells
  - Intercalated cells
- The medullary collecting duct has important transport functions for urea, Na^+, NH_3, and water.

Note energy for filtration is from cardiac mechanical energy sustaining blood whereas tubule energetics emanate from electrochemical gradients set up by adenosine triphosphatases (ATPases).

SYSTEM FUNCTION: REABSORPTION AND SECRETION

To understand the epithelial secretion and reabsorption that are critical to the homeostasis of the body, we must first review the concept of mass balance.

This concept, which relates to the net results of secretion and reabsorption, prepares the way for a discussion of the more minute mechanisms of secretion and reabsorption and the specialization of transport in the different segments of the tubule.

Mass Balance

Mass balance is a straightforward and intuitive principle: what goes in must come out.

- "What goes in" is the blood supplied to the kidney by the renal artery. This blood contains plasma, which consists of water, ions, proteins, and other solutes.
- "What comes out" is 2-fold: that which leaves the kidney via the renal vein and that which leaves the kidney via the urine (for the moment, we will assume no production or metabolism of a given solute).

The Fick equation is one way to express mass balance for any specific substance S:

$$\left(Q_{renal\,artery}\right)\left([solute]_{arterial\,blood}\right)$$
$$= (\dot{V})\left([solute]_{urine}\right) + \left(Q_{renal\,vein}\right)\left([solute]_{venous\,blood}\right)$$

The first term in the equation is the incoming mass of S:Q, the flow per minute through the renal artery, multiplied by the concentration of S in the artery.

- The terms on the other side of the equation represent the outgoing mass of S: the mass of S in urine plus the mass of S in the vein.
- The distribution of renal output between the vein and urine is determined by glomerular filtration, reabsorption, and secretion (see Fig. 17.7).

Tubular secretion refers to the transport of substances from the peritubular capillaries to the tubular lumen via the nephron's epithelial cells. Tubular reabsorption, the opposite of secretion, refers to the transport of substances from the tubular lumen to the interstitium.

It is important to remember the direction of solute movement attached to these terms. Secretion means transport to the lumen, and reabsorption implies reabsorption from the lumen.

Filtration and secretion can also be confused. Although they both refer to adding to the tubular lumen:

- Filtration only describes the bulk-flow process in the glomerulus.
- Secretion can and does happen all along the rest of the tubule.

Be aware, too, that some substances (such as K^+ and uric acid) are both secreted into and reabsorbed from the lumen in different segments of the tubule, but these terms usually refer to net secretion or net reabsorption.

Finally, a note of qualification about the mass balance equation: the equation assumes no consumption or creation of substances in the kidney, but consumption (metabolism) and creation of substances do occur in some cases. To account for this, the mass balance equation can be rewritten:

$$\left(Q_{renal\,artery}\right)\left([solute]_{arterial\,blood}\right)$$
$$+ mass\,of\,S\,produced\,by\,the\,kidney$$
$$= (\dot{V})\left([solute]_{urine}\right)\left(Q_{renal\,vein}\right)\left([solute]_{venous\,blood}\right)$$
$$- mass\,of\,S\,consumed\,by\,kidney.$$

Epithelial Transport

Recall that tight junctions separate the cell surface into an apical-luminal side and a basolateral side that faces the interstitium. To secrete or reabsorb, the nephron must convey substances across this boundary from lumen to interstitium or vice versa. It does so by various forms of epithelial transport, and there are two basic routes this transport can take.

- Paracellular transport (Fig. 18.3) is a passive process where solutes and ions can pass through the tight junctions between cells along their electrochemical gradient.
- Transcellular transport occurs with specific transporter proteins on the apical and basolateral membranes of the epithelial cells, which transport substances cross the apical membrane, through the cell, then across the basolateral membrane and vice versa. It can be either active or passive.

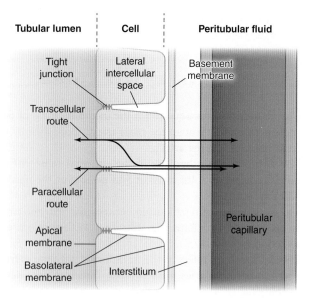

Fig. 18.3 Paracellular and transcellular transport routes across the wall of the renal tubule.

Most solute transport is essentially driven by the Na^+,K^+-ATPase in the basolateral membrane. When the ATPase pumps Na^+ out toward the interstitium in exchange for potassium and at the expense of adenosine triphosphate (ATP), it is conducting primary active transport (Fig. 18.4A). Specialized proteins then couple this Na^+ transport to the transport of other solutes. This process works in the following manner:

- Primary active transport of Na^+ out of the cell creates low intracellular $[Na^+]$
- Na^+ flows down favorable electrochemical gradient into the cell through apical Na^+ channels
- Apical symporters couple solute transport to Na^+ movement in the same direction
- Antiporters couple solute transport to Na^+ movement in the opposite direction
- This process is termed secondary active transport because there is an indirect requirement for ATP (Fig. 18.4B).

Transcellular transport may, in turn, drive paracellular transport. Transcellular translocation of cations and anions can create electrical and osmolar gradients across the tight junction that promote the movement of ions and water.

- For instance, if mostly cations have crossed transcellularly, an electrical gradient is set up that promotes the movement of anions (such as Cl^- or HCO_3^-) across the tubular epithelium via the paracellular route.
- Also as solutes cross the membrane, they establish an osmolar gradient; water then crosses the epithelium paracellularly.

While the entire tubule makes use of the transport mechanisms mentioned previously, each epithelial segment of the nephron has unique transport properties. This is because different parts of the tubule have various types of pumps and channels.

Reabsorption

Reabsorption is the transport of substances from the tubule lumen to the interstitium and peritubular capillary. Owing to the

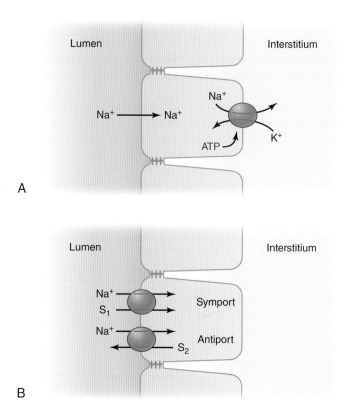

Fig. 18.4 Transcellular active transport. A, Primary active transport of Na^+ by the basolateral Na^+,K^+-ATPase. B, Secondary active transport of a solute S_1, coupled to Na^+ movement by a symporter, and another solute S_2, coupled to Na^+ movement by an antiporter. S_1 is actively reabsorbed, and S_2 is actively secreted.

large rate of filtration, there is a burden on the tubule to prevent valuable solutes, such as glucose and amino acids, from becoming lost in the urine. Consequently, the tubule must perform a large amount of reabsorption and must expend a great deal of energy doing so.

As a rule, solutes are initially reabsorbed in bulk, followed by a regulated titration, to achieve the urinary excretion required to maintain balance. An important aspect of bulk reabsorption is the concept of transport maximum (T_m).

- Simple diffusion across a membrane obeys the electrochemical gradient without limitation.
- Carrier-mediated diffusion, however, is limited by the capacity of the carrier proteins (transporters).
- As the concentration of a substance climbs, the transport rate for that substance climbs until the substance saturates its transport proteins, at which point the transport rate reaches its maximum, T_m (Fig. 18.5).

T_m is equivalent to V_{max} in Michaelis-Menten kinetics.

A substance's K_m is the concentration at which the transport rate is half-maximum (see Clinical Correlation Box 18.1). Note that in the saturable transport condition, for solute concentrations well below K_m, the transport is mostly unidirectional, but as the concentration increases, and the curve is clearly nonlinear, there starts to be more bidirectional until forward transport is halted (transporter saturation).

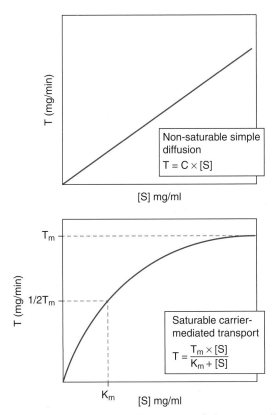

Fig. 18.5 Nonsaturable and saturable transport. *C*, A constant; K_m, the concentration of S at which the transport rate is half-maximum; [*S*], the concentration of substance S in the compartment from which S is being transported (e.g., the tubule lumen); *T*, transport rate; T_m, maximum transport rate for substance S.

Clinical Correlation Box 18.1

D-Glucose is a valuable solute that is almost completely reabsorbed under normal circumstances (zero clearance). In a person with a normal plasma glucose level, the amount of glucose filtered does not elevate the tubular glucose concentration high enough to saturate the glucose transporters; the tubular glucose transport rate is below transport maximum (T_m), and nearly all the glucose is reabsorbed. A patient with diabetes mellitus, however, has an abnormally high plasma glucose concentration, which leads to more filtered glucose, and a tubular glucose concentration that exceeds capacity; the transporters become saturated and cannot reabsorb all of the glucose. As a result, some glucose is excreted into urine, which can be seen on urine dipstick testing.

Whether a substance has a high or a low T_m may reflect whether the kidney regulates the level of that solute in the blood.

- For instance, phosphate has a lower T_m that is easily reached if plasma phosphate rises just slightly above normal. This creates de facto regulation of phosphate, for when plasma levels rise too high, transport capacity is exceeded and the excess phosphate is excreted into the urine.
- By contrast, the kidneys are not the primary regulator of glucose levels in the blood (that is accomplished by pancreatic insulin-secreting cells). (See Fast Fact Box 18.1 and Clinical Correlation Box 18.2).

Fast Fact Box 18.1

At normal glomerular filtration, spillage of glucose into the urine does not occur until the blood sugar exceeds approximately 180 mg/dL, a higher-than-normal fasting value.

Clinical Correlation Box 18.2

Sodium-Glucose Linked Transporter 2 Inhibitor

Sodium-glucose linked transporter 2 (SGLT2) is the glucose transporter responsible for the majority of glucose reabsorption in the proximal tubule. SGLT2 inhibitors, such as canagliflozin and dapagliflozin, are designed to treat type 2 diabetes by decreasing glucose reabsorption in the first segment of the proximal tubule. Effects of SGLT2 inhibitors also include weight loss (through calorie leakage into the urine) and lowering blood pressure (through osmotic diuresis). Osmotic diuresis occurs because the proximal tubule must reabsorb isosmotic fluid—sodium reabsorption rises as glucose reabsorption falls. Because of the increased sodium reabsorption in the earlier segments of proximal, leading to the fall of sodium in tubular fluid, fewer amounts of sodium and fluid are reabsorbed in the later segments of the tubule. The net effect is decreased sodium and water reabsorption leading to diuresis.

Secretion

Secretion is the process of transport of substances from the peritubular capillaries to the tubular lumen.

- Many substances that are freely filtered by the glomeruli—organic anions and metabolic products (such as choline and creatinine)—are also eliminated from the body by this route.
- Because substances that are highly protein-bound in the plasma will not be freely filtered by the glomerulus, these solutes need to be secreted to be cleared.
  - To be filtered or secreted, protein-bound solutes must coexist with an unbound or "free" component in the plasma.
  - The kidney also secretes H^+, K^+, and foreign compounds, such as drugs. Most substances, including H^+, are secreted in the proximal tubule, whereas H^+ and K^+ are secreted in the distal tubule and collecting ducts (information to follow).

Recall that one example of an exogenous substance that is actively secreted in the proximal tubule is the organic anion para-aminohippurate (PAH).

- Like glucose reabsorption, PAH secretion has a T_m. As long as T_m is not reached, virtually all PAH that reaches the kidney is secreted and thus excreted.
- Therefore the amount of plasma cleared of PAH is a good estimate of the renal plasma flow, as all the blood that passes through the kidney is cleared of PAH.

The Proximal Tubule

Now we will consider the specialized reabsorptive and secretory functions of each tubule segment (Fig. 18.6). Our journey begins in the proximal tubule, where two-thirds of Na^+ and H_2O reabsorption takes place.

Reabsorption in the Early Proximal Tubule

In the early proximal tubule, Na^+ reabsorption is coupled with the reabsorption of glucose, amino acids, lactate, and

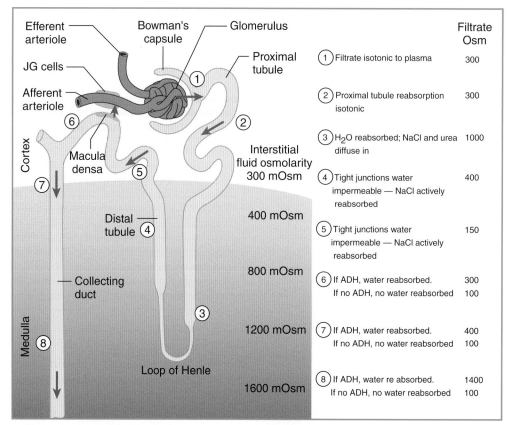

	Filtrate Osm
① Filtrate isotonic to plasma	300
② Proximal tubule reabsorption isotonic	300
③ H₂O reabsorbed; NaCl and urea diffuse in	1000
④ Tight junctions water impermeable — NaCl actively reabsorbed	400
⑤ Tight junctions water impermeable — NaCl actively reabsorbed	150
⑥ If ADH, water reabsorbed.	300
If no ADH, no water reabsorbed	100
⑦ If ADH, water reabsorbed.	400
If no ADH, no water reabsorbed	100
⑧ If ADH, water re absorbed.	1400
If no ADH, no water reabsorbed	100

Fig. 18.6 Key transporters along the renal tubule. (From Carroll R. *Elsevier's Integrated Physiology*. Philadelphia: Mosby Elsevier; 2007. Fig. 11.18.)

phosphate by apical symporters (also known as cotransporters) (Fig. 18.7A). Like glucose, the other solutes are almost completely reabsorbed from the lumen during the first half of the proximal tubule.

Na⁺ reabsorption in the early proximal tubule is also coupled to bicarbonate reabsorption in the early proximal tubule in a slightly more complex way (Fig. 18.7B):

- In addition to the symporters, Na⁺ is reabsorbed across an apical antiporter that secretes H⁺ ions from inside the cell to the tubular lumen (Na⁺/H⁺ exchange or NHE).
- Once the H⁺ is inside the tubular lumen, it combines with filtered bicarbonate to form H_2CO_3 (which then forms CO_2 and H_2O) via the carbonic anhydrase enzyme located on the apical brush border of the epithelium.
- CO_2 readily diffuses inside the cell and recombines with H_2O to form H⁺ and bicarbonate via carbonic anhydrase.
- Bicarbonate then crosses the basolateral membrane by secondary active transport, usually via a Na⁺/bicarbonate cotransporter. The energy driving this transport is the net electrochemical gradient, as the basolateral Na⁺,K⁺-ATPase and the cell membrane's permeability to K⁺ render the inside of the cell electronegative with a low Na⁺ concentration.
- As described previously, this draws Na⁺ across the apical membrane and the cell's electronegativity then propels 3 HCO_3^- with 1 Na⁺ across the basolateral membrane.
- Thus the net effect is the reabsorption of $NaHCO_3^-$ (see Fig. 18.7B). (See Clinical Correlation Box 18.3).

Clinical Correlation Box 18.3

Acetazolamide

Diuretics are drugs that can increase urine output, usually by directly or indirectly decreasing Na⁺ reabsorption. Acetazolamide is a weak diuretic that acts in the proximal tubule. It inhibits carbonic anhydrase in the cytoplasm and on the apical membrane of the epithelial cells (see Fig. 18.7B). This decreases the H⁺ gradient across the apical membrane, impedes Na⁺/H⁺ exchange and lowers bicarbonate resorption. The diuretic effect results from decreased Na⁺ reabsorption. Note that acetazolamide is less efficacious than thiazide or loop diuretics (see Clinical Application Box 18.3).

Water reabsorption occurs both in a paracellular and transcellular fashion. The former occurs via free flow via tight junctions, whereas the latter occurs via water channels on the apical/basolateral membranes.

- Because proximal water permeability is high, water follows the solute reabsorption freely, so the reabsorbed fluid is isosmotic to the filtrate. By the end of the early proximal tubule, a significant portion of water has been reabsorbed.
- This osmotic flow of water (both transcellular and paracellular) results in a solvent drag , in which additional solutes, such as Na⁺, Cl⁻, K⁺, Ca²⁺, and Mg²⁺, are carried by water flow into the interstitium.

Reabsorption in the Late Proximal Tubule

In the late proximal tubule, sodium and chloride are reabsorbed via both transcellular and paracellular pathways (Fig. 18.7C).

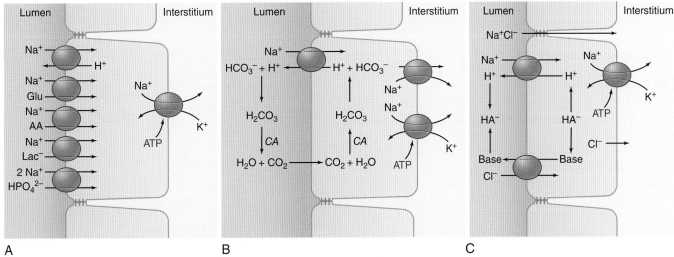

Fig. 18.7 Solutes transported in the proximal tubule. A, Early proximal tubule: glucose (*Glu*), amino acids (*AA*), lactate (*Lac⁻*), and phosphate (*HPO₄²⁻*) reabsorbed by Na⁺ symporters and extrusion of H⁺ by a Na⁺ antiporter. B, Early proximal tubule: bicarbonate (*HCO₃⁻*) reabsorbed via the Na⁺/H⁺ antiporter and carbonic anhydrase (*CA*). C, Late proximal tubule: chloride (*Cl⁻*) reabsorbed transcellularly via Cl⁻/anion (*A⁻*) antiporter and paracellularly by a chemical gradient.

- In the lumen of the late proximal tubule, there is very little glucose, amino acids, lactate, phosphate, and bicarbonate because of the reabsorption of these solutes in the early proximal tubule.
- The amount of water is also low because water has osmotically followed the proximal reabsorption of solutes.
- However, [Cl⁻] is higher in the late proximal tubule lumen as it was not actively reabsorbed earlier on. This creates a chemical gradient to drive Cl⁻ across the tight junctions and into the interstitium, where the chloride concentration approximates that of plasma.

Because Na⁺ has been reabsorbed in the early proximal tubule with HCO₃⁻, allowing the Cl⁻ concentration to rise, there is also an HCO₃⁻ gradient in the late proximal tubule such that interstitial HCO₃⁻ concentration exceeds the luminal concentration.

- The reflection coefficient for HCO₃⁻ exceeds that for Cl⁻, such that Cl⁻ preferentially moves from the lumen to the interstitium.
- Because the chemical gradient is large enough to drive the movement of Cl⁻ against its electrical gradient, the movement of Cl⁻ lowers the electrical potential of the interstitium and Na⁺ is drawn into the interstitium, restoring electroneutrality.

Transcellular Cl⁻ crossing in the late proximal tubule is possible via parallel operation of Na⁺/H⁺ and Cl⁻/A⁻ antiporters, where A⁻ represents anions, such as OH⁻, oxalate, or formate (HCO₂⁻).

- The secreted H⁺ and A⁻ combine in the tubular lumen to reform the weak acid (e.g., formic acid), and reenter the cell by diffusion, so the net effect is the reabsorption of NaCl⁻ into the cell.
- Na⁺ leaves the cell by the basolateral Na⁺,K⁺-ATPase pump, and Cl⁻ leaves by Cl⁻ channels along a favorable chloride concentration gradient.

Reabsorption of Proteins in the Proximal Tubule

The glomerular filtration of proteins is normally small, but in total, it adds up to a significant daily filtered load.

- If the tubule were unable to reabsorb the filtered protein, the body would lose a considerable amount of it.
- Enzymes, including peptidases and proteinases, on the apical surface of the proximal tubule lumen can partially degrade these polypeptides and proteins, which are then taken up by endocytosis and digested into amino acids, which diffuse back to the bloodstream via basolateral channels.

Secretion in the Proximal Tubule

The proximal tubule also secretes organic anions and cations, especially those that are bound to plasma proteins and are thus not easily filtered by the glomerulus. The secretion rates of these substances are high, as indicated by the fact that the kidney can completely clear many organic ions and some drugs from the plasma.

Organic anion secretion is best illustrated by the secretion of PAH.

- PAH crosses the basolateral membrane against its chemical gradient by a PAH-di/tricarboxylate antiporter.
- The dicarboxylates and tricarboxylates are recycled back into the cell via a basolateral di/tricarboxylate-Na⁺ symporter.
- These combined actions result in a high intracellular concentration of PAH, which can now drive PAH across the apical membrane into the tubular lumen via a PAH/A⁻ antiporter.

This organic anion transport system is not specific, so many organic anions compete for these transporters; increasing the plasma concentration of a single one can inhibit the secretion of other anions.

For organic cations, there are also secretory pathways. Organic cations enter the cell across the basolateral membrane via facilitated diffusion and exit across the apical membrane via an organic cation/H^+ antiport.

The Loop of Henle

Whereas the proximal tubule reabsorbs water and NaCl simultaneously as an isosmotic fluid, the loop of Henle splits the reabsorption of water and NaCl. This is critical for generating the salt gradient in the kidney, where osmolality increases with descent into the renal medulla.

- Recall that the descending limb of Henle is permeable to water but not to NaCl. As the filtrate passes down the descending limb, water is reabsorbed (another 20% on top of the proximal tubule's 67%), and the filtrate becomes concentrated in salt.
- The thin ascending limb is impermeable to water but permeable to NaCl. This allows the thin ascending limb to gradually unload its concentrated salt into the medullary interstitium, maintaining the medullary salt gradient.
  - This salt gradient, along with a urea gradient, is necessary for the regulated reabsorption of water from the collecting duct, a topic to which we will return.
- Upon reaching the thick ascending limb (also permeable to salt but not water), approximately 25% more of the filtered Na^+, K^+, and Cl^- load is actively reabsorbed.
  - The main energy source is the basolateral Na^+,K^+-ATPase pump, which establishes a low intracellular $[Na^+]$, rendering the filtrate that leaves the loop hypoosmotic to plasma.
  - In the thick ascending limb, the Na^+ is reabsorbed across the apical membrane by a $Na^+/K^+/2Cl^-$ symporter—different from the symporters found in the proximal tubule.
- Cl^- ions leave passively via a basolateral Cl^- channel, whereas K^+ ions can leave via K^+ channels located on both the apical and the basolateral sides.
- Because intracellular K^+ and Cl^- both leave via the basolateral side, but only K^+ can exit the apical side, the tubular lumen becomes positively charged relative to the interstitium.
  - This positive electrical potential drives paracellular diffusion of Na^+, K^+, Ca^{2+}, and Mg^{2+}.
- Na^+ also enters the cell via a Na^+/H^+ antiporter, which results in the ultimate reabsorption of HCO_3^- across the basolateral membrane (Fig. 18.8). (See Clinical Correlation Box 18.4).

Clinical Correlation Box 18.4

The diuretic furosemide inhibits one of the Cl^- sites on the $Na^+/K^+/2Cl^-$ cotransporter, which in turn decreases K^+ uptake and therefore recycling of K^+ back to the lumen. As a result, the lumen is less positively charged and Ca^{2+} and Mg^{2+} reabsorption is diminished. Furosemide therefore has an effect to increase Ca^{2+} excretion. In another setting, when blood Ca^{2+} is high, Ca^{2+} binds to a basolateral membrane Ca^{2+} receptor, which leads to an inhibition of apical $Na^+/K^+/2Cl^-$ transport and decreased Ca^{2+} reabsorption.

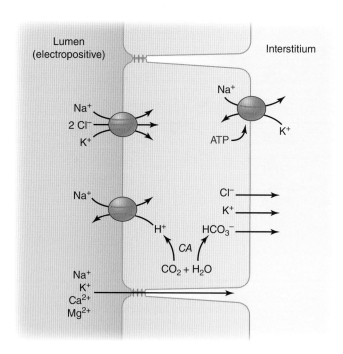

Fig. 18.8 Reabsorption in the thick ascending limb of the loop of Henle. Salt is actively reabsorbed without water, unlike the isosmotic reabsorption in the proximal tubule. Bicarbonate is reabsorbed here as well. Na^+, K^+, Mg^{2+}, and Ca^{2+} are reabsorbed paracellularly by electrical gradient.

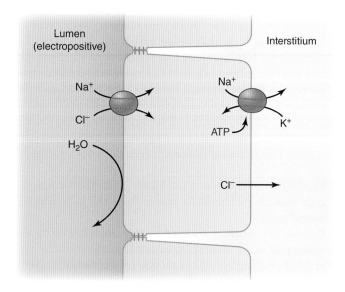

Fig. 18.9 Reabsorption in the early distal tubule. Salt (but not water) is reabsorbed, similar to the situation in the ascending limb of the loop of Henle.

The Distal Tubule and Collecting Duct

The distal tubule is divided into two segments with very different properties:

- Early distal tubule extends from the juxtaglomerular apparatus to the middle of the distal convolution (Fig. 18.9)

- Late distal tubule continues from there to the cortical collecting duct and is morphologically and functionally similar to the collecting duct

The Early Distal Tubule

The early distal tubule is impermeable to water, but can reabsorb Na$^+$, Cl$^-$, and Ca^{2+}. This acts to dilute the tubular fluid.

- Na$^+$ and Cl$^-$ enter the cell across the apical membrane via the Na$^+$/Cl$^-$ cotransporter.
- Once in the cell, Na$^+$ exits to the blood via the Na$^+$,K$^+$-ATPase, and Cl$^-$ diffuses across the basolateral membrane via a Cl$^-$ channel (see Clinical Correlation Box 18.5).

Clinical Correlation Box 18.5

Loop Diuretics and Thiazide Diuretics

A commonly used class of diuretics is the loop diuretics, such as furosemide and bumetanide, which work by directly inhibiting the Na$^+$/K$^+$/2Cl$^-$ symporter in the thick ascending limb of the loop of Henle. This keeps the medullary interstitium less hypertonic and thus prevents water reabsorption in the collecting ducts, leading to a large diuresis. Because of the inhibition of the Na$^+$/K$^+$/2Cl$^-$ symporter, less K$^+$ reenter the lumen to drive Ca^{2+} reabsorption (see Fig. 18.8). This causes an increased net excretion of Ca^{2+}, which can be exploited in the treatment of hypercalcemia in selected patients.

Thiazide diuretics, such as hydrochlorothiazide and chlorthalidone, target the Na$^+$/Cl$^-$ cotransporter in the distal tubule. Unlike furosemide, which increases Ca^{2+} excretion, thiazides increase calcium reabsorption. Two mechanism have been proposed: (1) volume depletion leads to increased passive Ca^{2+} reabsorption, (2) decreased Na$^+$ in tubular cells enhances Na$^+$/Ca^{2+} exchange in the basolateral membrane and thus increase Ca^{2+} diffusion across the apical membrane. Thiazide's ability to lower luminal Ca^{2+} is useful in the management of patients with calcium kidney stones.

Compared with these diuretics that act more distally, proximal tubule diuretics do not work as well, because there is some reserve capacity of the thick ascending limb to reabsorb more Na$^+$ to compensate when proximal Na$^+$ reabsorption is blocked.

The Late Distal Tubule and Collecting Duct

The late distal tubule or connecting tubule and the collecting ducts have two types of cells (Fig. 18.10):

- Intercalated cells
  - The alpha-intercalated cells secrete H$^+$ and reabsorb HCO$_3^-$ independently of Na$^+$ transport, which is important in the regulation of blood pH.
  - The beta-intercalated cells secrete HCO$_3^-$ ions into the lumen. Intercalated cells also reabsorb K$^+$ by a mechanism involving H$^+$/K$^+$-ATPase. These transporters will be discussed in subsequent chapters.
- Principal cells contain the widespread basolateral Na$^+$,K$^+$-ATPase pump, reabsorb Na$^+$, and secrete K$^+$ across the apical membrane through protein channels in the membrane. K$^+$ also flows out of the cell down its chemical gradient via channels on the basolateral membrane (see Genetics Box 18.1, Pharmacology Box 18.1, Development Box 18.1, and Fast Fact Box 18.2).

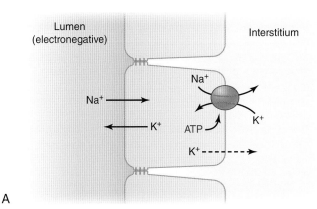

A

B

Fig. 18.10 Reabsorption and secretion in the late distal tubule and collecting duct. A, Transport in a principal cell. B, Transport in an intercalated cell.

🧬 GENETICS BOX 18.1

Gordon syndrome, also called pseudohypoaldosteronism type 2 or familial hyperkalemic hypertension, is an inherited cause of type 4 renal tubular acidosis. It is caused by mutations in genes, such as WNK1 and WNK4. WNK4 mutations lead to excess expression of the distal tubule NaCl symporter and decreased expression of K$^+$ channels, leading to increased NaCl resorption (thus hypertension) and decreased K$^+$ excretion. Normal WNK1 inhibits the WNK4 protein, so WNK1 gain of function mutations lead to the disease.

💊 PHARMACOLOGY BOX 18.1

In addition to adopting a reduced sodium and potassium diet, patients with pseudohypoaldosteronism type 2 can be treated with thiazide diuretics that inhibit the overexpressed NaCl symporter.

🛡 DEVELOPMENT BOX 18.1

Despite having normal renal function, patients with pseudohypoaldosteronism type 2 have hyperkalemia, hypertension, hyperchloremic metabolic acidosis, and occasionally hypercalciuria. The age of symptom onset is highly variable, although elevated K$^+$ typically precedes elevations in blood pressure. Symptoms include fatigue, weakness, nausea, and vomiting.

When Na^+ is reabsorbed across the apical membrane, a negative charge is left in the lumen, which creates an electrical gradient favorable to K^+ secretion.

- In addition, the passage of tubular fluid through the collecting duct has the effect of sweeping away the K^+ secreted by the principal cell.
- This keeps the luminal $[K^+]$ low outside the principal cell and maintains a favorable chemical gradient for K^+ secretion.
- Together, these processes allow K^+ secretion to take place (see Clinical Correlation Box 18.6).

Clinical Correlation Box 18.6

Potassium-Sparing Diuretics

The apical Na^+ channels found on principal cells are blocked by diuretics, such as amiloride and triamterene. These drugs are not as effective at increasing natriuresis as diuretics that work on earlier segments of the nephron, because most of the Na^+ has already been reabsorbed by the time the filtrate has reached the late distal tubules and collecting ducts. By blocking the reabsorption of Na^+, these diuretics reduce the negative charge in the lumen, which decreases the electrical driving force for the secretion of K^+. Thus they are known as potassium-sparing diuretics. Spironolactone is another potassium-sparing diuretic that acts on the principal cell of the collecting duct. It inhibits the action of aldosterone and therefore on epithelium sodium channel (ENaC) and the Na^+,K^+-ATPase, preventing both Na^+ reabsorption and K^+ secretion.

Water channels called aquaporins are thought to be present in all cell types that routinely conduct osmosis.

- The collecting duct, however, does not express aquaporins on its surface until stimulated to do so by antidiuretic hormone (ADH).
- In the presence of ADH, water is passively reabsorbed from the collecting duct, owing to the medullary osmotic gradient created by the loop of Henle.
- Differing water permeabilities exist along the nephron because of nonregulated aquaporin-1 channels in the leaky proximal epithelium and ADH regulated aquaporin-2 channels in the distal tight epithelia which is the most water impermeable segment.

Fractional Excretion

The fractional excretion (FE) of a solute can tell us to what extent a solute has been reabsorbed or secreted. FE equals the quantity of solute excreted divided by the quantity of solute filtered:

$$FE = \text{amount in urine/amount filtered}$$
$$= \{[\text{solute}]_{urine} \times \dot{V}\}/\{[\text{solute}]_{plasma} \times GFR\}$$

As explained in Chapter 17, glomerular filtration rate (GFR) is equal to the clearance of creatinine.

$$GFR = \text{clearance of creatinine}$$
$$= \dot{V} \times [\text{creatinine}]_{urine}/[\text{creatinine}]_{plasma}$$

We can substitute the clearance of creatinine into the equation for FE to come up with the following equation for FE.

$$FE = \{[\text{solute}]_{urine} \times [\text{creatinine}]_{plasma}\}/$$
$$\{[\text{solute}]_{plasma} \times [\text{creatinine}]_{urine}\}$$

OR

$$FE = \{[\text{solute}]_{urine}/[\text{solute}]_{plasma}\}/$$
$$\{[\text{creatinine}]_{urine}/[\text{creatinine}]_{plasma}\}$$

(The latter expression of FE reveals an important clinical feature of FE—namely, that it describes the renal handling of a solute more specifically than does a simple measurement of solute concentration in urine. A solute concentration in the urine can be affected by reabsorption of the solute and by the reabsorption of water. The denominator of FE corrects for water reabsorption, which is the only factor that alters the urine-to-plasma [creatinine] ratio.)

The FE of Na^+, called FeNa in clinical contexts, is a clinically relevant calculation in patients who have a low urine output and acute renal failure.

- A patient with renal failure owing to volume depletion but intact tubular function would have a high fractional reabsorption of Na^+—usually greater than 99%. This means that less than 1% of filtered Na^+ would be excreted (FeNa$^+$ <1%).
- In acute tubular necrosis (ATN), another cause of renal failure in which tubular function is abnormal, Na^+ reabsorption is impaired and a value for FeNa would be greater than 2%.
- In the context of a normal individual with high GFR, however, a low FeNa does not indicate an abnormality. For example, in someone in balance on a 100 mEq/day Na^+ intake (or 100 mEq/day Na^+ excretion) who has a GFR of 180 L/day and a plasma Na^+ of 140 mEq/L, the FeNa is 100 divided by the product of 180 times 140, or 0.4%.

Glomerular-Tubular Balance

Recall from Chapter 17 that tubuloglomerular feedback is a form of autoregulation that stabilizes GFR and renal blood flow through compensatory mechanisms.

Glomerular-tubular (G-T) balance refers to the relationship between the load delivered to a tubule segment and reabsorption by that segment.

- Without G-T balance, an increase in GFR would result in large volumes of water loss and solute loss in the urine because an increase in GFR means that more solute, such as Na$^+$, and more water are filtered into the tubule lumen.

- If the proximal tubules merely reabsorbed a fixed amount of Na$^+$ under these circumstances, there would be a greater than normal excretion of Na$^+$.
- The proximal tubules do not reabsorb a constant amount of Na$^+$ and other solutes, however. Instead, they reabsorb a fairly constant percentage of the filtered load.

A higher GFR is met with more tubular reabsorption of solute and water. There are probably two mechanisms for G-T balance.

- The first mechanism for G-T balance is caused by changes in pressure in the efferent arteriole and peritubular capillaries.
  - A higher GFR means more plasma water will be filtered, leaving behind a higher oncotic pressure in the efferent arteriole and peritubular capillary.
  - If the rise in GFR is caused by increased resistance in the efferent arteriole (relative to the resistance in the afferent arteriole), then the peritubular capillary downstream of the arteriole will also have lower hydrostatic pressure.
  - The combination of increased oncotic "pull" and decreased hydrostatic pressure in the peritubular capillary shifts the Starling forces in favor of an increased reabsorption of Na$^+$ and water from the lumen of the proximal tubule by way of the interstitium (Fig. 18.11).
- The second mechanism follows from the fact that flow rate and reabsorptive rate are linked.
  - An increased GFR results in a greater filtered load not only of Na$^+$ but also of all other normally filtered substances.
  - Many of these substances cotransport with Na$^+$ in the proximal tubule, and this increased delivery of cotransported

solutes increases the amount of Na$^+$ that can be cotransported across the membranes.

PATHOPHYSIOLOGY OF THE KIDNEY TUBULE

An understanding of the consequences of renal disease follows logically from an understanding of the normal physiology of the kidney and the normal functions of the nephron, which include:

- Essential homeostatic functions, including electrolyte and water balance
- Nitrogenous waste removal
- Reabsorption of valuable substances

It therefore follows that disorders of the tubule compromise these homeostatic functions. Disorders can lead to retention of unwanted substances and fluid or the loss of valuable substances.

Kidney disease specific to the tubule falls into two broad categories:

- Disorders that adversely affect the tubular transport proteins without killing the tubule cells
- Disorders that kill the tubule cells, leading to a specific scenario known as ATN, which is the common terminus of many sorts of acute insults to the kidney.

Disorders of the Tubular Transport Proteins

Disorders that affect the tubular transport proteins without causing acute cell death may result from:

- Hereditary factors: generally rare.
- Toxicity: a more common cause of tubular dysfunction. The renal tubule is particularly vulnerable to toxins because many of these substances are transported by the tubular epithelium.
- Ischemia: although ischemia often leads to ATN, it may also impair transport without causing cell death by splitting the tight junctions.
  - The kidney is highly sensitive to ischemia, possibly because the oxygen tension in the medulla is quite low.
  - This sensitivity is caused by the medulla's lesser degree of perfusion and the anatomy of the vasa recta, which is not favorable to oxygen delivery.
  - The outer medulla, particularly the late proximal tubule, is most susceptible to ischemic injury because the proximal tubule cannot perform anaerobic glycolysis.

Tubular dysfunction can also occur secondary to chronic glomerular disease, as the excess protein filtered in glomerular disorders over years can cause tubular injury.

Because each part of the tubule has a distinct function, pathologic transport has different sequelae depending on the tubule segment affected. We will discuss examples of transport derangements in each one, proceeding from the proximal tubule onward.

Disorders of Transport in the Proximal Tubule

A host of rare genetic disorders disrupt the proximal tubule's capacity to reabsorb many small molecules, such as glucose, amino acids, phosphate, and bicarbonate.

- Renal glucosuria is a benign tubular disorder that is characterized by normal levels of glucose in the blood, but high

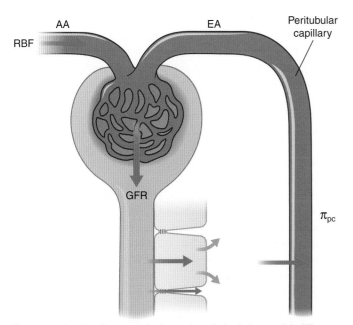

Fig. 18.11 Starling forces and glomerular-tubular balance. *AA,* Afferent arteriole; *EA,* efferent arteriole; π_{pc}, oncotic pressure in the peritubular capillary. *GFR,* Glomerular Filtration Rate; *RBF,* Renal Blood Flow.

levels of glucose in the urine. It results from faulty glucose transport mechanisms, resulting in impaired glucose reabsorption.

- Defects in amino acid transport systems may result in a generalized aminoaciduria, where all amino acids are not reabsorbed, or in failure to reabsorb specific amino acids, such as cysteine and glycine.
- Gout, a common disease of increased plasma urate level, may be caused by an inherited defect that increases proximal tubular reabsorption of urate by acquired renal disease or by nonrenal factors (see Clinical Correlation Box 18.7).

Clinical Correlation Box 18.7

What Is Gout?

A 69-year-old man calls his internist complaining that he was awakened at night by severe hot pain in his left big toe. The toe has been so painful it will not tolerate even the pressure of a bed sheet. In the office, the patient reports he has never suffered joint pain and has never been diagnosed with arthritis. History reveals a diet high in meat and daily light alcohol consumption (one beer with dinner). Aspiration of the left first metatarsal-phalangeal joint relieves the pain to some extent, and examination of the aspirate under the microscope reveals abundant urate crystals. The internist administers a corticosteroid shot in the affected joint, prescribes indomethacin, a nonsteroidal antiinflammatory drug (NSAID), and recommends the reduction of meat and beer intake. The diagnosis is gout.

Uric acid is a nitrogenous end-product of purine metabolism that cannot be further catabolized by the body. Consequently, uric acid accumulates if the kidney is unable to excrete it in amounts that match production. In gout, either an overproduction of uric acid or decreased renal excretion of uric acid leads to a high level of uric acid in the plasma (hyperuricemia). In cases when the kidney fails to excrete uric acid, the problem seems to be in the proximal tubule. For reasons that are not well understood, the proximal tubule has the ability to both actively secrete and reabsorb urate, the anion of uric acid, and in some individuals, the reabsorption of urate by the proximal tubule is excessive. Various types of intrinsic renal disease and some drugs, such as pyrazinamide, can decrease urate excretion. Other drugs are uricosuric, for example, probenizid, which inhibits uric acid reabsorption.

As the concentration of urate in the plasma reaches the limits of its solubility, uric acid crystals begin to precipitate, forming inflammatory deposits, usually in the joints. Gout attacks tend to be sudden in onset and frequently affect a peripheral joint in the lower extremities, often in the big toe. Treatment includes corticosteroids, NSAIDs, colchicine (which inhibits neutrophils' phagocytosis of urate crystals), and dietary modification. Underlying causes of hyperuricemia should be addressed, and drugs are also available to decrease the plasma urate level. Uricosuric drugs increase renal excretion of urate, and xanthine oxidase inhibitors block the final step in the production of urate.

We mentioned previously that the nephron is vulnerable to toxic injury. Because the proximal tubule is located next to the glomerulus, where plasma is filtered and because of its extensive reuptake of filtered substances, the proximal tubule is particularly susceptible to this type of injury.

- In lead nephropathy, a condition in which lead toxicity impairs proximal tubular reabsorption, loss of glucose in the urine (glucosuria) and loss of amino acids in the urine (aminoaciduria) occurs. In addition, because the proximal tubule is responsible for reabsorbing phosphates, low levels of phosphates are found in the serum (hypophosphatemia).
- Another important function of the proximal tubule is to reabsorb bicarbonate. When this function is compromised, the serum pH decreases; therefore lead toxicity may lead to acidosis.

Such clinical findings of general proximal tubule failure are described as Fanconi syndrome. Fanconi syndrome may also be inherited or may be caused by toxic exposure to other agents.

Disorders of Transport in the Loop of Henle

Recall that the loop of Henle is essential for the concentration of urine and the reabsorption of water from the collecting duct. It also reabsorbs the majority of the sodium, potassium, and chloride not reabsorbed in the proximal tubule (see Clinical Correlation Box 18.8).

Clinical Correlation Box 18.8

In an uncommon genetic disorder known as Bartter syndrome, sodium, potassium, and chloride are not reabsorbed, and the ability of the kidney to concentrate urine and reabsorb water in the collecting duct is consequently impaired. As a result, large volumes of urine are formed. The patient develops thirst, takes in more fluids, and as a result, may maintain a high urine output. Because of the resultant volume depletion, the renin-angiotensin-aldosterone system is activated, resulting in an increase in Na^+ reabsorption and increased H^+ and K^+ excretion. The ultimate result is severe volume depletion, low serum concentrations of potassium (hypokalemia) and chloride (hypochloremia, and oversecretion of acid, which creates a metabolic alkalosis.

Disorders of Transport in the Distal Tubule and Collecting Duct

The distal tubule normally reabsorbs Na^+ and Cl^-. Although infrequently observed clinically, mutations can occur in the Na^+/Cl^- cotransporter located in the distal tubule. Na^+, Cl^-, and consequently, water, are wasted in the urine, and volume depletion can occur.

In addition to regulating water reabsorption, the distal tubule and collecting duct fine-tune the amount of Na^+ reabsorbed by the kidney and secrete K^+ and H^+.

- When the transport capabilities of the collecting duct are impaired, Na^+ wasting, hyperkalemia, and acidosis can occur.
- When transport in the distal tubule and collecting duct is overactive, just the opposite occurs. Under conditions in which too much aldosterone is secreted (e.g., by an adrenal tumor), then too much Na^+ is reabsorbed and too much K^+ and H^+ are secreted, resulting in mild hypernatremia, hypokalemia, and alkalosis.

Under the control of ADH, water reabsorption also occurs in the collecting duct.

- If ADH is not secreted or if the tubules are not responsive to ADH, as in diabetes insipidus, water will not be reabsorbed properly.

- Conversely, if excess ADH is inappropriately secreted, then the collecting duct will reabsorb too much water, lowering the concentration of the serum electrolytes.

Acute Tubular Necrosis

Whatever the cause, the common pathway of ATN starts with a depletion of tubular cell ATP and damage to the tubular cell membranes. This leads to increasing intracellular calcium, activation of proteases and lipases, and eventual cell death. The dead tubular cells slough off, form aggregates called casts, and block the tubules. Blockage of the tubules ultimately results in a decrease in GFR and backup of filtered fluid. ATN is therefore classified as a major cause of intrinsic renal failure (i.e., acute renal failure originating within the renal parenchyma).

ATN may result from:

- Ischemic injury
  - Severe hypotension—as seen in septic shock, hemorrhage, or shock during major surgery—causes insufficient perfusion of the tubules and is the predominant cause of ischemic tubular injury and ischemic ATN.
  - The ischemic insult to the tubules can also be exacerbated by toxic mediators that are present because of tissue damage or sepsis.
  - As alluded to previously, the outer medulla is especially susceptible to ischemic injuries.
- Toxic injury
  - Because toxins can reach high concentrations in the tubular epithelial cells, the kidney is also very susceptible to damage by a broad range of toxins, including both exogenous and endogenous substances.
  - Exogenous substances frequently implicated in nephrotoxic ATN include antibiotics, such as aminoglycosides or amphotericin B, chemotherapeutic agents like cisplatin, heavy metals, or radiocontrast agents.
  - Endogenous toxins include myoglobin, which is released after muscle breakdown because of crush injuries or pressure sores, and hemoglobin in the context of a transfusion reaction.
- Inflammatory injury (see Clinical Correlation Box 18.9)

Clinical Correlation Box 18.9

Because severe ischemia often causes acute tubular necrosis (ATN), the prerenal failure (because of sudden reduction in blood flow to the kidney) of ischemia and the intrinsic renal failure of ATN may be seen together. Furthermore, given that they both reduce the glomerular filtration rate (GFR), they share certain clinical signs, such as elevated plasma creatinine and urea. Many clinical signs differentiate the two, which is important in the differential diagnosis of acute renal failure. For example, the ratio of plasma urea to creatinine is higher in prerenal failure, the fractional excretion of sodium (FeNa) is elevated only in intrinsic renal failure, and muddy granular casts are not seen in the urine unless ATN is present.

The prognosis for patients who have had ATN without any other serious medical problems is good and the tubular cells regenerate; however, these patients may have some degree of prolonged renal impairment. For patients with preexisting renal disease or serious comorbid conditions, such as sepsis, the mortality rate can be high.

SUMMARY

- The renal tubule has three main sections: the proximal tubule, where the bulk of salt, water, and other solutes are reabsorbed; the loop of Henle, where salt is concentrated in the medulla; and the distal tubule and collecting duct, where water reabsorption is regulated to control serum osmolality.
- A mass balance equation describes the allocation of renal arterial contents between the urine and the renal vein:

$$\left(\dot{V}_{renal\ artery}\right)\left(\left[solute\right]_{arterial\ blood}\right)$$
$$= \left(\dot{V}_{urine}\right)\left(\left[solute\right]_{urine}\right) + \left(\dot{V}_{renal\ vein}\right)\left(\left[solute\right]_{venous\ blood}\right)$$

- The processes of filtration, reabsorption, and secretion determine how a given substance will be divided between urine and venous blood.
- Solutes and water may cross from tubule lumen to the interstitium by a transcellular route or a paracellular route.
- The Na$^+$,K$^+$-ATPase pump drives all reabsorption and secretion across the tubule wall. Na$^+$ is reabsorbed by primary active transport, whereas other solutes are moved by secondary active transport; that is, they are indirectly coupled to the movement of sodium.
- The tubule reabsorbs 99% of Na$^+$, 100% of glucose, and the majority of Mg^{2+}, Ca^{2+}, K$^+$, phosphate, and amino acids. The bulk (about two-thirds) of the reabsorption takes place in the proximal tubule, but the "fine-tuning" of the amounts of each solute to be conserved or excreted takes place in the distal portions of the nephron. Thus, the percentages reabsorbed in the distal portions will change depending on dietary intake and other mechanisms.
- Na$^+$ reabsorption in the early proximal tubule takes place via cotransport with glucose, amino acids, lactate, phosphate, and bicarbonate and in the late proximal tubule with Cl$^-$. Because water osmotically follows these solutes, 67% of water is reabsorbed isosmotically in the proximal tubule; solvent drag also contributes to the reabsorption of Na$^+$, Cl$^-$, K$^+$, Ca^{2+}, and Mg^{2+}.
- Substances that require elimination but could not be filtered are often secreted. Many organic anions and cations are completely cleared via proximal tubule secretion.
- Overall, the loop of Henle reabsorbs 20% of the filtered load of Na$^+$, Cl$^-$, Ca^{2+}, and Mg^{2+}. It also reabsorbs about 20% of the filtered water, which occurs in the descending limb of Henle. The active pumping of salts along the thick ascending limb makes the tubular fluid hypoosmotic, with an osmolarity less than 150 mOsm/kg H$_2$O.
- In the late distal tubule and collecting duct, principal cells actively reabsorb Na$^+$ and secrete K$^+$. Intercalated cells secrete H$^+$ and reabsorb bicarbonate.

- FE = amount in urine/amount filtered = $\{[\text{solute}]_{\text{urine}} \times [\text{creatinine}]_{\text{plasma}}\}/\{[\text{solute}]_{\text{plasma}} \times [\text{creatinine}]_{\text{urine}}\}$
- G-T balance yields proportional changes in Na^+ reabsorption with changes in GFR.

- Tubular dysfunction may disrupt transport without killing tubular cells or may involve ATN.
- ATN is caused by ischemia or toxicity and results in derangements of tubular transport and decreased GFR.

REVIEW QUESTIONS

Directions: Each of the numbered items or incomplete statements in this section is followed by answers or by completions of the statement. Select the one lettered answer or completion that is best in each case.

1. A 65-year-old man underwent surgery for the repair of an abdominal aortic aneurysm. In the postoperative period, he was noted to have decreased urine output. His blood urea nitrogen (BUN) and creatinine were 29 and 1.9 mg/dL, indicating a decreased GFR. His fractional excretion of sodium was 4.2%. Muddy brown granular casts were observed on urinalysis, indicating tubular necrosis. His increased fractional excretion of sodium is likely caused by:
   A. Increased filtration of sodium
   B. Increased filtration of glucose
   C. Decreased reabsorption of sodium
   D. Increased secretion of chloride
   E. Increased secretion of sodium

2. A 34-year-old woman being treated for a urinary tract infection is diagnosed with diabetes mellitus after urinalysis shows glucose in her urine and blood tests confirm hyperglycemia. The likely cause of her glucosuria is
   A. A decreased glucose T_m in the proximal tubule
   B. Saturation of the Na^+/glucose cotransporters
   C. Severely decreased Na^+ reabsorption
   D. An elevated GFR
   E. Backflow of glucose across faulty tight junctions

3. A 72-year-old man with congestive heart failure because of idiopathic dilated cardiomyopathy was placed on furosemide to help alleviate his peripheral edema. Which of the following electrolyte abnormalities may result from his use of this drug?
   A. Hyponatremia
   B. Hypocalcemia
   C. Hypermagnesemia
   D. Hypokalemia
   E. Two of the above

ANSWERS TO REVIEW QUESTIONS

1. **The answer is C.** The renal tubule normally reabsorbs 99% or more of the filtered sodium, but in this patient, ATN has interfered with the tubule's ability to reabsorb sodium, leaving excess sodium in the urine and increasing the FeNa above its normal limit of 1%. Although increased filtration of sodium would increase the tubular sodium load, we know that in this case, the GFR is low and that sodium filtration is actually decreased; furthermore, a normally functioning tubule would still reabsorb the increased load of sodium. Increased filtration of glucose is not present because GFR is decreased; moreover, increased filtration of glucose promotes sodium reabsorption—this is one of the mechanisms of G-T balance. The kidney does not secrete either sodium or chloride; it only reabsorbs them.

2. **The answer is B.** In diabetes mellitus, a high serum glucose level (hyperglycemia) leads to an abnormally high filtered load of glucose. The Na^+/glucose transporters become saturated and cannot reabsorb all the filtered glucose; the rest is lost to the urine. Normally, all the glucose is reabsorbed. An inherited disorder can lower the glucose transport maximum (T_m) and can cause glucosuria in the context of normal serum glucose, but the patient's serum glucose is not normal in this case. Severely decreased Na^+ reabsorption would decrease glucose reabsorption because glucose is cotransported with Na^+, but this is not the cause of glucosuria in diabetes mellitus. Increased GFR can contribute to splay and faulty tight junctions would interfere with solute reabsorption, but these are not contributors to diabetic glucosuria.

3. **The answer is D.** Furosemide can cause hypokalemia because inhibition of salt reabsorption in the thick limb results in increased delivery of Na^+ to the collecting duct, where K^+ is secreted. That is why potassium-sparing diuretics are useful adjuncts in the treatment of the edematous patient. Although furosemide increases urinary calcium and magnesium excretion, hypocalcemia is unusual because the blood calcium is closely regulated by hormonal influences. Hypomagnesemia, on the other hand, is not unusual. Hypermagnesemia is not a feature of furosemide treatment. The drug causes diuresis through the inhibition of the Na^+/K^+/$2Cl^-$ reabsorptive symporter in the thick ascending limb of the loop of Henle. This prevents dilution of the tubular fluid, which is necessary for water reabsorption in the collecting duct, and induces a higher urine volume. Inhibition of K^+ reabsorption may lead to hypokalemia as a side effect. Under normal circumstances, the Na^+/K^+/$2Cl^-$ symporter and the distribution of ion channels in the thick ascending limb also lead to an electropositive tubule lumen that drives the paracellular reabsorption of Ca^{2+} and Mg^{2+}. Inhibition of the symporter disrupts the establishment of a net positive charge on the inside of the tubule lumen and the driving force for reabsorption of Ca^{++} and Mg^{++} is diminished, resulting in hypercalcuria and magnesuria. Loop diuretics do not usually create hyponatremia by themselves because they lead to the excretion of hypotonic urine. They would only cause hyponatremia if the patent ingested more free water while the diuretic caused sodium depletion.

19

The Regulation of Blood Pressure and Extracellular Fluid Volume

INTRODUCTION

Organ perfusion, and therefore function, is dependent on blood pressure (BP). The cardiovascular system does not govern BP by itself; equally important to the regulation of BP is the kidney's control over the volume of the extracellular fluid (ECF).

- Recall that systemic blood pressure (SBP) is equal to the product of cardiac output (CO) and systemic vascular resistance (SVR).

$$SBP = CO \times SVR$$

Note that this is analogous to Ohm's law in electrical systems.

- The cardiovascular system affects BP by adjusting CO and SVR at the level of the heart and the arterioles, respectively.
- The kidney affects BP by adjusting the size of the ECF compartment, which affects the heart's preload and CO.
- The cardiovascular and renal effectors of BP homeostasis act in concert, and the nervous system coordinates their efforts.

The kidneys control volume in the same way that they control the level of solutes in the bloodstream—by modifying the reabsorption of solutes and water filtered into the tubule.

SYSTEM STRUCTURE: BODY FLUID COMPARTMENTS

Recall that body fluid is divided into two spaces, extracellular and intracellular.

- ECF is divided into intravascular and interstitial compartments that are separated by capillary endothelium, which is freely permeable to water and small ions but not to proteins.
- Intracellular fluid (ICF) is the fluid contained inside all the cells of the body. The amount of solutes, predominantly ionic in nature, in the intracellular versus extracellular compartments determines the volume of fluid in each space.

Also remember from previous chapters that Na^+ (sodium) is the major cation of the ECF, and K^+ (potassium) is the major cation of the ICF (Fig. 19.1).

- The Na^+,K^+-adenosine triphosphatase (ATPase) pump that operates in all body tissues segregates Na^+ and K^+ to the outside and the inside of cells, respectively.
  - Na^+ is therefore primarily responsible for creating the osmotic pressure that holds water (and volume) in the extracellular space.

- K^+ is primarily responsible for the osmotic pressure that holds water in the intracellular space. (See Ch. 1 for more discussion of osmotic pressure and fluid shifts.)
- Changes in the Na^+ concentration of the ECF alter the osmotic pressure of the ECF.
- If Na^+ is added to the ECF—for example, by eating a salty meal and absorbing salt into the blood from the intestines—the osmotic pressure of the ECF will increase, and water will move from the ICF into the ECF, thereby increasing the ECF volume.

The kidney makes use of this principle when it alters the volume of the ECF.

- By adjusting the amount of Na^+ reabsorbed from the nephron tubule, the kidney adjusts the osmotic gradient for water reabsorption from the tubule, and thereby adjusts the amount of water and volume reabsorbed from the tubule back into the bloodstream.
- The point here is not that water reabsorption always follows salt reabsorption in the kidney; in fact, in certain parts of the tubule, salt reabsorption without water is essential to kidney function.
- The kidney does not control ECF volume by hydrostatically pumping filtered water back into the bloodstream; instead, it does so by creating osmotic gradients with Na^+, the major ECF cationic osmole (Fig. 19.2).

SYSTEM FUNCTION: BLOOD PRESSURE HOMEOSTASIS

The kidneys maintain BP and perfusion pressure by increasing the ECF volume when perfusion pressure is low and decreasing ECF volume when perfusion pressure is high. Perfusion pressure refers to the local arterial BPs at particular organs, such as the brain or the kidneys, as opposed to the average systemic BP.

Fig. 19.3 breaks down renal and cardiovascular regulation of perfusion pressure into homeostatic elements.

Cardiovascular and Renal Regulation of Perfusion Pressure

The cardiovascular and renal regulation share similar sensors but use different effector mechanisms. As we shall see, renal and cardiovascular regulation are intimately connected.

In both systems, BP regulation begins with the baroreceptors, which sense changes in perfusion pressure. The term "baroreceptor reflex" is used to describe the feedback loop by which the nervous system responds to changes in perfusion pressure.

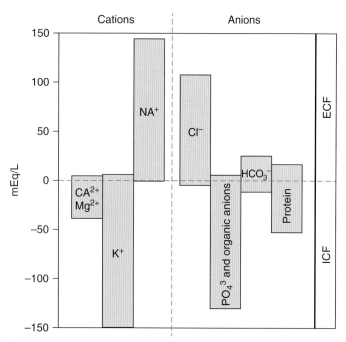

Fig. 19.1 Major cations and anions of the extracellular fluid (*ECF*) and intracellular fluid (*ICF*). Na^+ and Cl^- are the major ions of the ECF. K^+ and a variety of anions, including PO_4^{3-}, are the major ions of the ICF.

Cardiovascular Regulation

Cardiovascular regulation is initiated by baroreceptors in the heart, lungs, and carotid arteries. On the basis of information it receives from the baroreceptors, the brain discharges impulses through the sympathetic nervous system and parasympathetic nervous system to control heart rate, heart contractility, and resistance of the blood vessels. The sympathetic outflow also impinges on the kidney to regulate proximal reabsorption, renin secretion, and renal vascular resistance.
- More sympathetic output raises BP and heart rate.
- More parasympathetic output slows the heart rate and lowers BP.

Renal Regulation

Three main feedback loops constitute the renal regulation of BP.
1. BP changes within the renal microcirculation stimulate the juxtaglomerular apparatus (JGA) in the afferent arterioles, which in turn leads to changes in renin secretion which affect the renin-angiotensin-aldosterone (RAA) hormonal cascade.
   a. Production of renin -> production of angiotensin II -> adrenal release of aldosterone.
   b. Angiotensin II and aldosterone increase sodium (and thus) reabsorption from the renal tubules to increase intravascular volume, which increases systemic BP.
   c. Angiotensin II also increases vascular resistance systemically, which increases systemic BP.
2. Atrial and ventricular receptors can sense stretch and alter the release of atrial natriuretic peptide (ANP), a 28-amino acid peptide stored in granules of the myocytes and brain natriuretic peptide (BNP). These peptides act as systemic vasodilators and reduce tubular salt/fluid reabsorption, which decreases BP.

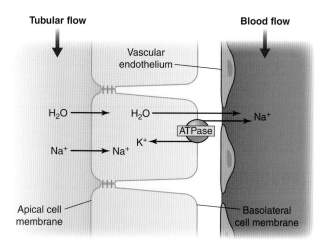

Fig. 19.2 Water and salt reabsorption in the kidney. Water follows salt. *ATPase,* Adenosine triphosphatase.

3. Baroreceptors stimulate the secretion of antidiuretic hormone (ADH) in the setting of hypotension, which increases the reabsorption of water from the tubule and leads to increased systemic BP.

Fig. 19.4 provides an overview of the homeostatic responses to changes in perfusion pressure.

Sensors in Regulation of Perfusion Pressure

BP changes throughout the day in accordance with numerous stimuli including:
- Stress
- Exertion
- Variations in dietary salt and water intake
- Fluid losses
- Many pathologic states, such as hemorrhage
Baroreceptors signal the brain in response to stretch in blood vessel walls.
- Baroreceptor cells "sense" stretch from the transmural pressure gradients across the vessel wall.
- When increased perfusion pressure distends the vessel wall, the baroreceptor increases its rate of firing.
- For example, the myocytes containing ANP and BNP stretch in response to a pressure gradient between the atrial cavity and the intrathoracic space (see Fast Fact Box 19.1).

Fast Fact Box 19.1

As mentioned in Chapter 10, a perfusion pressure or driving pressure is the gradient of pressures between two locations within the circulation. The actual pressure at one site in the circulation contributes *both* to the transmural pressure across the vessel wall and the driving pressure forward through the circulation. Therefore the actual pressure at a site in the circulation where the peripheral or atrial mechanoreceptors exist contributes to a transmural distending pressure.

Baroreceptors exist in low-pressure and high-pressure areas of vasculature:
- Low-pressure baroreceptors:
  - Cardiac atria
  - Pulmonary vessels

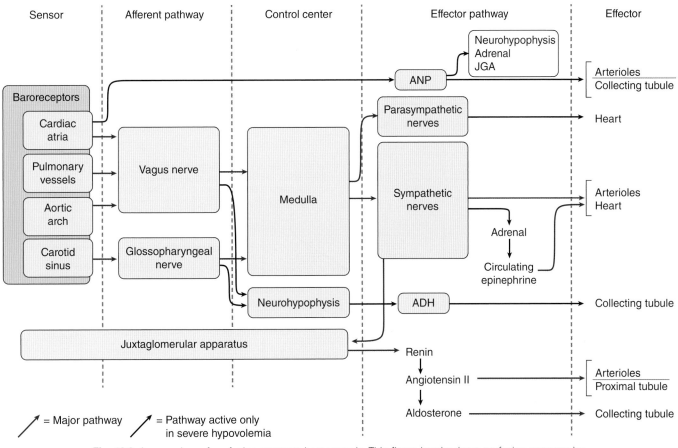

Fig. 19.3 An overview of perfusion pressure homeostasis. This figure breaks down perfusion pressure homeostasis into the classic homeostatic elements: sensors, afferent transmission pathways, control centers, efferent transmission pathways, and effectors. *ADH*, Antidiuretic hormone; *ANP*, atrial natriuretic peptide; *JGA*, juxtaglomerular apparatus.

- High-pressure baroreceptors:
  - Aortic arch
  - Carotid sinus
  - JGA in the afferent arterioles of the kidney (see Clinical Correlation Box 19.1 and Clinical Correlation Box 19.2)

Remember that although ECF volume and perfusion pressure are related, they are not the same. Despite the fact that the kidney affects perfusion pressure by altering ECF volume, the kidney senses only arterial perfusion pressure to the kidney (see Clinical Correlation Box 19.3).

Many texts use the term effective circulating volume (ECV) to address this concept of perfusion pressure in contrast with extracellular volume. The idea is that only some of the high fluid volume in the body is "effective"; that is, only some of the volume is actively perfusing the tissues while the rest remains pooled in the veins or sitting in the interstitium, effectively out of circulation. Alterations in ECV, not total ECF volume, drive the baroreceptor reflex.

Afferent Pathways in Regulation of Perfusion Pressure

The baroreceptors in the atria and pulmonary vessels communicate with the medulla in the brain via the vagus nerve (CNX). The aortic arch and carotid sinus baroreceptors transmit information to the medulla as well—the aortic arch through the vagus nerve (CNX) and the carotid sinus through the glossopharyngeal nerve (CNIX).
- Higher perfusion pressure leads to more stimulation from peripheral baroreceptors, which in turn signals the body to lower the BP through its effector mechanisms.
- Lower perfusion pressure and less stimulation of the baroreceptors and medulla tells the body's effectors to do the opposite.

In contrast, the JGA is its own control center. It alters its renin secretion in direct response to stimulation by changes in stretch at the afferent arteriole of the nephrons.

Clinical Correlate Box 19.1

In some pathologic conditions, the extracellular fluid (ECF) volume may be high (hypervolemia) while the perfusion pressures are low. In congestive heart failure, fluid pools in the veins and cardiac output falls owing to poor heart pumping ability. Because the homeostatic sensors respond to perfusion pressure, which will be low in the poor cardiac output state, they trigger changes in ECF volume. This added fluid collects in the high-capacitance veins and eventually leaks out into the interstitium from the peripheral capillary, causing swelling in the tissues. Clinically, this increase in volume is seen as pitting edema.

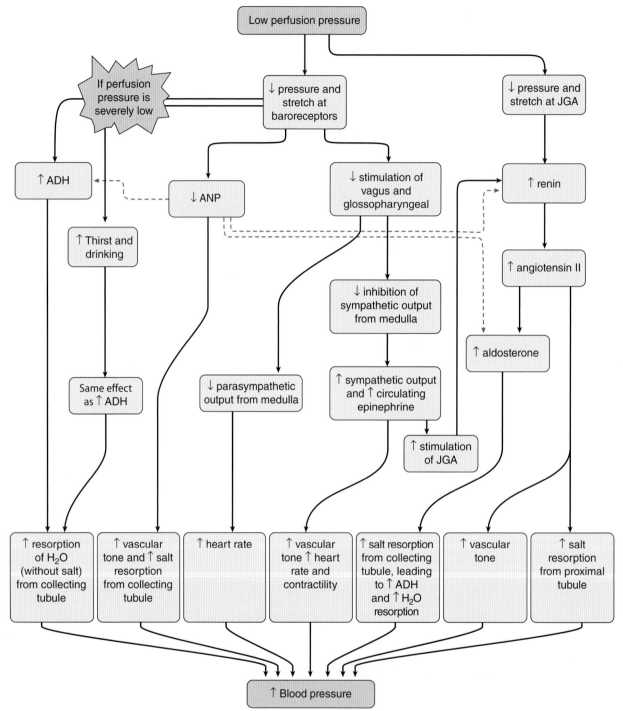

Fig. 19.4 Homeostatic responses to changes in perfusion pressure. This chart shows all the parallel pathways that are activated in the response to changes in perfusion pressure, as well as the horizontal interactions between pathways. As we discuss each individual efferent pathway, we will reproduce this figure with the relevant pathway highlighted. Note that only the response to low perfusion pressure is depicted in this figure and in each of the related highlighted figures. High perfusion pressure produces effects through the exact same pathways and with all the same interactions, but the changes are in the opposite direction. The baroreceptors detect increased stretch, ANP and BNP secretion goes up, vagal stimulation goes up, sympathetic inhibition goes up, renin secretion goes down, and finally, blood pressure is decreased. *ADH*, Antidiuretic hormone; *ANP*, atrial natriuretic peptide; *JGA*, juxtaglomerular apparatus.

Clinical Correlation Box 19.2

Diuretics

Diuretics are drugs used to elevate urine volume and decrease extracellular fluid volume. They are most often used to treat hypertension or congestive heart failure. There are four kinds of diuretics: loop diuretics, thiazide-type diuretics, K$^+$-sparing diuretics, and carbonic anhydrase inhibitors (see Figure below). Loop diuretics inhibit the Na/K/2Cl cotransporter in the loop of Henle, impeding salt reabsorption. Thiazide diuretics bind the Na/Cl cotransporter in the distal tubule, inhibiting salt reabsorption there. Loop and thiazide diuretics can promote K$^+$ wasting because they increase tubular flow to the K$^+$ secretion site in the collecting duct. Increased flow keeps the tubule [K$^+$] down and improves the gradient for K$^+$ secretion. K$^+$-sparing diuretics inhibit salt reabsorption where salt reabsorption is coupled with K$^+$ secretion (i.e., they inhibit aldosterone), thereby preserving serum K$^+$. Carbonic anhydrase inhibition in the proximal tubule cells inhibits bicarbonate reabsorption and thereby osmotically promotes diuresis. See Chapter 18 for additional details.

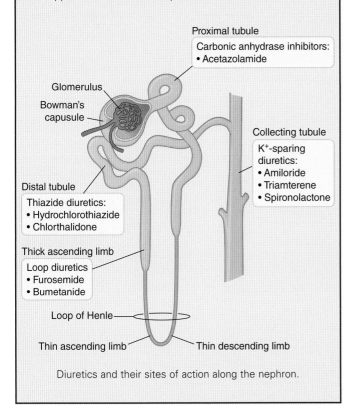

Diuretics and their sites of action along the nephron.

Clinical Correlation Box 19.3

In the case of renal artery stenosis, the juxtaglomerular apparatus senses a decrease in perfusion pressure at the afferent arteriole and increase the secretion of renin. The activation of the renin-angiotensin-aldosterone cascade leads to increase in volume, vasoconstriction, and finally hypertension.

Efferent Pathways in Regulation of Perfusion Pressure

Neural Pathways

The sympathetic nerves are a major route of efferent transmission, extending from the medulla to peripheral arterioles

throughout the body. The sympathetic nerves also synapse with the adrenal gland and help to govern the secretion of epinephrine from the adrenal gland into the bloodstream.

The medulla also sends out signals along the parasympathetic efferent fibers in the vagus nerve. Under normal circumstances, there is always some amount of output from the medulla along sympathetic and parasympathetic nerves. This output is called sympathetic tone and parasympathetic tone. Parasympathetic output works reciprocally with sympathetic output.

- When perfusion pressure is high, the body decreases sympathetic tone and increases parasympathetic tone. In response to increased perfusion pressure, the parasympathetic tone acts mainly as a negative chronotrope at the heart (meaning it lowers the heart rate) to reduce CO and BP. Reduced sympathetic tone decreases the BP and the ECF volume.
- Increased sympathetic tone raises the BP and the ECF volume.
- Sympathetic nerves also synapse with the JGA, augmenting the stimulation from the JGA's own sensors (Fig. 19.5).

Hormonal Pathways

Circulating epinephrine acts as an efferent mechanism that reinforces the effects of stimulation by the sympathetic nerves.

Additionally, the JGA transmits information to the hormonal effectors of the RAA system.

- When perfusion pressure is low, the JGA is stimulated to secrete more renin.
- When perfusion pressure is high, the JGA is stimulated to secrete less renin.
- Renin converts angiotensinogen (produced in the liver) to angiotensin I, and angiotensin I is converted in the lung to its active form, angiotensin II, with the help of angiotensin-converting enzyme (ACE) (Fig. 19.6).
- ACE is found in large quantities on the endothelial surfaces of the pulmonary vasculature. Because angiotensinogen and ACE are readily available in high concentrations, renin secretion yields rapid production of angiotensin II.
- Angiotensin II acts directly on the kidney and blood vessels to increase blood volume and pressure, and also acts on the zona glomerulosa of the adrenal cortex, promoting the aldosterone secretion.
- Aldosterone is a steroid hormone (a mineralocorticoid as opposed to a glucocorticoid) that acts on the kidney to increase blood volume by means that will be discussed later in this chapter.

Fig. 19.7 highlights the role of the RAA system in responding to changes in perfusion pressure. The RAA system is a vital component of the rapid response to depleted intravascular volume and pressure, as might occur with hemorrhage (see Clinical Correlation Box 19.4).

Clinical Correlation Box 19.4

In some disease states, the renin-angiotensin-aldosterone system may act to increase blood pressure and blood volume inappropriately. This can occur with tumors of the kidney that secrete renin or of the adrenal gland where aldosterone is overproduced.

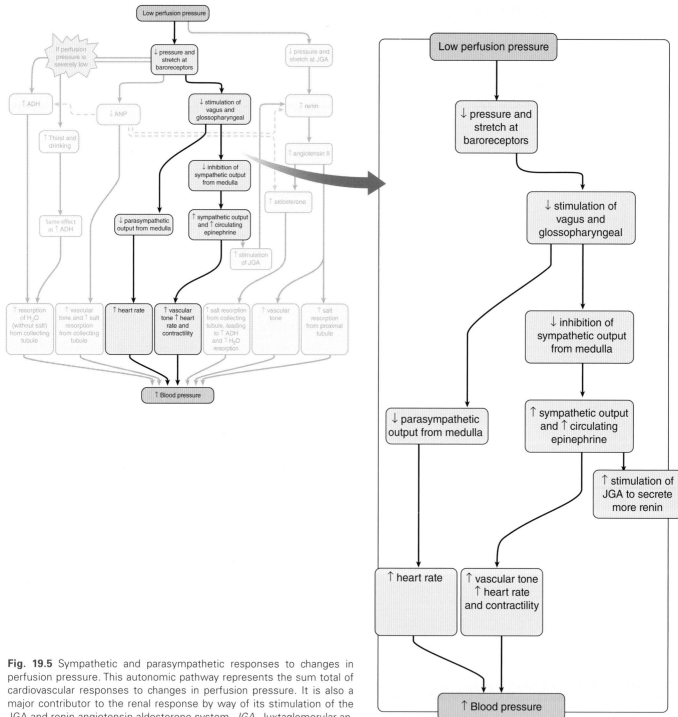

Fig. 19.5 Sympathetic and parasympathetic responses to changes in perfusion pressure. This autonomic pathway represents the sum total of cardiovascular responses to changes in perfusion pressure. It is also a major contributor to the renal response by way of its stimulation of the JGA and renin-angiotensin-aldosterone system. *JGA,* Juxtaglomerular apparatus.

The atrial baroreceptor, in addition to transmitting information via the autonomic nerves, also secretes the hormone ANP.

- ANP is secreted in response to high perfusion pressure.
- ANP acts to decrease the blood volume by means that will be discussed later, and decreases systemic vascular resistance (SVR), thereby lowering BP.
- Fig. 19.8 summarizes the role of ANP in responding to changes in perfusion pressure.

Finally, ADH is secreted from the posterior pituitary as an agent of efferent transmission.

- The baroreceptors send signals directly to ADH secretory cells in the posterior pituitary gland. This process is known as baroreceptor control of ADH, in contrast with osmoreceptor control of ADH, the usual mode of ADH control.
- Normally, the role of ADH is in connection with regulating plasma osmolality (see Ch. 20).
  - When plasma osmolality is high, ADH acts at the kidney to promote the reabsorption of water without solute,

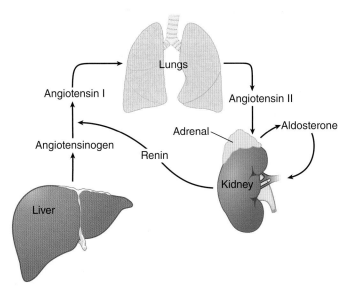

Fig. 19.6 Components of the renin-angiotensin-aldosterone system. The liver produces angiotensinogen to maintain a constant level of it in the bloodstream. The liver does not participate in the homeostatic response to changes in perfusion pressure.

thereby reducing the plasma osmolality. In severe blood volume depletion, however, the baroreceptors stimulate ADH secretion (Fig. 19.9).
- The baroreceptor system is less sensitive than the osmoreceptor system for ADH secretion, and the baroreceptors require a 5% to 10% reduction in BP before inducing ADH secretion.
- Once the less sensitive baroreceptor control of ADH is activated, however, baroreceptor control overrides osmoreceptor control. In the case when large volumes of water are ingested at a time of extreme hypotension, the baroreceptor-mediated increase in ADH predominates over the osmoreceptor-mediated decrease. The result is water retention and a low body fluid osmolality until the intravascular volume is replenished (see Clinical Correlation Box 19.5).

Not only does reduced aortic arch and carotid sinus baroreceptor stimulation lead to the hypothalamic production of ADH; it also contributes to the thirst response, which will be described in more detail in Chapter 20 (see Fast Fact Box 19.2).

Fast Fact Box 19.2

Baroreceptor input to the hypothalamus can reduce the hypothalamic set point for osmotic antidiuretic hormone (ADH) secretion. The consequence is that in hypotensive patients, lower levels of plasma osmolality will stimulate ADH, and, in fact, such patients may become severely hyponatremic.

Effector Mechanisms in Regulation of Perfusion Pressure

Once a change in perfusion pressure has been sensed and the control center has sent out a signal along the efferent pathways, effector mechanisms return the perfusion pressure to its desired level. The effectors are best discussed by grouping them under the efferent pathway that triggers them.

Sympathetic Nervous System

The sympathetic nerves convey signals to the heart and arterioles throughout the body, and also indirectly stimulate angiotensin II through sympathetic stimulation of the JGA.
- Sympathetic constriction of vascular beds throughout the body increases SVR and raises BP. (See Ch. 4 for more information on how increased SVR affects BP.)
- This is achieved via synaptic secretion of norepinephrine onto blood vessels, as well as the adrenal medulla to produce circulating epinephrine.

It should be noted, however, that arterioles supplying active skeletal muscle beds do not constrict. When exercised, active muscle, in fact, produces local vasodilation and blood flow increases to the active muscle. This is because local vasodilating metabolites override the sympathetic vasoconstriction.
- Resting muscle during exercise maintains vasoconstrictor tone, allowing active muscle to receive greater blood flow.

Clinical Correlation Box 19.5

The Effect of an Angiotensin-Converting Enzyme Inhibitor on a Patient With Volume Depletion

A 59-year-old man has congestive heart failure, and his medications include an angiotensin-converting enzyme (ACE) inhibitor. He was doing well until he developed severe diarrhea after dining at an all-you-can-eat buffet. He presented to his primary care physician, having lost 10 pounds in 2 days. His diarrhea is resolving, but he is concerned because he has not urinated since the previous day. On examination, his oral mucosa is dry, his skin turgor is poor, and he has orthostatic hypotension, all of which are physical signs of volume depletion.

He is admitted to the hospital for rehydration and further management. His admission serum creatinine is 3 mg/dL, which is elevated from his baseline of 1 mg/dL. He is rehydrated with intravenous fluids, and his ACE inhibitor is stopped. Over the next several days, his weight returns to his baseline, his urine output increases, and his serum creatinine decreases to 1.5 mg/dL.

This scenario illustrates the importance of the renin-angiotensin system in maintaining adequate glomerular filtration rate (GFR) in a state of volume depletion. ACE inhibitors block the formation of angiotensin II and therefore block the blood pressure-raising effects of angiotensin II. ACE inhibitors also block angiotensin II's ability to preserve GFR in face of decreased renal plasma flow. The patient's diarrhea-induced volume depletion would normally trigger an increase in the level of angiotensin II, but his ACE inhibitor prevents that. Consequently, he cannot as effectively restore lost blood volume and his GFR is not preserved in the event of decreased renal blood flow. Urine output falls and serum creatinine rises, although he has no glomerular or tubular damage. Once the ACE inhibitor is stopped, his renin-angiotensin system can respond appropriately, and with rehydration, his kidney function returns to normal.

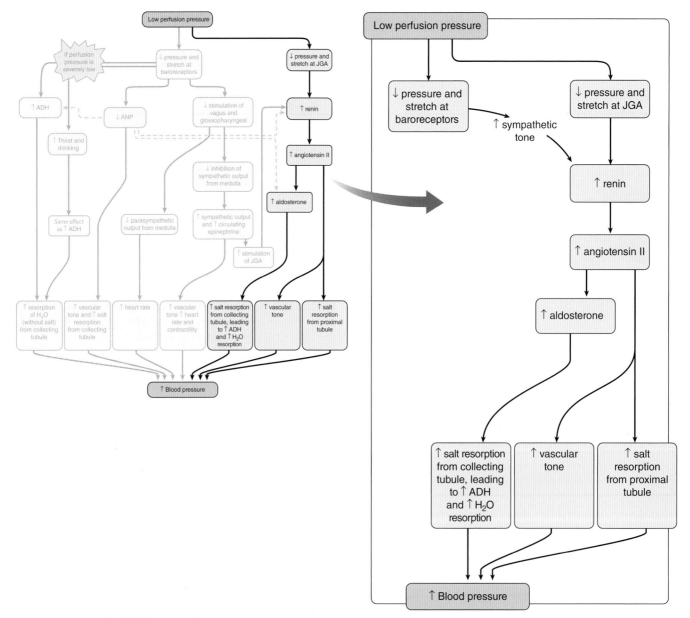

Fig. 19.7 The role of the renin-angiotensin-aldosterone system in response to changes in perfusion pressure. *ADH*, Antidiuretic hormone; *JGA*, juxtaglomerular apparatus.

• Thereby, sympathetic vasoconstriction does not impede muscular action during the "fight-or-flight" response.

Constriction of the afferent and efferent arterioles at the kidney nephrons has special consequences, as this leads to decreased renal blood flow (RBF), which reduces the glomerular filtration rate (GFR). In turn, decreased GFR means a slightly higher percentage of plasma volume and salt is retained in the blood vessels. However, this is not the most important determinant of ECF volume—tubular reabsorption of salt far exceeds filtration in importance.

At the heart, sympathetic stimulation increases the heart rate and contractility, which increases stroke volume.

Stroke volume × heart rate (HR) = cardiac output (CO)

Increased CO means increased BP, according to the Ohm's law analogy. When perfusion pressure is low and sympathetic tone is high, parasympathetic tone is conversely low, lessening the inhibition of the heart rate.

Angiotensin II

The RAA system controls BP via the arterioles and renal tubules.

• When low perfusion pressure stimulates the JGA, renin is released, yielding angiotensin II and aldosterone, as described previously (see Fig. 19.6).
• Angiotensin II has two direct effects on perfusion pressure:
  • It acts as a vasoconstrictor on arterioles throughout the body, raising the SVR.

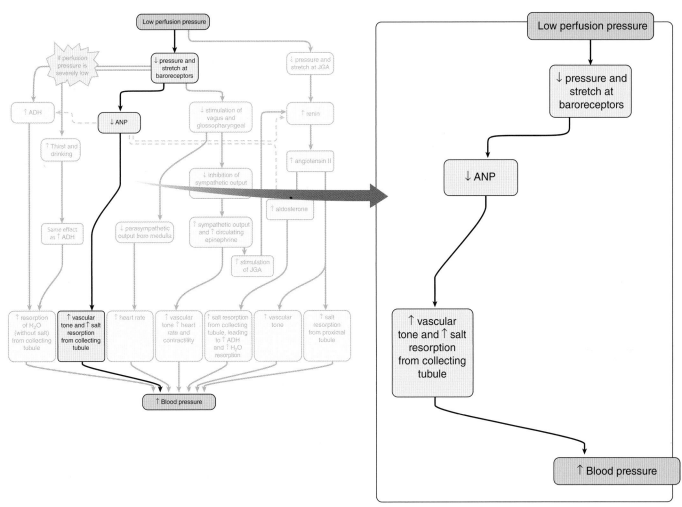

Fig. 19.8 The role of atrial natriuretic peptide (*ANP*) in response to changes in perfusion pressure.

- It stimulates increased salt reabsorption in the proximal tubule.

Furthermore, angiotensin II is part of the autoregulatory machinery that preserves GFR even as the renal blood flow is reduced.

- Angiotensin II raises efferent arteriolar resistance more than afferent, maintaining the hydrostatic pressure in the glomerulus to preserve filtration. Absolute glomerular filtration may not be increased, but does fall in proportion to renal blood flow (Fig. 19.10):
  - This varied effect on afferent versus efferent arteriole may be caused by differences in type of AII receptors or receptor densities.
  - Alternatively, this may be caused by difference in arteriolar lumen size at baseline. The efferent arteriole is smaller, so when vessels constrict because of angiotensin II, the same percent change in radius yields a greater increase in the resistance of the efferent arteriole. (Recall, the Poiseuille relationship in which resistance is inversely proportional to the radius to the fourth power (Fig. 19.11).

- Efferent arteriolar constriction not only preserves GFR but also augments fluid reabsorption into the peritubular capillaries by two mechanisms (Fig. 19.12):
  - Lowering the hydrostatic pressure in the peritubular capillary.
  - Because the filtration fraction has gone up, the oncotic pressure in the peritubular capillaries is greater, because a greater proportion of protein-free filtrate has been removed at the glomeruli.

How Angiotensin II Expands Extracellular Fluid Volume

To understand how angiotensin II acts to increase salt reabsorption in the proximal tubule to expand the ECF volume, we must first understand the features of the proximal tubule wall and its contents.

- The proximal tubule wall is permeable to water and salt and contains basolateral Na^+,K^+-ATPase pumps that drive Na^+ reabsorption (Fig. 19.13).
- The proximal tubule contents are isotonic to plasma, because the glomerulus filters solution isotonic to plasma.
- Therefore when the proximal tubule pumps Na^+ out of the tubule lumen and into the interstitium, water passively follows by

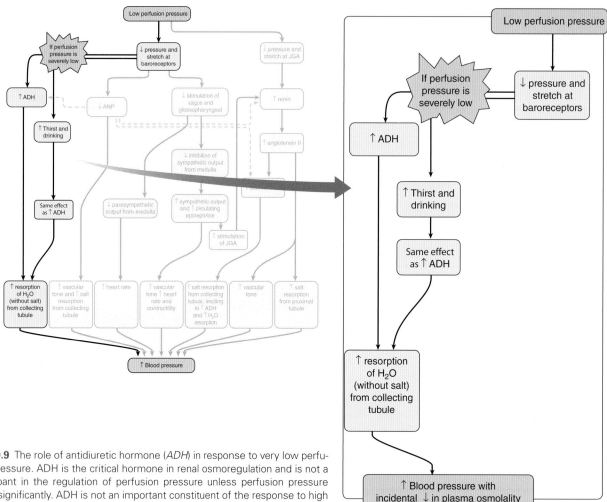

Fig. 19.9 The role of antidiuretic hormone (*ADH*) in response to very low perfusion pressure. ADH is the critical hormone in renal osmoregulation and is not a participant in the regulation of perfusion pressure unless perfusion pressure drops significantly. ADH is not an important constituent of the response to high perfusion pressure.

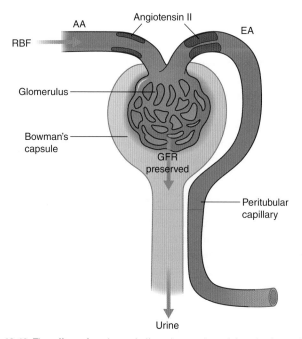

Fig. 19.10 The effect of angiotensin II on the renal arterioles. Angiotensin II decreases renal blood flow while preserving glomerular filtration rate. *AA,* Afferent arteriole; *EA,* efferent arteriole; *GFR,* glomerular filtration rate; *RBF,* renal blood flow.

osmosis, and a saltwater solution isotonic to plasma is reabsorbed and added back to the plasma of the peritubular capillary.

Why is it important that the kidney adds isotonic fluid back to the bloodstream in its efforts to boost ECF volume?

- If it added hypotonic fluid, much of the added fluid would osmotically redistribute into the ICF space, thus failing to raise ECF volume as much.

Why is it important that the proximal tubule reabsorb an isotonic sodium salt solution?

- Na^+ is the major effective osmole in the ECF space. The proximal tubule reabsorbs K^+ in proportion to Na^+, but because reabsorbed Na^+ stays in the ECF space as an effective osmole, the water (and hence, the volume) stays in the ECF space.

Given the information in the previous paragraph, we should not be surprised that when angiotensin II prompts increased activity of the apical Na^+/H^+ antiporter, the ECF expands. Increased activity of the Na^+/H^+ antiporter drives more Na^+ into the cell, in turn driving more Na^+ across the basolateral membrane by the Na^+,K^+-ATPase—that is, driving more salt reabsorption—and adding more isotonic fluid to the ECF space.

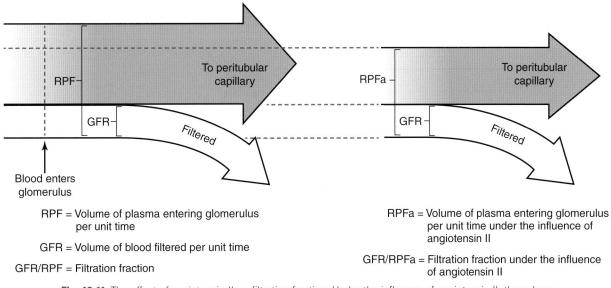

RPF = Volume of plasma entering glomerulus
per unit time

GFR = Volume of blood filtered per unit time

GFR/RPF = Filtration fraction

RPFa = Volume of plasma entering glomerulus
per unit time under the influence of
angiotensin II

GFR/RPFa = Filtration fraction under the influence
of angiotensin II

Fig. 19.11 The effect of angiotensin II on filtration fraction. Under the influence of angiotensin II, the volume of plasma entering the glomerulus per unit time falls while the glomerular filtration rate (*GFR*) remains roughly the same. Therefore GFR/RPF$_a$ > GFR/RPF; the filtration fraction rises under the influence of angiotensin II. RPF = renal plasma flow.

The Indirect Effects of Angiotensin II on Perfusion Pressure

In addition, angiotensin II has two indirect effects on perfusion pressure:
- Stimulates aldosterone secretion from the adrenal gland, and, alongside the baroreceptor control of ADH.
- Stimulates the secretion of ADH at very low blood volumes.

The Effects of Aldosterone

Aldosterone controls BP via the principal cells of the cortical collecting tubule (Fig. 19.14A):
- It transduces its signal like all steroids, by binding to an intracellular receptor that turns on protein synthesis.
- Aldosterone triggers protein synthesis that yields more Na$^+$,K$^+$-ATPase and more Na$^+$ channels, increasing salt reabsorption. As

in the proximal tubule, the reabsorption of salt leads to expansion of the ECF volume.

The expansion caused by aldosterone action is not a simple case of adding isotonic saline solution to the ECF, however. Fluid in the collecting duct is not isotonic to plasma, and the collecting duct is not permeable to water unless ADH is present.
- Aldosterone may prompt the reabsorption of Na$^+$ without water, and the water may follow only after osmoreceptors in the brain have detected an increase in osmolality and prompted the secretion of ADH.
- Then, water can be osmotically reabsorbed after the salt, producing a net effect of salt, water, and hence volume addition to the ECF (Fig. 19.14B). (See Physiology Integration Box 19.1, Development Box 19.2, Pharmacology Box 19.2, and Genetics Box 19.2).

Physiology Integration Box 19.1

How Aldosterone Links Extracellular Fluid Volume, K$^+$, and H$^+$ Balance

In addition to its effects on extracellular fluid (ECF) volume, aldosterone governs K$^+$ balance and affects acid-base balance. As aldosterone upregulates the activity of the Na$^+$,K$^+$-ATPase to pump Na$^+$ into the interstitium from the tubule lumen, it concurrently pumps K$^+$ from the blood and interstitium into the lumen for excretion. Not only does this occur as an incidental result of efforts to restore ECF volume, the adrenal gland actually senses the plasma [K$^+$] and releases aldosterone in response to high [K$^+$]. Aldosterone also has an effect on acid excretion because it stimulates the activity of the H$^+$-ATPase in the intercalated cells of the collecting duct thereby increasing acid excretion in urine. As a result of these multiple roles, ECF volume status, K$^+$ balance, and acid-base balance are interrelated. Decreases in perfusion pressure that prompt the release of aldosterone may also drive down the plasma [K$^+$] and raise the plasma pH. (The latter situation is sometimes called a contraction

alkalosis because contracted ECF volume drives aldosterone release and consequent H$^+$ excretion.) Increases in [K$^+$] that prompt the release of aldosterone may promote salt reabsorption and volume expansion,

Why should one hormone, aldosterone, participate in more than one homeostatic system? One possible reason is that this situation creates negative feedback to avoid either too much volume expansion or too much K$^+$ secretion. When a lot of volume has been retained, the zona glomerulosa of the adrenal gland will sense low [K$^+$] and scale down its production of aldosterone, preventing further volume expansion and hypokalemia. Both the homeostatic system governing ECF volume and that governing [K$^+$] use other, more important, sources of negative feedback; however, the body typically involves redundant systems as backup mechanisms. We will discuss potassium and ECF volume homeostasis in greater detail in Chapter 21.

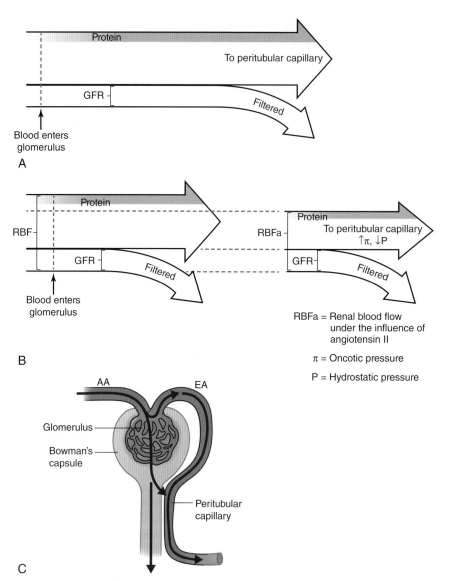

Fig. 19.12 The impact of increased filtration fraction on peritubular reabsorption. A, The oncotic pressure goes up in the postfiltration fluid of the efferent arteriole. Owing to the lower fluid volume in the efferent fluid, there is also less hydrostatic pressure. B, Increased filtration fraction under the influence of angiotensin II results in an even higher oncotic pressure in the efferent peritubular fluid. C, This increased peritubular oncotic pressure and decreased hydrostatic pressure under the influence of angiotensin II means that there will be more fluid reabsorption by the peritubular capillary. *AA,* Afferent arteriole; *EA,* efferent arteriole; *GFR,* glomerular filtration rate.

DEVELOPMENT BOX 19.1

Patients with Liddle syndrome often present with hypertension as children. As it recapitulates aspects of hyperaldosteronism, affected individuals may also have hypokalemia and metabolic alkalosis. The most serious complications of unrecognized or untreated hypertension are cardiac and cerebrovascular disease, such as myocardial infarction and stroke. Patients have low plasma renin and aldosterone levels as negative feedback loops try to compensate for the excess collecting duct cell membrane epithelial sodium channels (ENaCs).

GENETICS BOX 19.1

Liddle syndrome is an autosomal dominant familial hypertension caused by mutations in the SCNN1B or SCNN1G genes. These genes encode the β and γ chains of the aldosterone regulated epithelial sodium channel (ENaC) in collecting duct cells. Normally, ENaC is removed from cell membrane when aldosterone concentrations decrease, but mutations in the β or γ chains can disrupt this removal process, leading to persistent, high concentrations of ENaC and thus Na$^+$ resorption, extracellular fluid expansion, and hypertension.

Atrial Natriuretic Peptide

ANP and BNP both act to reduce BP. They achieve salt excretion in three ways:

- Directly inhibit salt reabsorption in the collecting duct
- Inhibit the release of aldosterone from the adrenal gland
- Inhibit renin release from the JGA

PHARMACOLOGY BOX 19.1

Patients with Liddle syndrome can be treated with the potassium-sparing diuretics triamterene or amiloride, which antagonize the epithelial sodium channel (ENaC).

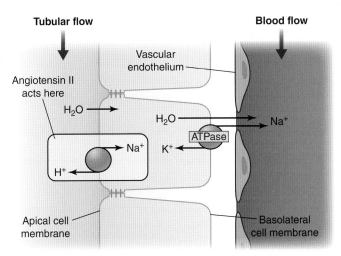

Fig. 19.13 Angiotensin II action in the proximal tubule. Angiotensin II increases the activity of the apical Na^+/H^+ antiporter. *ATPase,* Adenosine triphosphatase.

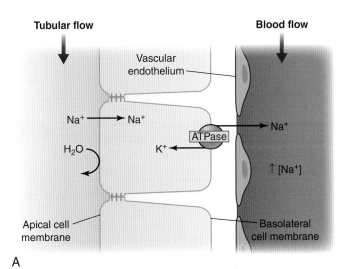

A

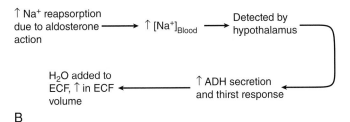

B

Fig. 19.14 Aldosterone action in the cortical collecting duct. A, Aldosterone increases the number of Na^+,K^+-ATPases on the basolateral membrane and the number of Na^+ channels on the apical side. Water cannot directly follow salt here. B, Aldosterone mediated increases in Na^+ reabsorption alter osmolality and lead to antidiuretic hormone (*ADH*) secretion. Aldosterone can raise the extracellular fluid volume only through ADH secretion. *ATPase,* Adenosine triphosphatase; *ECF,* extracellular fluid.

Decreasing salt absorption from the tubule increases the percentage of the filtered volume that is lost to urine, and therefore leads to reduced ECF volume.

Furthermore, ANP and BNP also reduce perfusion pressure in the following mechanisms:

- Promote the loss of water without salt to some degree, by inhibiting the secretion of ADH from the posterior pituitary and inhibiting ADH action on the collecting duct.
- Act on the arterioles throughout the body to vasodilate, thus lowering systemic vascular resistance.
- Reduce ECF volume in concert with the lowering of sympathetic tone and the reduction of renin output.

Antidiuretic Hormone

ADH controls BP via the collecting duct in the nephron.

- ADH promotes water reabsorption without solute by binding to a G-protein coupled receptor, using cyclic adenosine monophosphate as a second messenger and inserts water channels (aquaporin-2) into the apical membrane. (See Ch. 20).
- Adding pure water to the ECF is not as effective as adding isotonic saline; furthermore, under normal circumstances, the body deploys ADH to lower plasma osmolality and not to correct low perfusion pressure.

ADH secretion in response to baroreceptor stimulation is a type of last resort for raising perfusion pressure in very low volume states (see Fast Fact Box 19.3).

Fast Fact Box 19.3

At very high levels, antidiuretic hormone also has a systemic vasoconstrictive effect, which accounts for its alternate name, vasopressin. In fact, vasopressin infusions are used clinically to raise blood pressure in critically ill patients with hypotension.

Other Mediators of Perfusion Pressure

The majority of perfusion pressure regulation is achieved via the sympathetic nerves, the RAA system, ANP, BNP, and ADH. However, there are other mediators that are not involved with the homeostatic response to changes in BP, but can nonetheless have dramatic effects on BP.

- Cortisol potentiates the constrictive action of catecholamines, decreases the permeability of the vascular endothelium to keep fluid inside the vascular tree, and enhances myocardial function.
  - Cortisol generates a constant level of vessel tone, and, once again, does not respond to changes in BP.
- Estrogen has a number of less critical effects on BP. It is thought to raise BP by increasing salt retention and RAA activity from an increased production of angiotensinogen and to have a vasodilatory effect through the stimulation of nitric oxide (NO) synthase.

In addition to the systemically acting mediators, there are vasoactive mediators produced by endothelial cells that act locally.

- Mediators acting at their site of origin are called autocrine.
- Mediators acting near their site of origin are called paracrine.

In response to a variety of stimuli, endothelial cells produce vasodilators, such as NO and prostaglandin, and vasoconstrictors, such as endothelin.

- NO's potent vasodilatory effect works through a cyclic guanosine monophosphate mechanism. Many vascular beds can synthesize NO locally for regulation of blood flow.
- The vasodilatory effects of some prostaglandins serve to dampen the response to low perfusion pressure.

Table 19.1 summarizes key regulators of renal blood flow and tubular transport.

PATHOPHYSIOLOGY

Dietary variations in salt and water intake produce daily fluctuations in ECF volume. These fluctuations must be corrected to keep ECF volume high enough for adequate perfusion and to keep ECF volume low enough to avoid edema and hypertensive complications.

Normally, the kidneys can handle these fluctuations in salt and water intake without difficulty. In fact, on average, Americans consume more than 20 times the salt they need every day, and the majority stay free of hypertension, as long as they have normal renal function. Various conditions may either overwhelm or impair the kidney's ability to maintain normal ECF volume, however.

Although this chapter discussed homeostatic regulation of BP in general, the pathophysiology section is limited to derangements of fluid volume. It does not discuss the very important topic of essential hypertension—that is, hypertension at normal fluid volumes.

Disorders of Extracellular Fluid Volume

There are three main types of disorders of ECF volume:

- Hypovolemia with low intravascular volume and therefore low perfusion pressure.
- Hypervolemia with normal or high intravascular volume and therefore high perfusion pressure.
- Hypervolemia with low intravascular volume and therefore low perfusion pressure (Table 19.2).

Hypovolemia with high perfusion pressure is infrequent, but in cases of malignant hypertension (extreme hypertension caused by factors other than ECF volume), hypovolemia and hypertension may be seen together.

Hypovolemia

Causes of hypovolemia, or low ECF volume, include:

- Hemorrhage
- Vomiting
- Diarrhea
- Poor fluid intake
- Many conditions that lead to polyuria (diabetes mellitus, diabetes insipidus, iatrogenic overtreatment with diuretics, and hypercalcemia)

TABLE 19.1	**Physiologic and Pharmacologic Influences on Glomerular Hemodynamics**					
	ARTERIOLAR RESISTANCE		Renal Blood	Net Ultrafiltration		
	Afferent	Efferent	Flow	Pressure	K_{uf}	GFR
Renal sympathetic nerves	↑↑	↑	↓	↓	↓	↓
Hormonal physiologic influences in normal circumstances						
Epinephrine	↑	↑	↓	→	?	↓
Angiotensin II	↑	↑↑	↓	↑	↓	↓→
ANP (high dose)	↓	→	↑	↑	↑	↑
Autocrine and paracrine mediators						
Adenosine endothelin-1	↑	↑↑	↓	↑	↓	↓
Nitric oxide	↓	↓	↑	?	↑	↑ (?)
PGE₂/PGI₂	↓	↓ (?)	↑	↑	?	↑
Diet						
High-protein diet	↓	→	↑	↑	→	↑
Drugs						
Cyclosporine	↑	→	↓	↓	?	↑
NSAIDs	↑↑	↑	↓	↓	?	↓
Calcium-channel blockers	↓	→	↑	↑	?	↑
ACE inhibitors/ARBs	↓	↓↓	↑	↓	↑	?[a]

[a]In clinical practice, GFR is usually either decreased or unaffected.
The overall effect on glomerular filtration rate (GFR) will depend on renal blood flow, net ultrafiltration pressure, and the ultrafiltration coefficient (K_{uf}), which is controlled by mesangial cell contraction and relaxation. The effects shown are those seen when the agents are applied (or inhibited) in isolation; the actual changes that occur are dose dependent and are modulated by other agents. Effectors like hypoxemia, angiotensin II, and hypercalcemia can constrict mesangial cells within the glomerular tuft, decreasing the surface area for filtration and therefore the K_{uf} and GFR.
ACE, Angiotensin-converting enzyme; *ANP*, atrial natriuretic peptide; *ARBs*, angiotensin receptor blockers; *NSAIDs*, nonsteroidal antiinflammatory drugs; *PGE 2/PGI 2*, prostaglandins E 2 and I 2.
(From Bailey MA, Unwin RJ. Renal physiology. In: *Comprehensive Clinical Nephrology*, 2nd Edition. p. 14-28.e1. Table 2.1.)

TABLE 19.2 Disorders of Extracellular Fluid Volume

Disorders	Causes
Hypovolemia	Hemorrhage
	Vomiting
	Diarrhea
	Poor fluid intake
	Polyuria
	Diabetes mellitus
	Diabetes insipidus
	Iatrogenic overtreatment with diuretics
	Hypercalcemia
Hypervolemia with normal or high perfusion pressure	Advanced renal failure
	Nephrotic syndrome
Hypervolemia with low perfusion pressure	Congestive heart failure
	Nephrotic syndrome with severe proteinuria

In these situations, the baroreceptors sense low perfusion pressure, which leads to increased sympathetic tone and renin secretion as the body attempts to reverse the low BP.

Signs and symptoms of hypovolemia may include:
- Dry mucous membranes (e.g., lips)
- Fainting (syncope)
- Orthostatic hypotension
- Elevated blood urea nitrogen (BUN)/creatinine (Cr) ratio

All of these signs and symptoms reflect inadequate perfusion; in syncope, it is a case of poor perfusion of the brain (see Clinical Correlation Box 19.6 and Clinical Correlation Box 19.7).

Clinical Correlation Box 19.6

In people with hypovolemia, venous return to the heart drops when they change from a sitting or lying position to a standing position. The drop in venous return to the heart causes a decrease in blood pressure and a compensatory rise in heart rate (tachycardia). Measuring blood pressure and heart rate in the supine position and then in the standing position (sometimes referred to in the hospital as performing "orthostatics") is often a part of assessing a patient with syncope.

Clinical Correlation Box 19.7

The Vasovagal Response

People with no disturbance of their extracellular fluid volume can faint from low blood pressure, too. In the vasovagal response, anxiety may trigger vigorous sympathetic-mediated ventricular contraction leading to parasympathetic output, which decreases cardiac output and causes syncope. Micturition syncope is another form of vasovagal response. In this case, the parasympathetic output associated with urination decreases cardiac output and causes syncope.

The elevated BUN/Cr ratio in hypovolemia reflects the way that urea and creatinine are cleared from the blood.
- Creatinine is filtered, but not reabsorbed and secreted only to a small extent.
- Urea is filtered and reabsorbed.

- The increased tubular reabsorption of fluid associated with hypovolemia (affected by the mechanisms described previously) increases the reabsorption of urea in the proximal tubule and medullary collecting duct, but not that of creatinine. Hypovolemia (decreased ECV) with poor renal perfusion is one cause of acute kidney injury. An elevated BUN/Cr ratio (usually >20:1) is sometimes called a "prerenal" condition. As discussed in Chapter 17:
- "Prerenal failure" refers to disturbances in renal perfusion, characterized by oliguria, decreased excretion rates of sodium and water, and production of urine concentration greater than plasma.
- "Intrarenal failure" indicate damage to the kidneys
- "Postrenal failure" is caused by problems with urinary outflow, usually because of obstruction. These terms refer to anatomic location of the disturbances, not different stages of renal failure.

Hypervolemia With Normal or High Perfusion Pressure

Hypervolemia is high ECF volume. Diseases that significantly decrease renal Na^+ excretion lead to significant water retention, hypervolemia, and generalized edema. The two major examples are advanced renal failure and many cases of nephrotic syndrome.
- In advanced renal failure when the GFR is very low, little salt and water are delivered to the tubule to allow excretion.
- Nephrotic syndrome refers to a group of disorders that increase glomerular permeability to protein. For reasons not well understood, an increase in collecting duct reabsorption of salt is associated with the nephrotic syndrome, which expands the ECF volume.

When salt and water retention expand the ECF volume, the hydrostatic pressure created in the capillaries by the volume expansion leads to leakage from the capillaries into the interstitium. This is generalized edema, a general swelling of the tissues (see Clinical Correlation Box 19.8 and Clinical Correlation Box 19.9).

Clinical Correlation Box 19.8

What Is Nephrotic Syndrome?

A 15-year-old boy goes to see the pediatrician with a complaint of swelling around the ankles of several months' duration. Aside from some pitting edema of the lower extremities, he has a normal physical exam and a blood pressure of 130/80 mm Hg. Lab tests reveal 3.5 g of albumin in the 24-hour urine (normally <30 mg per day) and a low serum albumin of 3.0 g/dL (normal is 3.5–5 g/dL). The pediatrician suspects nephrotic syndrome.

Nephrotic syndrome is caused by damage to the glomerulus and is characterized clinically by heavy proteinuria, hypoalbuminemia, and edema. The most common underlying pathology in children is minimal change disease (so called because the damage to the glomeruli cannot be visualized under light microscopy), but this disease also affects adults. Other causes include focal and segmental glomerular sclerosis, membranous glomerulonephritis, diabetic nephropathy, amyloidosis, and preeclampsia. In these conditions, the glomerulus becomes permeable to protein macromolecules. Damage to the renal tubule leads to salt retention and hence edema. When the hypoalbuminemia associated with the disease is more severe, the oncotic gradient decreases between the intravascular space and the interstitium, promoting more edema. Minimal change disease responds very well to treatment with glucocorticoids and rarely progresses to renal failure.

As explained in the text, some cases of nephrotic syndrome lead to hypervolemia with high perfusion pressure, and some lead to hypervolemia with low perfusion pressure. When should we expect normal or high pressure with edema from salt and water retention (overflow edema), and when should we expect normal or low pressure with edema from proteinuria and low oncotic pressure (edema from underfilling of the vasculature)?

When hypoalbuminemia is less severe, we should expect to see hypervolemia with high intravascular volume and pressure. Even though proteinuria has decreased the intravascular oncotic pressure, why does the oncotic pressure gradient not favor extravasation of fluid from the vessels? The hypoalbuminemia has caused the oncotic pressure of the interstitium to drop in proportion to that of the vessels. Remember that it is the oncotic pressure of the vessels relative to the interstitium, the oncotic gradient, which drives the movement of fluid. In this case, there is no oncotic gradient.

When the hypoalbuminemia becomes more severe (e.g., <2.5 g/dL), however, the oncotic pressure gradient does begin to favor extravasation of fluid. The protein level of the interstitium reaches a minimum below which it cannot sink. As the intravascular protein level continues to fall, its oncotic pressure falls relative to the interstitial oncotic pressure. The vessels lose fluid to the interstitium, creating edema from underfilling of the vascular space, and as in cirrhosis and congestive heart failure, hypervolemia with low pressure ensues. The baroreceptors worsen the problem by signaling the kidneys to hold onto more salt and fluid, which is immediately third spaced.

Hypervolemia With Low Perfusion Pressure

In some states of increased ECF volume (often referred to clinically as volume-expanded states), the volume and pressure in the arterial system may be low. Important examples are congestive heart failure (CHF), cirrhosis, and severe nephrotic syndrome.

- In CHF, the heart's failure to pump blood from the low-pressure veins into the higher-pressure arteries leads to venous pooling. Hydrostatic pressure builds in the veins and fluid leaks from the veins into the interstitium, causing edema.
- In cirrhosis (liver failure), the liver's failure to produce albumin lowers the oncotic pressure of the plasma, and fluid is lost from the intravascular space to the interstitium. Also,

scarring in the liver obstructs the passage of plasma through the portal venous system. Hydrostatic pressure builds in the liver and in the portal system (portal hypertension), and fluid leaks into the peritoneum. The accumulation of fluid here is known as ascites.

- In severe cases of nephrotic syndrome, the loss of albumin (the major protein in blood) to the urine from damaged glomeruli may also lower oncotic pressure and cause a loss of fluid to the interstitium, leading to generalized edema with low perfusion pressure.

When fluid builds up in the ECF space but outside of the vasculature, clinicians sometimes call this third-spacing because the fluid is not in the vessels and not in the cells, but in a third space—the interstitium, or a potential space similar to the peritoneum that is not normally filled with fluid.

- When a large amount of ECF is sequestered in a third space and the intravascular volume and BP are low, the baroreceptors cause more salt and water reabsorption. Much of the added fluid is merely lost to the third space, however, worsening the edema and/or ascites.
- In the supine position during sleep, fluid accumulated in the lower extremities returns to the vasculature (increased venous return) and transiently decreases the salt and water retaining neurohumeral effectors and together with the improved renal perfusion pressure, increases salt and water excretion.

Why is interstitial swelling (third-spacing) a problem?
- First, third-spacing means fluid is being lost from the intravascular volume, and the patient may be hypotensive.
- Second, third-spacing leads to organ dysfunction.
  - Congestion in the lungs—pulmonary edema—compromises respiratory function.
  - Congestion of the liver farther down the venous circuit can lead to liver dysfunction.
  - Generalized edema is also extremely uncomfortable, as is ascites, and the ascites fluid can become infected.

The BUN/Cr ratio will also be elevated in hypervolemia with low perfusion pressure. This is because the BUN/Cr ratio reflects the adequacy of kidney perfusion rather than reflecting the ECF volume.

SUMMARY

- The volume of the ECF is controlled by the renal handling of Na^+.
- The cardiovascular and renal organ systems together accomplish the baroreceptor reflex, which ensures BP homeostasis.
- In response to baroreceptor detection of changes in perfusion pressure, the cardiovascular organ system alters SVR and CO through the autonomic nervous system.
- In response to baroreceptor detection of changes in perfusion pressure, the renal organ system alters SVR through the RAA system, and alters ECF volume (which in turn alters CO) through the RAA system, ANP, BNP, and ADH.
- The sensors of perfusion pressure are the baroreceptors and JGA.
- The afferent pathways of transmission are the vagus and glossopharyngeal cranial nerves.

- The control centers are the medulla and JGA.
- The efferent pathways of transmission are the neural and hormonal activation of effectors— sympathetic nerves, circulating epinephrine and parasympathetic nerves, RAA system, ANP, BNP, and ADH.
- The effectors in the regulation of perfusion pressure are the systemic arterioles, the heart, and the salt-reabsorbing elements in the nephron tubule.
- A wide array of other mediators affects BP without participating directly in its homeostasis. These mediators are important to consider when evaluating derangements in BP.
- Disorders of ECF volume fall into one of three categories: hypovolemia, hypervolemia with normal or high intravascular volume, and hypervolemia with low intravascular volume.

REVIEW QUESTIONS

Directions: Each of the numbered items or incomplete statements in this section is followed by answers or by completions of the statement. Select the one lettered answer or completion that is best in each case.

1. An 84-year-old man is admitted to the intensive care unit with a mean arterial blood pressure of 60 mm Hg and a pulse of 130 beats per minute. A Swann-Ganz catheter is placed, and his cardiac output is determined to be 2 L/min. The right atrial pressure is 20 mm Hg. His total peripheral resistance is:
   A. 20 mm Hg/L per min
   B. 30 mm Hg/L per min
   C. 200 mm Hg/L per min
   D. 300 mm Hg/L per min
   E. 2000 mm Hg/L per min
   F. 3000 mm Hg/L per min

2. A 28-year-old woman is involved in a motor vehicle accident and suffers serious blood loss. With activation of the compensatory mechanisms to maintain her blood pressure, which of the following serum factors is likely to be low?
   A. Natriuretic peptides
   B. Renin
   C. Angiotensin II
   D. Aldosterone
   E. Antidiuretic hormone (ADH)

3. A patient with primary aldosteronism (excess serum concentrations of aldosterone) will have which of the following?
   A. Hypotension (low blood pressure)
   B. Bradycardia (low heart rate)
   C. Hyponatremia (low serum sodium concentration)
   D. Hypokalemia (low serum potassium concentration)
   E. Hypovolemia (low ECF volume)

ANSWERS TO REVIEW QUESTIONS

1. **The answer is A.** Mean systemic blood pressure is the product of the cardiac output (CO) in liters per minute and the systemic vascular resistance (SVR), expressed as a restatement of Ohm's law: SVR = (MAP – RAP)/CO, where MAP = mean arterial pressure (in mm Hg) and RAP = right atrial pressure (in mm Hg). SVR in units of mm Hg/L per min may be converted to a standard unit of measurement of resistance in dynes $\times$ cm^{-5} by multiplying by 80.

   (60 – 20) mm Hg/2 L per min = 20 mm Hg/L per min, or 1600 dynes $\times$ cm^{-5}

   This patient has a low systemic blood pressure and a low cardiac output, consistent with a number of diseases. Because the heart rate (pulse) is elevated and the cardiac output is low, the stroke volume must also be small: (2000 mL/min)/(130 beats/min) = 15.4 mL/beat. The situation reflects profound intravascular volume depletion with an elevated SVR.

2. **The answer is A.** With the rapid loss of ECF (and intravascular) volume from hemorrhage, the baroreceptors throughout the vascular tree signal to the kidneys to conserve volume and to the brain to increase volume intake and maintain blood pressure, respectively. The kidneys activate the RAA system, so all of these factors should increase in concentration. Likewise, the production and release of ADH should increase to: (1) promote thirst so the patient will drink (if able), (2) retain free water at the kidney, and (3) vasoconstrict. (Recall that ADH is also called vasopressin for its vasoconstrictive effects, which increase SVR and, thus, blood pressure.) Concentrations of ANP and BNP, however, should drop because this agent causes the kidneys to decrease sodium reabsorption and decrease ECF volume, which would be maladaptive in these circumstances.

3. **The answer is D.** Excess aldosterone causes the kidney to reabsorb more sodium from the renal tubule than is necessary. Because water follows sodium in this case, the ECF volume increases (hypervolemia, not hypovolemia), and with the increase in intravascular volume, the blood pressure increases (hypertension, not hypotension). A typical cardiac response to hypervolemia is an increase in heart rate (tachycardia, not bradycardia). The serum sodium does not drop profoundly unless extenuating circumstances (such as increased free water intake) intervene, but aldosterone causes the kidney to save sodium by exchanging it for potassium. Thus, the kidneys excrete large amounts of potassium, and the serum potassium drops (hypokalemia).

20

Osmoregulation

INTRODUCTION

Osmolality (or concentration of the solutes in the body fluids) is critical to organ function and must be closely regulated.
- Disturbances in the osmolality of the body fluids arise from the gain or loss of water, or from the gain or loss of osmoles (glucose, urea, salts).
- Accordingly, normal plasma osmolality is restored by:
  - Excretion of extra water
  - Replenishment of lost water
  - Restoration of normal amounts of solutes in the body

SYSTEM STRUCTURE: BODY FLUID COMPARTMENTS

Osmoregulation is coupled to the regulation of perfusion pressure, both of which are affected by shifts between the body's fluid compartments. Instead of modulating the volume of the extracellular fluid (ECF) through variations in Na^+ reabsorption, however, the osmoregulatory apparatus modulates the Na^+ *i* the ECF by varying the amount of water within the total body water space. For the purposes of osmoregulation, the total body water is the compartment of interest, because water can freely move between cells and the ECF (see Fast Fact Box 20.1).

Fast Fact Box 20.1
Recall that in the adult, approximately 50% to 60% of body weight is water and that two-thirds of the water is within cells (the intracellular water), whereas one-third is in the extracellular fluid (ECF). The plasma volume is 1/4 of the ECF and is the most important determinant of blood pressure.

The anatomic elements that constitute the homeostatic feedback loop are fewer than those in the loop that controls ECF volume and blood pressure. The organs involved in osmoregulation are the brain and the kidney, and to a lesser extent, the intestines and the circulatory system, which act as conduits.

SYSTEM FUNCTION: HOMEOSTASIS OF SODIUM CONCENTRATION

Before detailing the governance of Na^+ concentration, it is first necessary to establish the physiologic importance of a stable Na^+ concentration and the challenges to the stability of plasma $[Na^+]$. To do that, we should review the concept of osmolality and reexamine the constitution of the body fluid compartments.

Osmolality, Osmosis, and Fluid Shifts Between Body Fluid Compartments

Recall that molarity and molality both describe the concentration of solute in a solution, but in different units of measurement.
- Molarity: the units of molarity are mol solute/L solution. Because volume changes with temperature, molarity is temperature-dependent.
- Molality: the units of molality are mol solute/kg solvent. Molality is independent of temperature because it is relative to mass of solvent (see Fast Fact 20.2).

Fast Fact Box 20.2
Osmolarity and osmolality reflect the number of moles of solute particles in a solution, as opposed to moles of compound in a solution. So, if a solution contained 140 mmol NaCl per 1 kg water, its molality would be 140 mmol/kg. Its *os*molality would be 280 mOsm/kg because we would count the free-floating ions Na^+ and Cl^- separately.

Also recall that osmosis is the diffusion of water (as solvent) across a membrane from an area of low-solute concentration to an area of high-solute concentration (i.e., along a concentration gradient).
- It is a passive process that occurs only in liquids, not gases, and obeys the second law of thermodynamics, the law of entropy.
- The random molecular motion of the water molecules causes them to traverse the membrane in both directions. Molecules starting on the high-solute concentration side of the membrane and moving toward the membrane for crossover are obstructed in their progress by their "sticky" interactions with the excess solute.
- Fewer water molecules make it across from the high-solute concentration side than do molecules from the low-solute concentration side. A net influx of water molecules onto the high-solute concentration side occurs.
- The influx of water from the high-solute concentration side stops when the solute concentrations on each side are equal—that is, when the amount of solute obstructing water efflux is equal on both sides. The rate of efflux is the same on both sides, and osmotic equilibrium is reached.

Osmotic Pressure

The osmolarity or osmolality of the compartments on either side of a membrane is what determines the compartments' osmotic pressure, which is a reflection of how much water that compartment will draw into it through osmosis.

- With 1 mmol/kg of glucose on one side of a membrane and 1 mmol/kg NaCl on the other, water will diffuse into the NaCl side because that side's osmolality is twice as high.
- Osmosis is sensitive to the number of free dissolved particles and does not distinguish between different molecular species like Na^+ and Cl^-.

Effective Osmoles

Note that in the situations considered in the preceding paragraph, the osmoles of solute may or may not be able to cross the membrane. If the osmoles of solute could cross the membrane freely, as water does, the solute would distribute evenly, and there would no longer be a concentration gradient to drive osmosis. Such solutes (e.g., ethanol and urea) are not effective osmoles because they do not create osmotic pressure.

Effective osmoles cannot freely diffuse across membranes; their movement is determined by the presence of pumps and the distribution of channels.

- Examples of effective osmoles are the solutes Na^+, K^+, and Cl^-.
- The pumps and channels keep Na^+ mostly outside of cells and K^+ mostly inside of cells as effective osmoles (see Fig. 1.5) (see Clinical Correlation Box 20.1).

Clinical Correlation Box 20.1

In a diabetic patient, when glucose cannot freely enter cells because of low insulin levels, glucose becomes an effective osmole, attracting water from cells to the extracellular fluid (ECF).

Aquaporins

It is also important to note that just as the body limits the diffusion of solutes, in some cases, it can limit the diffusion of its primary solvent; although water freely crosses most cell membranes in the body, this is not the case universally.

- The default state of the cell membrane is relatively low permeability to water.
  - Recall that the interior of the cell membrane phospholipid bilayer is nonpolar and hydrophobic.
- Consequently, ions can cross membranes only via channels, and a polar molecule like H_2O only crosses the membrane to a limited extent without a channel.
  - The permeability of cells to water is greatly increased by water channels called *aquaporins* in the membrane.
  - Permeability to water increases in proportion to the number of these channels.
  - Different tissues have various densities and types of aquaporins, so their cells may be more or less water permeable than others.

The proximal tubule, descending limb of Henle, has high water permeability at all times associated with aquaporin-1.

Cells in the tip of Henle's loop, transitioning from descending to ascending limb, abruptly lose aquaporin-1 in the lumenal membranes.

Some tissues are practically impermeable to water, like the ascending limb of Henle's loop, and some have a low permeability, greatly augmented by vasopressin through the type 2 vasopressin receptor which regulates the insertion and removal of aquaporin-2 into the lumenal membrane of distal nephron cells after the distal convoluted tubule.

Fluid Shifts

What are the implications of the fact that the body fluid compartments (ECF and intracellular fluid [ICF]; see Fig. 8.1) are in general freely permeable to water and contain effective osmoles Na^+ in the ECF and K^+ in the ICF?

- First, the free movement of water means that the ECF and ICF always come to osmotic equilibrium and achieve equal osmolality, because when the osmolality changes on one side of the membrane, water shifts until the solute concentrations are equal.
- Second, the presence of effective osmoles means that osmotic pressure can be created on one side of the membrane. An increase or decrease in [Na^+] in the ECF will cause fluid shifts between ECF and ICF.
- Ingesting a salty meal adds salt to the ECF, raising the ECF osmolality. Fluid moves from the ICF into the ECF, shrinking the ICF volume and expanding the ECF volume.
- Adding isotonic saline to the ECF (i.e., adding NaCl in solution with the same osmolality as the ECF) will increase the size of the ECF but no fluid shift will occur, so ICF volume will stay the same.
- Drinking water adds pure water to the ECF, dropping the ECF osmolality, so some fluid will shift from the ECF to the ICF. ECF and ICF volume both expand slightly (in proportion to the relative volume of ICF and ECF). Because only changes in the level of effective osmoles in the ECF can produce such fluid shifts, fluid shifts do not necessarily correlate with the total osmolality of the ECF, but only with the osmolality of the effective osmoles, most importantly Na^+.

Tonicity refers to the effect that a particular solute concentration has on cell volume.

- Hypertonic ECF will lead to cell shrinkage, an isotonic ECF no change at all in ICF.
- Hypotonic ECF will expand cell volume.

The Physiologic Importance of Maintaining Constant Plasma Osmolality

The body encounters daily changes in ECF osmolality relative to ICF as a consequence of variations in water elimination and intake.

- If the body had no means of regulating the plasma osmolality, fluid shifts would occur unopposed between the ECF and ICF.

The body would not be able to tolerate those fluid shifts, which create swelling or shrinkage of the ICF volume and hence, of the cells. This can be catastrophic, particularly in the brain.

Thus when the body's sensors detect that a fluid shift has begun to occur, which indicates a change in ECF osmolality, effector mechanisms restore normal ECF osmolality. This reverses the fluid shift and protects the ICF from expansion or contraction.

Physiologic Challenges to Osmolality Homeostasis

In the normal state, fluids lost from or added to the ECF are usually hypotonic.

- When hypotonic fluid is lost, water is lost in excess of solute and the plasma solute concentration increases.
- When hypotonic fluid is added to the plasma, its solute concentration decreases.

The osmoregulatory apparatus of the kidney and brain modulates water elimination and intake to maintain constant osmolality.

A variety of physiologic processes involve exchanges of hypotonic fluid with the external environment (Table 20.1). Water may be lost in:

- Excess of solute in the stool.
- Evaporation from the respiratory tract (in this case, the loss is all water and no solute).
- Hypotonic fluid of sweat, which is produced in connection with the hypothalamic regulation of body temperature
- Excretion of nitrogenous wastes requires a minimal level of urinary water loss that concentrates the plasma.

Unregulated additions of water to the ECF occur through drinking and the ingestion of food, which has a water content that can approach 1 L/day.

- The water inside dietary food is sometimes called preformed water.
- Unregulated additions of water to the ECF also occur metabolically. Recall from biochemistry that oxidative phosphorylation is the means by which the reduced cofactors of the citric acid cycle are aerobically transduced to adenosine triphosphate (ATP). This process consumes oxygen and yields H_2O on an ongoing basis in every aerobic cell. Water produced from oxidative phosphorylation is sometimes called metabolic water (see Fast Fact 20.3).

Fast Fact Box 20.3

Approximately 20 mol of water (and CO_2) may be produced per day normally in an adult. Because water is 55 mol/L, water production is approximately 20/55 of a liter, or close to 400 mL/day.

Obligatory Water Loss in the Excretion of Nitrogenous Wastes

It may not seem immediately obvious why urinary excretion of nitrogenous wastes causes an obligatory concentration of the plasma. If the urine is even more concentrated than the blood (plasma osmolality is around 280 mOsm/kg, whereas maximum

TABLE 20.1   Physiologic Challenges to Osmolality Homeostasis[a]

Source of Unregulated Water Loss From ECF		Volume
Stool		200 mL/day
Respiratory tract		400 mL/day
Urine		500 mL/day is the minimum loss of water to urine for excretion of nitrogenous wastes.
Skin	Evaporation	500 mL/day evaporates from skin and mucous membranes under any circumstances.
	Sweat	under circumstances of elevated body temperature, up to 7000 mL water/day or more can be lost to sweat.
Source of Unregulated Water Addition to ECF		**Volume (mL/day)**
Dietary	Habitual drinking	1000[b]
	Eating (preformed water)	850
Metabolic (oxidative phosphorylation)		350

[a] The table does not include urinary losses of hypotonic fluid that occur as a part of osmoregulation, as those losses respond to the unregulated additions of water to the ECF. The table also does not include ADH-mediated additions to the ECF, or water ingested due to thirst, because these additions respond to, and should be differentiated from, the unregulated losses from the ECF.

[b] Obviously, habitual and social water ingestion is highly variable from person to person. It is also difficult to distinguish habitual drinking from osmoregulatory (thirst-stimulated) drinking quantitatively.

Rose and Post estimate total average water consumption at 400 to 1400 mL/day.

Adopted from Rose BD, Post TW. *Clinical Physiology of Acid-Base and Elecirolyte Disorders*. 5th Edition. New York: McGraw-Hill; 2001. Table 9-1. The figure 7000 mL/day comes from Smith H., p. 161.

urine concentration is around 1200 mOsm/kg), how can hypotonic fluid be lost in the urine?

To understand this better, we must first understand the obligation to excrete nitrogenous wastes.

- The digestion of dietary proteins yields amino acids.
- Some of these amino acids are used in protein synthesis, whereas others are metabolized to nitrogen-free compounds (such as pyruvate) that may yield energy through the citric acid cycle.
- Hence metabolism of amino acids requires their deamination and yields the toxic substance, ammonia (NH_3).
- The liver combines NH_3 with CO_2 to make the less-toxic substance, urea (NH_2-CO-NH_2), but urea must also be eliminated, lest it have toxic effects, particularly on the brain.
- One of the kidney's important functions is to excrete urea.

If urea is to be excreted from the body in solution, it must be transported in a certain amount of water donated from the plasma.

- The plasma must donate a hypotonic volume of water for this purpose so that this volume of water can be loaded with osmoles of urea.
- If the plasma donated an isotonic volume of water, the body would waste excess salt in urea excretion and compromise extracellular fluid volume.
- The maximal osmolality of human urine is about 1200 mOsm/kg; 600 mOsm can be excreted in a half liter of water. About half of this amount of normal osmole excretion is urea.
- Thus the plasma must donate a minimum level of hypotonic fluid to urine to excrete urea in solution. Around 10 mL of water is required for every gram of metabolized protein, meaning that a minimum of approximately 500 mL water/day must be lost to the urine.

Low-protein diets can help reduce this obligatory urinary water loss. Even on a protein-free diet, however, the kidney has excretory duties that require water to transport wastes from the body. The absolute lower limit of obligatory water loss on a protein-free diet is about 300 mL water/day.

Control of Extracellular Fluid Osmolality

Together, the brain and kidney maintain a steady plasma osmolality through two effector mechanisms.

The principal effector mechanism involves a hormone introduced in Chapter 19, antidiuretic hormone (ADH), also known as vasopressin.

- An increased level of ADH increases the reabsorption of water without solute in the kidney (thus lowering urine volume, i.e., opposing diuresis). This in turn dilutes ECF Na^+ and lowers plasma osmolality.
- A decreased level of ADH decreases reabsorption of water without solute in the kidney (thus increasing the urine volume, i.e., creating a diuresis). This excretion of water without solute drains the pool of water around the Na^+ and raises plasma osmolality.

The second important homeostatic response to plasma osmolality is thirst. The higher the plasma osmolality is relative to the ICF, the greater the perception of thirst will be, which in turn leads to behavior (drinking) that will add water to the ECF.

Like other homeostatic systems, the osmoregulatory system is composed of sensors, a control center, and effectors. The ADH and thirst mechanisms for altering ECF osmolality share a similar sensor and control center, which we will now consider.

Osmoreceptors

The sensors involved in the regulation of ECF osmolality are each located in the diencephalon in the brain (Fig. 20.1):

- When changes in osmolality drive fluid shifts, osmoreceptor cells in the hypothalamus and in related structures swell or shrink.
- Just like many other cells in the body, they swell in response to decreased plasma osmolality and shrink in the presence of increased plasma osmolality.
- Unlike other cells, however, shrinkage in osmoreceptor cells depolarizes the cells by stimulating mechanosensitive channels in the cell membrane.
  - The stimulation results in an increased cationic conductance and the cations raise the intracellular electrical potential, thus initiating an action potential or predisposing the cell toward an action potential.
- Conversely, swelling inhibits these channels, decreasing cationic conductance and hyperpolarizing the cell, thus inhibiting action potentials.

Some of the osmoreceptor cells are magnocellular neurons located in the supraoptic and paraventricular nuclei of the hypothalamus.

- The axons of these cells project directly into the posterior pituitary.
- Action potentials traveling down these axons to their termini in the pituitary then cause Ca^{2+}-dependent release of ADH into the bloodstream by exocytosis of ADH granules.

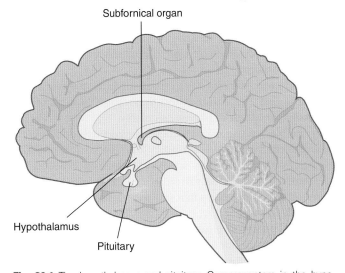

Fig. 20.1 The hypothalamus and pituitary. Osmoreceptors in the hypothalamus project their axons into the posterior pituitary, also known as the neurohypophysis. The termini of these axons secrete antidiuretic hormone. Circumventricular organs, such as the subfornical organ, also participate in osmoreception and thirst generation. (Modified from Nolte J. *Elsevier's Integrated Neuroscience*. Philadelphia, PA: Elsevier; 2007. Fig. 5-15.)

Other osmoreceptor cells are thought to exist in *circumventricular organs* nearby: the subfornical organ, the organum vasculosum of the lamina terminalis, and others.

- These centers may augment or modulate the excitement of the magnocellular osmoreceptors. Some investigators refer to the entire group as an *osmoreceptor complex*.
- Although the neurophysiology is incompletely understood, it is clear that the osmoreceptor complex not only drives increased ADH secretion, but it also helps generate the thirst sensation and drinking behavior.

Although one might think that osmoreceptors respond directly to the total osmolality of the ECF, they cannot and do not. Only a change in the level of effective osmoles in the ECF relative to the ICF can swell or shrink cells, and osmoreceptors are no different in this respect from other cells.

- They respond to changes in the effective osmolality of the plasma. Accordingly, the ineffective osmoles of solutes that can pass freely from ECF to ICF, such as urea, cannot affect the osmoreceptors, so a high plasma urea concentration (uremia) does not drive an osmoregulatory response.
- The hypothalamus is, however, quite sensitive to changes in effective osmolality, with changes as small as 1% producing a secretory response (Fig. 20.2A).

Recent research suggests that peripheral osmoreceptors located in the oropharynx may also contribute to the ADH response.

- Evidence indicates that oropharyngeal exposure to hypertonic fluid may increase the ADH level independent of any increase in plasma osmolality.
- These oropharyngeal receptors are thought to be NaCl-sensitive.

Baroreceptors

Recall from Chapter 19 that in addition to osmoreceptor control of ADH secretion, the baroreceptors also exert some influence over ADH secretion.

- Under circumstances of severe volume depletion, baroreceptors trigger the secretion of ADH to raise ECF volume. (Keep in mind that an addition of water without solute raises both ECF and ICF volume.)
- Secretion of ADH for the purposes of ECF volume control means that the baroreceptors can cause dilution of the plasma regardless of plasma osmolality.
- If the plasma osmolality is normal and the blood volume is extremely low, the baroreceptors' invocation of ADH secretion may cause an undesired hypoosmolality in the plasma, if dilute fluids are ingested (Fig. 20.2B). This is important clinically when evaluating possible causes of low plasma [Na$^+$].
- The baroreceptors also stimulate the hypothalamus to produce a thirst response in severe volume depletion.

The baroreceptors appear to influence the osmoreceptor complex via the vagus nerve, which synapses in the medulla. Neurons in that area project into the hypothalamus.

The Set Point

The hypothalamus functions as a control center in osmoregulation.

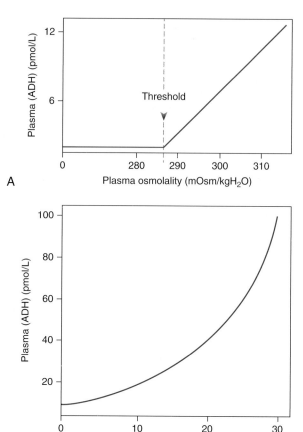

Fig. 20.2 Correlations between antidiuretic hormone (*ADH*) secretion and its provoking factors. A, Osmoreceptor control of ADH. Although the graph does not reflect it, regulation occurs by increasing or decreasing ADH levels, not by turning ADH secretion completely on or completely off. B, Baroreceptor control of ADH. Severe decreases in blood volume and pressure prompt ADH secretion. ADH secretion in response to hypovolemia is not significant until a 10% drop in blood pressure has occurred.

The maximum level of osmolality tolerated before ADH is secreted is known as the osmolal set point.

- Beyond this threshold of approximately 280 or 285 mOsm/kg H$_2$O, the hypothalamus signals ADH release.
- The osmolal set point for thirst is higher than that for ADH secretion by about 10 mOsm/kg. Thus the usual plasma Na$^+$ concentration is closer to the ADH set point, which gives humans the ability to concentrate urine without thirst. This ability is well adapted to life without constant drinking behavior.

The set point can be lowered under certain circumstances, such as under baroreceptor stimulation or during pregnancy.

- A lowered set point means ADH will start being secreted at a lower plasma osmolality.
- Consequently, when the baroreceptors respond to severe volume depletion by stimulating the osmoreceptors, not only do they promote ADH secretion, but they also lower the threshold for ADH secretion in response to plasma osmolality.

Thirst as an Effector Mechanism

Physiologists and neuroscientists still have much to learn about how increased osmolality leads to thirst and drinking behavior, but it is clear that thirst serves, along with ADH, to decrease plasma osmolality and increase ECF volume.

- The absorption of ingested water from the intestines adds this water without solute to the ECF in the same way that the kidney adds water under the influence of ADH.
- Thirst, like ADH, thereby expands ECF volume and dilutes the plasma osmoles, which in turn reverses the fluid shift caused by high plasma osmolality and prevents shrinkage of the ICF.

Both central and oropharyngeal osmoreceptors trigger thirst through stimulation of the osmoreceptor complex. The thirst sensation may arise in connection with increased plasma osmolality, but it dissipates long before normal plasma osmolality is restored. It takes only a short time to consume the appropriate amount of water to correct plasma osmolality.

- It takes longer for the plasma osmolality to actually correct, as the water must first be absorbed from the intestines and distributed into the ECF.
- If thirst and drinking were only to stop when plasma osmolality had corrected, one would overshoot one's water needs and become hypoosmolar.

The body possibly avoids such a dysfunctional means of thirst termination through the oropharyngeal osmoreceptors. The application of water to the oropharynx may relieve the peripheral receptors of salt stimulation and help abolish thirst long before the intestines absorb the water and the plasma osmolality is corrected (see Clinical Correlation Box 20.2).

Clinical Correlation Box 20.2

Alternatives to Thirst in the Animal Kingdom

Thirst is not universal in the animal kingdom. All animals do require a supply of water without solute to correct increases in plasma osmolality (if dilution is unneeded or if concentration of plasma is needed, free water can then be purged in urine); however, evolution has devised myriad strategies in addition to drinking for the acquisition of free water. The cartilaginous marine fish maintain a high urea level in the blood to extract free water osmotically from the sea. In arid climates, preformed water and metabolic water may be the only sources of solute-free water. Some moths and beetles subsist wholly on metabolic water and can live in a nearly anhydrous environment. Finally, marine mammals do not drink either because highly concentrated seawater is the only water supply available to them and would leave them unable to dilute their plasma effectively. Marine mammals derive all their water from preformed sources (i.e., food) and from metabolism.

Antidiuretic Hormone Action as an Effector Mechanism

Once secreted, ADH travels via the blood circulation to the kidney. ADH diffuses out of the peritubular capillary to act on the basolateral side of the tubule. It acts in two places:

- Thick ascending limb, where it promotes salt reabsorption
- Collecting duct, where it increases permeability of the duct to water, facilitating water reabsorption

The mechanism of ADH action in the thick ascending limb is unclear; however, the activity of the $Na^+/K^+/2Cl^-$ symporter is known to increase in animals in the presence of ADH. In the collecting duct, ADH binds G-protein coupled receptors (predominantly vasopressin receptor type 2) that triggers a cyclic adenosine

monophosphate (cAMP)-mediated signal transduction cascade. The end result is the insertion of aquaporins in the otherwise poorly permeable collecting duct apical surface (Fig. 20.3).

The effect of ADH is to increase water permeability approximately 100-fold. Now we turn to the following question: How exactly do the actions of ADH account for the tubular reabsorption of water and its subsequent addition to the ECF? (See Genetics Box 20.1, Development Box 20.1 and Pharmacology Box 20.1).

GENETICS BOX 20.1

Although the collecting duct is a critical site for osmoregulation because of the effects of antidiuretic hormone (ADH), cells in this section of the nephron also express the epithelial sodium channel (ENaC) that resorbs NaCl. Patients with a mutation in the SCNN1A gene produce a mutant ENaC ß chain, which renders the channel nonfunctional and results in significant Na^+ loss and subsequent hyponatremia, hyperkalemia because of reduced K^+ excretion, and volume depletion. This condition is known as autosomal recessive pseudohypoaldosteronism type 1 (PHA1).

DEVELOPMENT BOX 20.1

Manifestations of autosomal recessive pseudohypoaldosteronism type 1 (PHA1) appear in infancy and include failure to thrive, hyponatremia, hyperkalemia, and volume depletion. These symptoms and sign tend not to improve with age alone. Affected patients have high levels of circulating aldosterone which, because of the dysfunction of the the epithelial sodium channel (ENaC), cannot stem the loss of Na^+.

PHARMACOLOGY BOX 20.1

PHA1 is first treated with a high sodium diet to compensate for renal Na^+ losses. If this is ineffective, fludrocortisone or carbenoxolone can help limit Na^+ wasting and ameliorate hyponatremia and volume depletion.

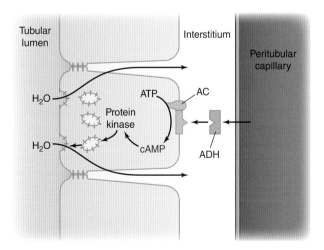

Fig. 20.3 Cyclic adenosine monophosphate (*cAMP*)-mediated insertion of vesicles carrying aquaporins. Antidiuretic hormone (*ADH*) triggers a cAMP-mediated signal transduction cascade. For simplicity, the diagram shows adenylyl cyclase directly attached to the ADH receptor. In fact, adenylyl cyclase is a membrane-bound enzyme and is dependent on a G protein for connection with the receptor and for signal transduction from receptor to adenylyl cyclase. *AC*, Adenylyl cyclase; *R*, ADH receptor. *ATP*, Adenosine triphosphate.

Countercurrent Multiplication in the Loop of Henle

We established earlier that water moves passively across tubule walls only in accordance with osmotic gradients. Consequently, without an osmotic gradient favoring the reabsorption of water, the ADH-dependent increase in the water permeability of the collecting duct would not move any water by itself.

- In the proximal tubule, water reabsorption occurs through an active pumping of solute, causing water to follow solute out of the tubule and into the interstitium.
- In the collecting duct, water reabsorption can far exceed the level accounted for by its reabsorption of solute.
- Thus to reabsorb water in this part of the tubule, the kidney must use a different mechanism to create an osmotic gradient that would cause water to flow out of the collecting duct and into the surrounding tissue in the presence of aquaporins.

That mechanism is called countercurrent multiplication in the loop of Henle, a system that maintains high solute concentration in the renal medulla. Countercurrent multiplication requires a particular tubular anatomy and special tubular transport properties:

- The loop of Henle is a U-shaped segment of the nephron composed of:
  - Thin descending limb, which is permeable to water but has low permeability to salt.
  - Thin ascending limb, which is permeable to salt but not to water.
- Thick ascending limb, which reabsorbs salt by active transport and is impermeable to water.
- This arrangement generates an increasing salt concentration with descent into the medullary interstitium (Fig. 20.4).

Countercurrent Multiplication as a Form of Countercurrent Exchange

Although the concentrating function of the loop of Henle is called countercurrent multiplication, it is, underneath, just a slightly more complicated form of countercurrent exchange.

- A simpler example of countercurrent exchange is that of heat exchange between arteries and veins in the extremities (Fig. 20.5).
  - Arteries carry blood from the heart, and also consequently carry heat away from the body core.
  - Veins, by contrast, carry blood from the less well-insulated and hence cooler extremities.
  - Because the arteries and veins of the extremities run in parallel, they are subject to transverse heat exchange from hot artery to cool vein.

The physiology of the loop of Henle is analogous to heat exchange in an extremity. The hairpin turn at the bottom of the loop is analogous to the body core, and salt concentration is analogous to heat (Fig. 20.6A).

- The fluid entering the descending limb is isotonic to plasma (less salt-concentrated than the base), so the descending limb is like the cool vein.

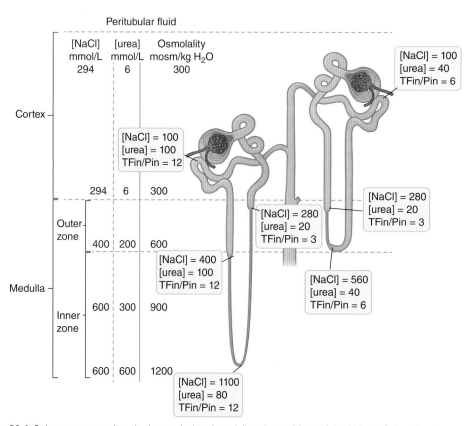

Fig. 20.4 Solute concentrations in the cortical and medullary interstitium of the kidney. Salt and urea concentrations rise with descent into the medulla. Urea accounts for a larger percentage of total osmolality deep in the inner medulla.

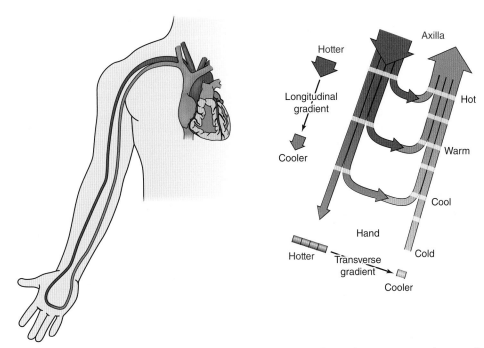

Fig. 20.5 Countercurrent heat exchange in the upper extremity. Heat flows along a transverse heat gradient from artery to vein to create a longitudinal heat gradient from axilla to hand. The process is analogous to countercurrent multiplication in the loop of Henle.

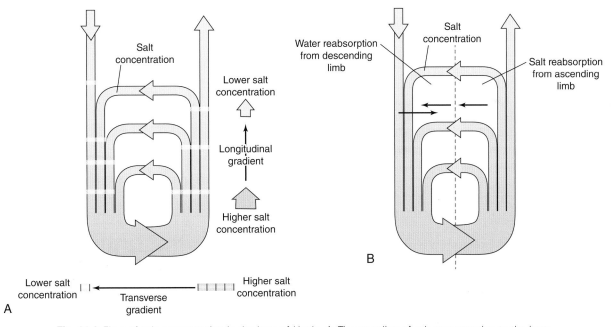

Fig. 20.6 Flow of salt concentration in the loop of Henle. A, The recycling of salt concentration to the base of the loop. The flow of salt concentration along transverse concentration gradients from ascending to descending limb creates a longitudinal concentration gradient from renal cortex to inner medulla. B, Two constituents of the leftward flow of salt concentration. Salt reabsorption to the left and water reabsorption to the right both affect salt concentration flow to the left.

- The ascending limb, loaded with fluid containing a high salt concentration, is like the hot artery.
  - NaCl in the ascending limb is reabsorbed transversely (without water), and the salt concentration progressively rises in the fluid of the descending limb.
  - Salt concentration is thus recycled to the inner medulla, maintaining a high inner medullary salt concentration.

- When ADH increases the water permeability of the collecting duct, water can flow down its osmotic gradient into the medullary interstitium.

One matter complicating the analogy to heat exchange in the extremities is that although salt is reabsorbed by the ascending limb, salt is not secreted into the descending limb in the same way that heat is transferred directly into the vein. Rather, the

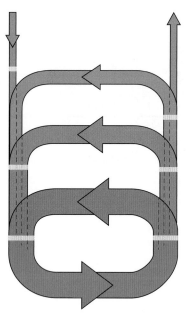

Fig. 20.7 Interstitial salt concentration as a result of salt flow concentration in the loop of Henle. Unlike in heat exchange, a flow of salt concentration means that the interstitium must acquire the same salt concentration as the ascending limb, and the descending limb must acquire the same salt concentration as the interstitium.

fluid of the descending limb acquires a higher salt concentration through the descending limb's reabsorption of water.

- The ascending limb reabsorbs salt without water into the interstitium, raising the osmolality of the interstitium.
- The increased osmolality of the interstitium draws water without salt from the tubule lumen, concentrating the fluid of the descending limb.
- Thus although salt itself does not pass all the way from the ascending limb to the descending limb, salt concentration does in a manner analogous to heat exchange (Fig. 20.6B).

The difference between heat transfer and the flow of salt concentration does, however, have a critical functional ramification.

- In heat exchange, an absolute quantity is passed transversely.
- In the exchange of salt concentration, only a ratio (mOsm of salt to kilograms of water) is passed transversely.

Consequently, the interstitium is not just a passageway for small amounts of salt; rather, the interstitium acquires a high salt concentration.

- The high salt concentration of the interstitium is necessary osmotically to draw water from the descending limb.
- Furthermore, a high salt concentration in the interstitium is necessary to compel water reabsorption from the collecting duct, which is the purpose of the apparatus.
- The transverse flow of salt concentration in the loop of Henle accounts for the high interstitial salt concentration of the medulla.
- Fig. 20.7 amends Fig. 20.8 to reflect the fact that the interstitium shares the same high salt concentration as the tubular fluid. Clinical Correlation Box 20.3 provides another way of illustrating this concept.

Clinical Correlation Box 20.3
Countercurrent Exchange Demonstration

1. Gather 7 participants and at least 15 pennies.
2. Seat the 7 participants around a table, 3 on each side and 1 at the head of the table (Fig. 20.10). Participants 1–3 are analogous to the descending limp, while participants 5–7 act as the ascending limb.
3. For each turn:
   a. Participants 5–7 hand 1 penny across the table (this is analogous to salt absorption in the ascending limb).
   b. Participants 1–3 takes 1 penny from the supply.
   c. Each participant hands everything they have to the person sitting to their right (this mimics the flow of the tubular fluid).
   d. The leader passes 1 penny at each turn to participant #1, acting like the proximal tubule delivery. Note that at the start participants may not have any pennies to either move across or move downstream. Patience is required as the steady state is achieved.
4. Keep taking turns until participant #7 acquires a penny to discard and steady state is established.
5. All participants then reveal how many pennies they have in their possession.

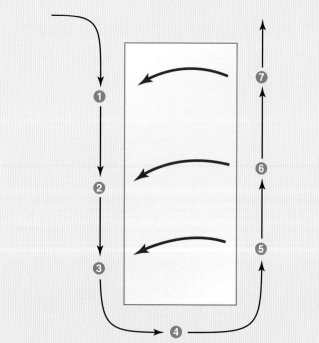

Fig. 20.10 A game with pennies that illustrates the basic mechanism of the countercurrent multiplier, which in turn depends on the mass balance of solute and water.

The Ultimate Origin of the High Salt Concentration Entering the Ascending Limb: the Na⁺,K⁺-ATPase Versus Urea

A final matter complicating the analogy between heat exchange and countercurrent multiplication is that of origins.

- Heat in the artery comes from metabolism in the body core, a process external to heat exchange.
- In the loop of Henle, however, the high salt concentration entering the ascending limb appears to depend on the function of the loop itself (see Fig. 20.8).
  - The ascending limb receives tubular fluid high in salt concentration from the descending limb.

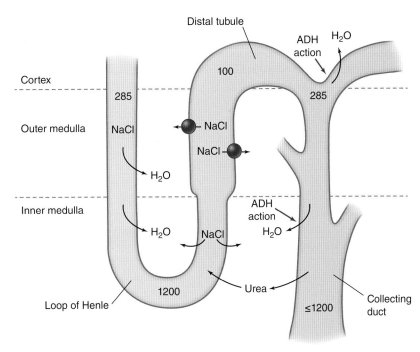

Fig. 20.8 Handling of salt, water, and urea in the loop of Henle and collecting duct.

- The descending limb in turn has a high salt concentration because water has diffused out of the tubule into the interstitium, which is highly concentrated in salt.
- Meanwhile, the interstitium is highly concentrated in salt because of salt reabsorption from the highly concentrated ascending limb.

Werner Kuhn, who proposed the countercurrent multiplication hypothesis in 1942, believed that active transport of Na^+ from the ascending limb into the interstitium was the point of origin in the cycle that creates high interstitial salt concentration.

- By actively pumping salt into the interstitium, the descending limb could be secondarily concentrated through water reabsorption, thus delivering highly concentrated fluid to the ascending limb.
- This would enable the ascending limb to deliver even more solute to the interstitium in a self-amplifying process.
- The theoretically self-amplifying character of the process is what led Kuhn to give it the name multiplication.

The mechanism for active Na^+ reabsorption in the thick ascending limb of Henle is the Na^+,K^+-ATPase on the basolateral membrane and the apical $Na^+/K^+/2Cl^-$ cotransporter. However, whereas the thick ascending limb does have Na^+,K^+-ATPase pumps, the thin ascending limb does not appear to have these pumps.

Thus how the inner medullary interstitium acquires its high salt concentration remains an unsolved problem. One possible explanation is that much of the interstitial osmolality at the base of the loop of Henle is accounted for by urea and not salt.

- If the descending limb were largely impermeable to urea, the interstitial urea concentration could draw water from the descending limb, thus delivering fluid high in salt concentration to the thin ascending limb.
- Then, the high luminal NaCl could passively be reabsorbed in this segment.

The question then remains, of course, where did the medullary urea come from?

- An incomplete answer is that urea is reabsorbed from the medullary collecting duct and secreted in the loop of Henle; urea thereby follows a circular path through the nephron and the interstitial tissue within the inner medulla.
- Consequently, urea remains trapped deep in the medullary interstitium in steady concentrations. This phenomenon is known as *urea trapping*.

On the whole, it can be safely stated that recycling of salt and urea through the medullary interstitium accounts for the high osmolality of the inner medulla, and that the thick ascending limb Na^+,K^+-ATPase and luminal $Na^+/K^+/2Cl^-$ cotransporter render the fluid entering the distal tubule and collecting duct hypotonic (see Fig. 20.8).

Countercurrent Exchange in the Vasa Recta

Once ADH has enabled the reabsorption of water into the interstitium, the water must find its way back into the bloodstream to reduce plasma osmolality.

- Recall that the peritubular vasa recta has a high oncotic pressure owing to the previous loss of protein-free fluid to glomerular filtration.
- The high oncotic pressure of the vasa recta reabsorbs this water, and carries it away into the renal vein. The vasa recta also absorbs some solute.
- Thus countercurrent multiplication does not accumulate salt and water indefinitely in the interstitium, and a steady state is achieved.

Why does the vasa recta not completely dissipate the salt gradient concentrated here by the loop of Henle? The vasa recta runs in parallel to the loop of Henle and shares its U-shape (Fig. 20.9).

As the vasa recta runs down into the increasingly salty medulla, it loses water and absorbs solute, gaining in osmolality.

- It seems counterintuitive that the descending vasa recta (DVR), with its high oncotic pressure, would actually lose some of its water to the surrounding interstitial fluid (ISF).
- As the DVR enters the high salt environment of the medullary ISF, however, the driving force for osmotic water flow from the capillary into the high NaCl ISF exceeds the oncotic forces favoring water moving into the capillary.
- This is the only place in the body where osmotic pressure overpowers oncotic pressure.

As the ascending vasa recta (AVR) flows into the less-concentrated portions of the medullary interstitium, it gains water and loses solute.

- If the vasa recta took a straight path through the medulla, it would certainly dissipate the gradient.
  - With its U-shape, it keeps the medullary salt gradient intact and absorbs any excess water or solute.
  - The volume flow of the AVR exceeds that of the entering DVR by the amount of volume reabsorbed by the descending limb and the collecting duct.
  - Once again, this is a form of countercurrent exchange; the vasa recta transversely cycles solute from ascending to descending limb, thereby conserving osmolality in the inner medulla.

The vasa recta capillaries also bring with them red blood cells (RBCs). The RBCs play an important role in the ability to concentrate urine.

- Given the high urea concentration, RBCs in the DVR could potentially lose enough water to shrink to the point of hemolysis.
- An RBC membrane urea transporter with high capacity ensures the rapid equilibration of urea into the RBC, preventing this shrinkage. The transporter also allows the rapid efflux of urea.

- If that urea could not exit the AVR rapidly as it flows toward the cortex, the RBC would swell to the point of hypotonic lysis. Furthermore, it would be impossible to excrete urea because the RBC would carry urea that came from filtration back to the renal vein.

Urine Osmolality

When ADH enables water reabsorption back into plasma, and the dilution of plasma, it consequently leaves the fluid of the collecting duct concentrated with solute.

- Normally, when plasma osmolality rises, urine osmolality rises, and vice versa.
- The urine, however, can never be more concentrated than the medullary interstitium, because water diffuses through aquaporins until osmolality is equal on both sides of the tubule membrane.
- Urine osmolality peaks, therefore around 1200 mOsm/kg, the maximum osmolality achieved in the medullary interstitium. The minimum urine osmolality is 50 to 75 mOsm/kg. It is less than the 100 mOsm/kg leaving the loop because some salt reabsorption does occur in the collecting duct.
- Recall that this aldosterone-influenced Na^+ reabsorption is one of the means of governance over the ECF volume.
- The removal of this salt can further dilute the tubular fluid.

Free Water Clearance

Free water clearance (C_{H20}) is an index of how much water free of solute has been cleared from the body.

- The free water clearance is normally only a positive number in hypoosmotic situations (e.g., after one drinks water), when the suppression of ADH causes "free water" to be excreted from the tubule in hypoosmotic urine, thus returning the plasma osmolality to normal.

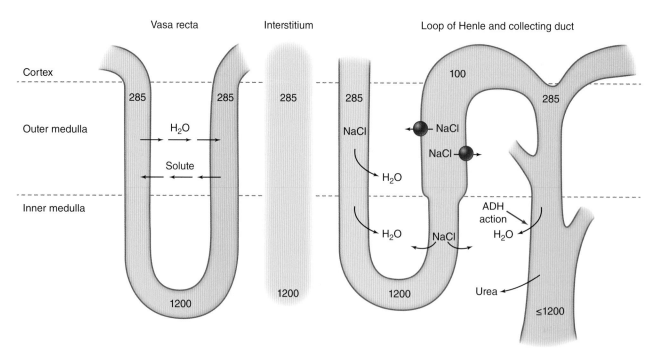

Fig. 20.9 The vasa recta.

- When ADH causes free water to be reabsorbed and added to plasma, there is either no free water clearance or there may be a negative C_{H20}.
- Free water clearance is a different concept from urine osmolality, as the former is quantitative rather than qualitative.

The calculation of free water clearance is relatively straightforward. Free water clearance equals the urine volume per time, V, minus the osmolar clearance (C_{osm}):

$$C_{H20} = \dot{V} - C_{osm}$$

C_{osm} is defined in accordance with the standard clearance equation:

$$C_{osm} = \left(\dot{U}_{osm}\dot{V}\right)/P_{osm}$$

Total osmolar clearance equals urine osmolality times the urine flow rate divided by the plasma osmolality. Putting the two equations together, we have an equation for free water clearance as follows:

$$C_{H20} = \dot{V} - \left(\dot{U}_{osm}\right)\left(\dot{V}\right)/P_{osm}$$

In accordance with the definition of clearance and mass balance (see Ch. 18), the osmoles in the volume of plasma cleared must equal the osmoles that show up in the urine.

- Filtration at the glomerulus is isoosmotic.
- If the tubule did not alter the tubular fluid solute concentration, the urine volume would equal the volume of plasma cleared of solute.

- In that case, the plasma volume cleared would have been filtered and excreted with no net reabsorption of water or secretion of solute.
- If the urine volume carrying the excreted solute is larger than the volume of plasma cleared, we know that there was a net "addition" of free water to the tubular fluid before it left the collecting duct and entered the urinary collecting space.
  - Therefore the free water added to the tubule for excretion—the free water clearance—is defined as the urine volume minus the volume of plasma cleared of solute. Because water is not secreted, this "additional" free water could only be formed from reabsorption of solute without water.

This ability to dilute the tubular fluid is a property of the thick ascending limb of Henle and the cortical distal tubule. The process is known as separation and requires impermeability of the cells to water. The impermeability is always present in the thick limb, but in the distal tubule and collecting duct it is only present when ADH is decreased.

To produce maximum amounts of dilute urine, three aspects of integrated tubular function are required:

- There must be adequate delivery of isotonic fluid from the proximal tubule.
- The thick ascending limb and distal tubule, as diluting segments, must be able to reabsorb NaCl: the separation step.
- ADH must be low, so that water is not reabsorbed with NaCl in the distal tubule, and the collecting duct remains relatively impermeable to water: the regulation step.

TABLE 20.2   **Responses to Physiologic and Pathophysiologic Challenges to Osmolality Homeostasis**

Challenge	Δ in ECF/ICF Vol.	Δ in Plasma Osmolality	Main Homeostatic Response
Addition of isotonic saline to ECF	↑ ECF volume	No Δ in Plasma osmolality	↓ Salt and water reabsorption
	No Δ in ICF		↑ Iso-osmotic urine output
			↓ ECF Volume
Addition of water or hypotonic fluid to ECF	↑ ECF volume, then shift into ICF	↓ Plasma osmolality	↑ Free water clearance (i.e. ↑ hypo-osmotic urine output)
	Net Δ: some ↑ ECF, some ↑ ICF		↑ Plasma osmolality
			↓ ECF Volume
Addition of salt to ECF	Fluid shifts from ICF to ECF, ↑ ECF, ↓ ICF	↑ Plasma osmolality	↓ Free water clearance (i.e. ↓ urine volume)
			↑ Urine osmolality
			↓ Plasma osmolality
			↑ ECF Volume
Loss of isotonic fluid, as in hemorrhage	↓ ECF	No Δ in Plasma osmolality	↑ Salt and water reabsorption
	No Δ in ICF		↓ Iso-osmotic urine output
			↑ ECF Volume
Loss of hypotonic fluid, such as sweat	↓ ECF	↑ Plasma osmolality	↑ Salt and water reabsorption
	↓ ICF fluid shifts from ICF to ECF		↑ Free water clearance
			↓ Urine volume
			↑ Urine osmolality
			↓ Plasma osmolality
			↑ ECF Volume

Synthesis of Volume and Osmolality Control

Now that we have been introduced to the body's interrelated mechanisms for ECF volume and osmolality homeostasis, we can predict the body's response to a number of different homeostatic challenges (Table 20.2).

- The osmolality of fluids added to or lost from the ECF affects the ECF volume.
- Likewise, the regulation and treatment of ECF volume has implications for the plasma osmolality (see Clinical Correlation Box 20.4).

Clinical Correlation Box 20.4
Fluid Management

With an understanding of what happens in the body in response to various homeostatic challenges, we can make more informed clinical decisions regarding the appropriate fluids for treating patients. By considering volume status, blood pressure, and plasma osmolality in the context of the disorder present, we can best judge whether the patient needs volume added or subtracted from the extracellular fluid (ECF)—and whether this fluid should be hypotonic or isotonic. In cases of dramatic hypotension, as in hemorrhage or shock, 1 to 2 L of isotonic saline or Ringer's lactate (which is also isotonic to plasma) may be administered rapidly through a large bore catheter. The choice of isotonic fluids avoids changes in body fluid osmolality. One of the reasons paramedics and physicians are so quick to establish an intravenous line in emergency situations is to gain control over the ECF volume and thereby over the perfusion pressure.

PATHOPHYSIOLOGY: DISORDERS OF SERUM OSMOLALITY AND THEIR SEQUELAE

Plasma osmolality, or serum osmolality, may be calculated using the following equation:

$$P_{osm} = 2\left(\left[Na^+\right]\right) + \left[glucose\right]/18 + \left(\text{blood urea nitrogen }\left[BUN\right]\right)/2.8$$

The term $2\left(\left[Na^+\right]\right)$ represents Na^+ and its anions, primarily Cl^- and HCO_3^-. These are the major extracellular ions.

- The divisors for glucose and urea (BUN) are conversions from mg/dL to mmol/L.
- Normally, P_{osm}= 280 mOsm/kg to 290 mOsm/kg.

Disorders That Affect Plasma Osmolality

Various conditions may cause abnormal deviations from the normal P_{osm}. Most of these conditions do so by disturbing the body's osmoregulatory function and causing the kidney to reabsorb too much or too little water, lowering or raising the plasma $[Na^+]$. Thus common endpoints of osmoregulation disorders are:

- Hyponatremia: low plasma Na^+
- Hypernatremia: high plasma Na^+

First, we will briefly summarize how some conditions derange plasma osmolality (see Clinical Correlation Box 20.5).

Clinical Correlation Box 20.5
The Osmolal Gap

The osmolar gap, which is the measured osmolality minus the osmolality calculated from serum electrolytes is often increased by toxic alcohols such as methanol, ethanol, and ethylene glycol. In those cases, the osmolar gap is widened by the presence of the neural alcohol that affects the measured osmolality but not included in the calculation, hence the gap. The equation for calculating plasma osmolality describes the main physiologic contributors to plasma osmolality: Na^+, Cl^-, glucose, and urea. In some conditions, such as methanol intoxication, the concentration of other solutes not included in the equation rises, thus contributing to plasma osmolality. In such cases, P_{osm} measured by freezing point depression will differ from the calculated P_{osm}:

$$P_{osm} = 2\left(\left[Na^+\right]\frac{mmol}{L}\right) + \left(\frac{\frac{\left[glucose\right]mg}{dL}}{\frac{180\,mg/mmol}{10\,dL/L}}\right) + \left(\frac{\left[BUN\right]mg/dL}{\frac{28\,mg/mmol}{10\,dL/L}}\right)$$

The difference between measured and calculated P_{osm} is called the osmolal gap. Note that by custom the glucose and BUN concentrations are expressed in units of md/dL so to make the dimensional analysis accurate in units of mmol/L, those concentrations must be divided by the gram molecular weight (for glucose 180 mg/mmol, and for urea nitrogen 28 mg/mmol) divided by 10.

In many instances of osmolal gap, an acidosis or other more prominent findings lead the way to the diagnosis. An anion gap is created not by *osmoles* unaccounted for in physiologic calculation but by anions unaccounted for by physiologic calculation. Many acidoses create an anion gap, and many neutral solutes can cause an osmolal gap and an anion gap because of the presence of anionic metabolites. Ethanol is one substance that can create an osmolal gap without creating an anion

---

Diabetes Mellitus

In diabetes mellitus (DM), the plasma glucose concentration is abnormally elevated, which directly raises the plasma osmolality by the equation shown previously.

- Glucose, acting as an effective osmole, causes water to leave cells and enter the ECF.
- The result will be a dilution of the serum sodium concentration despite the high osmolality.
- Elevated plasma glucose concentration also raises the osmolality in another way—by creating an osmotic diuresis.
  - The high plasma glucose concentration overwhelms the reabsorptive capacity of the tubule and the intratubular glucose concentration goes up.
  - This increases the osmotic pressure in the tubule and impairs water reabsorption.
  - ADH is unable to successfully increase water reabsorption and correct the hyperosmolality.
  - The plasma $[Na^+]$ therefore begins to rise, and eventually, hypernatremia may be observed. The osmotic diuresis accounts for the increased urination (polyuria) observed in DM, and the hyperosmolality accounts for the thirst and increased drinking (polydipsia).

Diabetes Insipidus

Diabetes insipidus (DI) is a disorder in which the brain produces too little ADH (central DI) or when the kidney fails to respond to circulating ADH (nephrogenic DI).

- Central DI may be caused by damage to the pituitary or hypothalamus, as in head trauma, surgery, or global chemical derangements that affect the brain, such as hypoxia.

- Nephrogenic DI is associated with chronic lithium use (for bipolar disorder) or hypercalcemia. When ADH cannot act, water cannot be reabsorbed normally to correct hyperosmolality, and hypernatremia and polyuria ensue.

Syndrome of Inappropriate Secretion of Antidiuretic Hormone

Like central DI, the syndrome of inappropriate secretion of ADH (SIADH) appears in connection with disorders that affect the pituitary and hypothalamus. In this case, the problem is too much ADH action, as opposed to too little.

- The kidney absorbs excess water (decreased or negative free water clearance), and hyponatremia follows.
- One of the most common causes of this syndrome is the secretion of ADH by tumors, particularly certain lung cancers. Hypoxia and pulmonary infections can also cause ADH secretion.
- Tolvaptan, a vasopressin receptor 2 antagonist, is used to treat SIADH (see Clinical Correlation Box 20.6).

Clinical Correlation Box 20.6

Tolvaptan

Tolvaptan is an example of an orally active vasopressin receptor 2 (V2) antagonist. By competitively inhibiting the V2 receptor of the distal nephron, tolvaptan increases the excreting of solute-free water and increases blood osmolality. In other words, Tolvaptan opposes the action of antidiuretic hormone (ADH). Clinically, Tolvaptan is effective in increasing serum sodium concentration in patients with euvolemic or hypervolemic hyponatremia (serum Na$^+$ concentration <135 mmol/L) associated with congestive heart failure, cirrhosis, and the syndrome of inappropriate antidiuretic hormone (SIADH).

Extracellular Fluid Volume Depletion

As described previously and in Chapter 19, very low intravascular pressures trigger the baroreceptors to signal ADH release from the brain, regardless of the plasma osmolality. The kidney reabsorbs more water than the plasma osmolality requires, the plasma osmolality drops, and hyponatremia follows.

Consequences of Osmolar Disturbances: Hypernatremia and Hyponatremia

Earlier, we stated that osmoregulation is necessary to prevent the fluid shifts associated with changes in ECF osmolality.

- Hypernatremia (e.g., because of DM or DI) causes fluid to shift from ICF to ECF, shrinking the cells.
- Hyponatremia causes fluid to shift from ECF to ICF, swelling the cells (see Clinical Correlation Box 20.7).

Cellular shrinkage and swelling are particularly dangerous for the brain.

- Cerebral shrinkage and cerebral edema may lead to altered mental status, seizures, or coma.
- These symptoms occur only in acute cases of hypo- or hypernatremia (within a day or two).

When plasma osmolality changes gradually, brain tissue adapts to minimize fluid shifts.

- It does so by modulating the level of intracellular organic solutes, such as inositol, glutamine, and taurine.

Clinical Application Box 20.7

Pseudohyponatremia

In some disease states, *hyperlipidemia*, excess lipids, or *hyperproteinemia*, excess proteins, can reduce the percentage of plasma that is water. Recall that blood is composed of red blood cells and plasma. Plasma is composed of plasma water and solids. Plasma is 93% water. Hyperlipidemia or hyperproteinemia, the excess solids can drive plasma water down below 75%. In such a case, lab tests will reveal hyponatremia because they measure the [Na$^+$] in the plasma, not just in the plasma water. The osmolality and [Na$^+$] of the plasma water remains normal, however, and the tissues are not exposed to any osmotic stress. The appropriate treatment would focus on the hyperlipidemia or hyperproteinemia and not the hyponatremia, because it is a false finding (thus the name *pseudo*hyponatremia). Multiple myeloma is a common cause of hyperproteinemia and pseudohyponatremia. A direct measurement using an ion-selective electrode in an undiluted plasma sample will get around this artifact.

- The concentrations of these organic osmolytes are reduced in the case of hyponatremia, and are increased in the case of hypernatremia, to lessen the osmotic pressure gradient that drives a fluid shift
- Recall that the cells of the renal medulla make use of osmolytes to prevent cell shrinkage in instances of very high ECF salt concentrations.

Because of adapted osmolyte levels in chronic hypo- or hypernatremia, cell volume is normal despite the abnormal osmolality. Therefore it is important not to try to rapidly reverse the chronic disturbance in plasma osmolality (see Clinical Correlation Box 20.8).

Clinical Correlation Box 20.8

A rapid reversal of chronic hyponatremia causes cell shrinkage from the reduced osmolyte levels. Likewise, a rapid reversal of hypernatremia causes cerebral edema. As water is added, it will enter the brain cells, which will expand starting from an adapted normal volume.

The Contribution of Potassium to Body Fluid Osmolality

Because one observes solute concentrations through routine blood tests in practice, the window into body fluid osmolality is the ECF. Therefore sodium is of major importance.

- If one were to sample intracellular water, the major osmolyte would be potassium, with its accompanying anions.
- In fact, in determining the total body osmolality, both Na$^+$ and K$^+$ are important.
  - Consider a loss of K$^+$ from the body, as might occur in diarrhea or in the urine.
  - As cells become depleted in K$^+$, Na$^+$ may enter cells and give the appearance of hyponatremia.
  - Similarly, if a concentrated KCl solution were given, K$^+$ would move into cells with water, resulting in hypernatremia.

For these reasons, it is necessary to consider the osmotic impact of both Na$^+$ and K$^+$ in intravenous fluids and when assessing urinary free water clearance.

SUMMARY

- Na^+ is the major cation of the ECF. Therefore $[Na^+]$ is the main determinant of ECF osmolality.
- Na^+ is an effective osmole, meaning that it cannot freely diffuse out of the ECF, and that it creates osmotic pressure in the ECF.
- Changes in ECF $[Na^+]$ relative to the ICF osmolality cause fluid shifts between ECF and ICF, leading to cellular swelling or shrinkage. Cellular swelling and shrinkage are unfavorable for physiologic functioning.
- The brain and kidney regulate the ECF $[Na^+]$ to protect the ICF from fluid shifts.
- Osmoreceptors in the hypothalamus and circumventricular organs shrink and swell like other cells in response to changes in the effective osmolality of the ECF. In addition, osmoreceptors respond to shrinkage and swelling by modulating ADH secretion and thirst.
- During severe volume depletion, baroreceptors will trigger the hypothalamus to release ADH, thus boosting ECF volume at the expense of strict osmoregulation.
- ADH promotes the insertion of aquaporins in the collecting duct, increasing its permeability to water. Signal transduction is cAMP-mediated.
- Increased water permeability in the collecting duct can only promote water reabsorption, given a favorable osmotic gradient for water reabsorption in this part of the nephron. The favorable gradient is established by countercurrent multiplication in the loop of Henle, which maintains a high solute concentration in the renal medulla.
- Water reabsorption without solute in the descending limb of the loop of Henle concentrates the solute in the descending limb. NaCl reabsorption without water in the ascending limb concentrates the medullary interstitium and renders the tubular fluid low in solute concentration.
- Urea trapping contributes to the high medullary osmolality that enables water reabsorption from the collecting duct.

- When ADH prompts the reabsorption of water into the interstitium, the vasa recta are responsible for absorbing this water into the bloodstream. The vasa recta avoid dissipating the medullary solute gradient by countercurrent exchange.
- When plasma osmolality goes up and the ADH adds water to the ECF, urine osmolality goes up. When plasma osmolality goes down and excess water is excreted from the ECF, urine osmolality goes down. The maximum urine osmolality = medullary interstitial osmolality = 1200 mOsm/kg.
- Free water clearance equals the urine volume per time, V, minus osmolar clearance (C_{osm}):

$$C_{H20} = \dot{V} - C_{osm}$$

- Cosm is defined in accordance with the standard clearance equation:

$$C_{osm} = (\dot{U}_{osm})(\dot{V})/P_{osm}$$

- Plasma osmolality, or serum osmolality, may be calculated using the following equation:

$$P_{osm} = 2([Na^+]) + [glucose]/18 + BUN/2.8$$

- DM causes osmotic diuresis and may cause hypernatremia.
- DI causes increased free water clearance and may cause hypernatremia.
- SIADH and ECF volume depletion may cause hyponatremia.
- Hypernatremia causes shrinkage of brain cells, and hyponatremia causes swelling. Osmolyte levels in the brain are increased in response to chronic hypernatremia and are decreased in response to chronic hyponatremia. A rapid reversal of chronic hypernatremia or hyponatremia thus poses a threat to the patient.

REVIEW QUESTIONS

Directions: Each of the numbered items or incomplete statements in this section is followed by answers or by completions of the statement. Select the one lettered answer or completion that is best in each case.

1. A 25-year-old psychiatric patient drinks huge quantities of water because he is worried that he is losing excessive fluid from his body. Drinking large amounts of water may result in which of the following acute changes?
   A. Hyperosmolality in ECF
   B. Hypoosmolality in ECF
   C. Decreased ECF volume
   D. Decreased ICF volume
   E. No change in ICF volume

2. A 15-year-old boy has a mutation that interferes with the action of ADH in the collecting duct. If he feasts on a salty meal, he might have difficulty with hypernatremia for which of the following reasons?
   A. Enhanced urea reabsorption
   B. Failure of salt reabsorption
   C. Enhanced salt reabsorption
   D. Failure of water reabsorption
   E. Enhanced water reabsorption

3. A 65-year-old man with a pituitary tumor is found to be hyponatremic. His hyponatremia may be the result of which of the following?
   A. Elevated plasma glucose
   B. Cerebral edema
   C. Central DI
   D. Nephrogenic DI
   E. Excess secretion of ADH

ANSWERS TO REVIEW QUESTIONS

1. **The answer is B.** Drinking excessive quantities of free water, as might occur in a patient such as this with psychogenic polydipsia, leads to the addition of water to the ECF. This leads to a drop in ECF osmolality, which will then trigger a fluid shift of water from the ECF to the ICF, expanding the ICF volume, until the ECF and ICF are isotonic once more.

2. **The answer is D.** The action of ADH in the collection duct results in the insertion of aquaporins into the apical surface of the collecting duct. This results in enhanced water reabsorption, which would increase ECF fluid levels and act to decrease plasma osmolality. ADH enhances salt reabsorption in the thick ascending limb, which functions as part of the loop of Henle's countercurrent multiplication system to enhance the reabsorption of pure water.

3. **The answer is E.** Pituitary pathology may lead to central DI or SIADH. We know that SIADH (excess secretion of ADH) is present because of the hyponatremia. In patients with excess secretion of ADH, excessive water reabsorption by the kidney dilutes the ECF fluid and leads to hyponatremia. Hyponatremia, in turn, may lead to cerebral edema by the shift of fluid from the ECF to the ICF; the edema is therefore not the cause but the effect of the hyponatremia. Elevated plasma glucose, as seen in DM, would result in impaired water reabsorption and hypernatremia. Likewise, in either central or nephrogenic DI, there is inadequate water reabsorption, and *hypernatremia* can occur.

21

The Regulation of Potassium Balance

INTRODUCTION

In the past few chapters, we made several observations about extracellular fluid (ECF) volume and osmolality:

- The stability of these parameters is critical for normal physiologic functioning
- These parameters are subject to daily changes
- The kidney counters these changes to preserve stable ECF volume and osmolality.

In this chapter and the next, we will see that the same principles apply to two other critical physiologic parameters: the plasma potassium, or $[K^+]$, and the plasma acidity, or pH.

K^+ is present in human tissues at an overall concentration of about 50 mEq/kg body weight. Because plant and animal cells are filled with K^+, it is also ingested daily in dietary vegetables, fruits, and meats, which adds K^+ to the plasma through the intestines, raising plasma $[K^+]$ (Fig. 21.1).

The kidney modulates excretion of this daily K^+ load to keep the plasma $[K^+]$ stable, which in turn maintains the special distribution of K^+ between the intracellular fluid (ICF) and the ECF. Without this special distribution of K^+, the basic functions of most tissues would not be possible.

SYSTEM STRUCTURE: THE DISTRIBUTION OF POTASSIUM

Just as Na^+ is the major cation of the ECF, K^+ is the major cation of the ICF.

- Roughly 98% of total body K^+ resides in the ICF, with 2% in the ECF.
- In absolute terms, this represents a total of 3500 mEq of potassium in the ICF and 70 mEq in the ECF in the average person (Table 21.1).
- The Na^+,K^+-adenosine triphosphatase (ATPase) pumps that drive Na^+ out of cells and K^+ into cells create this distribution.

The two basic homeostatic elements in the regulation of the potassium distribution are:

- The sensors of plasma $[K^+]$
  - The K^+ sensors are thought to be located in the adrenal gland, perhaps in the zona glomerulosa, where aldosterone is secreted.
  - Recall that aldosterone indirectly regulates K^+ excretion in the late distal tubule and collecting duct.
- The effectors of regulatory K^+
  - The proximal tubule conducts a great deal of K^+ reabsorption on an unregulated basis, that is, it reabsorbs K^+ regardless of the plasma $[K^+]$.

SYSTEM FUNCTION: POTASSIUM HOMEOSTASIS

Why is a stable distribution of potassium physiologically important?

Recall that the segregation of K^+ inside cells is the chief determinant of the resting cell membrane potential, and that the resting membrane potential accounts for the excitability of nervous and muscle tissue. Without the potassium distribution, muscles could not contract, and neurons could not generate or transmit action potentials.

The distribution of potassium accounts for tissue excitability in the following way:

- The Na^+,K^+-ATPase pump creates a large $[K^+]$ gradient between the interior and exterior of cells.
- The high density of K^+ channels in most cell membranes (high K^+ permeability) allows K^+ to flow down that concentration gradient, from interior to exterior. The migration of positively charged K^+ ions out of the cell renders the intracellular side of the membrane electronegative (polarized).
- When a neurotransmitter stimulates an influx of Na^+ down its concentration gradient, the electrical potential inside of the cell increases (depolarizing the cell), and this change in transmembrane voltage triggers the opening of more epithelial sodium channels (ENaC).
- As the membrane depolarizes, more K^+ channels also open, leading to an efflux of K^+. If the initial neurotransmitted stimulus is strong enough, the influx of Na^+ continues to depolarize the cell, which opens more ENaCs.
- The Na^+ influx continues to build until the Na^+ influx surpasses the K^+ efflux, giving the inside of the cell a positive electrical potential, or action potential.
- The threshold potential is the minimum initial depolarized potential that the neurotransmitter must achieve to send the cell into the self-amplifying ascent toward action potential.

The K^+ distribution thus establishes the electrophysiologic ground upon which action potentials can occur. More generally, a high intracellular $[K^+]$ is necessary for a wide variety of enzymatic cell functions, including the regulation of protein synthesis, cell growth and division, and glycogen synthesis.

Disturbances in K^+ distribution, reflected in high or low plasma $[K^+]$, therefore threaten vital tissue functions. Consequently, many mechanisms are brought to bear upon the plasma $[K^+]$ to keep it within tight bounds.

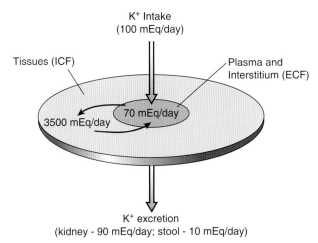

K⁺ Intake
(100 mEq/day)

Tissues (ICF)

Plasma and
Interstitium (ECF)

3500 mEq/day

70 mEq/day

K⁺ excretion
(kidney - 90 mEq/day; stool - 10 mEq/day)

Fig. 21.1 Potassium intake, excretion, and body stores. The values are totals, not concentrations, and are meant to represent averages for a 70-kg person. The *arrows* reflect the fact that K⁺ moves across the cell membranes. *ECF*, Extracellular fluid.

TABLE 21.1 The Normal Distribution of Potassium

	Intracellular Fluid	Extracellular Fluid
Total value	–3500 mEq	–70 mEq
Percentage of total	98%	2%
[K⁺]	140 mEq/L	4–5 mEq/L

TABLE 21.2 Sources of Unregulated Potassium Additions and Losses

Factors That ↑ Plasma [K⁺]	Factors That ↓ Plasma [K⁺]
Diet	Losses in stool
Cellular breakdown	Cellular uptake

This table does not include disturbances in the mechanisms that regulate [K⁺], although such disturbances are the most common causes of derangements in plasma [K⁺]. Rather, the table is meant to show the types of challenges that may confront the physiologic regulatory apparatus.

Challenges to Stable Transmembrane Potassium Distribution

The main source of K⁺ is the diet (Table 21.2). However, many different processes can lead to fluctuations in the plasma [K⁺]:

- Cellular breakdown on a massive scale, as in crush injuries, can also release potassium into the bloodstream in significant amounts.
- Unregulated potassium losses occur in the stool and in a variety of disease states.
- Increased cellular production, which traps large amounts of potassium inside cells, can also result in increased uptake of potassium, which lowers the plasma [K⁺].
- Pregnant mothers may also experience a drop in their plasma [K⁺] as the growing fetus traps potassium inside its cells.

Because the precise transmembrane potassium gradient is so critical to neuromuscular function, disturbances in the distribution can create life-threatening cardiac arrhythmias. Consequently, dietary loads of potassium must be removed from the ECF immediately.

- The renal excretion of dietary potassium takes place over hours—a time frame that is too slow to protect cardiac functioning.
- Intracellular storage of the potassium absorbed from the intestines serves as a temporary measure until renal mechanisms can eliminate the excess potassium.

Intracellular Storage: The Rapid Phase of Normalization

Within minutes of an increase in plasma [K⁺], K⁺ is stored inside cells. This occurs via various mechanisms, which will now be discussed (see Fast Fact Box 21.1).

Fast Fact Box 21.1

Without storage, one meal's addition of 50 mEq of K⁺ to the roughly 14 L extracellular fluid would double the normal plasma [K⁺] of 4 mEq/L. This change in plasma [K⁺] would significantly alter the resting membrane potential.

Plasma Potassium Concentration

The problem of increased plasma [K⁺] is partly self-correcting, as some of the K⁺ storage occurs unassisted. This is because the increased ECF [K⁺] favors K⁺ entry into the cell and opposes its egress.

- Some of the added K⁺ is pumped into the cells as the altered gradient facilitates the work of the Na⁺,K⁺-ATPase.
- The proportionate distribution of some of the added K⁺ between the ICF and ECF thus preserves the membrane potential in part and mitigates the problem of increased plasma [K⁺].

The Na⁺,K⁺-ATPase appears not to be able to normalize the potassium distribution (and hence the tissue membrane potential) by itself. Therefore other rapid defenses are in place in addition to slow renal excretion to lower the plasma [K⁺] by intracellular storage.

Insulin and Catecholamines

Intracellular potassium storage is also facilitated by two hormones.

The main function of insulin is to store glucose inside cells in response to high glucose levels and to promote anabolic pathways for the cellular storage of carbohydrate energy.

- After a meal, intestinal absorption yields a load of both glucose and potassium together. Insulin's linkage with the blood glucose level therefore indirectly yokes the hormone's secretion to the K⁺ level.
- Insulin is sometimes administered therapeutically to lower the plasma [K⁺] (see Genetics Box 21.1, Development Box 21.1, Environmental Box 21.1, and Pharmacology Box 21.1).

GENETICS BOX 21.1

Periodic hypokalemic paralysis (PHP) is an autosomal dominant disease in which affected individuals experience the sudden onset of severe arm and leg muscle weakness or even paralysis (as the name suggests) that can last from minutes to days. Mutations in the CACNA1S gene that encodes a skeletal muscle Ca^{2+} channel α chain or in the SCN4A gene that encodes a skeletal muscle Na^+ channel are responsible for this disease, although the mechanisms by which they do so are incompletely understood.

DEVELOPMENT BOX 21.1

Attacks of periodic hypokalemic paralysis (PHP) generally start in childhood or adolescence. As patients age, the attacks may decrease in frequency, but many develop a proximal limb myopathy of variable severity.

ENVIRONMENTAL BOX 21.1

Precipitants of attacks can be difficult to identify, but in some patients rest after exercise and ingestion of high carbohydrate meals are implicated. This latter observation suggests that insulin secretion might cause acute K^+ shifts related to paralytic attacks. It has been reported that use of the albuterol β agonist inhaler caused weakness in one affected individual.

PHARMACOLOGY BOX 21.1

Acute attacks are treated by administering intravenous potassium chloride (KCl). Attacks can be prevented with KCl supplementation, the carbonic anhydrase inhibitor acetazolamide, or the potassium sparing diuretics triamterene and spironolactone.

The catecholamines (the most important examples outside the brain are epinephrine [adrenalin] and norepinephrine) are secreted at a basal level and are increased in response to stress. They have a wide variety of effects, including an increase in cardiac output and blood pressure.

- Increased catecholamines lead to increased potassium uptake into the cell.
- The catecholamines are not thought to regulate plasma $[K^+]$, but only to lower it as an incidental effect.

- β_2-adrenergic agonists, such as salbutamol, can also be used in the treatment of high plasma $[K^+]$ (see Clinical Correlation Box 21.1).

Plasma pH

The cellular uptake and release of potassium is also important for the rapid handling of acid loads.

When the $[H^+]$ rises in the blood—for example, because of the metabolism of digested proteins—H^+ diffuses into cells.

- The migration of the positive charge inward results in an efflux of positively charged Na^+ and K^+, resulting in a rising plasma $[K^+]$ (Fig. 21.2).
- In fact, 60% of acid loads are "buffered" by cellular uptake. The rest of the load is buffered by bicarbonate in solution in the blood (see Ch. 22).

When the $[H^+]$ falls, H^+ migrates out of the cell, and K^+ shifts inward toward the negative charge left behind by the H^+.

- The plasma $[K^+]$ therefore falls.
- The rise in pH, however, does not lower the $[K^+]$ to the same extent that low pH raises the plasma $[K^+]$. The reasons for this are not entirely clear.

This inverse relationship between $[H^+]$ and $[K^+]$ is also seen in the cells of the late distal tubule and collecting duct, as will be discussed later.

Renal Handling: The Slow Phase of Normalization

Whereas intracellular storage takes place in minutes, it represents only a temporary solution to the problem of excess K^+. Without actual elimination of K^+ from the body, the plasma $[K^+]$ would continue to rise and the transmembrane distribution (and potential) would be increasingly disturbed.

Consequently, renal excretion of K^+ is critical to avoid life-threatening increases in the plasma $[K^+]$.

- When plasma $[K^+]$ is low, nearly all filtered K^+ may be reabsorbed, but the kidney always excretes some K^+ in the urine—regulation simply determines how much is excreted.
- As with other parameters under renal control, the kidney adjusts excretion or clearance (and hence the plasma $[K^+]$) through adjustments in tubular reabsorption and secretion.

Clinical Correlation Box 21.1

Exercise and β-Blockade

In addition to the primary factors mentioned in the text, secondary factors affect the plasma $[K^+]$. Two examples are exercise and drugs called β-blockers. Such factors do not normally cause pathogenic disturbances in the plasma $[K^+]$, but they can do so in the context of another underlying disturbance in potassium homeostasis. Therefore they can be important clinical considerations.

Exercise may transiently increase the plasma $[K^+]$. The adenosine triphosphate (ATP) depletion that occurs during exercise and muscle contraction may open ATP-dependent potassium channels, increasing permeability to potassium in the muscle cells. Given that efflux of potassium follows muscular contraction in the repolarization period, one might think that muscular action potentials themselves would contribute to the increased plasma $[K^+]$. This is not the case,

because the number of mEq of K^+ exchanged during and after the action potential is extremely small and does not affect the overall plasma $[K^+]$.

β2-blockers like propranolol are competitive antagonists for adrenergic β-receptors. They inhibit the binding of epinephrine and norepinephrine and interfere with the actions of those hormones, such as increasing heart rate and cardiac output. They are therefore used to treat hypertension. Because the catecholamines also promote the cellular uptake of K^+, these drugs may also increase the plasma $[K^+]$. When these drugs are administered in the context of another aggravating factor, they may cause hyperkalemia—pathologically high plasma $[K^+]$, >5 mEq/L. Hyperkalemia may have very serious consequences for cardiac function if left untreated.

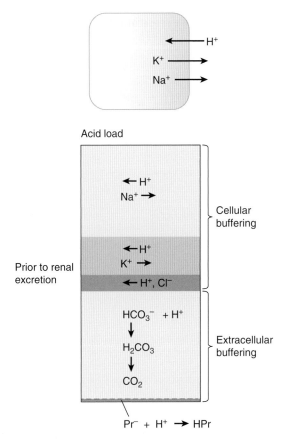

Acid load

Cellular buffering

Prior to renal excretion

Extracellular buffering

$$HCO_3^- + H^+$$
$$\downarrow$$
$$H_2CO_3$$
$$\downarrow$$
$$CO_2$$

$$Pr^- + H^+ \rightarrow HPr$$

Fig. 21.2 Intracellular buffering of acid loads. This figure shows that in addition to the exchange of H^+ for Na^+ and K^+, H^+ migration into cells draws a small amount of Cl^-. The protonation of plasma proteins is a minimal contributor to buffering. *Pr*, Plasma protein.

- Under normal circumstances of adequate amounts of dietary potassium, secretion predominates and can lower the plasma $[K^+]$ in a time frame of hours.

To understand the renal regulation of plasma $[K^+]$, we must first review the tubular transport of K^+.

Renal Potassium Transport

Potassium is reabsorbed in bulk in the proximal tubule and loop of Henle, while regulation of potassium balance takes place in the late distal tubule and collecting duct.

- In these late tubule segments, various amounts of K^+ are reabsorbed or secreted under the control of regulatory mechanisms.
- Roughly 80% of K^+ is reabsorbed in the proximal tubule, and 10% is reabsorbed in the loop of Henle (Fig. 21.3).
- Although the thick ascending limb of Henle may reabsorb 10% of the filtered K^+, a significant amount of K^+ reabsorbed via the NaK2Cl cotransporter is recycled back to the lumen, a process that maximizes NaCl reabsorption in that segment.

Although the proximal tubule cells are rich with basolateral Na^+,K^+-ATPases that drive K^+ from the interstitium into the cells, most of renal K^+ reabsorption occurs here. How can this be, given the ATPase-governed movement of K^+ away from the interstitium?

- The proximal tubular K^+ reabsorption is thought to be mainly paracellular.

- Two forces may drive paracellular K^+ reabsorption.
  - This first means of K^+ reabsorption is known as solvent drag, and it occurs not through the genesis of an electrical or chemical gradient for K^+ but merely because the flowing water imparts kinetic energy to the K^+ ions.
  - A second driving force is the electropositivity of the late proximal tubule lumen.
    Recall that the cotransport of Na^+ with a variety of non-Cl^- anions in the early proximal tubule raises the $[Cl^-]$ in the luminal fluid. This action creates a concentration gradient for paracellular Cl^- reabsorption in the late proximal tubule, and the migration of negatively charged Cl^- anions from lumen to interstitium raises the electrical potential of the lumen.
    This, in turn, may provide an electrical driving force for the paracellular reabsorption of K^+ (as it does for Na^+).

The reabsorption of K^+ in the thick ascending limb of the loop of Henle also occurs paracellularly because of a positively charged tubule lumen.

- Recall that the Na^+,K^+-ATPase drives Na^+ across the basolateral and hence the apical membrane of the tubule cells.
- The apical translocation of Na^+ across the $Na^+/K^+/2Cl^-$ symporter drives the reabsorption of K^+ and Cl^-. Chloride is reabsorbed across the basolateral membrane into the interstitium.
- Potassium, which is also driven inside the cell by the Na^+,K^+-ATPase, can escape either through basolateral channels into the interstitium or through apical channels back into the tubule lumen.
- Apical recycling of the K^+ without Cl^- renders the tubule electropositive and drives the paracellular reabsorption of K^+ and other cations.

Potassium may be either reabsorbed or secreted by the late distal tubule and collecting duct (Fig. 21.4). In some types of intercalated cells, the H^+/K^+-ATPase may drive transcellular K^+ reabsorption in exchange for H^+ secretion.

Potassium secretion takes place in principal cells of the late distal tubule and collecting duct and is driven by the Na^+,K^+-ATPase.

- The basolateral Na^+,K^+-ATPase pumps Na^+ from inside the cell to the interstitium, and K^+ from the interstitium into the cell.
- The high intracellular $[K^+]$ causes K^+ to flow down its concentration gradient across apical and basolateral K^+ channels.
- At the same time, the low intracellular $[Na^+]$ causes Na^+ reabsorption across the apical membrane from lumen to cytosol. Sodium reabsorption in excess of anions leaves the lumen negatively charged, however.
- Consequently, the electronegative tubule lumen favors net diffusion of K^+ across its apical channels and hence net secretion of K^+. The end result is that the Na^+,K^+-ATPase drives K^+ secretion in this part of the nephron.

Tubular flow promotes increased K^+ secretion by sweeping away luminal potassium in its forward flow and reducing the luminal $[K^+]$.

- This augments the concentration gradient for potassium diffusion into the tubule lumen.
- Increased tubular flow therefore increases potassium secretion and excretion.

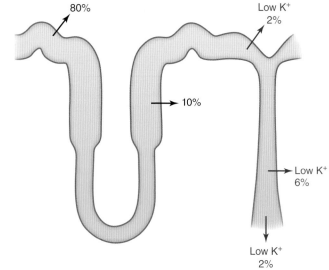

Under normal to high extracellular [K⁺] conditions

80%

Normal/ high K⁺
10–50%

10%

Normal/
high K⁺
5–30%

Normal/
high K⁺
10–80%

A

Under low extracellular [K⁺] conditions

80%

Low K⁺
2%

10%

Low K⁺
6%

Low K⁺
2%

B

Fig. 21.3 Potassium transport along the renal tubule. Reabsorption in the proximal tubule and loop of Henle are obligatory. In response to potassium status, net excretion is determined by regulated reabsorption and secretion in the late distal tubule and collecting duct. Part A shows the tubular handling of K⁺ when [K⁺] is normal to elevated and part B shows the handling when [K⁺] is low.

The 80% reabsorption of filtered K⁺ in the proximal tubule and the 10% reabsorption in the thick ascending limb allows for almost complete reabsortion of filtered K⁺ by the time the fluid arrives at the late distal nephron and collecting duct. At that site, particularly in collecting duct principal cells, regulated K⁺ secretion (A) or further reabsorption (B) will occur. Therefore, the K⁺ excreted during high body [K⁺] may greatly exceed the K⁺ filtered in order to maintain [K⁺] homeostasis (A). In the less common situation when the body [K⁺] is depleted, K⁺ secretion is suppressed and the K⁺/H⁺ ATPase of the intercalated cells of the collecting duct increase further reabsorption of filtered K⁺, which can markedly lower the urinary [K⁺] to as low as 2% of the filtered amount (B).

Because of the normal countercurrent mechanism, K⁺ reabsorbed in the thick ascending limb via the NKCC2 transporter concentrates in the renal medulla. This process leads to a gradient of higher K⁺ in the interstitium than in the lumen of the collecting duct. Under conditions of high body K⁺, the usual state on a well balanced diet, this gradient opposes the backleak of K⁺ from the lumen of the collecting duct back into the interstitium to aid K⁺ excretion. In contrast, under the less common state of K⁺ depletion, the K⁺ gradient between the medullary interstitium and the collecting duct lumen results in a small amount of backleak into the lumen from the interstitium, explaining the obligatory loss of a small amount of K⁺, so K⁺ conservation in humans is not as great as Na⁺ conservation.

Another mechanism by which increased flow increases potassium excretion is that of increased sodium delivery to the distal tubule.

- Increased sodium delivery increases sodium reabsorption here, which drives potassium secretion by the mechanisms described previously.
- Increased tubular flow in this region of the tubule is sometimes called distal flow.

Regulatory Factors in Renal Potassium Excretion

Aldosterone serves as the primary regular of renal K⁺ excretion. It promotes K⁺ secretion from principal cells in the late distal tubule and collecting duct.

- It does so by diffusing out of the peritubular capillaries and acting on the nuclei of principal cells to modulate deoxyribonucleic acid transcription, producing several end results via messenger proteins.
- Primarily, aldosterone enhances the performance of the Na⁺,K⁺-ATPase in the basolateral membrane.
  - This increases the tubular intracellular [K⁺], but importantly, it stimulates increased Na⁺ uptake from the tubule lumen. (Recall that aldosterone is also an important hormone in the regulation of Na⁺ reabsorption and ECF volume.)

- Increased Na⁺ uptake increases the electronegativity of the tubule lumen and promotes paracellular K⁺ secretion by electrostatic force.
- Aldosterone also increases the apical permeability to Na⁺ by causing the principal cell to insert more channels into its apical membrane and by opening silent Na⁺ channels. This further increases Na⁺ uptake and hence K⁺ secretion (Fig. 21.5) (see Fast Fact Box 21.2).

Fast Fact Box 21.2

Aldosterone has a cytoplasmic receptor that also recognizes cortisol, which is in greater concentration, yet cortisol has little effect on potassium, sodium, and hydrogen transport. The reason is that the collecting duct cell has an enzyme, 11-beta OH steroid dehydrogenase, which converts cortisol to inactive cortisone. There is an ingredient of natural licorice that inhibits the enzyme, causing hypertension (Na⁺ retention), hypokalemia (K secretion), and alkalosis (H⁺ secretion).

Aldosterone secretion is thought to be controlled by two different homeostatic systems:

- Blood pressure
  - Recall that low blood pressure stimulates aldosterone secretion through the renin-angiotensin-aldosterone system.

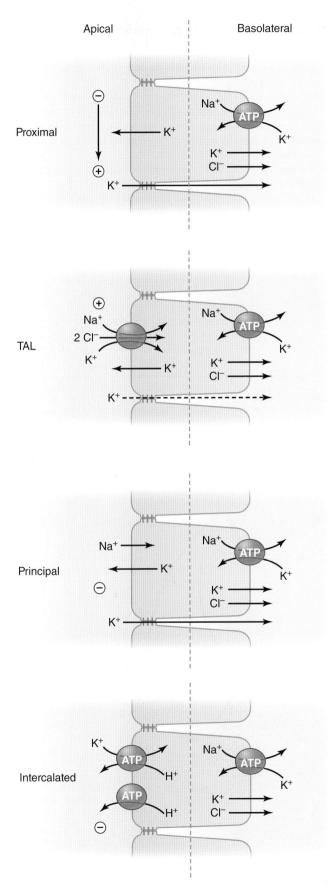

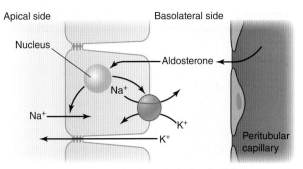

Fig. 21.5 Aldosterone action in the principal cell. Aldosterone stimulates the production of proteins that stimulate the basolateral Na^+,K^+-ATPase and that upregulate the number and the activity of apical Na^+ channels. It also increases K^+ conductance.

Fig. 21.4 Pumps and channels participating in K^+ transport. *ATP,* Adenosine triphosphatase; *TAL,* Thick Ascending Limb.

- Plasma $[K^+]$
  - High plasma $[K^+]$ stimulates the secretion of aldosterone, perhaps by stimulating K^+ sensors in the zona glomerulosa.

Depending on the stimulus and the presence of other regulators, aldosterone can selectively decrease Na^+ excretion (correct hypovolemia and low blood pressure) or increase K^+ excretion (correct hyperkalemia). (See Clinical Correlation Box 21.2.)

Fig. 21.6 summarizes the hormonal influences on plasma $[K^+]$, for both intracellular storage and renal excretion.

PATHOPHYSIOLOGY: DISORDERS OF PLASMA $[K^+]$ REGULATION

Hyperkalemia is pathologically high plasma $[K^+]$, and it is usually defined as a plasma $[K^+]$ greater than 5.5 mEq/L. Hypokalemia is pathologically low plasma $[K^+]$, and it is usually defined as a plasma $[K^+]$ less than 3.5 mEq/L.

Pathologic derangements in plasma $[K^+]$ are usually caused by defects or alterations in the regulatory apparatus itself.

Membrane excitability is determined by the difference between the negative resting potential and the less-negative threshold potential. (Recall that the threshold potential is the minimum depolarizing potential that is necessary from a synaptic stimulus to trigger an action potential.)

- If the resting potential (e.g., –70 mV in most neurons) is close to the threshold potential (e.g., –60 mV), a smaller stimulus may bump up the electrical potential inside the cell enough to achieve the threshold potential of –60 mV and send the cell over the edge to an eventual action potential.
- If the resting potential (again, suppose –70 mV) is farther from the threshold potential (e.g., –50 mV), a larger amount of depolarization is necessary to reach the threshold potential.
- When the resting and threshold potentials are close together and action potentials are achievable with smaller stimuli, the membrane is considered more excitable. When the membrane requires larger stimuli for an action potential, the membrane is said to be less excitable.

Because the plasma $[K^+]$ determines the resting potential, alterations in plasma $[K^+]$ alter the resting potential, and consequently can alter membrane excitability.

- Hyperkalemia will impede the resting efflux of potassium and render the resting potential less negative, or closer to threshold.

Clinical Correlation Box 21.2

Potassium and Extracellular Fluid (ECF) Volume Homeostasis

Because aldosterone helps regulate both plasma [K⁺] and ECF volume, how does the body avoid disturbing plasma [K⁺] when it seeks to correct ECF volume? How does it preserve ECF volume when aldosterone is being secreted to correct plasma [K⁺]? This creates the so called "aldosterone paradox." A key factor in this regulation system is WNK (with no lysine = K) kinase, a class of serine threonine kinases that have among their myriad functions the modulation of transporter functions along the renal tubule.

When ECF volume is decreased, angiotensin II and aldosterone increase Na⁺ reabsorption in the proximal tubule and late distal tubule/collecting duct, respectively. In the presence of angiotensin II, aldosterone also increases Na⁺ reabsorption (Na⁺-Cl⁻ transporter) in early distal convoluted tubule (via WNK-SPAK pathway). Through unknown mechanisms, K⁺ transport is inhibited although increased WNK1 signaling (increase in WNK1/KS-WNK1 ratio; KS-WNK1 acts as a dominant-negative inhibitor of WNK1). This results in increased net Na⁺ reabsorption without affecting serum K⁺.

In contrast, the main response of hyperaldosteronemia in the context of hyperkalemia (and baseline angiotensin II level) is to increase K⁺ excretion. Both aldosterone and hyperkalemia increase K⁺ channel activity despite decreased WNK1 signaling. Aldosterone still stimulate the reabsorption of Na⁺ in the late distal tubule/collecting duct; however, without angiotensin II, the Na⁺-Cl⁻ transporter that was activated in the presence of aldosterone and angiotensin II is actually inhibited.

Familial hyperkalemic hypertension (PHHt, also known as Gordon syndrome or pseudohypoaldosteronism) represents a dysfunction of this homeostatic mechanism. It is characterized by hypertension, hyperkalemia, hypercalciuria, and metabolic acidosis. Because of mutations in different WNK kinases, the Na⁺-Cl⁻ transporter activity in the early distal tubule increases. PHHt responds to thiazide which inhibits this Na⁺-Cl⁻ transporter. The details of this disease are still under active investigation.

	Angiotensin II + Aldo	Hyperkalemia + Aldo
Proximal tubule	^ Na⁺/H⁺ exchanger —> ^ Na⁺ reabsorption	No change
Early distal tubule	^ Na⁺-Cl⁻ transporter —> ^ Na⁺ reabsorption No ^K⁺ excretion	No change ^ K⁺ channel —> ^ K⁺ excretion
Late distal Tubule	^ Na⁺ channel —> ^ Na⁺ reabsorption No ^K⁺ excretion	^ Na⁺ channel —> ^ Na⁺ reabsorption ^ K⁺ channel —> ^ K⁺ excretion

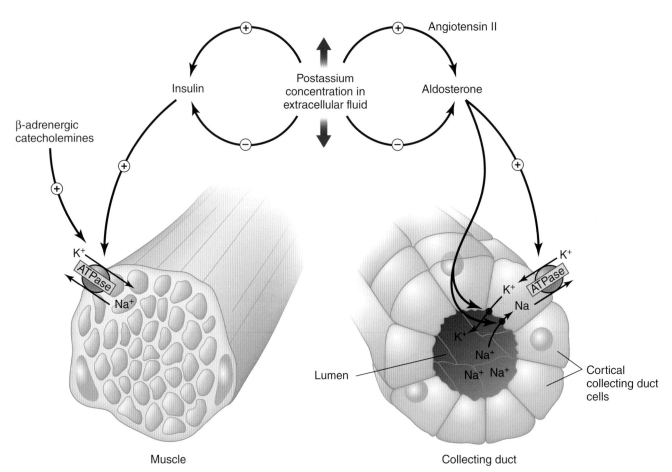

Fig. 21.6 A summary of hormonal influences on plasma [K⁺]. Although the figure suggests insulin secretion is promoted by high plasma [K⁺] and vice versa, this is a matter of controversy. Some investigators believe catecholamine-stimulated K⁺ uptake to be mediated by β-receptors.

- Hypokalemia does the reverse. Therefore hyperkalemia should render cell membranes more excitable and hypokalemia less excitable (see Clinical Correlation Box 21.3 and Fast Fact Box 21.3).

Fast Fact Box 21.3

The actual situation is slightly more complicated, however. Prolonged exposure to disturbances in plasma [K⁺] may actually produce the opposite effects, with hyperkalemia leading to decreased excitability and hypokalemia to increased excitability. This may occur through effects on Na^+ channel inactivation.

HYPERKALEMIA

The primary cause of hyperkalemia is decreased renal excretion, with two minor causes, including increased dietary intake and increased cellular release.

The two main causes of decreased renal excretion are as follows:

- Decreased filtration
  - Decreased glomerular filtration is called renal failure. Acute renal failure is probably the most common cause of hyperkalemia.
  - Whereas 90% of filtered K⁺ is usually reabsorbed, decreased glomerular filtration rate (GFR) prohibits the elimination of the remaining 10% and also interferes with secretion.
- Decreased secretion
  - Secretion depends on a good distal flow rate and when GFR is reduced, the distal flow rate is reduced.
  - Decreased secretion may occur independently of decreased GFR in the case of hypoaldosteronism and medication side effects.

    Hypoaldosteronism is decreased aldosterone secretion, which may occur in Addison disease (primary adrenal insufficiency), in hyporeninemia (low levels of renin in the blood) secondary to various types of kidney disease, or as an idiopathic effect (having an unknown cause).
  - A variety of drugs impair K⁺ secretion, including potassium-sparing diuretics and nonsteroidal antiinflammatory drugs.

In the context of renal failure, a large dietary potassium load may overwhelm whatever secretory capacities remain in the kidney, thereby leading to hyperkalemia. Likewise, an increased release of K⁺ from cellular breakdown in the context of renal failure may cause persistent hyperkalemia.

- If renal failure is not present, these conditions may cause transient hyperkalemia.
- Three examples of increased cellular breakdown are:
  - tumor lysis syndrome, wherein cancer chemotherapy leads to widespread cell death.
  - rhabdomyolysis, massive tissue breakdown, as in crush injuries.

- hemolysis, the rupture of red blood cells, as in transfusion reactions or vasculitis, where inflammation in the blood vessels damages the red blood cells.
- The release of potassium from cells by way of transmembrane shifting may also cause hyperkalemia. Metabolic acidosis and the administration of ß₂-blockers may create hyperkalemia this way, especially in the context of renal failure (see Clinical Correlation Box 21.4).

Clinical Correlation Box 21.4

What is Rhabdomyolysis?

A 19-year-old male is rushed by ambulance from the scene of a motor vehicle accident. He has sustained massive crush injuries to his lower extremities, but he is breathing, has a pulse of 130 bpm and a BP of 80/50 mm Hg, is alert and oriented, and his pupils are equally round and reactive to light. History taking reveals the boy was trapped in his car for over an hour. Shortly after arrival in the emergency room, the patient develops a cardiac arrhythmia with QRS complexes that are wide and low in amplitude. He loses consciousness and goes into cardiac arrest. After cardiopulmonary resuscitation and an intravenous (IV) push of calcium gluconate, he recovers. He receives IV glucose, insulin, and salbutamol. Laboratory values show an initial serum K⁺ of 10 mEq/L, confirming the diagnosis of hyperkalemia secondary to rhabdomyolysis.

Rhabdomyolysis is widespread breakdown of muscle tissue. It may occur in crush injuries, because of large pressure sores from immobility, in circumstances of heat and exertion, in the context of illicit drug use, including cocaine and ecstasy, and in other scenarios. In addition to releasing large amounts of potassium into the bloodstream, rhabdomyolysis also dumps large amounts of myoglobin (a protein that serves as an oxygen reservoir in muscle tissues) into the bloodstream. When myoglobin is filtered in the kidney, it can cause intrinsic renal failure. The combination of acute renal failure and release of K⁺ from the cells makes rhabdomyolysis especially predisposing toward hyperkalemia.

Immediate treatment should be directed at the respiration and circulation, including hemostasis, if hemorrhaging is present; the administration of calcium gluconate should be provided to stabilize the membrane potential of excitable tissue exposed to hyperkalemia; and drugs, such as insulin and β2 agonists should be used to reduce the plasma [K⁺] if hyperkalemia and cardiac arrhythmias are present. Treatment should next focus on preserving renal function with IV hydration and, if necessary, dialysis.

Hyperkalemia is more imminently life-threatening than hypokalemia. The signs and symptoms of hyperkalemia include:

- Cardiac arrhythmias (and accompanying abnormalities on electrocardiogram)
- Muscle weakness or paralysis
- Paresthesias (tingling or other unusual peripheral sensations)
- Metabolic acidosis

For plasma [K⁺] values of less than 7 mEq/L, treatment with Kayexalate (sodium polystyrene sulfonate) may be sufficient. However, many additional treatments are available.

- Kayexalate is an orally administered ion exchange resin that draws excess K⁺ into the intestinal lumen, leading to excretion in the stool.
- Severe hyperkalemia (>7 mEq/L) should be treated with intravenous calcium gluconate, which helps restore the normal level of excitability of the myocardium.
- Glucose and insulin may be administered together—the insulin to shift the K⁺ rapidly inside the cells, and the glucose to prevent hypoglycemia (low blood sugar) because of the insulin.

- Salbutamol, a β-adrenergic agonist, may also be administered to shift K$^+$ rapidly into cells.
- Finally, dialysis may be used to reverse hyperkalemia.

HYPOKALEMIA

In 1998 the *New England Journal of Medicine* reported that hypokalemia may be the electrolyte abnormality most commonly seen in clinical practice. Hypokalemia is, however, not as life-threatening as hyperkalemia.

- When mild, it may in fact produce no symptoms at all
- When more severe, it may cause:
  - Muscle weakness
  - Paresthesias
  - Muscle necrosis
  - Impaired renal function
  - Cardiac arrhythmias

Hypokalemia can occur by a number of different mechanisms:

- Excess urinary losses
  - Thiazide and loop diuretics cause excess K$^+$ secretion by increasing distal flow.
  - Other causes of increased tubular flow may lead to potassium wasting as well.
    For example, glucosuria in diabetes mellitus causes an osmotic diuresis that can result in excess K$^+$ secretion in the distal nephron.

Hyperaldosteronism, which occurs in some adrenal tumors, may lead to an excess loss of K$^+$.

- Excess stool losses
  - Any cause of diarrhea may lead to hypokalemia.
    In patients with eating disorders, for example, chronic diarrhea caused by laxative abuse may lead to hypokalemia. This may be worsened by decreased dietary intake of potassium.
  - Gastrointestinal losses are especially threatening in the context of renal potassium wasting, as the kidney can usually compensate for losses with increased reabsorption.
- Increased cellular uptake
  - An increased plasma pH will cause H$^+$ to shift out of cells and K$^+$ into cells, leading to decreased plasma [K$^+$]. β-adrenergic agonists, which are used in treating asthma to dilate the bronchioles, may also shift potassium into cells by mimicking the action of catecholamines.
  - Vitamin B12 therapy for anemia may promote cell growth and trap potassium inside cells.
  - Other conditions of rapid cell growth, such as pregnancy, may drop the plasma [K$^+$].

The treatment for hypokalemia, in addition to addressing the underlying cause, is repletion of body K$^+$. Repletion should be done slowly, preferably with oral potassium chloride (KCl) supplements. Among naturally occurring foods, dried figs, molasses, and seaweed have the highest concentration of potassium.

SUMMARY

- Body potassium is 98% intracellular and 2% extracellular.
- This distribution is critical to establishing the resting membrane potential in excitable cells, such as muscle and nervous tissue. It is also important to the performance of many internal cell functions.
- The body faces constant challenges to the physiologic distribution of potassium between the ICF and ECF, including dietary intake and the loss of K$^+$ in the stool.
- The body normalizes the plasma [K$^+$] after a dietary load with rapid mechanisms and slower mechanisms.
- The rapid mechanisms for normalizing plasma [K$^+$] after a dietary load involve intracellular storage of K$^+$. The slower mechanisms involve increased renal excretion of K$^+$.
- The factors promoting intracellular potassium storage are high plasma [K$^+$] and the secretion of insulin and catecholamines.
- Low plasma pH (high [H$^+$]) causes H$^+$ to shift inside body cells in exchange for potassium, raising the plasma [K$^+$].
- About 65% of filtered K$^+$ is reabsorbed in the proximal tubule, and another 25% is reabsorbed in the loop of Henle; the remaining 10% is usually excreted.

- Under normal circumstances, in addition to excreting 10% of filtered potassium, the distal tubule and collecting duct secrete potassium to eliminate the rest of the excess plasma potassium.
- Regulatory factors control potassium secretion in the distal segments of the tubule. High plasma [K$^+$] and aldosterone promote distal potassium secretion, as does increased distal flow.
- Disorders of potassium level are almost always caused by disturbances in renal secretion.
- Hyperkalemia, high plasma [K$^+$], is most often caused by decreased renal secretion of potassium because of renal failure. It causes life-threatening cardiac arrhythmias and is treated with calcium gluconate, Kayexalate, glucose and insulin, beta-2 agonists, and dialysis.
- Hypokalemia, low plasma [K$^+$], is most often caused by excess potassium secretion in the distal nephron because of the administration of diuretics. It is associated with less morbidity and mortality than hyperkalemia but is far more common. It is treated with potassium repletion, usually oral KCl.

REVIEW QUESTIONS

Directions: Each of the numbered items or incomplete statements in this section is followed by answers or by completions of the statement. Select the one lettered answer or completion that is best in each case.

1. An 80-year-old woman is treated for congestive heart failure with the loop diuretic, furosemide. After com-

plaining of fatigue, she is found to have a low serum K$^+$ level of 2.6 mEq/L. Her hypokalemia is caused by which of the following mechanisms?

A. Increased activity of the distal Na$^+$,K$^+$-ATPase

B. Increased glomerular filtration

C. Increased distal flow

D. Decreased proximal K$^+$ reabsorption
E. Decreased K$^+$ reabsorption in the loop of Henle

2. A 28-year-old human immunodeficiency virus-positive man with a recent history of pulmonary tuberculosis presents with loss of energy and a dark pigmentation to his skin. He is found to have low blood pressure, low blood glucose, and an elevated plasma [K$^+$]. Further lab studies are likely to show:
A. Low serum [Na$^+$]
B. Low serum ACTH
C. Low serum renin
D. Low hematocrit

E. Low serum aldosterone

3. A 45-year-old woman with a long history of asthma runs a 10-km race on a cold October morning and has to stop several times to use her albuterol inhaler (a β2-adrenergic agonist). If she has inadvertently dropped her serum [K$^+$], the reason could be:
A. Exercise
B. Transmembrane K$^+$ shift
C. Osmotic diuresis
D. Hyperaldosteronism
E. Inhibition of the Na$^+$/K$^+$/2Cl$^-$ symporter

ANSWERS TO REVIEW QUESTIONS

1. **The answer is C.** The loop diuretic furosemide (Lasix) can cause hypokalemia by increasing tubular flow. It does so by inhibiting Na$^+$ reabsorption in the loop of Henle (which in turn inhibits water reabsorption from the collecting duct). Increased flow in the distal segments of the tubule washes away tubular K$^+$ and creates a favorable gradient for potassium secretion. Increased Na$^+$ delivery results in more Na$^+$ reabsorption here and an electrical gradient for paracellular potassium secretion. Although increased activity of the distal Na$^+$,K$^+$-ATPase would result in increased potassium secretion, the scenario stated that the drug in question acts in the loop of Henle and not distally; furosemide does not act in the distal segments. Furthermore, increased Na$^+$,K$^+$-ATPase activity would have an antidiuretic effect. Spironolactone, a "potassium-sparing" diuretic that acts on the distal Na$^+$,K$^+$-ATPase, inhibits this ATPase and conserves potassium. Increased GFR could increase potassium secretion by increasing tubular flow, but there is no reason to suspect an increased GFR. In a patient with congestive heart failure, in fact, the GFR would likely be normal or low because of decreased renal blood flow, but likely not high. Decreased proximal reabsorption would also lead to potassium wasting, but neither congestive heart failure per se nor furosemide action in the loop of Henle cause decreased proximal tubular reabsorption. Finally, furosemide does inhibit the Na$^+$/K$^+$/2Cl$^-$ symporter in the loop of Henle and may impede potassium reabsorption here, but this is not the direct mechanism of potassium loss with loop diuretics. If potassium loss in the loop of Henle were the only mechanism of excess potassium excretion, the distal segments of the tubule could make up for it with increased reabsorption. Because increased distal flow accelerates distal potassium secretion, no such compensation can occur.

2. **The answer is E.** The patient has Addison disease, probably because of a tubercular infection of the adrenal glands. Addison disease is primary adrenal failure, in this case, because of infectious destruction of the glands. Addison disease results in a failure to secrete glucocorticoids and the mineralocorticoid, aldosterone. (Failure of the adrenal medulla may also occur, but this does not produce significant symptoms, as the sympathetic nervous system compensates.) Lack of glucocorticoids results in hypoglycemia and low blood pressure, and lack of aldosterone results in decreased distal Na$^+$ and water reabsorption (leading to low blood pressure) and decreased K$^+$ secretion (leading to hyperkalemia). Although less Na$^+$ is reabsorbed distally in the absence of aldosterone, this would not decrease the plasma [Na$^+$]. Remember that the amount of distal free water reabsorption determines the [Na$^+$] and that free water reabsorption is determined by antidiuretic hormone, not aldosterone. Adrenocorticotropic hormone (ACTH) is not low but high in Addison disease. With no negative feedback from adrenal hormone secretion, the pituitary secretes more ACTH, not less. If the problem were a lack of central endocrine stimulation to the adrenal from the pituitary (hypopituitarism), we might still expect aldosterone secretion to occur as part of the renin-angiotensin-aldosterone system and in response to high plasma [K$^+$], because neither plasma [K$^+$] nor blood pressure is regulated through the pituitary. Hyperpigmentation can occur in Addison disease caused by the increased levels of ACTH and melanocyte-stimulating hormone, MSH. Low renin would explain the hypoaldosteronism and low blood pressure but not the other clinical signs. In fact, in Addison disease, renin is likely to be high to counteract the low blood pressure. Low hematocrit can be associated with transient hyperkalemia if the hyperkalemia is caused by hemolysis. There is nothing to suggest hemolysis in this case, nor would hemolysis explain the other findings.

3. **The answer is B.** The woman has suffered a transmembrane shift of potassium cations from ECF to ICF from her use of a β2-agonist with sympathomimetic effects (i.e., effects mimicking the sympathetic catecholamine neurotransmitters, epinephrine, and norepinephrine) that shift potassium intracellularly. Exercise does not decrease plasma [K$^+$] but transiently increases it by opening ATP-dependent potassium channels and enabling more potassium flow out of cells. An osmotic diuresis, if it occurred, could cause distal potassium wasting by increasing distal flow, but osmotic or any other diuresis is not relevant to this scenario. Hyperaldosteronism would increase potassium secretion and decrease the plasma [K$^+$], but again, it is not relevant to this case. Inhibition of the Na$^+$/K$^+$/2Cl$^-$ symporter would, like osmotic diuresis, increase potassium secretion by increasing distal flow. This is the mechanism of action of loop diuretics, such as furosemide, but it has nothing to do with this case.

22

Acid-Base Homeostasis

INTRODUCTION

Bodily processes are exquisitely sensitive to pH. Deviations from the normal range of blood pH of 7.35 to 7.45 may have serious consequences.

- Low pH (<7.2) causes significant clinical manifestations, including impaired growth, decreased cardiac output, decreased blood pressure, insulin resistance, and hyperkalemia.
- High pH (>7.6) is equally destructive, producing disturbances in heart rhythm and tetany from low free calcium.

This pH sensitivity reflects the chemical reactivity of free protons. Inappropriate protonation and deprotonation of proteins caused by abnormal pH can dramatically alter protein structure and render the proteins less functional.

Because biochemical processes cannot tolerate marked changes in pH, the body has an elaborate system to ensure pH regulation. Most of our view of acid base balance pertains to the blood and thus extracellular fluid (ECF), but also important is the regulation of pH by various cells of the body and the brain.

- The brain uses sensitive transport and metabolic mechanisms to closely maintain its pH.
- Intracellular pH is usually lower than that of the ECF because the cells are electronegative with respect to the ECF.
- Most cells have H^+ secretory mechanisms, such as H^+-adenosine triphosphatases (ATPases) and Na^+/H^+ exchangers that provide the housekeeping function of pH regulation for the metabolically active cell.

SYSTEM STRUCTURE: COMPONENTS OF THE pH REGULATORY APPARATUS AND THE DISTRIBUTION OF BODY ACID

The components of the acid-base homeostatic system include:
- Body fluid buffers
- Kidneys
- Lungs

Carbonic acid (H_2CO_3) and its two breakdown products (bicarbonate [HCO_3^-] and carbon dioxide [CO_2]) constitute the most important buffer in the blood. These breakdown products exist in relationship to one another in the blood, as described by the following equation:

$$CO_3 + H_2O \leftrightarrow H_2CO_3 \leftrightarrow H^+ + HCO_3^-$$

The HCO_3^- buffer opposes dramatic changes in the concentration of H^+ (denoted [H^+]) by titrating acid loads added to the blood. The HCO_3^- cannot work alone to keep pH stable, however.

Although the HCO_3^- lessens the change in [H^+] caused by acid loads, it does not eliminate the change. Therefore the lung and the kidney modulate the elements of the buffer equilibrium to oppose the changes in [H^+].

- The lungs eliminate CO_2, lowering the partial pressure of CO_2 (PCO_2) to shift the reaction to the left, thus reducing the [H^+]. When the arterial PCO_2 rises above about 40 mm Hg, the respiratory centers drive more ventilation to drop the arterial PCO_2.
- The kidneys excrete protons and make new bicarbonate to reduce the [H^+]. The kidneys respond directly to increases in [H^+]. When the blood pH dips under 7.4, the kidneys eliminate acid in the urine and manufacture new bicarbonate.

In addition, the brain and its chemosensors play a role in acid-base balance.

Neural Structures in the Regulation of Acid-Base Balance

The central nervous system (CNS) is responsible for the total body content of CO_2, achieved as a result of the modulation of both voluntary and involuntary respiration.

- Voluntary respiration, as well as the hyperventilation seen in anxiety and certain primary CNS lesions, are determined by higher cortical centers.
- Involuntary respiration is controlled by areas in the brain stem and depends on input from both central and peripheral sensory receptors that respond to the concentrations of hydrogen ion, PCO_2, and partial pressure of oxygen (PO_2) of the blood and cerebrospinal fluid (CSF).

The central component in involuntary ventilatory control is the respiratory control center in the medulla oblongata, which is composed of several nuclei. The medulla is responsible for establishing the basic respiratory pattern and integrates input from multiple sources, including higher brain centers, central and peripheral chemoreceptors, and baroreceptors.

Central chemoreceptors are distinct from the respiratory control center, but are located adjacent to it at the ventrolateral surface of the medulla.

- Two areas of chemosensation have been identified in this region, one caudal and one rostral, which sense changes in the pH and PCO_2 of the brain stem interstitial fluid (ISF).
- Gap junctions in the pia may permit mixing of the brain ISF and CSF, allowing the chemosensitive areas to sense

changes in the pH, PCO_2, and bicarbonate concentrations of the CSF.

- The central chemoreceptors are relatively insensitive to changes in PO_2 except in cases of severe hypoxia.

Peripheral sensory input is contributed by pulmonary stretch receptors and carotid sinus and aortic arch chemo- and baroreceptors.

- The most important for maintenance of systemic acid-base balance is the carotid chemoreceptors.
- The carotid bodies, surrounded by a capillary plexus affording close proximity to systemic blood, respond to hypercapnia (high PCO_2) and hydrogen ion concentrations.
- Their response to both PCO_2 and to hydrogen ion concentration is virtually linear in the range of PCO_2 from 25 to 65 mm Hg and a hydrogen ion concentration of 25 to 60 mEq/L.
- The carotid chemosensor is less sensitive to hypoxia with a PO_2 of less than 60 mm Hg required for stimulation. Recall that at these PO_2 levels, hemoglobin desaturation becomes significant.
- The carotid chemoreceptors' sensitivity to combined hypoxia and hypercapnia exceeds the additive effect of the response to each stimulus individually: hypoxia renders the chemoreceptors more sensitive to hypercapnia, and vice versa.

An important concept in understanding the regulation of ventilation is that CO_2 permeates into the CNS across the blood-brain barrier more quickly than HCO_3^-. Therefore sudden increases in PCO_2 peripherally will cause CO_2 to enter and acidify the brain ISF and promote hyperventilation. A sudden decrease in PCO_2 will allow CO_2 to leave the CNS, giving a transient alkalinization of the brain ISF, depressing ventilation.

SYSTEM FUNCTION: THE VARIATION AND CONTROL OF pH

Before beginning to learn more about the acid loads that vary the plasma pH and about the mechanisms that counter those variations to serve homeostasis, it is first necessary to have a good understanding of the physiologic buffers. The simplest way to understand physiologic buffers is to review the basic chemistry.

A Review of Chemical Equilibria and Buffers

When we first learn about chemical reactions, we hear about reactants and products, and we learn that some reactions can proceed in reverse as well as forward.

- Forward reaction between molecules of reactants occurs much more easily and frequently than the reverse reaction between molecules of products (Fig. 22.1).
- The reverse reaction may still occur on a smaller scale and does so at the same time that the forward reaction proceeds. In this equation, the two-way arrow denotes reversibility.

$$A + B \leftrightarrow C + D$$

Also recall that in first-order kinetics, the rate of the forward reaction is proportional to the concentration of the reactants in solution. Conversely, the rate of the reverse reaction is proportional to the concentration of the products.

- The more reactant molecules there are, the more forward reaction occurs per unit time.
- In a forward reaction that is energetically favorable, the reactants convert to products until the reactant concentrations have dropped considerably. In turn, the product concentrations have risen.
- The rate of the forward fast reaction decreases along with the dropping reactant concentration, and the rate of the reverse slow reaction climbs along with rising product concentration.
- When the forward and reverse rates meet and become equal, the concentrations of reactants and products can no longer change, and chemical equilibrium is reached.

Most metabolic reactions and drug metabolic processes occur with first-order kinetics, but recall that in some cases, the rate of product formation is independent of reactant concentration, and therefore linear (zero order, as in the case of alcohol metabolism when excess alcohol has saturated the enzyme alcohol dehydrogenase). In other cases, the reaction rate is related to the square of the reactant concentration (second-order kinetics).

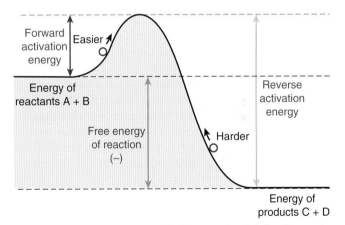

Fig. 22.1 Forward and reverse activation energies. A ball rolling up the curve toward the right is the forward reaction, and the reverse reaction is a ball rolling up the curve toward the left. The forward reaction requires less kinetic energy to make it over the hump from reactants to products than the reverse reaction requires to clear the hill from products to reactants. Because of the greater energy requirement for the reverse reaction, if reactant and product concentrations are equal, fewer reverse balls will clear the hill and go to reactants. The reverse rate will therefore be slower than the forward rate. The passage of balls (reactions) over the hill will be net in a forward direction. Once the number of product molecules becomes large enough, however, the rate of passage over the hill from right to left will grow. The energy requirement has not changed; the number of molecules (balls) attempting the hill from right to left has increased. Even if the same low percentage of balls clears the hill, the total number of balls clearing the hill has risen. When the rate of passage of balls (reactions) is equal in both directions, equilibrium has been reached. The longer the ascent is from right to left, the more products there will have to be before the rate of passage from right to left increases. This means K as a ratio of products over reactants will be larger. Therefore a larger K means a more favorable forward reaction.

If the energetics favor the forward reaction, the equilibrium is pushed "to the right," toward the products.

- When the forward reaction is very energetically favorable, the product concentration must build up quite high before forward and reverse reactions have an equal rate and equilibrium is reached.
- The more favorable the forward reaction is, the larger the ratio of products to reactants at equilibrium will be.
- This equilibrium ratio of products to reactants is described by the equilibrium constant expression:

$$K = [C][D]/[A][B]$$

K is the equilibrium constant, which reflects the ratio of forward to reverse rate constants of the reaction. The more favorable the forward reaction is, the higher K will be.

The opposite holds for a reaction in which the energetics are more favorable to the reverse reaction. Then the equilibrium is pushed "to the left," toward the reactants.

- This implies that the K ratio of products to reactants at equilibrium must be lower.
- An irreversible reaction is one in which the reactants completely disappear as products appear; consequently, the K is infinite.

Adding to or subtracting from the concentrations of the reactants or products in equilibrium will cause a shift in the concentrations of reactants and products until they again reach equilibrium, where the ratio of products to reactants is again, K.

In Fig. 22.1, if more A is added, for example, the forward reaction rate climbs, and more product is made.

- The forward rate then falls, and the reverse rate climbs, until equilibrium ratio K is again achieved.
- If D is subtracted (e.g., by reaction with another chemical species), the reverse reaction rate falls, and net product is made until the forward and reverse rates are again equal.

Equilibrium equations are also written for dissociation reactions, such as when an acid HA (considered the reactant) dissociates into products H^+ and an anionic conjugate base A^-:

$$HA \leftrightarrow H^+ + A^- \quad K = [H^+][A^-]/[HA]$$

Acids are defined as strong acids or weak acids, depending on their tendency to dissociate into H^+ and A-. Stronger acids are more inclined toward dissociation and therefore have larger Ks, and weaker acids are less inclined toward dissociation and have smaller Ks.

Buffer solutions are solutions in which a weak acid (reactant) and conjugate base (product) are present together in similar concentrations at equilibrium.

- When a strong base is added, swallowing up protons, more net weak acid dissociates, producing more H^+ and A^- until the equilibrium ratio of products to reactants is recovered, and the weak acid therefore acts as a reservoir for protons to restore the $[H^+]$.
- When a strong acid is added, raising $[H^+]$, the conjugate base associates with added free H^+, producing more HA until recovery of the equilibrium ratio, and the conjugate base thus acts as a sponge for protons.

- In an unbuffered solution, adding acid will increase the free proton concentration dramatically, causing a steep drop in the pH. Adding base to an unbuffered solution will decrease the free proton concentration dramatically, causing a steep rise in pH.

It is important to understand that buffers lessen changes in pH but do not eradicate them.

The Bicarbonate Buffer in the Blood

The most important extracellular buffer in body fluids is the bicarbonate/CO_2 system.

$$CO_2 + H_2O \leftrightarrow H_2CO_3 \leftrightarrow HCO_3^- + H^+$$

The buffer is composed of a weak acid, carbonic acid ($H_2CO_3^-$), and a conjugate base, bicarbonate (HCO_3^-). Because of the rapid interconversion of CO_2 and HCO_3^-, we sometimes ignore the presence of H_2CO_3 in the reaction sequence shown previously, and instead write:

$$CO_2 + H_2O \leftrightarrow HCO_3^- + H^+$$

The equilibrium equation is the following, with α equal to 0.03 mmol/L per mm Hg, the constant that accounts for dissolved CO_2 and H_2CO_3 in solution:

$$K = 1 \times 10^{-6.1} = [HCO_3^-][H^+]/\alpha PCO_2$$

The bicarbonate buffer behaves in accordance with the description of buffers just shown.

- When protons are added, most of them will react with bicarbonate to form CO_2, as dictated by the buffer's equilibrium constant.
- Proton losses will cause CO_2 to combine with water, and then break down into HCO_3^- and H^+, thus restoring some of the lost H^+ and preventing a severe change in pH.
- Increases in bicarbonate consume some protons and raise the pH to a limited extent.
- Loss of bicarbonate will cause a shift to the right in the reaction. More CO_2 will dissociate into H^+ and HCO_3^-, and the increase in H^+ means a drop in pH. Because it is a buffer system, the equilibrium constant dictates that much of the acid (CO_2) stays as CO_2, and therefore the pH drop is limited.
- Increases in CO_2 will also shift the reaction to the right, elevating the free $[H^+]$, but again, the equilibrium constant dictates that much of the added CO_2 stay as CO_2.
- Decreases in CO_2 cause protons and bicarbonate to react to replace the lost CO_2, raising the pH to a limited extent.

In considering the bicarbonate buffer relationships, physiologists use a more convenient form of the equilibrium equation, called the Henderson-Hasselbalch equation. It relates pH directly to the PCO_2 and $[HCO_3^-]$, mathematically summarizing the notion that increases in CO_2 drop the pH (and vice versa) and decreases in $[HCO_3^-]$ drop the pH (and vice versa):

$$pH = 6.1 + \log\{HCO_3^-]/[0.03] \times [PCO_2]\}$$
(see Fast Fact Box 22.1)

Fast Fact 22.1
By measuring arterial partial pressure of CO_2 (PCO_2) and serum bicarbonate level and inserting them into this simple equation, we can rapidly calculate the pH of the blood. Under normal physiologic conditions, with $[HCO_3^-]$ = 24 mmol/L and arterial PCO_2 = 40 mm Hg, the ratio of HCO_3^-/0.03(PCO_2) is 20/1:
pH = 6.1 + log [24/(0.03) × (40)] = 7.4
The normal physiologic pH of the blood is thus in the range of 7.40.

Because the best buffers are those that have a pK close to the pH of body fluids (ratio of base-to-acid close to 1), one might expect the HCO_3^-/CO_2 buffer pair not to be a good buffer with its pK of 6.1, far from the normal pH of 7.4.

- The reason that HCO_3 is considered a good buffer at physiologic pH, is because the system works in an "open" fashion in which CO_2 is allowed to escape from the system via ventilation (as opposed to a "closed" container).
- The lungs prevent buildup of acid and CO_2 when an excess of H^+ is added to the body.

Other Buffers in the Body

In addition to the bicarbonate buffer system, there are other buffers in the ECF and the ICF. The same body fluid H^+ concentration is simultaneously in equilibrium with multiple buffer pairs, the importance of each depending on their pK and the amount of buffer present.

This isohydric principle allows for the acid-base status to be examined by close evaluation of a single buffer pair, such as HCO_3^-/PCO_2.

- Protein and phosphates both act as weak acid buffers inside and outside of cells.
- Buffering inside cells by protein and phosphate takes place when an increase in the extracellular $[H^+]$ leads to the diffusion of protons into cells. (In red blood cells, hemoglobin is a protein that buffers $[H^+]$ changes intracellularly.)

Intracellular buffering may account for half or more than half of the buffering of acid loads

- When increased plasma $[H^+]$ shifts from the ECF to the intracellular fluid (ICF), important changes occur in the levels of other cations in the blood.
- When the protons diffuse into the cell, there is an increase in the positive charge inside the cell, slightly depolarizing the membrane, and thus reducing the electrical gradient that opposes K^+ efflux from the cell.
- The net result is that H^+ enters the cell and K^+ leaves, raising the plasma $[K^+]$.
- This is why acidemia (low serum pH) is often associated with hyperkalemia (high serum $[K^+]$), as discussed in Chapter 21.

Acid Loads

Metabolically generated acid can be divided into two main groups:

Gaseous or volatile acid (CO_2) is produced by oxidative metabolism of carbohydrates and fats, on the order of 15,000 to 20,000 mmol/day.

- The production of CO_2 raises PCO_2, raises $[H^+]$, and lowers blood pH, in accordance with the equilibrium equation described previously.
- The kidneys respond to the acidity, and the lungs respond to the increased CO_2 (and to the acidity) to counter the drop in pH.
- CO_2 accounts for the vast majority of acid produced by the body (see Fast Fact Box 22.2).

Fast Fact 22.2
The molecular weight of water is 18 g/mol, and there are 1000 g of water in a liter (density is 1000 g/L), so the molarity of water is 55 mol/L.
Therefore the production of 20 mol of water (with the 20 mol of CO_2) adds about 364 mL of water daily to the body fluids. Still, this is less than the water lost in sweat and via the respiratory tree, so that there is a net loss of water per day amounting to about 500 mL. Usually, this is incorporated into the so called insensible losses (sweat and respiratory tree). The total (insensible plus urinary) loss of water per day is approximately 1.45 mL/min, so that the total daily losses are (1.45 mL/min*1440 min/day) = 2,088 mL/day. The gain of water is diet dependent. Carbohydrates lead to more generation of water than fat. This is on the order of approximately 500mL/day and when this is subtracted from the total water loss, you get to approximately 1.5L per day, which is the intake obligated for humans to remain in water balance.

The metabolism of amino acids, nucleic acids, and other compounds releases acidic and alkaline byproducts that are not gaseous (nonvolatile), sometimes called fixed acids and bases.

- The breakdown of sulfur-containing amino acids, such as cysteine and methionine, yields acid sulfates, whereas lysine, arginine, and histidine are often hydrochlorides.
- The digestion of organic phosphorus-containing compounds gives rise to acid phosphates.
- Alkaline byproducts come from the metabolism of anionic amino acids, such as aspartate and glutamate, with accompanying strong cations, such as Na^+, K^+, and Ca^{2+}.
- The normal, high-protein American diet yields a greater quantity of acid than base. On average, a net of 1 mEq/kg per day of nonvolatile organic and inorganic acids is produced.

Acid loads are buffered, but they still acidify the blood to some extent. The addition of H^+ to the blood raises $[H^+]$, lowers pH, and raises PCO_2 in accordance with the equilibrium equation. The kidneys respond to the acidity, and the lungs respond to the increased CO_2 (and to the acidity) to counter the drop in pH.

The Reabsorption of Filtered HCO_3^-

Before we consider the kidney's response to acid loads, we should consider the consequences of the fact that bicarbonate is freely filtered across the glomerulus.

The daily filtered HCO_3^- totaling about 4320 mEq of HCO_3^- (the product of a glomerular filtration rate of 180 L/day and an $[HCO_3^-]$ of 24 mEq/L) is presented to the tubules.

- Clearly, the first critical step confronting the tubule is to reabsorb this enormous filtered quantity, because loss of even a small fraction of that amount would result in severe acidosis.

- Therefore the kidney not only responds to acid loads by creating new bicarbonate and excreting acid, but must also first reabsorb all of the bicarbonate in the tubular filtrate to maintain the blood pH at normal levels.

How does the reabsorption of bicarbonate take place?

- Renal tubule cells do not have any apical transporters to reabsorb bicarbonate directly.
- Instead, the cells along the nephron use a more complex series of reactions to reabsorb the bicarbonate (Fig. 22.2).
- Although the actual reabsorption reactions are more involved than direct transport of bicarbonate, the end result is that bicarbonate is translocated from the tubule lumen into the bloodstream at the expense of adenosine triphosphate (ATP).

The Transport of Bicarbonate in the Proximal Tubule

The majority of bicarbonate reabsorption occurs in the proximal tubule. Note in Fig. 22.2 that the familiar reactions interconverting CO_2 and HCO_3^- recur.

- After passing through the glomerulus into the tubular fluid, the HCO_3^- molecule combines with H^+, which is continuously secreted by the proximal tubular cell.

- The H^+ secretion is driven by the basolateral Na^+,K^+-ATPase, which provides a gradient for apical Na^+ reabsorption across a Na^+/H^+ antiporter.
- An apical H^+-ATPase may have a lesser role here, as well. The continual secretion of H^+ raises the tubular $[H^+]$ and helps drive the reaction of H^+ and HCO_3^-, which produces water and CO_2.
- The presence of carbonic anhydrase in the luminal membranes greatly accelerates this reaction, keeping the luminal $[H^+]$ depressed and avoiding an unfavorable gradient for H^+ secretion into the lumen. Once formed, CO_2 rapidly diffuses into the cell, with a membrane that is highly permeable to the dissolved gas.

Inside the cell, the reverse reaction takes place, again catalyzed by carbonic anhydrase.

- CO_2 and H_2O combine to form HCO_3^- and H^+.
- The bicarbonate exits the basolateral membrane into the peritubular blood across an $Na^+/3HCO_3^-$ symporter, driven in part by the intracellular electronegativity created by the basolateral Na^+,K^+-ATPase and K^+ permeability.

The proportion of bicarbonate reabsorbed in each segment of the nephron is shown in Fig. 22.3.

- The proximal tubule accomplishes 80% to 90% of HCO_3^- reabsorption.
- The next 5% to 15% is reabsorbed in the thick ascending limb of the loop of Henle by the same mechanism as in the proximal tubule.
- The collecting duct reclaims the remaining 5%. Nearly all filtered bicarbonate is reabsorbed under normal conditions when the urine pH is less than 6.0.
- The range of urine pH is between 5.0 and 8.0, so that in circumstances when the more alkaline pH is reached, bicarbonate is present in the urine.

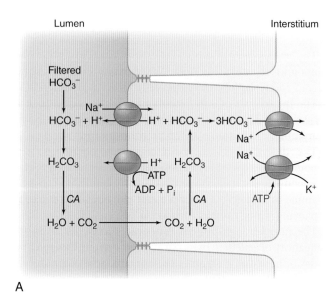

A

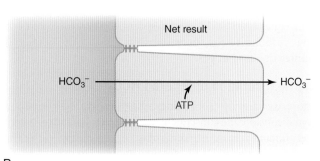

B

Fig. 22.2 The reabsorption of bicarbonate in the early proximal tubule A) detailed chemical transformations and molecular movements. B) net result without chemical details. *CA,* Carbonic anhydrase, the enzyme that facilitates interconversion between H_2CO_3 and CO_2 and H_2O^-. *ATP,* Adenosine triphosphate

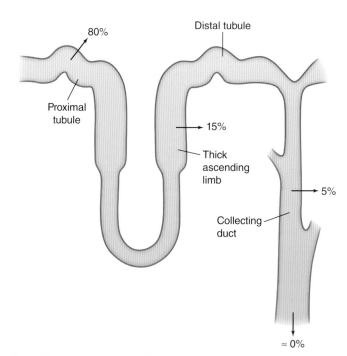

Fig. 22.3 The reabsorption of bicarbonate along the nephron. The majority of HCO_3^- reabsorption occurs in the proximal tubule.

The Transport of Bicarbonate in the Collecting Duct

Reabsorption in the collecting duct takes place through the intercalated cells in a manner slightly different from HCO_3^- reabsorption in earlier tubule segments (Fig. 22.4).

- There is no luminal carbonic anhydrase in the collecting duct, so the dehydration reaction of $H_2CO_3^-$ to CO_2 and water proceeds more slowly. This is in keeping with the decreased amount of HCO_3^- reabsorbed in these segments.
- The Na^+/H^+ exchanger of the proximal tubule is replaced by two types of active transporters.
  - H^+-ATPase, pumps out protons using energy from ATP hydrolysis.
  - H^+/K^+-ATPase, uses energy from ATP to secrete a proton for a potassium reabsorbed.
- Finally, the bicarbonate exits the cell into the blood using a different transporter: an HCO_3^-/Cl^- exchanger in the basolateral membrane.
  - Basolateral reabsorption results from the movement of Cl^- into the cell down a concentration gradient, extruding HCO_3^- via antiport.
  - In the collecting duct, where Na^+ concentration is less than that of the proximal tubule and pH is lower in the lumen compared with the proximal tubule, the driving forces available for an Na^+-H^+ exchange mechanism may not be adequate to accomplish acid secretion.
  - Under such circumstances, the ATP-dependent proton-secreting mechanisms have added importance.
  The predominant intercalated cell (alpha) has an apical H^+-ATPase and basolateral Cl^-/HCO_3^- exchanger, which functions in the setting of acid loads in need of excretion.
  An intercalated cell of reverse polarity (beta) in the cortical collecting duct, with basolateral H^+ pumps and apical Cl^-/HCO_3^- exchangers, is primed to secrete bicarbonate in the setting of an alkaline load. The number of each cell type may be dictated by the acid-base needs of the individual.

Although the individual transporters differ in the earlier and later segments of the nephron, the principles for HCO_3^- reabsorption are similar.

- In all locations, a secreted proton combines with a luminal HCO_3^-, converting it into CO_2, which diffuses into the cell.
- Bicarbonate is then reconstituted and passes across the basolateral membrane into the interstitium and on into the peritubular blood.

The Regulation of Acidity

In the absence of an acid load in the plasma, a certain amount of H^+ is secreted across the apical membranes.

- This H^+ escorts filtered HCO_3^- into the cell, is secreted again, escorts more HCO_3^- into the cell, is secreted again, and so on.
- Acidity is cycled back and forth across the apical membrane in the transcellular reabsorption of HCO_3^- back to the bloodstream.
- The kidney thus saves all the bicarbonate that had entered the tubule by filtration.

When the average daily acid load of 70 mEq H^+ acidifies the blood, chemical events change in the bicarbonate-reabsorbing cells of the proximal tubule and collecting duct.

- Instead of reabsorbing filtered HCO_3^- with no net secretion or reabsorption of H^+, the tubule cells secrete net H^+ and generate new HCO_3^- in addition to the HCO_3^- reabsorbed from the tubule lumen.
- The clearance of H^+ from the blood and the addition of HCO_3^- to the blood reverse the impact of the acid load on the blood buffer and on the blood pH.

Acidification of the Blood and the Tubular Cells

When protons are added to the blood, some of them remain free, which drops the pH, and others react with bicarbonate, which drops the $[HCO_3^-]$ and increases the PCO_2.

- These changes in the ECF pH then cause changes in the renal tubular intracellular pH.
- Increased PCO_2 leads to diffusion of CO_2 from the peritubular capillaries across the gas-permeable cell membranes of the tubule cells and increases PCO_2 in the cells.
- Decreased peritubular and interstitial $[HCO_3^-]$ alters the basolateral transmembrane $[HCO_3^-]$ gradient in favor of reabsorption of HCO_3^- into the interstitium. Increased reabsorption of HCO_3^- drops the intracellular $[HCO_3^-]$.

Increased PCO_2 and decreased $[HCO_3^-]$ in the tubule cells pushes the buffer reaction rightward, leading to an increase in $[H^+]$ and therefore a drop in intracellular pH. Under normal dietary conditions, changes in ECF pH are minimal.

Unless the secretory and reabsorptive functions of the cell are impaired, the renal tubular cells will respond to pathologic increases in acidity in the same way that they respond to physiologic acid loads. Only when an acid load exceeds the capacity

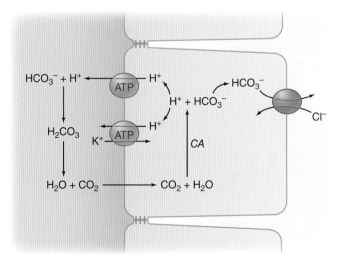

Fig. 22.4 The reabsorption of bicarbonate in the intercalated cell of the collecting duct. Bicarbonate reabsorption in this part of the tubule does not occur via Na^+ reabsorption but by active H^+ secretion and HCO_3^-/Cl^- antiport driven by Cl^- diffusion down its concentration gradient. *ATP,* Adenosine triphosphate.

of the kidney to excrete that load does systemic pH noticeably change.

Renal Acid Secretion

In both the proximal tubule and the collecting duct, increased intracellular acidity stimulates an increase in H^+ secretion through active and passive mechanisms.

- In the proximal tubule cell, the increased intracellular $[H^+]$ drives more H^+ down its concentration gradient across the apical Na^+/H^+ exchanger and into the tubule lumen.
- The performance of the exchanger is also enhanced by low pH, as is that of the proximal tubular H^+-ATPase.
- In the collecting duct, more H^+-ATPase is inserted into the apical membrane by a process of exocytosis, thereby increasing H^+ secretion.

With increased H^+ secretion, H^+ is now secreted in excess of the amounts required for complete bicarbonate reabsorption.

- Increased H^+ secretion accelerates HCO_3^- reabsorption as luminal CO_2 is produced at a higher rate.
- H^+ is secreted in excess of luminal HCO_3^-, and thus a certain amount remains in the urine where it will be excreted after combining with the urinary buffers, particularly ammonia (NH_3) and phosphate.

H^+ secretion is more exaggerated in the distal tubule segments than in the proximal tubule.

- Excess CO_2 in the blood diffuses into the tubular cell, and the HCO_3^- deficit in the blood leads to high basolateral HCO_3^- reabsorption in the proximal tubule.
- The high basal level of HCO_3^- reabsorption in the proximal tubule leads to higher PCO_2 of the proximal tubular cells compared with other parts of the tubule. This leads to reduced CO_2 diffusion from the blood into the tubular cell.
- The proximal tubular cell is therefore less easily acidified by acid loads than is the distal tubular cell, which is not engaged in as much basal HCO_3^- reabsorption.

The Generation of New Bicarbonate

When an acid load in the plasma acidifies the tubular cells—by increased PCO_2 and decreased intracellular $[HCO_3^-]$ —this pushes the buffer reaction rightward, yielding new intracellular H^+ and new HCO_3^-.

- Increased $[H^+]$ leads to increased H^+ secretion, which exceeds the amount required for HCO_3^- reabsorption.
- New HCO_3^- replaces that which was lost from the cell when the bicarbonate-poor plasma in the peritubular capillary absorbed more HCO_3^- across the basolateral membrane.
- With intracellular $[HCO_3^-]$ partially replenished, the bicarbonate-poor blood can continue to extract increased amounts of HCO_3^- from the tubular cells.
- H^+ secretion in excess of luminal HCO_3^- increases the generation of new HCO_3^- because secreting H^+ keeps the buffer relation at a rightward tilt, which generates more HCO_3^-.

- For new bicarbonate to be generated, the secreted H^+ combines in the lumen with phosphate and NH_3 buffers rather than filtered bicarbonate.

The distal tubule cells, which are more acidified and which achieve more net H^+ excretion, produce more new HCO_3^- compared with the proximal tubule cells.

The Restoration of Normal Plasma Acidity: Effects of the Kidneys and Lungs

The peritubular capillaries are the site where the acid load's alterations in the blood buffer are relieved.

- Excess CO_2 diffuses out of the blood and the kidney takes on the acidic burden.
- The tubular cells dispense with this burden through increased H^+ secretion and generation of new HCO_3^-.

The ability of renal tubular cells to secrete and excrete H^+ and to generate new HCO_3^- without increasing their own acidity allows the peritubular blood to continue to deliver CO_2 and to reabsorb HCO_3^- from the kidney. The decrease in plasma PCO_2 and increase in plasma $[HCO_3^-]$ reverses the changes imposed by the acid load.

The lungs, meanwhile, contribute to handling of the acid load as well.

- The central chemoreceptors detect increased PCO_2 and the peripheral chemoreceptors detect increased acidity (decreased pH).
- In response, they increase lung ventilation to reduce the plasma PCO_2, shifting the buffer relation leftward and consuming H^+.

Through pulmonary regulation of ventilation, renal modulation of acid excretion, and new bicarbonate formation, all acting in concert, the body counters changes in blood pH.

A simple stoichiometric way to think about renal handling of acid loads is to focus on what happens to CO_2 in the kidney.

- In the reabsorption of filtered HCO_3^-, no net CO_2 is consumed.
- The intracellular CO_2 that is hydrated and breaks down to give H^+ and HCO_3^- was first created in the tubule lumen by H^+ secretion.
- The net effect is the translocation of HCO_3^- from the tubule lumen to the blood with no net increase or decrease in the PCO_2 of the tubular cell.
  - When an acid load acidifies the tubular cell, however, CO_2 is hydrated and broken down to H^+ and HCO_3^- in excess of the CO_2 delivered from luminal HCO_3^- reabsorption.
- The new H^+ is excreted, and the HCO_3^- is transferred to the blood—a new HCO_3^- at the cost of a CO_2.

Urinary Titration of Excreted Acid

When H^+ is secreted in excess of luminal HCO_3^-, it remains in the urine, where it will be excreted. This is because there is not enough HCO_3^- to react with the H^+ in the tubule lumen.

- Although the protons lost in the urine do not react with bicarbonate, they cannot remain free in the tubular fluid.
- If the protons remained free in the lumen, the luminal pH would rapidly drop, and the high concentration of luminal protons would produce a large lumen-to-cell proton gradient.
  - At a certain point, the pumps responsible for secreting protons would not be able to function against this gradient.

- This point corresponds to a urinary pH of around 4.5, or a free proton concentration of 0.03 mEq/L (see Fast Fact Box 22.3).

Fast Fact 22.3

To excrete enough free protons to counter the daily acid load and still keep the urine pH above 4.5, the kidney would have to produce more than 2000 L of urine a day!

- The kidneys use buffers to avoid a luminal buildup of H^+ and maintain the luminal pH above 4.5.

The two most important urinary buffers are phosphate and ammonia (Fig. 22.5). The availability of these buffers determines the capacity for urinary acid excretion and bicarbonate creation.

The Phosphate Buffer: $HPO_4^{2-}/H_2PO_4^{2-}$

The phosphate available for buffering depends primarily on the dietary intake of phosphate-containing compounds.

- Phosphate is filtered through the glomerulus and then partially reabsorbed proximally.
- The remaining 10% to 20% of the phosphate serves to buffer urinary protons.
- Because the pK for the reaction $HPO_4^{2-} + H^+ <-> H_2PO_4^-$ is 6.8, phosphate is a good urinary buffer.
- Two-thirds of the phosphate buffer is consumed by acidity because of HCO_3^- reabsorption and excess H^+ secretion in the proximal tubule.

Because most of the excess H^+ secretion takes place distally, the quantity of phosphate buffer is clearly insufficient by itself to handle excreted protons.

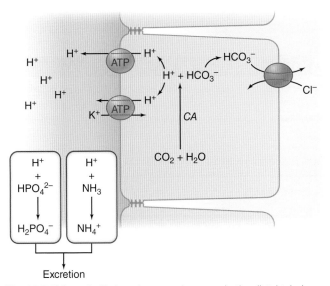

Fig. 22.5 Urinary buffering of secreted protons in the distal tubule segments. Some buffering by phosphate also occurs in the proximal tubule. *ATP*, Adenosine triphosphate.

The Ammonia Buffer: NH_3/NH_4^+

The most important urinary buffer is NH_3/NH_4^+. NH_3 is produced by the metabolism of amino acids, purines, pyrimidines, and other nitrogen-containing compounds in many body tissues, especially the liver and kidney.

The primary site of ammonia production is the proximal tubule mitochondria. The proximal tubule cells express high levels of the enzyme glutaminase, which helps convert glutamine to glutamate, liberating an NH_4^+.

- The enzyme glutamate dehydrogenase converts glutamate to α-ketoglutarate and a second NH_4^+ (Fig. 22.6).
- The consumption of glutamine by this pathway leads to increased uptake of glutamine from the bloodstream, which supplies the pathway with constant substrate. Under conditions of increased acid loads, more glutamine is transported into the proximal cell and the glutaminase activity is increased.

Once produced, the NH_4^+ is secreted into the proximal tubule lumen, putatively across the Na^+/H^+ antiporter, with NH_4^+ in place of H^+ (Fig. 22.7).

- NH_4^+ cannot leave the lumen, which is impermeable to this cation, until it reaches the thick ascending limb of the loop of Henle.
- NH_4^+ is then actively reabsorbed in the thick ascending limb, via the K^+ locus in the $Na^+/K^+/2Cl^-$ symporter.
- The H^+ is secreted into the loop of Henle tubule lumen in exchange for Na^+, where it serves HCO_3^- reabsorption.
- Meanwhile, the NH_3, to which only the basolateral membrane is permeable, diffuses into the interstitium.
- In this way, through countercurrent exchange, a medullary interstitial NH_3 gradient is maintained and ammonia is prevented from reaching the highly vascular renal cortex, where it could diffuse into the systemic blood.

The high medullary interstitial NH_3 drives the diffusion of NH_3 into the collecting duct.

- If an acid load has acidified the tubular intercalated cells, the cells are secreting acid in excess of HCO_3^- reabsorption.
- The NH_3 binds this excess H^+, keeping the luminal $[H^+]$ low so that H^+ secretion can continue unopposed.
- Once the NH_3 has bound H^+ and formed NH_4^+, it is trapped in the lumen because the cell membranes are less permeable to it. This is known as ammonium trapping, and results in excretion of excess acid in the titrated form of NH_4^+.

Not only does ammonium account for the majority of urinary H^+ excretion, but it is also another means of regulating H^+ excretion. Whereas the phosphate buffering capacity of the urine is relatively fixed and largely determined by body phosphate balance, the amount of ammonia available can be regulated by the kidney to match demands for acidification.

Increased NH_3 production is a major regulatory response to increased plasma acidity alongside increased H^+ secretion/HCO_3^- creation.

- When NH_4^+ production goes up, more NH_3 accumulates in the interstitium and more NH_3 diffuses into the collecting duct.
- This lowers the luminal $[H^+]$ and allows more H^+ secretion and excretion and hence more HCO_3^- production. Recent

studies also suggest that NH_3 directly stimulates distal H^+ secretion in intercalated cells of the collecting duct by promoting the insertion of H^+/K^+-ATPase into the apical membrane of these cells.

- Acid loads, both nonvolatile and because of elevated PCO_2, increase ammonia production.

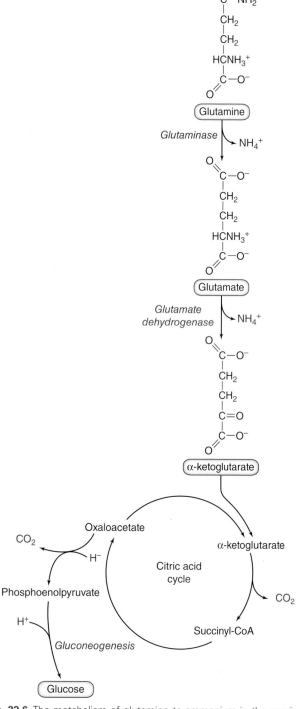

Fig. 22.6 The metabolism of glutamine to ammonium in the proximal tubule cell. Increased ammonia (NH_4^+) production helps to buffer urinary H^+, thereby increasing the amount of H^+ that may be secreted and excreted. This diagram also shows the fate of α-ketoglutarate.

The Influence of Volume and Potassium Homeostasis on Renal Acid Excretion

We have already seen that the intracellular pH of the renal tubular cells is the most important afferent input in the homeostatic regulation of renal acid excretion.

When blood pressure is low and angiotensin II stimulates increased proximal Na^+ (and hence water) reabsorption, the activity of the Na^+/H^+ exchanger is enhanced.

- More H^+ is secreted.
- HCO_3^- reabsorption is enhanced, and proximal H^+ excretion is increased.
- As a result, low blood volume and pressure (hypovolemia) can perpetuate an underlying alkalosis by increasing HCO_3^- reabsorption and H^+ excretion. This condition is sometimes called a contraction alkalosis because the alkalosis is maintained by contracted blood volume.

Aldosterone also contributes to this phenomenon by increasing the activity of the distal apical Na^+ channel and Na^+,K^+ exchanger in principal cells, thereby increasing distal Na^+ reabsorption.

- This leaves the tubule lumen more electronegative and promotes H^+ secretion from the intercalated cells.
- Furthermore, aldosterone stimulates the H^+-ATPase.

Overall, through the actions of angiotensin II and aldosterone, low blood volume increases bicarbonate reabsorption and may increase acid excretion (see Environment Box 22.1, Genetics Box 22.1, Development Box 22.1, and Pharmacology Box 22.1).

🏠 ENVIRONMENT BOX 22.1

Licorice contains glycyrrhetinic acid, a steroid that suppressed expression of the HSD11B2 gene and the function of the 11 β-hydroxysteroid type 2 enzymes. Licorice can thus recapitulate the manifestations of apparent mineralocorticoid excess (AME), but this typically only occurs when a person eats a significant amount of licorice daily for weeks.

🧬 GENETICS BOX 22.1

Apparent mineralocorticoid excess (AME) is an autosomal recessive disease causing metabolic alkalosis and severe hypertension in children. It is the result of mutation in the HSD11B2 gene that encodes the 11 β-hydroxysteroid dehydrogenase type 2 enzyme that normally converts cortisol (which binds to and activates renal cell aldosterone receptors and thus has mineralocorticoid effects) to cortisone (which has no mineralocorticoid effects).

DEVELOPMENT BOX 22.1

Apparent mineralocorticoid excess (AME) affects patients even before birth, as evidenced by low birth weight. Infants display failure to thrive, metabolic alkalosis, sever hypertension, and hypokalemia—all the expected effects of increased aldosterone activity, but in the absence of high concentrations of aldosterone. With time, patients develop renal failure and end organ damage.

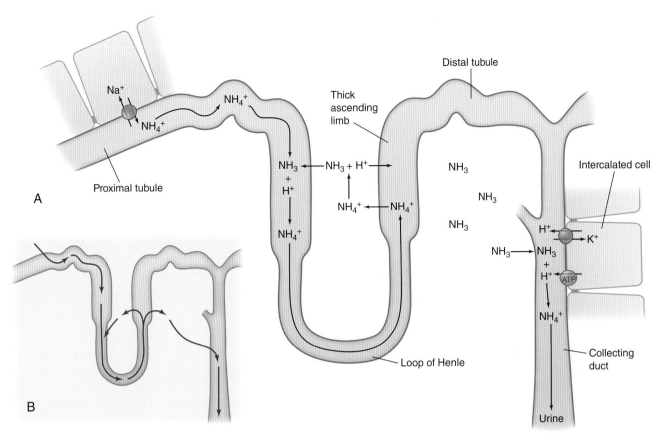

Fig. 22.7 Ammonia secretion and excretion in the renal tubule. A, Ammonia transport and trapping. B, The overall pathway of ammonia through the tubule.

Low plasma [K^+] (hypokalemia) may lead to alkalosis. This relationship is caused by transmembrane shifting of H^+ and K^+ in the periphery and increased H^+ secretion in the proximal and distal tubule segments.

- Low [K^+] causes K^+ to shift out of cells, making the cell interior more negative, which draws in H^+, alkalinizing the blood pH. In the proximal tubule, there is increased Na^+-H^+ exchange activity and $Na^+HCO_3^-$ cotransport at the basolateral membrane.
- Hypokalemia also increases proximal ammonium production. In the collecting duct, increased K^+ reabsorption across the H^+/K^+-ATPase may drive excess H^+ secretion.
- The decreased K^+ secretion in the collecting duct may also fail to raise the electrical potential of the tubule lumen, creating an increased electrical gradient for H^+ secretion.
- Overall, hypokalemia leads to or maintains metabolic alkalosis.

PATHOPHYSIOLOGY: ACIDOSIS AND ALKALOSIS

Many disease states can cause derangements in blood pH. Such conditions alter the PCO_2, the [H^+], or the [HCO_3^-], pushing the pH out of normal bounds.

- A condition that lowers the pH level is classified as an acidosis.
- A condition that elevates the pH is classified as an alkalosis.
  The terms acidosis and alkalosis are technically distinct from acidemia and alkalemia.
- Acidemia—If the pH of the blood falls below the normal range (7.35–7.45).
- Alkalemia—If the pH is above the normal range.
  The terms acidosis and alkalosis, on the other hand, refer to processes that tend to lower or raise the blood pH.
- This is relevant when two processes are working at the same time to raise and/or to lower the blood pH.
- Both acidoses and alkaloses are divided into two major subcategories:
  - Respiratory: Processes that affect pulmonary ventilation and skew the PCO_2.
  - Metabolic: Processes that alter the [H^+] or the [HCO_3^-].
- There are four main types of acid-base disorders:
  - Respiratory acidosis
  - Respiratory alkalosis
  - Metabolic acidosis
  - Metabolic alkalosis

Respiratory Acidosis

A respiratory acidosis is an acidosis that derives from decreased pulmonary ventilation. Any condition that limits the ability of the lungs to ventilate will cause an accumulation of CO_2 in the blood. This leads to a fall in blood pH.

- When the lungs are unable to fully accomplish their task, the kidneys can partially compensate.
- By increasing the proton excretion and bicarbonate generation, the kidneys can oppose the pH change produced by the rising PCO_2.
- The kidney will also begin to increase NH_4^+ production in the proximal tubule, which will promote distal H^+ secretion by buffering more tubular acid and by direct stimulation of H^+ secretion (see Clinical Correlation Box 22.1).

Clinical Correlation Box 22.1

An example of respiratory acidosis is decreased central respiratory drive. The lungs regulate partial pressure of CO_2 (PCO_2) by adjusting alveolar ventilation to keep arterial PCO_2 at about 40 mm Hg. This requires intact central neurologic input to the pulmonary system. If the respiratory center is damaged by stroke or suppressed by drugs, such as opioids, ventilation will be inadequately stimulated and hypoventilation will set in. When ventilation falls, CO_2 will not be eliminated at a sufficient rate. This accumulation of CO_2 will lower the pH.

Respiratory Alkalosis

A respiratory alkalosis is an alkalosis that derives from increased pulmonary ventilation. If ventilation increases above the level necessary to keep CO_2 at 40 mm Hg, the PCO_2 will fall, and the pH will rise.

- In this case, to offset the decrease in PCO_2, the kidneys will trigger a decrease in plasma bicarbonate concentration.
- This is accomplished by both a reduction in bicarbonate reabsorption and actual bicarbonate secretion. Bicarbonate secretion occurs in certain subtypes of intercalated cells in the collecting duct.

Respiratory alkalosis is the most common acid-base disorder and is frequently benign (see Clinical Correlation Box 22.2).

Clinical Correlation Box 22.2

Conditions, such as pneumonia and pulmonary edema, can cause oxygen desaturation and hyperventilation, driving down the partial pressure of CO_2 (PCO_2). Respiratory alkalosis also occurs in the context of increased central respiratory drive. Some common causes are anxiety, fever, and pregnancy. In pregnancy, the high levels of progesterone stimulate the respiratory center to increase ventilation.

Metabolic Acidosis

Three types of processes result in metabolic acidosis (Table 22.1):
- Increased nonvolatile acid loads in the blood
- Decreased renal acid excretion
- Loss of bicarbonate in urine or stool

TABLE 21.1 The Normal Distribution of Potassium

	Increased Non-volatile Acid Load in Blood	Decreased Renal Acid Excretion	Loss of Bicarbonate
Increased anion gap	• Poisoning (aspirin, ethylene glycol, methanol etc.) • Ketoacidosis and lactic acidosis	• Renal failure	
Normal anion gap		• Type 1 (distal) tubular acidosis (RTA)[a] • Type 4 RTA (hypoaldosteronism)	• Diarrhea • Type 2 (proximal) RTA[a]

[a] Type 3 RTA is a rare combination of Types 1 and 2.
(Modified from Rose, Burton D, Rennke HG. *Renal Pathophysiology the Essentials*, Baltimore: Williams and Wilkins, 1994: p. 153, 163. With permission.)

The lowered pH in any of these situations will stimulate the respiratory center to increase ventilation, which in turn lowers PCO_2.
- This shifts the buffer reaction to the left, consuming H^+ and opposing the drop in pH.
- The deep hyperventilatory breathing sometimes observed in patients with metabolic acidoses is called Kussmaul's respiration.

The kidneys also make adjustments in response to increased acidity in the absence of primary kidney pathology (i.e., not in cases of decreased renal acid excretion).
- The kidneys will increase H^+ secretion and the generation of new bicarbonate, shifting the buffer reaction to the left.
- Prolonged metabolic acidosis will promote increased NH_4^+ production in the proximal tubule.

Metabolic acidosis is further subcategorized as an anion gap acidosis or a normal anion gap/hyperchloremic acidosis.
- All cases of increased nonvolatile acid loads are anion gap acidoses.
- Some cases of decreased renal acid excretion are anion gap and some present (manifest clinically) with a normal anion gap.
- All cases of lost bicarbonate present with a normal anion gap. What is an anion gap?
- The total number of cations and anions in the ECF must be equal because the blood is electrically neutral.
- Most of the cations in the ECF are sodium.
- The anions are bicarbonate, chloride, plasma proteins (mainly albumin), and to a lesser extent, phosphate, sulfate, and organic acid ions.
- Sodium, bicarbonate, and chloride are measurable ions. The other anions are not usually measured.

Therefore the sodium level minus bicarbonate and chloride levels yields a number equal to the concentration of unmeasured anions; this is the anion gap. The anion gap is present even under normal circumstances because of albumin and other unmeasured anions normally present in the blood.

$$Anion\,gap = [Na^+] - ([Cl^-] + [HCO_3^-])$$

Plugging in the normal values $[Na^+]$ = 140 mEq/L, $[Cl^-]$ = 106 mEq/L, and $[HCO_3^-]$ = 24 mEq/L, we can calculate the normal anion gap to be about 6 to 10 mEq/L.

Normal dietary nonvolatile acid loads and their unmeasured anionic conjugate bases do not cause significant increases in the anion gap under normal conditions. Pathologic acid loads and their anionic conjugate bases can raise the anion gap to a significant extent, however.

- Ethylene glycol is a poison that can cause an anion gap acidosis. The ethylene glycol is metabolized to glyoxalate and oxalic acid in the liver, lowering pH, and these anions account for the increased anion gap.

Two very clinically relevant examples of anion gap acidosis owing to the body's own pathologic products are ketoacidosis and lactic acidosis.

- Ketoacidosis follows from starvation metabolism, which occurs not only in starvation but also in diabetes mellitus. Starvation metabolism yields acid metabolites that have unmeasured anionic conjugate bases (such as b-hydroxybutyrate and acetoacetate).
- Lactic acidosis may occur in circulatory or respiratory failure, when the tissues are deprived of oxygen. Anaerobic metabolism of carbohydrates in the tissues yields lactic acid, and lactate is the unmeasured anion associated with the acidosis.

In renal failure, the kidney fails to excrete acid, owing to decreased NH_3 production, and to make bicarbonate. At the same time, they fail to clear the sulfate and phosphate that are the unmeasured anionic conjugate bases of dietary nonvolatile acid. This results in an anion gap acidosis.

Cases of decreased acid excretion other than renal failure—as in renal tubular acidosis—present with a normal anion gap.

- Inherited defects in tubular pumps and transporters, autoimmune injury to these membrane proteins, hormone deficiencies, drug effects, and so on, can impair H^+ secretion and hence HCO_3^- reabsorption.
- Impaired HCO_3^- reabsorption acidifies the plasma, and, unlike anion gap acidosis, represents a subtraction of bicarbonate, rather than an addition of H^+. This failure to reabsorb anionic HCO_3^- results in a charge separation that causes Cl^- to increase in place of HCO_3^-.
- This is why normal anion gap acidoses are also called hyperchloremic, because the plasma chloride level is high in these conditions.

Diarrhea is another form of normal anion gap/hyperchloremic acidosis—in this case, because of a loss of HCO_3^- through the intestines. The loss of Na^+ with the HCO_3^- leaves relatively more Cl^- behind in the ECF, giving a hyperchloremic acidosis.

Metabolic Alkalosis

Metabolic alkalosis refers to nonrespiratory causes of alkalemia. It results from:

- An excessive loss of acid, as in vomiting and in the use of loop or thiazide diuretics
- An excessive intake of alkali

The lungs will respond to elevated pH by decreasing ventilation. This compensatory mechanism is greatly limited by the need to ventilate to take up oxygen.

The kidneys also react to an increase in bicarbonate by reducing bicarbonate reabsorption along the nephron.

- In fact, the kidneys have an enormous capacity to excrete filtered bicarbonate in the urine.
- Therefore metabolic alkalosis requires situations that specifically limit this compensatory ability of the kidney.

The two factors that interfere with renal correction of metabolic alkalosis are:

- ECF volume depletion (hypovolemia)
  - In hypovolemia, angiotensin II stimulates the reabsorption of Na^+ via the Na^+/H^+ antiporter in the proximal tubule, and aldosterone stimulates H^+ secretion by the H^+-ATPase in the cortical collecting duct.
  - The increased acid excretion and bicarbonate reabsorption perpetuate the alkalosis—so-called contraction alkalosis, as just mentioned.
- Hypokalemia
  - Recall that hypokalemia also drops the plasma $[H^+]$ because K^+ shifts out of cells and H^+ shifts into them.
  - Hypokalemia also stimulates distal H^+ secretion.
  - Therefore hypokalemia exacerbates alkalosis.

Blood Gas Analysis

In medical practice, we use laboratory values as a window into physiologic processes. The information needed to analyze a patient's acid-base disorder can be obtained from a sample of arterial blood called an arterial blood gas (ABG).

- The blood is typically drawn from the radial artery near the wrist.
- In this sample, we can measure the three parameters critical to acid-base balance:
  - pH
  - PCO_2
  - HCO_3^-

Typical normal ranges for these tests are pH: 7.35 to 7.45, PCO_2: 38 to 42 mm Hg, and HCO_3^-: 22 to 28 mmol/L.

A systematic approach to the results of arterial blood gases is diagrammed in Fig. 22.8 and outlined in the following list.

1. Determine the pH. If the pH is below 7.4, there is an acidemia. If it is above 7.4, an alkalemia exists.
2. Determine what type of process produced the observed pH change. We must determine which type of alkalosis or acidosis is present.
   a. Acidemia: If the PCO_2 is elevated (>40 mm Hg) there must be a respiratory acidosis. If the HCO_3^- is depressed (<24 mEq/L) there is a metabolic acidosis.
   b. Alkalemia: If the PCO_2 is decreased (<40 mm Hg) a respiratory alkalosis is present. If $[HCO_3^-]$ is increased (>24 mEq/L) a metabolic alkalosis is present.
3. Determine whether there are any compensatory changes.
   a. We expect that any primary acid-base disturbance will induce compensatory alterations.
   b. If there is no compensation—that is, if both PCO_2 and $[HCO_3^-]$ push the blood pH in the same direction, then the patient may have a "mixed disorder," combining respiratory and metabolic etiologies. (See Clinical Correlation Box 22.3.)

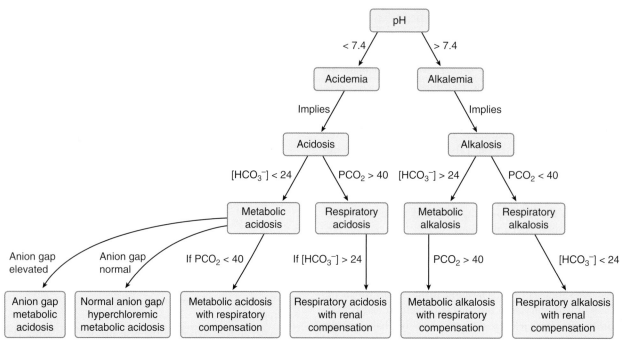

Fig. 22.8 A flow chart for the analysis of disturbances of blood pH.

Clinical Correlation Box 22.3

A Sample Analysis of an Acid-Base Disorder

A 12-year-old boy has had recent polyuria (increased urine volume) and polydipsia (increased thirst). He suddenly developed nausea, lethargy, weakness, and shortness of breath and was found to have hyperglycemia (high blood sugar), a blood pH of 7.25, a partial pressure of CO_2 (PCO_2) of 25 mm Hg, and a serum HCO_3^- of 10 mEq/L. The [Na^+] was 140 mEq/L (normal); [K^+] 3.5 mEq/L (normal); [Cl^-] 100 mEq/L (normal). The anion gap was increased to 30 mEq/L.

If we submit this case to the guidelines for the analysis of an acid base disorder, we begin with inspection of the blood pH. It is less than 7.4, which is acidemic, implying the presence of an acidosis. Next, we examine the PCO_2 and [HCO_3^-]. The PCO_2 is low (<40 mm Hg), which argues against a respiratory acidosis. The [HCO_3^-] is also low (<24 mEq/L), which supports the diagnosis of a metabolic acidosis. In addition to excluding a respiratory acidosis, the low PCO_2 also suggests that the metabolic acidosis is being partially compensated for by hyperventilation. Finally, the increased anion gap suggests this is an increased anion gap metabolic acidosis (sometimes called an

anion gap acidosis, for short). From Table 22.1, we might conclude that the patient has one of the following disorders: poisoning, ketoacidosis, lactic acidosis, or renal failure.

The answer comes from integrating the lab findings with the history. The polyuria, polydipsia, and hyperglycemia are highly suggestive of diabetes mellitus. In diabetes, a lack of insulin results in failure to transport glucose into cells. The liver is driven into a starvation metabolism in which it breaks down fats and proteins to make ketone bodies. Ketone bodies, namely β-hydroxybutyric acid and acetoacetic acid, accumulate in the blood until a gradient is established for continued diffusion of the ketone bodies into the starved body tissues. There, the ketones yield acetyl-CoA and provide an alternative source of energy to the citric acid cycle in the context of diminished glucose availability. The accumulation of these acids in the blood also drops the blood pH, binds HCO_3^- (dropping the [HCO_3^-]), and contributes unmeasured anions to the blood (β-hydroxybutyrate and acetoacetate), creating an increased anion gap. This condition is called diabetic ketoacidosis, and it is a medical emergency requiring intravenous insulin.

Respiratory compensation occurs in metabolic disorders such that a change in bicarbonate concentration is met with a change in PCO_2 in the same direction (e.g., decreased bicarbonate leads to decreased PCO_2).
- Note that this brings the ratio of HCO_3^-/PCO_2 back toward normal.

- From the Henderson-Hasselbalch relationship, normalization of the ratio brings the pH toward normal. Likewise, in primary respiratory disorders, changes in PCO_2 are met with changes in HCO_3^- concentration via renal mechanisms, in the same direction to partially correct the pH.
- In general, pH does not completely correct through compensation, and the degree of compensation is predictable.

SUMMARY

- Stable pH is critical to physiologic functioning because protonation or deprotonation of proteins alters their charge, shape, and therefore their function.
- The first line of defense against changes of pH inside the body is the bicarbonate buffer. The following three equations describe the bicarbonate buffer equilibrium.

$$CO_2 + H_2O \leftrightarrow H_2CO_3 \leftrightarrow HCO_3^- + H^+$$

$$K = 1 \times 10^{-6.1} = [HCO_3^-][H^+]/\alpha PCO_2$$

$$pH = 6.1 + \log\{[HCO_3^-]/[0.03] \times [PCO_2]\}$$

- The last of the earlier equations is called the Henderson-Hasselbalch equation.
- HCO_3^- reabsorption takes place predominantly in the proximal tubule. Na^+-coupled H^+ secretion binds HCO_3^- in the proximal tubule lumen, forms CO_2 (expedited by carbonic anhydrase), and the CO_2 diffuses into the tubule cells, where it is rehydrated and dissociates into H^+ and HCO_3^-. The HCO_3^- is reabsorbed across a $Na^+/3\ HCO_3^-$ symporter, and the H^+ is secreted.
- Acid loads add H^+ to the blood buffer, which drops the blood pH, consumes HCO_3^-, and produces CO_2. The buffer mitigates the acidification, but the disturbance in blood pH must still be corrected. To reverse this disturbance in the blood pH, the lungs increase ventilation to blow off more CO_2, and the kidneys increase H^+ excretion in the proximal and distal tubules.
- The distal responses increase H^+ secretion in excess of luminal HCO_3^-. The excess H^+ binds to the remaining HPO_4^{2-} and to NH_3 and is ultimately excreted as $H_2PO_4^-$ and NH_4^+, accompanied by the acid anions, such as Cl^-.

- Net peritubular loss of H^+ and gain of HCO_3^- restores normal plasma pH after the disturbance of the acid load.
- Much more net acid excretion and HCO_3^- production occurs in the distal tubule segments. Even under circumstances of increased acidity, the proximal tubule serves primarily to reabsorb HCO_3^- and only secretes a proportionally small amount of excess H^+.
- There are four types of pathophysiologic derangements in pH: respiratory acidosis, respiratory alkalosis, metabolic acidosis, and metabolic alkalosis.
- The respiratory disorders alter pH through primary disturbances in ventilation and hence PCO_2. The metabolic disorders alter pH through primary disturbances in $[H^+]$ or $[HCO_3^-]$.
- The lungs can partially compensate for metabolic disturbances with changes in ventilation, and the kidneys can partially compensate for respiratory disturbances with changes in acid excretion and bicarbonate reabsorption.
- The normal anion gap, which reflects the presence of unmeasured anions in the blood (like albumin), is defined by the following equation:

$$Anion\ gap = [Na^+] - ([Cl^-] + [HCO_3^-])$$

- Some metabolic acidoses are associated with an increased anion gap. The excess unmeasured anions are the conjugate bases of the acids that have caused the metabolic acidosis.

REVIEW QUESTIONS

Directions: Each of the numbered items or incomplete statements in this section is followed by answers or by completions of the statement. Select the one lettered answer or completion that is best in each case.

1. A 21-year-old heroin addict overdoses and is found unresponsive and barely breathing at 4 breaths per minute. His body attempts to compensate for his acid-base imbalance by which of the following methods?
   A. Decreased proton secretion by the kidneys
   B. Decreased CO_2 exhalation by the lungs
   C. Increased CO_2 exhalation by the lungs
   D. Increased renal bicarbonate production
   E. Decreased renal bicarbonate reabsorption
   F. Decreased NH_4^+ production
2. A 3-year-old boy is found unresponsive in his parents' garage, and an empty bottle of antifreeze (ethylene glycol) is beside him. He is breathing with deep and long inspirations.

Which of the following clinical observations are likely to be made in this case?
   A. Increased plasma $[Cl^-]$
   B. $PCO_2 > 40$ mm Hg
   C. Increased anion gap
   D. $[HCO_3^-] > 24$ mEq/L
   E. Normal blood pH
3. A 14-year-old girl with violent bacterial food poisoning is found to have a metabolic alkalosis. Her acid-base disorder might result from which of the following?
   A. Decreased H^+ production
   B. Increased ventilation because of fever
   C. Compensatory hypoventilation
   D. Diarrhea
   E. Increased oral alkali intake
   F. Increased H^+ loss

ANSWERS TO REVIEW QUESTIONS

1. **The answer is D.** This patient's decreased central respiratory drive results in the accumulation of CO_2, which lowers blood pH, resulting in a respiratory acidosis. To compensate, the kidneys increase the production of bicarbonate and the excretion of protons. NH_4^+ production would be increased, not decreased, to further promote H^+ excretion.

2. **The answer is C.** A patient with ethylene glycol toxicity has an anion gap metabolic acidosis. The lowered pH stimulates increased respiratory drive to lower PCO_2 and consume H^+ by shifting the buffer reaction to the left, which will oppose the decreased pH. The kidneys will also increase bicarbonate reabsorption and production in an attempt to shift the buffer reaction to the left. The plasma $[HCO_3^-]$ will be low, however, because of the titration of the HCO_3^- buffer by added H^+ from the ethylene glycol. The plasma $[Cl^-]$ is elevated in normal anion gap/hyperchloremic acidosis, not in conditions like this one, in which the anion gap is elevated by the unmeasured anion, oxalate, derived from the ethylene glycol. Kussmaul's respiration is the term applied to the deep, rapid breathing observed in patients with metabolic acidosis.

3. **The answer is F.** Her metabolic alkalosis likely results from an increased loss of H^+, most likely secondary to vomiting, and a loss of HCl from her stomach as a result of her food poisoning. Although the central respiratory drive and hyperventilation can be caused by fever, the question states that the girl has a metabolic alkalosis. Febrile hyperventilation is a cause of primary respiratory alkalosis. Respiratory compensation does not cause metabolic alkalosis; rather, metabolic alkalosis causes compensatory decreased ventilation, which raises the blood PCO_2 and shifts the buffer reaction to the right, yielding H^+ and lowering pH. Diarrhea is often associated with food poisoning, and if Cl-rich, it may cause metabolic alkalosis, but more often it is a cause of metabolic acidosis owing to increased HCO_3^- loss in the stool. Increased alkali intake would cause metabolic alkalosis by elevating the $[HCO_3^-]$ in the plasma, but the patient's history is not suggestive of increased intake of alkali or any food. Although this girl does have an elevated $[HCO_3^-]$, the reason is likely to be vomiting and loss of H^+, shifting the buffer relation to the right.

23

Micturition

INTRODUCTION

Micturition is the process by which the urinary bladder empties its contents, and it is more commonly known as urination. This process involves two steps: (1) the bladder fills until wall tension exceeds a certain threshold level and (2) a nervous reflex known as the micturition reflex occurs, and the bladder empties. The micturition reflex is an autonomic spinal cord reflex, occurring independently of signals higher up in the central nervous system. Micturition can be inhibited or facilitated by centers in the cerebral cortex or the brain stem. An individual may consciously suppress the desire to urinate created by the micturition reflex or may attempt to urinate even without such a feeling of urgency.

SYSTEM STRUCTURE: ANATOMY OF THE URINARY SYSTEM

The fluid that pools in the renal calyces is the same urine that exits the body during micturition. No further reabsorption or secretion of solutes, and no further transport of water across cell membranes, occurs once the urine passes through the collecting ducts of the kidney. Urine is transported from the kidneys to the urinary bladder via two muscular tubes known as ureters (Fig. 23.1). The bladder is a smooth muscle chamber that has two main parts. The body, also known as the fundus, is the main part of the bladder and acts as a storage chamber for the urine. The bladder neck, also known as the posterior urethra, is a funnel-shaped-shaped extension of the body of the bladder. This extension continues as the urethra, which opens to the outside of the body.

The smooth muscle of the bladder is known as the detrusor muscle. These muscle fibers extend in all directions around the bladder—longitudinally, radially, and spirally—without distinct layers, and the muscle cells themselves are fused together, similar to the syncytium of cardiac muscle. These muscle patterns create low-resistance electrical pathways between the cells and allow for a given action potential to spread quickly throughout the entire detrusor muscle, thereby producing a synchronous bladder contraction for micturition.

The mucosa of the bladder consists of a transitional epithelium, which includes basal columnar cells on the outside, intermediate cuboidal cells, and superficial squamous cells on the inside (Fig. 23.2A). When the bladder is empty or underfilled, even the superficial cells are slightly rounded. When the bladder is filled, these superficial cells stretch and flatten into the classic squamous shape. In addition to this distensibility at the histologic level, the bladder mucosa also maintains an anatomic level of distensibility (Fig. 23.2B). The mucosal surface at rest is grossly folded into *rugae*, similar to that of the stomach, and can also stretch and flatten to accommodate increases in urine volume. These two levels of distensibility enable the bladder to expand in volume without significantly increasing the pressure inside.

Urine enters the bladder through two ureters and leaves through a single urethra. These three ports make up the angles of the trigone, a small triangular area on the posterior wall of the bladder immediately above the neck (see Figs. 23.1B and C). The mucosa of the trigone is distinct from that of the rest of the bladder. Whereas the majority of the bladder mucosa is folded into rugae, the trigone mucosa is smooth, regardless of the volume of urine. The ureters enter obliquely through the detrusor muscle, coursing 1 to 2 cm beneath the bladder mucosa before emptying into the bladder along the two upper angles of the trigone. This oblique extended course through the bladder wall helps prevent vesicoureteral reflux, the retrograde flow of urine from the bladder into the ureters. The posterior urethra constitutes the lowermost apex of the trigone. In the male, the posterior urethra leads to the anterior urethra, which extends through the penis before opening to the outside of the body at the external meatus. In the female, the urinary tract nearly ends with the posterior urethra as it leads almost directly to the outside of the body. Females have higher risk of urinary tract infections because of the short urethra (see Clinical Correlation Box 23.1).

Clinical Correlation Box 23.1

What is a Urinary Tract Infection?

Melissa, age 30 years, has no significant past medical history. She lives alone and does not smoke or drink. She reports to her doctor that she's been feeling "this burning when I go to the bathroom all day." The discomfort has worsened, and Melissa has also experienced increased urinary frequency and very small urine volumes. She complains of a vague discomfort in her lower abdomen immediately after she finishes urinating. She has no fever or chills and no tenderness at the costovertebral angles on the back (location of the kidneys). Examination of the urine reveals a high white blood cell count. The doctor prescribes a sulfa antibiotic for acute uncomplicated urinary tract infection (UTI).

A UTI is a bacterial infection of the urethra that spreads to the bladder, where it causes inflammation. (Inflammation of the bladder is called cystitis.) These infections may be complicated by ascent of the infection to the kidneys (pyelonephritis), and they may be chronic or recurring. Most often they are acute and uncomplicated. The cystitis causes increased detrusor contraction, leading to increased frequency and urgency. Urethritis and cystitis cause a burning sensation upon urination and pain in the area of the bladder.

Treatment is with antibiotics and sometimes with phenazopyridine, an analgesic that distributes well to the urinary space. Prophylaxis should address the risk factors for UTI. UTIs are often caused by *Escherichia coli* bacteria from the rectum. Consequently, women should wipe from front to back to avoid contaminating the urethra with rectal *E. coli*. Urination shortly after sexual intercourse may also decrease the risk of infection.

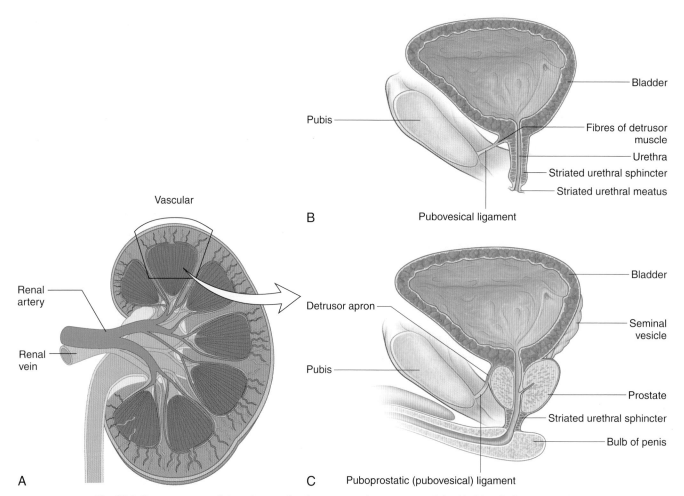

Fig. 23.1 Gross anatomy of the urinary collecting system, the ureters, and the bladder. **A,** A cross-sectional view of the kidney. **B,** The female bladder. **C,** The male bladder. (A, from Caroll. *Elsevier's Integrated Physiology*. Fig. 11.1. B and C with permission from Drake RL, Vogl AW, Mitchell A, Tibbitts R, Richardson P (eds). *Gray's Atlas of Anatomy*. Elsevier: Churchill Livingstone; 2008.)

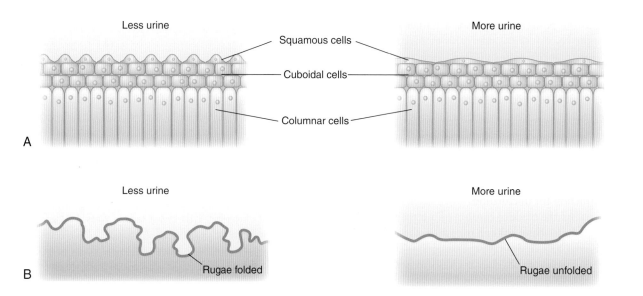

Fig. 23.2 Accommodating increased bladder volume. **A,** On the histologic level, the squamous cells flatten out to accommodate increased urine volume (bladder filling) and relieve tension in the bladder wall. **B,** On the anatomic level, the rugae flatten out to accommodate increased urine volume (bladder filling) and relieve tension in the bladder wall.

The bladder neck consists of the inferior 2 to 3 cm of the bladder. Its wall, like the wall of the bladder body, comprises the detrusor muscle; however, the muscle here is organized into distinct layers to form the internal sphincter of the bladder. Sympathetic tone supplied to the internal sphincter through the hypogastric nerve keeps the internal sphincter tonically contracted. Additional control of micturition is located beyond the bladder neck as the urethra passes through the urogenital diaphragm. Here, the external sphincter of the bladder, a voluntary muscle layer as opposed to the smooth muscle of the body and neck of the bladder, can be consciously controlled to prevent or interrupt urination (see Fig. 23.2).

Innervation of the Bladder

The bladder is innervated by the pelvic nerves, the hypogastric nerves, and the pudendal nerves (Fig. 23.3). These nerves provide parasympathetic, sympathetic, and somatic innervation, respectively. As a whole, they include afferent, as well as efferent fibers, and impart voluntary, as well as involuntary control of micturition. The nerves are wired to the spinal cord to participate in spinal reflex arcs. The spinal neurons receive input from the pontine micturition center in the brain stem, which in turn receives higher inputs from the diencephalon and cerebral cortex.

The pelvic nerves are the primary nerve supply of the bladder. Arising from the sacral spinal cord at levels S2, S3, and S4, the pelvic nerves contain both sensory and motor para-sympathetic fibers. The sensory fibers detect the degree of stretch in the bladder wall, and the motor fibers return the reflex signal and stimulate the bladder wall to contract for micturition.

The hypogastric nerves arise from the spinal cord mainly at L2 and pass through the sympathetic chain. These nerves then send sympathetic innervation to the bladder neck and induce closure of the internal sphincter, which facilitates urine storage in the bladder body and seals off the urinary tract during ejaculation. They play little role in the actual contraction of the bladder body for micturition. The hypogastric nerves also contain some sensory fibers, which sense fullness, as well as pain.

The pudendal nerves innervate the skeletal muscle of the external sphincter. The somatic motor fibers provide the signals for the sphincter to contract; thus cortical inhibition of the pudendal nerve leads to a voluntary relaxation of the external sphincter, allowing the bladder to empty.

SYSTEM FUNCTION: THE TRANSPORT OF URINE AND ITS NEURAL CONTROL

Urine from the collecting ducts of the kidneys is ready for elimination by the body. The basic function of the rest of the urinary tract is to transport the urine from the kidneys to the bladder and ultimately outside the body. Spinal reflexes and their conscious and unconscious modulation by the brain control this final step of voiding the bladder of urine.

The Transport of Urine From Kidney to Bladder

Whereas the hydrostatic pressure of filtration drives the urine into the renal calyces, from that area, urinary flow is assisted by the elasticity of the urinary conduit. As the urine pools in the renal calyces, the walls are stretched, initiating a series of

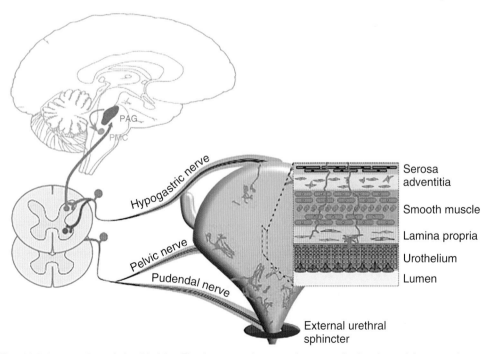

Fig. 23.3 Innervation of the bladder. The hypogastric nerve is sympathetic, the pelvic nerve is parasympathetic, and the pudendal nerve is somatic. The pudendal nerve alone stimulates the contraction of skeletal muscle. Afferent pathways are not shown in this figure. (From Umans BD, Liberles SD. Neural sensing of organ volume. *Trends Neurosci.* 2018;41(12): Fig. 3.)

peristaltic smooth muscle contractions, which spread to the renal pelvis and down the ureter. These contractions force the urine in the calyces toward the bladder for temporary storage before micturition.

For urine to enter the bladder, the pressure generated by the peristaltic wave in the ureter must exceed the pressure on the ureter caused by the inherent tone of the detrusor muscle of the bladder wall. This high pressure in the ureter pushes open the intravesical ureter and allows the urine to drain into the body of the bladder. (Vesical comes from the Latin *vesica* for bladder. Intravesical ureter refers to the segment of ureter passing through the bladder wall.) Remember that the ureters normally course at an oblique angle through the wall of the bladder. The bladder wall compresses the ureters and acts as a valve to prevent the backflow of urine. This mechanism is important when the pressure in the bladder increases with micturition or external compression. In fact, during bladder contraction, the detrusor muscle further compresses the intravesical ureters and occludes them to prevent the backflow of urine. Note that if the distance that one (or both) of the ureters courses through the bladder wall is less than normal (i.e., if the ureter courses at a less oblique, more direct angle), bladder contraction becomes less efficient at completely occluding that ureter and preventing backflow. The "valve" becomes leaky.

Vesicoureteral reflux is the pathologic backflow of urine and pressure. Chronic reflux can lead to enlargement of the affected ureter or ureters. If severe, it can lead to increased pressure in the renal calyces and ultimately damage the structures of the renal medulla.

The renal medulla is also protected from excess backflow by a reflex originating in the ureter. When an obstruction is sensed in the ureter, such as a kidney stone, the ureter undergoes an intense reflex constriction. This reflex is also associated with intense pain, because the ureters are well supplied with pain fibers by the pelvic nerves. This pain impulse precipitates a sympathetic reflex at the level of the kidney, decreasing urine output from the affected kidney (by increasing salt and water reabsorption), and minimizing the backflow of urine and pressure into the renal medulla. This protective reflex at the ureteral level is known as the ureterorenal reflex.

The Spinal Micturition Reflex

Remember that the bladder wall contains many folds known as rugae, thus creating a very distensible chamber. As the bladder fills with urine, the rugae smooth out and allow the volume inside the chamber to increase without increasing the pressure inside the chamber. Thus a normal bladder can fill to a volume of about 300 mL with only a small increase in intravesical pressure. Once this volume is reached, the inner wall of the bladder is smooth, and subsequent increases in total urine volume stretch the bladder wall like air blown into a balloon. Then after the body of the bladder is expanded, urine begins to fill the neck of the bladder. (Imagine that the neck of the bladder is equivalent to the tip of a balloon. The tip fills last; first the larger part of the balloon, which is nearer to the air inlet, fills and builds up a good deal of air under pressure.)

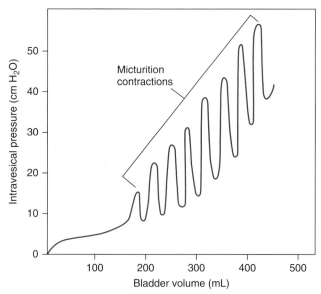

Fig. 23.4 Pressure in the bladder during filling. The micturition reflex creates spikes in pressure once the urine volume and pressure pass a certain threshold.

As the bladder continues to fill, sensory stretch receptors in the bladder wall are stimulated, sending signals along the pelvic nerves to the spinal cord. Such stretch receptors are especially numerous in the bladder neck, making the neck more sensitive to filling than the body. Similar to the patellar stretch reflex, this bladder stretch reflex returns to the bladder from the spinal cord via parasympathetic fibers of the pelvic nerve, resulting in an intense stimulation and contraction of the bladder wall's detrusor muscle. Remember that the individual muscle cells of the bladder wall are joined as a syncytium, and any stimulation for the contraction of a muscle fiber will cause the entire bladder to contract. The micturition reflex is initiated upon reaching threshold pressure.

When the bladder is only partly filled, the micturition contraction acutely increases the pressure inside the bladder and then spontaneously relaxes after a few seconds. The pressure inside the bladder subsequently falls back to the baseline tonic pressure from the total urine volume. This completes a single cycle of the micturition reflex (Fig. 23.4). The frequency of the micturition reflex increases with an increase in total urine volume (and increase in tonic pressure). Also, the reflex may be self-regenerative in that the micturition contraction also increases the pressure inside the bladder and stimulates additional sensory stretch receptors. As the bladder continues to fill, these reflexes increase in frequency and the micturition contractions increase in power and duration until a voluntary decision to urinate intervenes, allowing the micturition reflex to go uninhibited and the internal and external sphincters to relax. The voluntary decision inhibits the firing of the motor fibers in the pudendal nerve, eliminating its tonic contraction of the external sphincter, thereby relaxing it (Fig. 23.5; see also Clinical Correlation Box 23.2, Trauma Box 23.1 and Oncology Box 23.1).

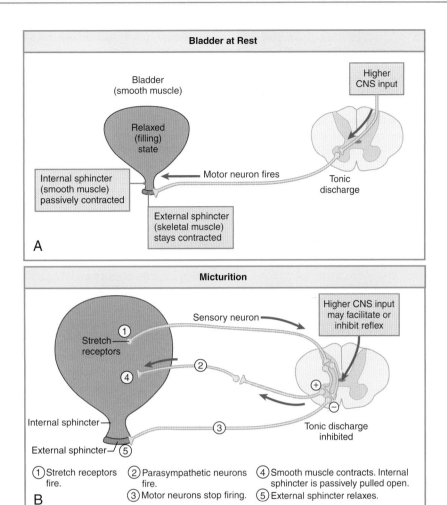

Fig. 23.5 The spinal micturition reflex. **A,** When the bladder is at rest, there is tonic contraction of the internal and external sphincters and the detrusor is relaxed during urine storage and before initiation of the reflex. **B,** During the micturition reflex, the detrusor contracts, and the sphincters relax. The external sphincter may be contracted or relaxed during the reflex, depending on cortical signals. The sympathetic reflex (afferent: pelvic, efferent: hypogastric) relaxes the internal sphincter. The parasympathetic reflex (afferent: pelvic, efferent: pelvic) contracts the detrusor and relaxes the internal sphincter. Cortical signals tonically inhibit the spinal micturition reflex. Conscious removal of this inhibition increases the strength of the spinal reflex and relieves the contraction of the external sphincter so that urination may begin. *CNS*, Central nervous system. (From Carroll R. *Elsevier's Integrated Physiology*. Philadelphia: Mosby Elsevier; 2007. Fig. 11.20.)

Clinical Correlation Box 23.2

What is Benign Prostatic Hyperplasia?

A 56-year-old man complains to his primary care physician that he is awakened several times a night with the need to urinate. Upon further questioning, he indicates that he often must strain slightly by tensing his abdominal muscles to initiate urination. He believes his urinary stream is "weaker than it used to be" and complains of a sensation of incomplete voiding after urination. He does not experience any burning sensation or pain during urination, and he has not noticed any blood or other discoloration of his urine. On conducting a rectal exam, the doctor finds an enlarged prostate.

As the name would suggest, benign prostatic hyperplasia (BPH) is a nonmalignant growth in the male prostate gland. Because of the prostate's anatomic location, it may create a urethral obstruction to outflow. This obstruction has several physiologic consequences. First, the obstruction means that higher intravesical pressures are necessary to drive the urine through the urethra. Patients may consequently complain of an inability to generate as strong a urinary stream as in their youth and may feel the need to push or strain to begin urination. Second, the higher pressure necessary for urination may lead to incomplete bladder emptying. Normal micturition usually leaves no more than 5 to 10 mL of urine remaining in the bladder; this volume is known as the postvoid residual (PVR). In BPH, the PVR is typically elevated. One can imagine that a high PVR decreases the interval of time that it takes the bladder to refill and therefore increases the frequency of urination.

Men with BPH often complain of nocturia (the need to urinate at night), as well as an increased frequency of urination throughout the day. They may notice that they void smaller amounts each time and may complain of a feeling of incomplete voiding (urinary retention). Many of these symptoms are at least partially relieved when the obstruction is reduced. For well over 50 years, a surgical procedure known as a transurethral resection of the prostate has been the mainstay of treatment, although medical therapy has been assuming increasing importance.

⚡ TRAUMA BOX 23.1

Spinal trauma, like compressive malignant growths (see Oncology Box 23.1), can damage the distal spinal cord at the conus medullaris or the cauda equine, resulting in bladder dysfunction and urinary retention. Urinary retention often leads to recurrent urinary tract infections in affected patients, especially as bladder decompression may need to be accomplished by insertion of a urinary catheter, and such instrumentation increases the risk of infection.

✳ ONCOLOGY BOX 23.1

Urinary retention may be a major component of the cauda equine syndrome and epidural spinal cord compression. Both or either alone can result from a malignancy that metastasizes to the spine or a primary spinal tumor that impinges on the distal spinal cord at the conus medullaris or the cauda equina just distal to it. Common tumors that do so are those of breast, lung, and prostate, as well as Hodgkin disease, non-Hodgkin lymphoma, and multiple myeloma.

PATHOPHYSIOLOGY: URINARY INCONTINENCE

Urinary incontinence, the loss of voluntary bladder control, affects millions of Americans of all ages. Approximately 50% of women experience occasional urinary incontinence. The incidence of urinary incontinence increases with age and its accompanying increase in pelvic relaxation. Urinary continence is possible because the intraurethral pressure exceeds the intravesical pressure. Tonic contraction of the internal and external sphincters are crucial mechanisms for preserving continence. The submucosal vasculature of the urethra also plays a role in maintaining urinary continence. Through a mechanism known as mucosal coaptation, the vasculature complex fills with blood, thus further increasing intraurethral pressure. In women, this mechanism is estrogen-sensitive, which partly explains why urinary incontinence occurs more frequently in postmenopausal women (Fig. 23.6).

Urinary incontinence can be categorized into four subgroups: stress incontinence, urge incontinence, total incontinence, and overflow incontinence. Stress incontinence involves the loss of urine with increased straining, usually in the setting of increased pelvic relaxation. The straining from activities, such as coughing, laughing, or exercising, increases abdominal pressure and allows the intravesical pressure to exceed the intraurethral pressure, resulting in stress incontinence.

Urge incontinence involves urine leakage because of uninhibited, involuntary bladder contraction, which increases intravesical pressure. This heightened micturition reflex overwhelms voluntary control. Such detrusor instability can result from urinary tract infections, bladder stones, cancer, diverticula, or neurologic disorders causing hyperreflexia, although many cases are idiopathic. Common urinary complaints in this setting include urgency and frequency (see Clinical Correlation Box 23.1).

The uninhibited neurogenic bladder is an example of how partial damage to the spinal cord or brain stem interrupts cortical inhibitory signals. Remember that these cortical signals keep the external sphincter voluntarily contracted, as well as curb the micturition reflex until micturition is voluntarily desired. Without these cortical signals, the sacral centers of micturition become overexcitable, such that even small amounts of urine in the bladder can elicit micturition reflexes and result in urinary frequency. Sometimes after spinal cord damage, spinal shock occurs, in which even the micturition reflex is suppressed. After a few days, and assuming that the bladder is protected from overstretching with artificial emptying—that is, catheterization—the micturition reflex gradually returns and at this point may become hyperreflexic because of lost inhibition from upper motor neurons. This condition is similar to the initial hyporeflexia or even areflexia followed by hyperreflexia of the patellar reflex with proximal spinal cord damage.

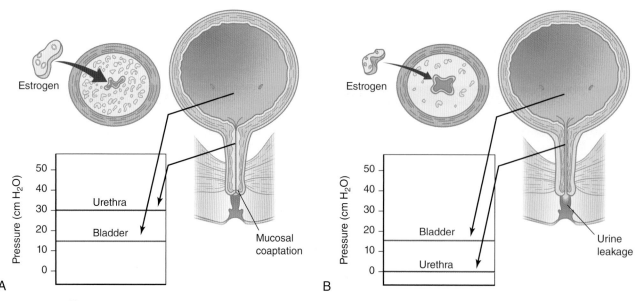

Fig. 23.6 Mucosal coaptation. **A,** Estrogen-dependent swelling of the female urethra helps maintain urinary continence by increasing urethral pressure. **B,** Estrogen deficiency results in decreased urethral pressure.

The restoration of the micturition reflex occurs without any voluntary control or sensation, thus resulting in periodic but unannounced bladder emptying. Some patients are able to learn new stimuli for the micturition reflex so that they can bring it on themselves and preempt unannounced micturition reflexes. Patients learn to associate local skin stimuli (i.e., scratching, tickling) with the micturition reflex. By stimulating their skin in the genital region, these patients are able to elicit an involuntary micturition reflex and empower themselves with a simulated voluntary control of micturition.

Total incontinence, in which urine leaks from the body as soon as it is delivered from the ureters, is typically the result of a urinary fistula. Connections between the bladder or urethra and the intestines are possible, as well as between the bladder or urethra and the vagina. Causes of these fistulae include pelvic radiation, pelvic surgery, and gastrointestinal diseases, such as diverticulitis, colon cancer, and Crohn disease. Treatment is typically surgical separation.

Overflow incontinence results from weak or absent bladder contractions, leading to urinary retention and overdistension of the bladder. The bladder empties only when its capacity is exceeded. Patients may present with a complaint of constant dribbling. This atonic bladder may result from afferent nerve fiber destruction, resulting in the lack of transmission of stretch signals from the bladder wall. Other causes include certain medications, outflow obstruction (as in benign prostatic hyperplasia [BPH]), or even postoperative overdistension. Self-catheterization may be necessary if medical management is not sufficient.

SUMMARY

- Urine is ready for excretion once it leaves the renal tubular collecting ducts. From the collecting ducts, it flows into the renal calyces, the renal pelvis, the ureter, and into the bladder.
- The calyces, pelvis, and ureter help push the urine down the ureter through elastic and peristaltic contraction. The muscular wall of the bladder compresses the ureters and acts as a one-way valve to prevent urinary backflow.
- The detrusor muscle in the bladder wall squeezes the urine during urination but is normally relaxed. The internal and external sphincters open during urination but are normally contracted.
- Three nerves mediate the spinal micturition reflex: hypogastric (sympathetic), pelvic (parasympathetic), and pudendal (somatic).
- Afferent signals detect stretch in the bladder walls when the bladder fills with urine. These signals travel via the pelvic nerve to the spinal cord and return efferent via the hypogastric and pelvic nerves. The efferent signals trigger detrusor contraction and sphincter relaxation.
- The reflex occurs intermittently, leading to spikes in intravesical (intrabladder) pressure. The spikes increase in amplitude and frequency as urine volume climbs.
- Firing from upper motor neurons inhibits the spinal micturition reflex and keeps the external sphincter contracted. The conscious reduction of upper motor neuron inhibition allows the micturition reflex to occur unimpeded, and urination occurs. Loss of upper motor neurons because of neurologic injury or disease can result in a hyperactive micturition reflex.
- Incontinence and other difficulties with urination may arise from neurologic or structural factors.
- The four varieties of incontinence are stress incontinence, urge incontinence, total incontinence, and overflow incontinence.

REVIEW QUESTIONS

Directions: Each of the numbered items or incomplete statements in this section is followed by answers or by completions of the statement. Select the one lettered answer or completion that is best in each case.

1. A 25-year-old man is stabbed multiple times in the lower back and pelvis, damaging one of the nerves that innervate the bladder. If he goes on to develop an atonic bladder and overflow incontinence, he is likely to have damaged neurons in which location?
   A. Pelvic nerves
   B. Hypogastric nerves
   C. Pudendal nerves
   D. Pontine micturition center
   E. Cerebral cortex

2. A 64-year-old postmenopausal woman with two grown children, both delivered vaginally, reports occasional incontinence after coughing or laughing. Her incontinence likely results from which of the following mechanisms?
   A. Involuntary bladder contraction
   B. Increased pelvic relaxation
   C. Neurogenic bladder
   D. Leakage from a urinary fistula
   E. Urinary retention because of obstruction

3. A 72-year-old man reports increased frequency of urination but decreased amounts of urine relative to several years ago. On urinary catheterization, he is found to have an increased postvoid residual, which might result from which of the following?
   A. Crohn disease
   B. Urinary tract infection
   C. Increased pelvic relaxation
   D. History of diverticulitis
   E. Prostate cancer

ANSWERS TO REVIEW QUESTIONS

1. **The answer is A.** The primary nerve supply of the bladder, the pelvic nerves, arises from the sacral plexus. Damage to these nerves would result in difficulty stimulating the contraction of the bladder wall for micturition. The hypogastric nerves are responsible for closure of the internal sphincter, which facilitates urine storage. The pudendal nerves are responsible for contracting the external sphincter. The cortex and pontine micturition center normally inhibit the micturition reflex and maintain contraction of the external sphincter. Voluntary removal of these inhibitory signals allows urination to occur.

2. **The answer is B.** This patient suffers from stress incontinence, which involves the leakage of urine in situations of increased straining or abdominal pressure. This often occurs in the setting of increased pelvic relaxation, which is a consequence of vaginal deliveries. Urge incontinence, which involves leakage secondary to uninhibited, involuntary bladder contraction, causes urinary urgency and increased frequency. Total incontinence is characterized by leakage of urine as soon as it enters the bladder, and typically results from a urinary fistula. Overflow incontinence may lead to constant urinary dribbling because of overdistention of the bladder, and may result from obstruction.

3. **The answer is E.** This patient's increased postvoid residual results from outflow obstruction, which might occur with prostate cancer in a male. Crohn disease and diverticulitis might predispose a patient to develop urinary fistulas, which would lead to urinary leakage, not retention. A urinary tract infection would be likely to result in frequent bladder emptying, not increased urinary retention. Increased pelvic relaxation is likely to result in stress incontinence, and is more frequent in women.

C.J. is a 52-year-old male with chronic hypertension (HTN) managed both with lifestyle changes and pharmacologically. He presented yesterday morning to an outside hospital with malignant HTN, headache, and complaints of "tearing" chest pain. His only past medical history is labile HTN and borderline type 2 diabetes, he has never had surgery.

PRESENTATION: HISTORY AND PHYSICAL EXAMINATION

In the morning while walking to the bathroom, C.J. began feeling a tightening followed by what he calls a "tearing" sensation between his shoulder blades. He does not endorse any pain in the left arm or up into the neck. He states that the pain was sudden and sharp and nothing he did would make it go away. He tried to sit down and relax but this did not help. He had not yet taken his morning medication of Metoprolol and Lisinopril, and thought perhaps that would help his symptoms. He waited 1 hour after taking the medication and with no remittance presented to the emergency department (ED). He further denies any abdominal pain, nausea, vomiting, recent fever or chills, shortness of breath, or any musculoskeletal pain. He has never experienced anything like this in the past, nor does he believe anyone in his family has ever experienced these symptoms.

He was evaluated by Vascular Surgery and admitted for further workup which included a computed tomography (CT) scan. As a member of the nephrology team, you were consulted after admission, laboratory evaluation, and imaging were complete.

On physical examination, C.J. is lying in bed, alert and oriented but in moderate distress. He is without any focal neurologic deficits, and auscultation reveals normal heart sounds, tachypnea, and normal lung sounds. His abdomen is soft, nondistended, and nontender to palpation in all four quadrants. He has 5/5 strength bilaterally and bounding 2+ pulses in his bilateral lower extremities, however his upper extremities differ with 2+ on the right and a diminished pulse on the left. His blood pressure is 176/96 mmHg, with a heart rate of 75 beats per minute, respirations of 22 breaths per minute, and a temperature of 37.0 °C. He is on supplemental oxygen via nasal cannula at 2L/min and has an oxygen saturation of 99%. Overnight he was given 3300 mL of continuous intravenous infusions, took in 880 mL of fluid by mouth, and received two 120-mL doses of radiocontrast for two separate CT scans. He is only making 10 to 15 mL of urine per hour and a bladder scan reveals only 30 mL of volume.

DISCUSSION

The history, review of systems, and physical examination are indicative of a patient at high risk for kidney injury. As discussed in Chapter 17, we can categorize the many causes of acute kidney injury into three locations of the primary process. Prerenal, defined as decreased glomerular filtration rate (GFR) owing to compromise in the blood flow to the kidney. Intrinsic, defined as disease involving any of the various components of the kidney—the glomerulus, the tubules, the interstitium, or the microvasculature—leading to decreased GFR. Postrenal, defined as obstructions of the urinary tract, anywhere from the renal pelvis to the urethra, resulting in kidney dysfunction by increasing hydrostatic pressure in Bowman's space, impeding glomerular filtration.

Prerenal injury can be caused by anything from gastrointestinal losses decreasing the amount of blood volume, reduced effective blood flow as seen in nephrotic syndrome or portal HTN, or even decreased cardiac output leading to hypoxia. In C.J., he was previously placed on an angiotensin-converting enzyme (ACE) inhibitor which can also lead to prerenal acute kidney injury in the right setting.

Intrinsic injury can be caused by vasculitis, postinfectious causes, or medications, such as the radiocontrast that C.J. received twice. The categories of intrinsic renal injury include acute tubular necrosis, glomerulonephritis, and tubulointerstitial nephritis.

Postrenal injury would be caused by something like an obstruction of a ureter by a renal stone that increases the pressure in Bowman's space and decreases the GFR. C.J. does not have a history or examination that raises clinical suspicion of this mechanism of kidney injury.

PRESENTATION: LABORATORY TESTS AND IMAGING

After attaining a thorough history and physical examination, C.J. was admitted to the hospital and underwent another CT angiogram of the thorax, abdomen, and pelvis. This revealed a large type B aortic dissection involving the left subclavian artery and extending down through the common iliac arteries bilaterally. The left kidney is found to be incorporated in the false lumen, however the mesenteric vessels and the right kidney continue to perfuse from the true lumen (Fig. 23.1.1).

Initial laboratory tests included a complete metabolic profile, a complete blood count, a type and cross, and a prothrombin time. The results for C.J. are:

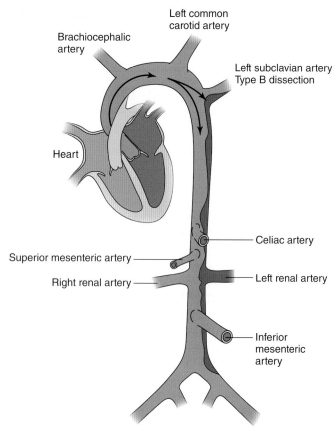

Fig. 23.1.1 Schematic diagram of a type B aortic dissection. The right renal artery is perfused by the true aortic lumen but the left renal artery branches off the false lumen.

Basic metabolic panel (BMP): Na 139 mEq/L, K 4.3 mEq/L, Cl 101 mEq/L, HCO$_3$ 26 mEq/L, blood urea nitrogen (BUN) 16 mg/dL, Cr 1.49 mg/dL, glucose 142 mg/dL, eGFR 49 mL/min/1.73 m^2 ("eGFR" is the estimated glomerular filtration rate, see Table 23.1.1)

Complete blood count (CBC): white blood cell (WBC) 17.48 cells/μL, hemoglobin (Hb) 15.2 g/dL, hematocrit (HCT) 45%, platelet 132,000/μL

TABLE 23.1.1   Stages of Chronic Kidney Disease

Stage	Description	GFR[a] mL/min/1.73 m^2
1	Slight kidney damage with normal or increased filtration	>90
2	Mild decrease in kidney function	60–89
3	Moderate decrease in kidney function	30–59
4	Severe decrease in kidney function	15–29
5	Kidney failure	<15 (or dialysis)

[a]GFR is glomerular filtration rate, a measure of the kidney's function. (From Eknoyan G, Levin A, Levin NW. Bone metabolism and disease in chronic kidney disease. *Am J Kidney Dis.* 2003;42(3):1-201. Table 1.)

Type and cross: ABO-A POS, antibody screen-negative
Prothrombin time (PT), international normalized ration (INR): PT 14.6 s, INR 1.4
Follow-up laboratory examination the next morning reveals:
BMP: Na 140 mEq/L, K 4.8 mEq/L, Cl 102 mEq/L, HCO$_3$ 23 mEq/L, BUN 18 mg/dL, Cr 1.92 mg/dL, glucose 141 mg/dL, eGFR 37 mL/min/1.73 m^2
CBC: WBC 13.62 cells/μL, Hgb 13.5 g/dL, HCT 41.1%, platelets 139,000/μL

DISCUSSION

C.J. is diagnosed with oliguric acute kidney injury stage 3 because of combination of contrast induced nephropathy and the type B dissection effectively occluding flow to the left kidney. Treatment includes further intravenous (IV) hydration with normal saline to help offset contrast exposure, a conversion of all medications to renal dosing, and a recommendation for no further contrast, gadolinium, ACE inhibitors, or nonsteroidal antiinflammatory drugs.

COURSE

Ultimately, C.J. underwent surgical management of his type B dissection which did not restore flow to his left kidney. His renal function continued to worsen postoperatively to a Cr of 2.89 mg/dL and an eGFR of 23 mL/min/1.73 m^2. This was compounded by the fact that he also was given IV antibiotics for a developing hospital acquired pneumonia. Fortunately, on hospital day 7 his GFR began to slowly improve. He did not require dialysis during his hospitalization; however if his renal function continued to worsen this was discussed as an option and C.J. was willing to undergo the intervention.

DISCUSSION

The indications for dialysis in acute kidney injury include fluid overload, metabolic acidosis, hyperkalemia, uremic pericarditis, severe hyperphosphatemia, and uremic symptoms. Upon admission, C.J. had a metabolic acidosis, and during his hospitalization he did become hyperkalemic and suffer uremic symptoms. Fortunately, these were able to be managed medically and did not require initiation of dialysis. There is one principal cause of hyperkalemia, namely decreased renal excretion.

The definitive treatment of hyperkalemia is typically a medical first approach followed by dialysis if needed emergently (see Box 23.1.1). The basis of treatment is the removal of potassium from the body, which can be accomplished by using a standard protocol. The acronym C BIG K Drop is frequently used. This

BOX 23.1.1   Indications for Dialysis

A acidosis
E electrolyte abnormalities
I intoxication/poisoning
0 fluid overload
U uremia symptoms/complications

stands for Calcium gluconate, Bicarbonate, Insulin and Glucose, Kayexalate (sodium polystyrene sulfonate), and Dialysis. The administration of a loop diuretic, such as furosemide, may increase urinary flow and excretion of potassium. Administering sodium polystyrene sulfonate (Kayexalate), a cationic exchange resin that lowers potassium by exchanging sodium for potassium in the colon. Calcium gluconate antagonizes the effects of hyperkalemia on cardiac function and bicarbonate may counter the metabolic acidosis that can accompany hyperkalemia. As discussed, emergent dialysis is a last resort.

Gastrointestinal Physiology

24

Nutrition, Digestion, and Absorption

INTRODUCTION

The gastrointestinal (GI) system supplies the fuel and the building blocks for the functioning of the body through the digestion and absorption of nutrients. Its machinery for doing so is the alimentary canal, also called the gastrointestinal tract, a highly specialized long tube that connects the mouth and the anus. While providing for the absorption of essential nutrients and elimination of waste products, the GI tract must also serve a critical barrier function in preventing the entry of toxic substances and organisms found in the environment (and therefore in the lumen of the digestive tract).

SYSTEM STRUCTURE

In general, the GI tract can be viewed as a hollow tube surrounded by a wall consisting of four layers starting from the inside (Fig. 24.1):
- The mucosa consists of an epithelial lining, a lamina propria (loose connective tissue, blood vessels, lymphatics), and a muscularis mucosae.
- The submucosa is similar to the lamina propria but its connective tissue is denser and it contains nerves.
- The muscularis propria contains two layers of smooth muscle.
  - The inner layer of smooth muscle is circular (muscle fibers are oriented around the circumference of the gut).
  - The outer layer of smooth muscle is arranged longitudinally (muscle fibers are oriented along the length of the gut).
  - Interposed between these two layers is the myenteric nerve plexus. The neural innervation of the GI tract will be discussed in detail in Chapter 25.
- The serosa is a thin layer of connective tissue consisting of blood vessels, lymphatics, adipose tissue, and a simple squamous epithelium, sometimes called a mesothelium.

In the intestine, the epithelial cells of the mucosa are called enterocytes. Enterocytes possess both a luminal (or apical) membrane, which faces the alimentary lumen, and a basolateral membrane, which faces the interstitial lamina propria and the blood supply.

Factors that aid in digestion are secreted across the luminal membrane, and nutrients are absorbed by facilitated diffusion and active transport across the luminal and then the basolateral membrane. Absorbed nutrients then enter the bloodstream and travel to the liver before they are distributed to the body tissues (see Fast Fact 24.1).

Fast Fact Box 24.1

This division of the intestinal epithelium into apical and basolateral membranes (with differing transporters on each side) is found in the epithelia of many organ systems. Other examples are the epithelium of the thyroid follicles and the epithelium of the renal tubules.

The abdominal portions of the digestive tract are supplied by the celiac and mesenteric arteries; venous blood collects into the portal vein, which then branches into a venous capillary bed within the liver. This is the portal circulation, which contain two capillary beds in sequence:
- The capillaries supplying arterial blood to the digestive tract
- The capillaries distributing the blood to the hepatic tissues for metabolism.

THE ORAL CAVITY

Digestion begins in the oral cavity, which contains:
- Tongue
- Teeth
- Salivary glands (Fig. 24.2). Three paired salivary glands are associated with the oral cavity—the parotid, submandibular, and sublingual glands—and smaller salivary glands are scattered throughout the mouth.
  - Within the glands are two types of secretory cells:
    Serous (protein-secreting)
    Mucous (mucus-secreting)

The Stomach

The pharynx is a transitional zone conveying food from the oral cavity to the esophagus.
- Food leaves the esophagus, passes through the lower esophageal sphincter, and enters the stomach.
- The stomach consists of four main regions (in proximal to distal order) (Fig. 24.3):
  - Cardia
  - Fundus
  - Body
  - Pylorus

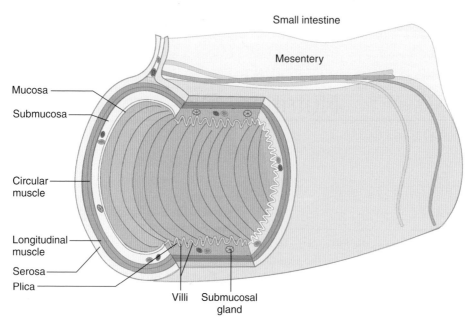

Fig. 24.1 Cutaway view of a segment of the gastrointestinal (GI) tract. The GI tract is essentially a hollow tube surrounded by a wall consisting of four main layers: from inside to out, the mucosa, submucosa, muscularis (composed of circular and longitudinal smooth muscle layers), and serosa. (From Carroll R. *Elsevier's Integrated Physiology.* Philadelphia: Mosby Elsevier; 2007. Fig. 12.1A.)

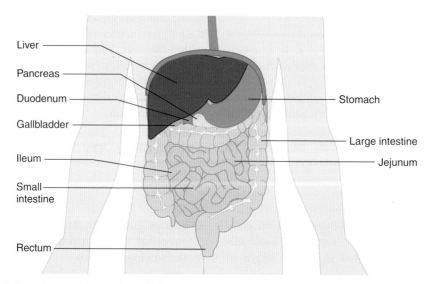

Fig. 24.2 Overview of the gastrointestinal tract organs and their roles. (From Carroll R. *Elsevier's Integrated Physiology.* Philadelphia: Mosby Elsevier; 2007. Fig. 12.1A.)

On the macroscopic level, the stomach's mucosa is bunched into ruggae (similar to the bladder), which increase the surface area of the stomach and allow for expansion and filling. On a microscopic level, the surface mucosa of the stomach invaginates to form gastric pits.

- Emptying into the gastric pits are branched tubular gastric glands, whose function is different in each region of the stomach.
  - The cardia, a narrow (<3 cm) band at the junction of the distal esophagus and stomach, contains glands that secrete mucus and lysozyme (which hydrolyzes bacterial cell walls).

- The glands of the fundus and body contain most of the stomach's parietal cells, which populate the upper half of the gastric glands, and chief cells which populate the lower half.

Parietal cells which secrete hydrochloric acid (HCl).

Chief cells produce and secrete enzymes for the digestion of protein and fat (pepsinogen and lipase, respectively).

A small amount of absorption takes place in the stomach. However, most absorption of nutrients takes place after the partially digested food, or chyme, passes beyond the pyloric sphincter, which divides the stomach from the small intestine.

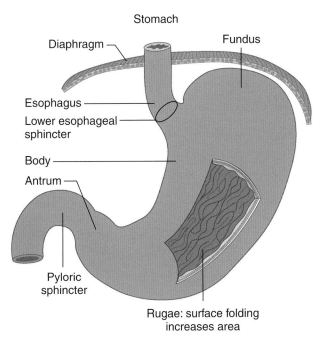

Fig. 24.3 Anatomy of the stomach. The lower esophageal sphincter separates the esophagus from the body of the stomach, whereas the pyloric sphincter separates the antrum of the stomach from the duodenum. (From Carroll R. *Elsevier's Integrated Physiology.* Philadelphia: Mosby Elsevier; 2007. Fig. 12.1A.)

The Small Intestine

The small intestine is the last and most important site of food digestion and food absorption (but not the last site of water absorption). It consists of three segments (in proximal to distal order):

- Duodenum
- Jejunum
- Ileum

These segments are coiled and tethered to the posterior wall of the abdominal cavity by the fatty mesentery, which contains the intestinal blood vessels.

The structure of the small intestine is well suited for digestion and absorption.

- Its great length (approximately 5 m) permits prolonged contact between food and enzymes and between digested foodstuffs and the absorptive lining.
- The small intestine also has a large surface area for digestion and absorption, achieved through numerous folds in the mucosa (Fig. 24.4).
  - The folds of the mucosa and submucosa are visible to the naked eye and are called plicae circulares.
    The plicae circulares are in turn ruffled into finger-shaped outgrowths of mucosa called villi, which are around 1 mm long. The plicae circulares are most prominent in the jejunum, and their presence triples the surface area of the intestine.
    Finally, microvilli are located on the luminal (apical) surface of absorptive cells in the small intestine. Each absorptive cell bears about 3000 microvilli (see Fast Fact Box 24.2).

Fast Fact Box 24.2

Each microvillus (1 μm tall by 0.1 μm in diameter) is a cylindrical protrusion of apical cytoplasm and cell membrane-enclosing actin filaments. The villi increase the surface area by approximately 10-fold and the microvilli by 20-fold.

Microvilli bear enzymes bound to their membranes. These enzymes hydrolyze complex carbohydrates and peptides into simple sugars and amino acids.

- In between the villi, tubular glands (also called the crypts of Lieberkuhn) open onto the intestinal lumen.
- The glands consist primarily of stem cells that divide and replace old epithelial cells and the other intestinal cells found on the villi:
  - Mucus-producing cells (goblet cells)
  - Lysozyme-producing cells (Paneth cells)
  - Enteroendocrine cells.

Carrier molecules are present in the apical membrane of intestinal enterocytes, as are Na^+,K^+-adenosine triphosphatase (ATPase) molecules. These proteins enable specific substances in the lumen to be absorbed into the enterocyte. In addition to absorption through the various carrier mechanisms, some nutrients or ions can be absorbed through the tight junctions between epithelial cells.

The blood vessels that remove the products of digestion from the small intestine penetrate the muscularis to form a submucosal capillary network. From there, branches of the plexus penetrate the muscularis mucosae and lamina propria to supply the villi.

- At the tip of each villus is a capillary network that drains into veins of the submucosal plexus (Fig. 24.5). (These veins drain into the mesenteric veins, which in turn empty into the portal vein that carries blood to the liver.)
- Lymphatics (lymph vessels), which are important for the absorption of lipids, are also located in each villus. Lymphatics begin as blind-ended vessels within the villus. These vessels join and are known as lacteals.
  - Lacteals anastomose to form the lymphatic drainage of the intestine, which eventually drains into the thoracic duct. The thoracic duct empties into the systemic venous circulation at the left subclavian and brachiocephalic veins.

The Pancreas, Liver, and Gallbladder

The pancreas and liver are important secretory organs that empty their products into the duodenum.

The pancreas is both an exocrine organ, secreting substances out of the body and into the GI lumen, and an endocrine organ-secreting hormones into the body via the bloodstream. The exocrine pancreas is the portion that participates in digestion.

- Like the parotid gland, the exocrine pancreas is organized into acini, which are small groups of serous (protein-secreting) cells clustered around a secretory duct.
- Pancreatic acinar cells contain granules loaded with inactive digestive enzyme precursors called zymogens.

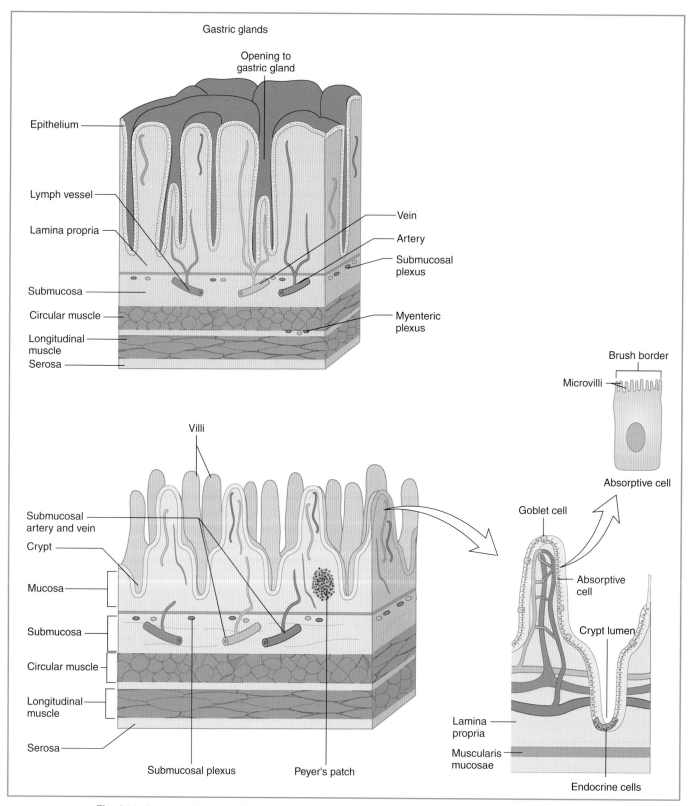

Fig. 24.4 Anatomy of the small intestine. The large surface area of the small intestine is imperative for absorption. (From Carroll R. *Elsevier's Integrated Physiology*. Philadelphia: Mosby Elsevier; 2007. Fig. 12.1B.)

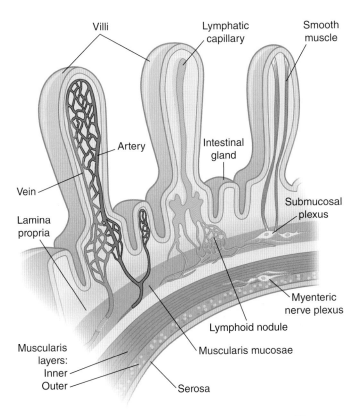

Fig. 24.5 Structure of the villi. Nutrients absorbed by the villi pass directly into the plasma through capillaries or into the lymphatic system, which empties its contents into the thoracic duct. The thoracic duct in turn empties into the subclavian vein.

- When stimulated, the acini dump their zymogens into the pancreatic duct, which empties into the ampulla of Vater.
- The ampulla in turn leads directly to the duodenum.

The liver also plays a key role in digestion, mainly through its production of *bile acids*, which are essential for the digestion of lipids.

- Once bile is produced, the gallbladder, a hollow pear-shaped organ on the undersurface of the liver, concentrates and stores it.
- Bile is collected from the liver into the common hepatic duct, which communicates with the gallbladder via the cystic duct. At the point where the cystic and hepatic ducts join, they are called the common bile duct.
- The common bile duct joins the pancreatic duct at the ampulla of Vater, which conducts bile and pancreatic secretions into the duodenum.
- Some of the other critical roles of the liver will be discussed in Chapter 26.

The Large Intestine

When all the foodstuffs that the body requires have been digested and absorbed, the remaining water, salt, and solids pass through the ileocecal valve into the large intestine (Fig. 24.6).

- The main function of the large intestine, also called the colon, is to absorb water and ions (Na^+, Cl^-) that escape absorption in the small intestine.

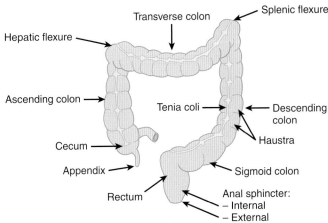

Fig. 24.6 Anatomy of the large intestine (colon). (From Carroll R. *Elsevier's Integrated Physiology.* Philadelphia: Mosby Elsevier; 2007. Fig. 12.6.)

- Once the process of absorption of salt and water is complete, feces are formed from dietary residua.

SYSTEM FUNCTION

A typical diet consists of carbohydrates, fats, and proteins, which are used to meet the maintenance, growth, and energy needs of the body. However, before the body is able to absorb and use what is ingested, these nutrients must first be broken down from macromolecules into their component building blocks. The process of breaking down ingested nutrients is called digestion.

- Polysaccharides and disaccharides are processed into monosaccharides.
- Triglycerides are digested into glycerol and fatty acids.
- Protein is digested into its component amino acids.
- Nucleic acids (deoxyribonucleic acid [DNA] and ribonucleic acid [RNA]) are degraded into their constituent bases, which in some cases are further modified.

Although different enzymes and different intestinal locations are involved in the digestion of the various classes of nutrients, one basic chemical process is used in the digestion of all the major types of food: hydrolysis.

The general formula for hydrolysis is as follows, where R represents an undefined organic group:

$$R'' - R' + H_2O \rightarrow R''OH + R'H$$

During this process, substrate-specific enzymes catalyze the addition of water to a macromolecule, leading to its breakdown. The chemical structure of macromolecules and the process of carbohydrate, protein, and lipid hydrolysis is shown in Fig. 24.7.

Digestion is followed by absorption, wherein nutrients are transferred from the intestinal lumen into the bloodstream for delivery to the periphery. There are several recurring absorptive mechanisms, including:

- Active transport: An energy-requiring process in which a substance is transported against its concentration gradient.
- Diffusion: A substance is transported along its concentration gradient, thus requiring no energy expenditure.

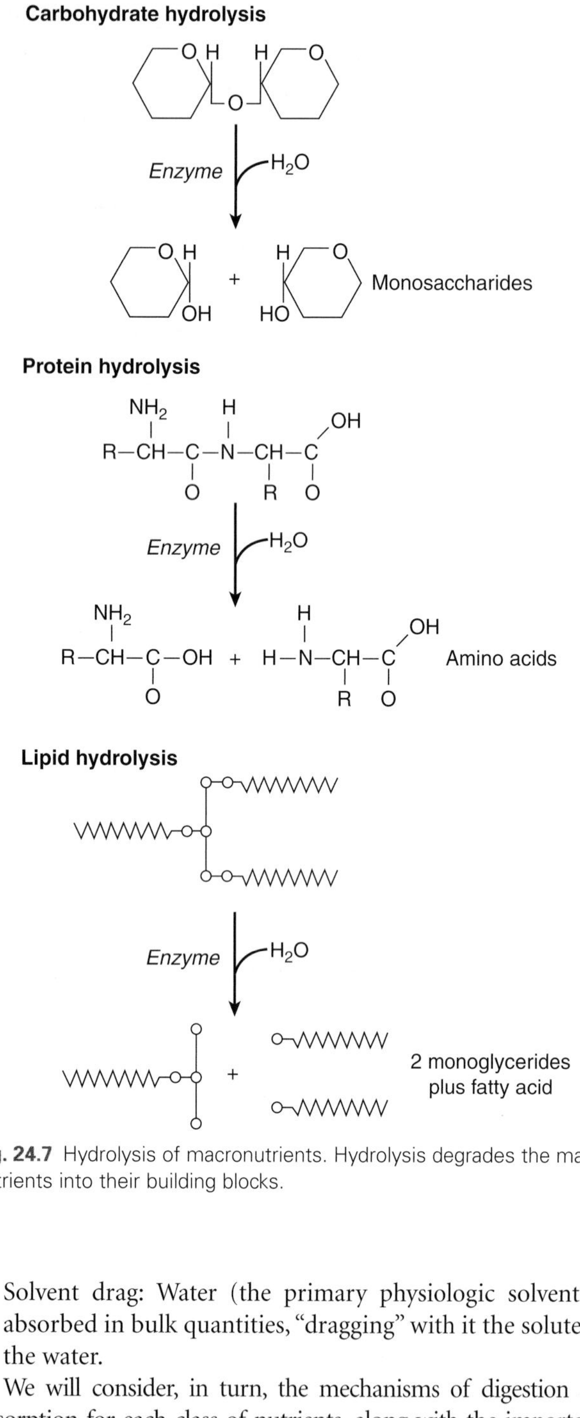

Carbohydrate hydrolysis

Protein hydrolysis

Lipid hydrolysis

Fig. 24.7 Hydrolysis of macronutrients. Hydrolysis degrades the macronutrients into their building blocks.

- Solvent drag: Water (the primary physiologic solvent) is absorbed in bulk quantities, "dragging" with it the solutes in the water.

We will consider, in turn, the mechanisms of digestion and absorption for each class of nutrients, along with the importance of nutrients to physiologic functioning and their sources in the diet.

Metabolism: The Reason We Eat

Metabolism encompasses the sum of all the energy transactions by which living tissues are produced and maintained. Metabolic processes are divided into two main categories:
- Anabolic reactions: The synthesis of macromolecules from building blocks, a process requiring energy
- Catabolic reactions: The breakdown of macromolecules into simpler substances, thereby releasing chemical energy which in turn fuels mechanical, heat, and electrical energy (see Fast Fact Box 24.3).

Fast Fact Box 24.3

Because the forms of energy are interchangeable, dietary energy is expressed in terms of heat—calories or kilocalories—even though most of that dietary chemical energy will be put to other uses. A **calorie** is defined as the amount of heat required to raise 1 g of water 1 °C in temperature. A **kilocalorie (kcal)** is defined as the amount of heat needed to raise 1 kg of water 1 °C in temperature.

All organisms store captured energy in various forms, such as starch (in plants) or glycogen and fat (in animals). If the diet does not provide enough calories to fuel metabolism, the body will catabolize these internal energy stores. When the internal energy stores are exhausted, metabolism will require catabolic breakdown of tissues that are not meant to store energy but nevertheless contain energy, such as the protein in muscle. Organic molecules yield energy in the following amounts:
- 1 g of protein yields 4 kcal
- 1 g of carbohydrate yields 4 kcal
- 1 g of fat yields 9 kcal
- 1 g of alcohol yields 7 kcal

Carbohydrates

Carbohydrates are a class of organic compounds made of carbon, hydrogen, and oxygen with hydrogen and oxygen present in the ratio of water (two atoms of hydrogen for each atom of oxygen).
- Carbohydrates are made from various species of monosaccharides, which often have six carbons and form a ring.
- Chains of monosaccharides are called polysaccharides.

Carbohydrates in the Diet

Carbohydrates are the major source of calories in a typical diet. Although oxidation of carbohydrates is the preferred mode of energy extraction, carbohydrates are not essential in the diet because they can be manufactured by the body.

Food often contains both digestible and nondigestible carbohydrates.
- The digestible dietary carbohydrates are starches, monosaccharides, and disaccharides (two monosaccharides linked together).
  - Starches are complex polysaccharides composed of long chains of glucose molecules linked by α-1,4 glycosidic bonds.
    The most abundant starch is amylopectin, a plant starch. Another dietary starch is glycogen, an animal starch.
  - The main monosaccharides in the diet are glucose and fructose, found in fruit, soft drinks, and processed foods.
  - Disaccharides include lactose (found in dairy products), maltose (found in beer), and sucrose (table sugar).
- Nondigestible carbohydrates, referred to collectively as dietary fiber, include cellulose, a β-1,4-linked glucose polymer.
- Cellulose is a major source of dietary fiber found in grasses and leaves.
- It is not digestible because the enzyme capable of hydrolyzing β-1,4 glucose linkages is not present in the human intestine.

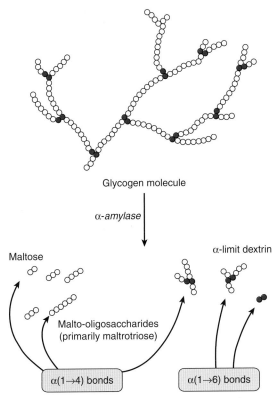

Fig. 24.8 Digestion of carbohydrates by α-amylase.

Carbohydrate Digestion

The digestion of carbohydrates is critical because the intestines can absorb only monosaccharides, such as glucose, galactose, and fructose.

Carbohydrate digestion begins in the mouth, where food is ground into smaller pieces by the action of the teeth and tongue.

- Salivary secretions contain salivary α-amylase, an enzyme that hydrolyzes α-1,4 glycosidic bonds (but not α-1,6 branchpoint linkages).
- Fig. 24.8 summarizes the digestion of carbohydrates by α-amylase. Before swallowing occurs, approximately 5% of dietary starch is digested.

Carbohydrate digestion continues in the stomach until salivary α-amylase is inactivated by the stomach's acidic environment.

- It is estimated that 30% to 40% of dietary starch is digested before food leaves the stomach.
- After leaving the stomach, the acidic and partially digested food and enzyme mixture called chyme enters the small intestine and mixes with pancreatic secretions containing pancreatic α-amylase, which is much more powerful than the salivary form.

Digestion to monosaccharides occurs in the duodenum and jejunum, which contain intestinal disaccharidases in the brush border of the epithelial membrane.

- The major brush border enzymes are α-dextrinase, maltase, sucrase, and lactase, which hydrolyze disaccharides to glucose, fructose, and galactose (Fig. 24.9).
- About 80% of ingested carbohydrates are digested to and absorbed as glucose.

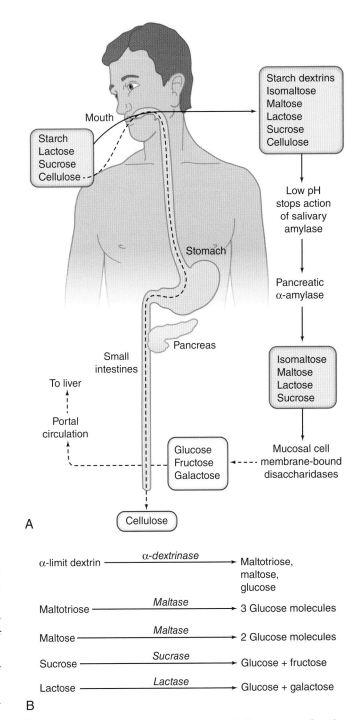

Fig. 24.9 Summary of carbohydrate digestion. **A,** Carbohydrate digestion at each location in the gastrointestinal tract. **B,** Hydrolytic reactions involved in carbohydrate digestion.

- Most carbohydrate absorption occurs in the upper small intestine (duodenum and upper jejunum).

Carbohydrate Absorption

The absorption of glucose and galactose occurs via a co-transport (or symport) mechanism linked to the absorption of sodium (Fig. 24.10).

- This is a form of secondary active transport. The process is considered "secondary" because the absorption of the

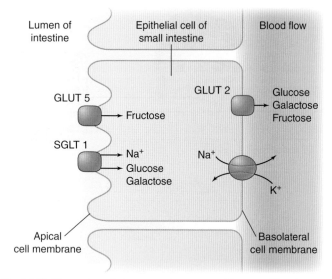

Fig. 24.10 Absorption of glucose, galactose, and fructose. The absorption of glucose and galactose but not fructose is sodium-coupled. *GLUT,* Glucose transporter; *SGLT,* sodium glucose transporter.

sugars is dependent on a sodium gradient established by the Na^+,K^+ pump, rather than adenosine triphosphate (ATP) directly.

- The process is considered "active" because ATP is required to fuel the pump that generates the Na^+ gradient.

The absorption of sodium can be thought of as occurring in two stages.

- In the first stage, an electrochemical gradient favoring absorption must be established before apical sodium can be absorbed. This is accomplished through the active transport of sodium from the enterocyte cytoplasm through the basolateral membrane and into interstitial fluid and the paracellular spaces by Na^+,K^+-ATPase molecules located in the basolateral membrane of the enterocyte.
- The second stage of intestinal glucose or galactose absorption involves the absorption of sodium from the lumen via facilitated diffusion. A carrier protein, the Na^+/glucose cotransporter (SGLT1), aids in ferrying both glucose (or galactose) and sodium into the cell. Sodium travels in a direction along its concentration gradient and provides the energy necessary to transport the sugar molecule in a direction opposite to its gradient.

If glucose is highly concentrated in the intestinal lumen, absorption can also occur via a solvent drag mechanism in addition to the Na^+-cotransport process.

- As glucose is absorbed by Na^+-cotransport, its concentration grows in the paracellular space.
- This increases the osmotic pressure in the paracellular space, which causes water to move from the intestinal lumen into the paracellular space. This movement of water occurs directly through intercellular junctions, bypassing the interior of the enterocyte.
- As fluid moves, glucose is "dragged" along with it (see Clinical Correlation Box 24.1).

Proteins

Proteins are composed of just a small number of subunits called amino acids linked by peptide bonds.

- With different linear combinations and permutations of amino acids, different protein structures and functions are possible.
- Although there are several hundred naturally occurring amino acids, mammals possess just 20.

Proteins in the Diet

The continuous breakdown of proteinaceous tissue in the body necessitates a fresh supply of amino acids to rebuild those tissues. This supply must come from the diet, because although amino acids can be metabolized to carbohydrates and fat, the reverse is not true.

There are nine essential amino acids that cannot be synthesized by the body and must be consumed directly. The remaining 11 are the nonessential amino acids.

- The bodily demand for nitrogen and essential amino acids necessitates an average protein intake of 1 g/kg of body weight per day.
- Anabolic states of growth (e.g., puberty, pregnancy, or wound healing) demand increased protein consumption.

Major sources of protein in the diet include meat, fish, eggs, dairy, and vegetables.

Protein Digestion

The digestion of protein begins in the stomach. Chief cells in the stomach secrete *pepsinogen*, which is converted to the active enzyme pepsin by gastric hydrochloric acid (HCl).

- HCl is secreted by parietal cells in the stomach by an H^+/K^+-ATPase pump.

- The optimum pH for pepsin is between 1 and 3 and when the pH rises to greater than 5, pepsin is denatured.
- Consequently, pepsin is active in the stomach but inactivated in the duodenum where the pH is higher.

Acidity in the stomach primarily serves to activate pepsin, but also serves as protection against microbial pathogens in food. Many bacteria cannot survive the acidity of the stomach. (See Clinical Correlation Box 24.2.)

Clinical Correlation Box 24.2

What is Peptic Ulcer Disease?

A 35-year-old man complains of "stomach pain" of several months' duration. The pain is described as a nagging ache or a burning sensation below the sternum. It is transiently relieved by taking Tums (a calcium carbonate antacid). The gastroenterologist performs an endoscopy with biopsy of the gastric and duodenal mucosa. The pathology reveals gastric metaplasia, ulceration of the duodenal epithelium, and colonization with the bacterium *Helicobacter pylori*. The diagnosis is peptic ulcer disease.

Peptic ulcer disease (PUD) affects 4 million Americans and costs the U.S. economy $20 billion annually. It can affect the gastric mucosa or the duodenal mucosa. In the United States, duodenal ulcers are more common, but in Japan, the reverse is true. Peptic ulcers represent breakdowns in the intestinal epithelium that result from excess secretion of acid and a failure of the barriers that normally protect the mucosa from acid injury.

Two major causes of weakened mucosal defenses against acid are infection with *H. pylori* and the use of nonsteroidal antiinflammatory drugs (NSAIDs). *H. pylori* is a bacterium that is adapted to life at low pH, such as in the human stomach. (It survives by hydrolyzing urea into ammonia to buffer the acidity.) Its presence causes inflammation that breaks down the protective mucosal barrier in the stomach. Injury to the duodenal wall (by acid hypersecretion) results in transformation of the duodenal epithelium into gastric mucosa (gastric metaplasia). This allows *H. pylori*, which is trophic for gastric tissue, to colonize the duodenum, worsening the duodenal injury.

NSAIDs interfere with prostaglandin-mediated defense mechanisms against gastric acidity: mucus production, bicarbonate secretion, and others. The most serious complications of PUD are hemorrhage and perforation of the digestive tract.

There are several different kinds of proteases (enzymes that break down proteins).
- Pepsin is an endopeptidase, meaning it can cleave peptide bonds in the middle of (endo-, inside of) a peptide polymer.
- Carboxypeptidases (C-terminal) and aminopeptidases (N-terminal) are enzymes that can cleave only a terminal peptide bond (i.e., one at the end of a polypeptide polymer)
- The actions of these enzymes are illustrated by the following equations, where A represents an amino acid with its amino terminus on the left:

$$A-A-A-A-A \xrightarrow{\text{endopeptidase}} A-A+A-A-A$$

$$A-A-A-A-A \xrightarrow{\text{aminopeptidase}} A+A-A-A-A$$

$$A-A-A-A-A \xrightarrow{\text{carboxypeptidase}} A-A-A-A+A$$

Approximately, 10% to 20% of total protein is digested in the stomach by pepsin. Most protein digestion occurs in the duodenum and jejunum, catalyzed by proteases secreted by the exocrine pancreas.
- The pancreas secretes the inactive zymogens (proenzymes) trypsinogen, chymotrypsinogen, procarboxypeptidases A and B, and proelastase into the pancreatic duct.
  - These forms are activated when they enter the intestine, where the duodenum and jejunum secrete the enzyme enterokinase.
  - Enterokinase converts trypsinogen to trypsin.
  - Trypsin then activates the other zymogens, as well as other molecules of trypsinogen.

The combined actions of the pancreas and small bowel break the polypeptides into shorter chains. Digestion continues in the small intestine with the action of peptidases on the brush border. These enzymes cleave the peptide fragments into smaller and smaller bits until they are single amino acids, dipeptides, and tripeptides.

The steps in protein digestion are summarized in Fig. 24.11.

Protein Absorption

In contrast with carbohydrates, which can be absorbed only as monosaccharides, proteins can be absorbed as amino acids,

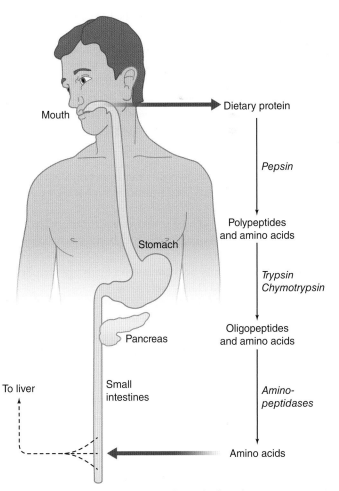

Fig. 24.11 Summary of protein digestion.

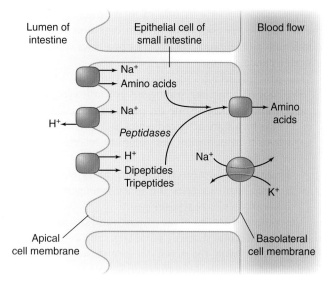

Fig. 24.12 Absorption of amino acids, dipeptides, and tripeptides. Sodium-dependent active transport facilitates the absorption of these molecules.

dipeptides, and tripeptides. This absorption occurs through a sodium-dependent secondary active transport mechanism analogous to the cotransport for glucose and galactose (Fig. 24.12).

- Na$^+$,K$^+$-ATPase pumps located in the basolateral membrane of enterocytes lower the intracellular concentration of sodium by transporting sodium into the paracellular spaces. This mechanism establishes a gradient favoring the transport of sodium from the intestinal lumen into the enterocytes.
- Carrier proteins (specific for neutral, acidic, basic, or imino amino acids) bind both sodium and a peptide or amino acid to cotransport them into the enterocyte.

Lipids

Lipids are hydrophobic molecules that generally contain fatty acids, which are straight-chain hydrocarbons having a carboxyl group at one end.

- A prevalent variety of lipid is triglyceride (or triacylglycerol), which is composed of a glycerol backbone attached to three fatty acid subunits.
- Other forms of fatty acid-containing lipids are glycolipids, phospholipids, and cholesterol esters.
- Fatty acids may also be present alone and as such are called free fatty acids.

Fatty acids are classified according to their size (short-, medium-, or long-chain) and according to the number of double bonds between carbons:

- Saturated: If the fatty acid has no double bonds
  - "Saturated" with hydrogens, because single bonds between carbon and hydrogen replace double bonds between carbons.
- Unsaturated: If the fatty acid contains one or more double bonds
  - If one double bond, then monounsaturated.
  - If more than one double bond, polyunsaturated.

Lipids, the major constituent of all cell membranes, are found in association with carbohydrates and proteins. Lipids are also stored in adipose tissue, where they act as an energy reserve for metabolism and as a thyroid-stimulated source of body heat. Dietary lipids are also important for the absorption of the fat-soluble vitamins A, D, E, and K.

Lipids in the Diet

About 98% of total dietary lipid is made up of triglycerides.

If triglycerides contain highly saturated fatty acids, they are called saturated fats.

- These fats contribute to cardiovascular risk by raising serum low-density lipoprotein (LDL) levels in both animals and humans.
- High levels of LDL are associated with atherosclerosis (fat deposition in arterial walls).

Triglycerides containing unsaturated fatty acids are called unsaturated fats.

A low-fat and low-cholesterol diet has been traditionally viewed as a way to lose weight and prevent cardiovascular disease. However, recent research shows that the type of fat that is consumed increases the risk for certain disease much more than the amount of fat in the diet.

- Saturated and trans fats (unsaturated fats with a trans-isomer fatty acid configuration) have been consistently shown to increase the risk of cardiovascular disease and consequently, the use of trans fats has been banned in many countries.
- On the other hand, monounsaturated and polyunsaturated fats have the opposite effect and are beneficial for the heart.
- Furthermore, the mix of fats in the diet has a greater influence on cholesterol in the bloodstream than does the amount of cholesterol consumed.

Unsaturated fats are found in olive and canola oil; almonds, hazelnuts, walnuts, and pecans; avocados; pumpkin, sesame, chia, and flax seeds; and fish. Saturated fats are found in cheese, pizza, whole milk, butter, meats (hamburgers, sausage, bacon, beef), ice cream, and many desserts.

Recent studies also show that consumption of omega-3 (polyunsaturated) fatty acids is associated with many health benefits, including protection against cardiovascular disease. The main types of omega-3 fatty acids in the diet are:

- Alpha-linolenic acid (ALA; found in vegetable oil and walnuts)
- Eicosapentaenoic acid (EPA, found in fatty fish, such as salmon)
- Docosahexaenoic acid (DHA, found in fatty fish, such as salmon)

Lipid Digestion

The digestion of lipids is complicated by the fact that lipids are insoluble in water, whereas the enzymes necessary for lipid digestion are water soluble. Therefore lipids and their breakdown products are emulsified in the GI tract.

Emulsification is a process whereby a water-insoluble oil is finely divided and mixed with water, sometimes with the help of an amphipathic substance, a substance that has both hydrophobic and hydrophilic properties—in other words, it possesses affinities for both oil and water. In the GI tract, emulsification increases the contact area of fat with water, thus increasing the size of the water-oil interface at which digestive enzymes act.

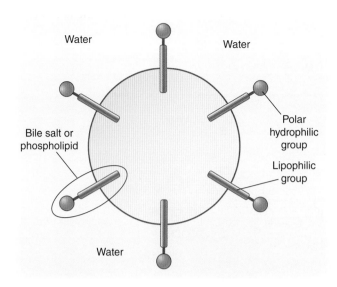

Fig. 24.13 Emulsification of fats in the small intestine. Emulsion droplets form when lipids first mix with bile. Pancreatic digestion follows.

Lipid digestion begins with the secretion of gastric lipase in the stomach.

- Lipase hydrolyzes and cleaves lipid bonds.
- The stomach also plays an important role in emulsification by mechanically agitating the food. This breaks fat into smaller globules, increasing the surface area for digestion. Lipids then pass from the stomach into the small intestine.
- Bile, produced in the liver and stored in the gallbladder, is secreted into the duodenum and acts as an emulsifier as it is composed of amphipathic substances—cholesterol-based bile salts and the phospholipid lecithin.
- The fat-soluble components of bile dissolve into the fat globules, whereas the hydrophilic components project outward into the surrounding water (Fig. 24.13).
- This increases the solubility of the lipids and lowers the surface tension of the fat globule. With lower surface tension and increased solubility, fragmentation into smaller emulsion droplets is possible.

Once the lipids have been emulsified, they are subject to the action of the powerful pancreatic enzymes that have been secreted into the duodenum. As the lipids in the emulsion droplet are cleaved, the products of cleavage drift away and fresh dietary lipids from within the hydrophobic core of the emulsion droplet rise to the surface, where they too are cleaved. Once inside the enterocytes, the cytoplasmic enzyme enteric lipase makes a small contribution to lipid digestion (Fig. 24.14).

Lipid Absorption

The process of lipid absorption begins when lipid cleavage products are released from the emulsion droplets. At this point, the cleavage products are organized into smaller emulsion droplets called micelles by the amphipathic bile salts (Fig. 24.15).

- The cholesterol portions of the bile salt molecules aggregate in the center of the micelle along with the products of lipid digestion and fat-soluble vitamins, as in the emulsion droplet.

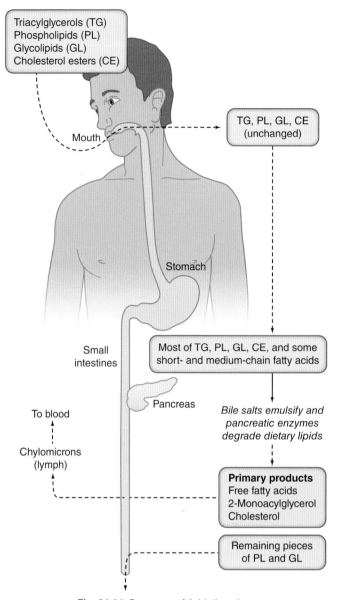

Fig. 24.14 Summary of lipid digestion.

- The outer surface of the micelle is covered with the polar groups of the bile salts, making the micelle water-soluble so it can interact with the enterocytes' brush border.
- After contacting the brush border, the lipid metabolism products diffuse freely from the micelle through the enterocytes' luminal plasma membrane and into the interior of the cells.
- Meanwhile, the bile salts of the emptied micelle return to the intestinal lumen to form new micelles loaded with fresh cleavage products. A critical mass of bile salts is necessary for micelle formation (see Clinical Correlation Box 24.3).

Clinical Correlation Box 24.3

Impairments in the production, delivery, or activity of bile salts result in impaired fat absorption and the excretion of excess fat in the stool (steatorrhea).

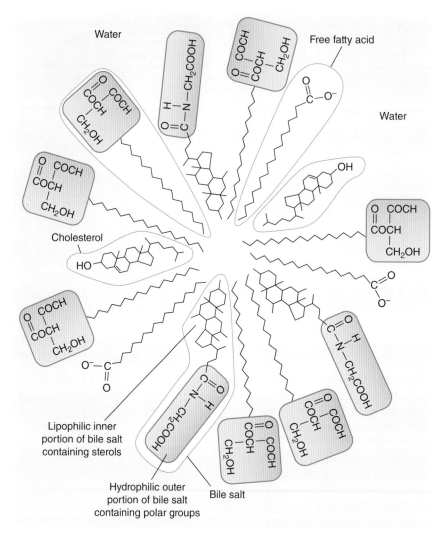

Fig. 24.15 Role of micelles. Micelles emulsify the products of pancreatic digestion and deliver them to enterocytes for absorption.

The rate-limiting step in the absorption of lipids is the diffusion of micelles through the unstirred layer, the fluid immediately surrounding the brush border (Fig. 24.16).

• This fluid does not mix readily with the rest of the lumen contents.

• However, a concentration gradient favors the passive diffusion of the lipid digestion products across the unstirred layer, toward the brush border, and into enterocytes.

A pH gradient also exists across the unstirred layer:

• The side closest to the brush border has a lower pH.

• This favors the protonation of free fatty acids, which enhances their rate of diffusion into the intestinal cells.

Once inside the enterocyte, the products of lipid digestion are transported to the smooth endoplasmic reticulum (ER), where they are reconstituted into their original forms by a series of reesterification reactions (Fig. 24.17).

• These reactions reattach the fatty acids that were cleaved in the emulsion droplets.

• Free fatty acids and 2-monoglycerides are reesterified to form new triglycerides.

• Lysophospholipid molecules and free fatty acids are reesterified into new phospholipid molecules.

• Free cholesterol molecules and free fatty acids are reesterified to form new cholesterol esters.

• In addition, after being absorbed, some of the 2-monoglyceride molecules are digested into glycerol and free fatty acids by intracellular lipases. Inside the ER, these free fatty acid molecules are also reconstituted into new triglycerides.

After the process of reesterification is complete, the new lipid particles aggregate in the Golgi apparatus and are processed to form lipoprotein spheres called chylomicrons.

• The chylomicron core contains cholesterol esters, triglycerides, and the hydrophobic fatty portions of the phospholipids.

• The chylomicron surface bears apoproteins, which serve as ligands that bind to specific receptors in other parts of the body and activate enzymes. In so doing, the chylomicron

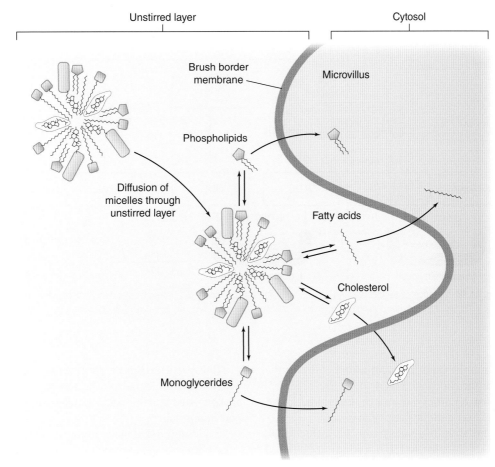

Fig. 24.16 Absorption of lipid cleavage products by enterocytes.

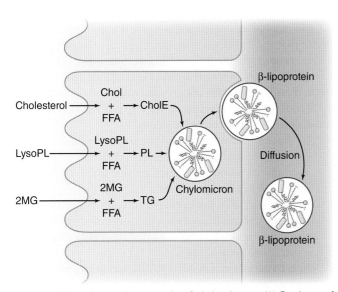

Fig. 24.17 Formation and exocytosis of chylomicrons. (1) Products of lipid digestion are reconstituted by reesterification, the reattachment of fatty acids. (2) The reconstituted fats are organized into chylomicrons. (3) Apoproteins are attached to the chylomicrons to allow exocytosis and entry into the lymphatic system.

apoproteins mediate the transfer of fats from one location to another.

The apoprotein *apoB-48* mediates the egress of chylomicrons from the enterocyte.

- *ApoB-48* attaches to sites on the basolateral enterocyte cell membrane, causing exocytosis of chylomicrons from the basolateral membrane.
- Chylomicrons are too large to enter capillaries. However, they can enter the lymphatics, whose endothelial cells are more widely spaced than those of capillaries.
- The chylomicrons then pass through the lymphatics to the thoracic duct and into the bloodstream via the left subclavian vein.

The vast majority of ingested lipid is absorbed in the form of chylomicrons.

Lipid Transport in the Blood

There are two lipid transport systems in the blood (Fig. 24.18), which both use lipoproteins as shuttles for the transport for fat.

- Exogenous system: processes lipids absorbed in the diet.
  - The lipoprotein shuttle for exogenous fat is the chylomicron, whose delivery of fat to the tissues is guided by

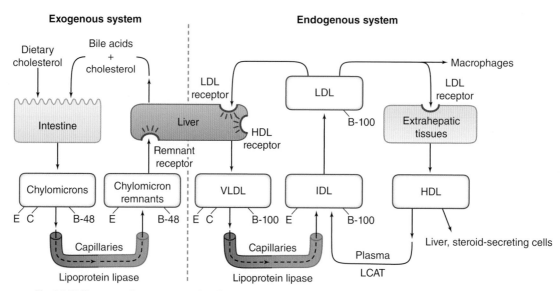

Fig. 24.18 Transport of exogenous and endogenous lipids in the blood. *IDL,* intermediate density lipoprotein; *LCAT,* lecithin:cholesterol acyltransferace; *LDL,* low-density lipoprotein; *VLDL,* very low-density lipoprotein.

interactions with the capillary endothelium and with the lipoproteins of the endogenous system.

- Endogenous system: shuttles fats and cholesterol back and forth between the liver and the peripheral tissues.
  - Lipoproteins for shuttling endogenous fat include LDL and high-density lipoprotein (HDL), which are released into the bloodstream by the liver and intestinal tissues.

The processing of exogenous fat begins with the action of lipoprotein lipase upon the chylomicron.

- Lipoprotein lipase is an enzyme found on the capillary walls of most tissues (but predominantly cardiac and skeletal muscle) and is activated by the apoprotein *apoCII* on the surface of the chylomicron.
- The capillary enzyme hydrolyzes triglycerides to monoglyceride, glycerol, and fatty acids.
- These digestion products are free to enter cells of the surrounding tissue.
- As the chylomicron circulates, more and more triglyceride is progressively removed, and thus the particle decreases in size and increases in density.
- The resulting *chylomicron remnant* is then removed from circulation by the liver (see Fig. 24.19).
- Inside the liver, the apoproteins, cholesterol esters, and other components are degraded to amino acids, free cholesterol, and fatty acids.

Endogenous fat that is stored in the liver and transported from the liver to other tissues by very-low-density lipoprotein (VLDL).

- Like chylomicrons, VLDLs bear apoCII and activate lipoprotein lipase, hydrolyzing triglycerides in their core to glycerol and fatty acids, which can then enter nearby cells.
- VLDL, which grows denser and changes from VLDL to LDL as it unloads fat, is much richer in cholesterol esters than chylomicrons and receives added cholesterol esters from HDL.

HDL particles shuttle cholesterol esters back to the liver, where they are degraded. The resulting cholesterol molecules are converted into bile acids, secreted into bile, or packaged into new lipoproteins.

- In addition, HDL plays an important role in the regulation of both endogenous and exogenous systems for lipid transport. It does so by delivering apoproteins to other lipoproteins and mediating the uptake and esterification of free cholesterol.
- Low levels of HDL and high levels of LDL both contribute to the risk of developing atherosclerosis.

Nucleic Acids

Nucleic acids—DNA and RNA—are composed of polymers of nucleotides bound together through phosphodiester linkages. Recall that nucleotides are molecules made of a pentose ring, a nitrogenous purine or pyrimidine base, and a group of phosphate esters. Since all animals and plants have DNA and RNA, these nucleic acids are present in all food.

Accordingly, the digestive tract has evolved the ability to break down and absorb nucleic acids.

- The digestion of nucleic acids begins in the small intestine, where pancreatic ribonucleases and deoxyribonucleases in pancreatic secretions hydrolyze phosphodiester bonds that link the nucleotides in a chain.
- The resulting oligonucleotides are further hydrolyzed by pancreatic phosphordiesterases to form a mixture of absorbable mononucleotides with a phosphate at either the 3′ or 5′ carbon of the pentose ring.
- These molecules can be further digested to free bases before absorption.
- Purine bases can also be converted to uric acid by enzymes found in the intestinal mucosa.
- The 3′ and 5′ mononucleotides and free bases are absorbed in the intestine through active transport.

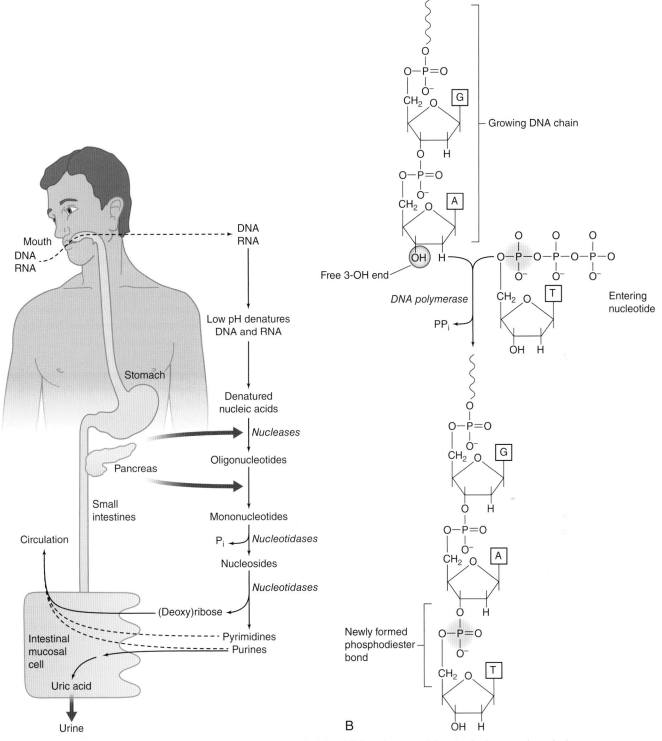

Fig. 24.19 Summary of nucleic acid digestion. **A,** Nucleic acid digestion at each location in the gastrointestinal tract. **B,** The structure of a nucleotide chain. The chain elongates when a phosphodiester forms between the free hydroxyl group of the nucleotide at the 3' end of the chain and the phosphate at the 5' end of the entering nucleotide. This bond is broken during digestion by various ribonucleases and deoxyribonucleases.

- In addition, uric acid is absorbed by enterocytes and excreted from the body in urine.
  Fig. 24.19 summarizes nucleic acid digestion and absorption.

Water and Electrolytes

The large intestine is the site of net water intake by the GI tract. Water absorption in the small intestine and colon is driven by solute absorption. In other words, the transport of electrolytes from the lumen into the blood results in an osmotic gradient, and water flows passively from the intestinal lumen into the bloodstream (see Fast Fact 24.4).

Fast Fact Box 24.4

Nearly 9 L of water passes through the digestive tract each day. Approximately 2 L of this fluid is ingested, and 7 L of water is contained in gastrointestinal secretions: 1500 mL in saliva, 2500 mL in gastric secretions, 500 mL in bile, 1500 mL in pancreatic secretions, and 1000 mL in intestinal secretions. The small intestine absorbs an amount roughly equal to that secreted (7 L), leaving 2 L to enter the large intestine (colon), which absorbs all but around 100 to 200 mL.

The reasons behind the body's need for a net absorption of 2 L of water per day lie in the governance of the osmolality (solute concentration) of the extracellular fluid volume (see Ch. 19).

- At least 1 L water is lost each day through evaporation from the skin and respiratory epithelium.
- About 500 L of water without salt is lost each day because of the excretion of nitrogenous wastes.
- This "free water" must be replaced by drinking. Otherwise, the plasma osmolality will rise, with adverse consequences for the brain and other body tissues.

Water Absorption

Water can be absorbed through one of two pathways:
- Cellular route: Through the plasma membrane.
- Paracellular route: Through tight junctions between intestinal epithelial cells.
  The principal mechanism for water absorption is via diffusion:
- The direction of the flow of water is determined by the concentration of solutes in the intestinal lumen versus that in the bloodstream.
- The chyme that is delivered into the duodenum from the stomach is hypertonic. Thus the net direction of water flow in the duodenum is from the blood into the lumen (secretion).
- As solutes are absorbed, however, the tonicity of chyme decreases. This causes a reversal in the direction of water flow, that is, net water absorption occurs in the remainder of the small intestine.
- In the colon, water follows the active absorption of sodium.

Sodium Absorption

Sodium is quantitatively the major cation present in the extracellular fluid, creating the osmotic pressure that holds water inside the extracellular space consisting of interstitial and plasma volume.

Sodium transport can occur by a variety of mechanisms.
- Active transport
  - The absorption of sodium in the small intestine occurs via the basolateral Na^+,K^+-ATPase in enterocytes pumps sodium across the basolateral membrane and into the interstitial fluid and the paracellular spaces.
  - Na^+ then diffuses down its concentration gradient into the cell.
  - It crosses the apical cell membrane through a variety of secondary active transporters, including SGLT1, Na^+-coupled amino acid transport, and Na^+/H^+ exchange.
- Sodium-solute symporters
  - High luminal concentrations of glucose and peptides drive sodium absorption by creating a gradient favorable to the functioning of the sodium-solute symporters.
  - Thus diffusion of glucose or amino acids into the enterocytes coupled to Na^+ can drive Na^+ absorption, in addition to the other way around.
  - In the ileum, the rate of sodium absorption decreases because the concentrations of sugars and amino acids are lower than in more proximal portions of the small intestine (see Clinical Correlation Box 24.4).

Clinical Correlation Box 24.4

Oral Rehydration Therapy

Some intestinal infections and the toxins they produce interfere with the active transport of sodium from the intestinal lumen and promote the secretion of chloride. This not only lessens the gradient for water absorption in the gastrointestinal tract, but also can cause the passive secretion of water from the blood into the intestinal lumen. With salt trapped in the intestines, the lumen solute concentration can exceed that of plasma, causing water to diffuse into the lumen. Diarrhea results. Drinking more water does not help, because without salt absorption there is no way for the water to enter the plasma. The water remains in the intestinal lumen, and the diarrhea intensifies. The ingestion of salty water exacerbates the problem. Without the capacity to absorb salt, the gradient for the secretion of water into the intestinal lumen is even worse.

Oral rehydration therapy, an important treatment for diarrhea, uses a different strategy to restore water absorption in the intestine. It makes use of glucose/sodium coupling in the small intestine. With oral administration of a solution with a high glucose concentration and some salt content (e.g., 20 g glucose and 3.5 g sodium chloride in 1 L of water), glucose may diffuse across the glucose/sodium symporter, bringing sodium along with it from intestinal lumen to the blood. This movement of solutes is followed by the diffusion of water into the bloodstream.

The importance of oral rehydration cannot be overstated, given that diarrhea with dehydration is the second greatest cause of infant mortality in the world and given that access to intravenous hydration is limited in most afflicted areas.

- Epithelial Na^+ channel (ENaC)
  - Found in the colon, as well as the renal collecting duct, action increased by the adrenal hormone aldosterone which is governed by the renin-angiotensin-aldosterone system.

Chloride and Bicarbonate Absorption and Secretion

The absorption of chloride is linked to that of Na^+.
- The absorption of sodium ions in the duodenum and jejunum creates a slightly electronegative potential in the intestinal

lumen, driving Cl⁻ across the lumen and into plasma. Most of the absorption of Cl⁻ ions is by passive diffusion via a paracellular route in accordance with this electrical gradient.

- In the ileum and colon, the main means of Cl⁻ absorption is by Cl⁻/HCO₃⁻ exchange.

Net Cl⁻ absorption also depends on how much Cl⁻ is secreted in pancreatic and other digestive fluids.

- The primary mechanism for Cl⁻ secretion in intestinal epithelia is the colonic apical membrane Cl⁻ conductance, mediated by the cystic fibrosis transmembrane conductance regulator (CFTR). CFTR is stimulated by cyclic nucleotides, in particular cyclic adenosine monophosphate and protein kinase A (basolateral adenyl cyclase receptor) and cyclic guanosine monophosphate (apical guanylate cyclase receptor).
- The basolateral Na⁺/K⁺/2Cl⁻ (NKCC) transporter allows Cl⁻ to enter the cell from extracellular fluid, driven by the inwardly directed Na⁺ gradient via the Na⁺,K⁺-ATPase.
- These steps provide the intracellular Cl⁻ and the intracellular negativity needed for a functioning CFTR to secrete Cl⁻ into the lumen (see Clinical Correlation Box 24.5).

Clinical Correlation Box 24.5

This pathway is important not only in cystic fibrosis, a disease characterized by abnormally low Cl⁻ secretions in various tissues, but also in many common diarrheal diseases.

- A mechanism by which cholera causes severe diarrhea is by activation of the alpha subunit of the G protein, Gₛ, resulting in increased cyclic adenosine monophosphate (cAMP). This results in increased Cl- secretion in the gut along with water efflux.
- Many common toxins associated with *Escherichia coli* overactivate either cAMP, which results in a mechanism similar to that of cholera toxin, or cyclic guanosine monophosphate, which results in decreased reabsorption of NaCl and water in the gut.
- *Clostridium difficile*, the cause of a common diarrheal disease in hospitalized patients, appears to increase intracellular Ca²⁺.

The transport of bicarbonate ions (HCO₃⁻) varies according to location in the GI tract.

- In the duodenum, HCO₃⁻ is secreted mainly through pancreatic and biliary fluids.
- In the jejunum, however, a large amount of luminal HCO₃⁻ is absorbed. This occurs mainly through the combination of luminal H⁺ and HCO₃⁻ to form carbonic acid (H₂CO₃⁻) (Fig. 24.20).
  - The carbonic acid dissociates to form H₂O and carbon dioxide (CO₂).
  - The CO₂ then diffuses through the apical cell membrane and dissociates into HCO₃⁻, which is then absorbed.
- In the ileum and colon, HCO₃⁻ is secreted into the lumen via Cl⁻/HCO₃⁻ exchange.

Potassium Absorption and Secretion

The absorption of potassium ions occurs by passive diffusion in the small intestine.

- As water is absorbed from the intestinal lumen, the concentration of luminal K⁺ increases.

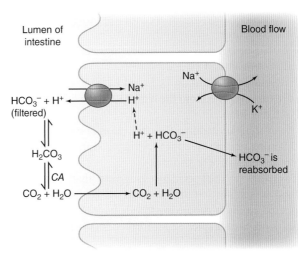

Fig. 24.20 Bicarbonate absorption in the jejunum.

- This increase establishes a driving force favoring the absorption of K⁺ through a paracellular route.

In the large intestine, K⁺ can be absorbed or secreted depending on the luminal concentration.

- When the luminal concentration is less than 25 mM, net secretion occurs; when luminal concentration is greater than 25 mM, net absorption occurs.
- A colonic H⁺/K⁺-ATPase, similar to the transporter in the renal collecting duct, is a mechanism that allows for K⁺ absorption, and may be increased by potassium depletion.
- The secretion of K⁺ is regulated by aldosterone, as it is in the distal nephron (see Environment Box 24.1).

🏠 ENVIRONMENT BOX 24.1

When malnourished individuals are given nutrition, there is a danger of precipitating refeeding syndrome. This occurs when patients who have depleted phosphate stores are abruptly given glucose or carbohydrates. This induces the release of insulin, which in turn promotes cellular uptake of extracellular phosphate, magnesium, and potassium, resulting in hypophosphatemia, hypomagnesemia, and hypokalemia. Patients may develop acute hemolysis, rhabdomyolysis (muscle cell lysis), congestive heart failure, peripheral edema, and seizures. If not treated, it can be fatal.

Vitamins and Minerals

Vitamins and minerals are micronutrients, constituents of the body tissues that make up a smaller percentage of the body weight than macronutrients (fats, proteins, and carbohydrates).

- Vitamins are organic compounds essential for many metabolic reactions in the body.
  - Unlike macronutrients, they do not yield energy; instead, most vitamins serve as coenzymes.
  - Coenzymes are separate molecules integrated into the structure of enzymes and necessary for enzymatic function.
- Minerals are inorganic elements, and like vitamins they do not furnish energy.
  - With a few exceptions—vitamin D, vitamin K, and biotin—humans cannot synthesize vitamins and minerals; we acquire them in the diet.

Vitamin D is synthesized from its precursor in human skin.

Vitamin K and biotin are produced by symbiotic microorganisms living in the intestines.

Vitamins are classified as fat-soluble or water-soluble. Table 24.1 lists the essential vitamins and minerals.

- Fat-soluble vitamins: A, D, E, and K, are present in micelles. They are absorbed into the lymph with the other products of lipid digestion.
- Water-soluble vitamins: The absorption of most water-soluble vitamins occurs by either facilitated diffusion or sodium-dependent active transport.

Growing research evidence suggests that vitamin D in particular is important for bone and muscle health and that an estimated 1 billion people worldwide have inadequate levels in their blood. See Chapter 32 for further detail on vitamin D and its effects on the body.

TABLE 24.1 Vitamins and Minerals

Vitamins

Fat-Soluble Vitamins	Water-Soluble Vitamins
A (retinol, carotenes)	C (ascorbic acid)
D (cholecalciferol)	B_1 (thiamine)
E (tocopherols)	B_2 (riboflavin)
K (phylloquinones, menaquinone, menadione)	B_3 (niacin)
	B_5 (pantothenic acid)
	B_6 (pyridoxine)
	B_{12} (cobalamin)
	Folate (folic acid)
	Biotin

Minerals

Macrominerals (>0.005% body weight)	Microminerals (<0.005% body weight)
Sodium	Chromium
Chloride	Cobalt
Calcium	Copper
Phosphate	Fluoride
Potassium	Iodine
Magnesium	Iron
Sulfur	Manganese
	Molybdenum
	Selenium
	Zinc
	Arsenic[a]
	Boron[a]
	Cadmium[a]
	Lithium[a]
	Nickel[a]
	Silicone[a]
	Tin[a]
	Vanadium[a]

[a]Physiologic role has not been established.

Vitamin B_{12} Absorption

The absorption of vitamin B_{12} (cobalamin) is unique in that it occurs in two phases and requires the presence of a cofactor known as intrinsic factor (IF). Without IF, only 1% to 2% of the ingested amount of vitamin B_{12} is absorbed. Most of the ingested B_{12} is bound to proteins.

- In the first phase of absorption, the gastric phase, the low pH of the stomach and the presence of pepsin cause the release of B_{12} from these proteins.
  - At this point, vitamin B_{12} binds to glycoproteins from the saliva and gastric secretions known as R proteins.
  - In the stomach, IF is secreted by parietal cells. IF binds to vitamin B with less affinity than the R proteins.
- In the second phase of vitamin B_{12} absorption, the intestinal phase, the B_{12} complexes are released into the duodenum where they are digested by pancreatic proteases.
  - Vitamin B_{12} is then transferred to IF, and IF/B_{12} complexes are resistant to proteases.
  - The absorption of vitamin B_{12} occurs in the terminal ileum, which contains receptors for IF/B_{12} complexes.

After binding of the complexes to the receptors, the vitamin B12 is absorbed, exits the basolateral membrane, and enters the portal bloodstream.

- Within the portal system, vitamin B_{12} binds to *transcobalamin II*, a protein synthesized by the liver and intestinal epithelium.
- Transcobalamin II/B_{12} complexes are then taken into hepatocytes via receptor-mediated endocytosis (see Clinical Correlation Box 24.6).

Clinical Correlation Box 24.6

Vitamin B_{12} is required for the normal development of red blood cells. Without B_{12}, pernicious anemia results. Apart from anemia, neurologic abnormalities and dementia are part of the clinical syndrome of B_{12} deficiency. Pernicious anemia can be caused by:

- insufficient B_{12}, as in gastrectomy, gastric atrophy, and in the presence of antibodies to intrinsic factor
- the lack of pancreatic enzymes to digest R protein/B_{12} complexes, as in pancreatic insufficiency
- the lack of a functioning terminal ileum, as might occur with surgical resection of the small intestine

Iron Absorption

The absorption of iron is critical to maintaining a steady level of iron at approximately 4 g in a healthy adult (see Fast Fact Box 24.5).

Fast Fact 24.5

Iron losses of approximately 1 to 2 mg/day occur through the sloughing of cells from skin and the gastrointestinal tract; in women, losses secondary to menstrual bleeding occur. The recommended daily intake of iron is 20 mg/day. However, only 0.5 to 1.0 mg/day is absorbed by healthy men, and in women only 1.0 to 1.5 mg/day is absorbed.

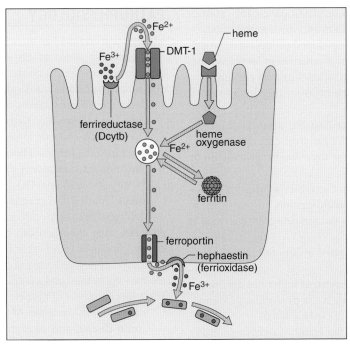

Fig. 24.21 Iron absorption in the duodenum. Heme is transported via the heme transporter (HT) and heme oxygenase then separates Fe^{2+} from the heme porphyrin ring. Ferric (Fe^{3+}) iron is reduced to the ferrous (Fe^{2+}) form using ferric reductase. Fe^{2+} is then transported through the brush border using divalent metal transporter 1 (*DMT1*). Cytosolic Fe^{2+} can be stored by binding to ferritin or transported through the basolateral border using ferroportin 1 (FP) and the associated hephaestin (Hp) protein. In the blood, Fe^{2+} is converted to Fe^{3+} and bound to the iron transport protein transferrin (TF). (From Hypochromic anemias. In: Hoffbrand V, Pettit JE, and Vyas P. *Color Atlas of Clinical Hematology*, 4th ed. Chapter 5, p. 75–91. Fig. 5.3.)

The majority of dietary iron is absorbed by the enterocytes of the duodenum.

- Dietary iron is mostly in the ferric (Fe^{3+}) form, yet the ferrous (Fe^{2+}) form is absorbed.
- Ferric iron is reduced to the ferrous form by ferric reductase at the brush border (Fig. 24.21).
- The iron transporter divalent metal transporter 1 (DMT1) then transports Fe^{2+} into the enterocyte at the apical membrane.

Iron can also be absorbed in the form of heme (iron in the center of a porphyrin ring, as is present in the oxygen-carrying blood protein hemoglobin). Heme is absorbed by intestinal cells via a separate heme transporter (HT).

- Once inside cells, the iron (Fe^{2+}) is released from the heme molecule by the action of heme oxygenase (HO_2).
- Some of the intracellular Fe^{2+} is stored and the rest is transported out of enterocytes by ferroportin 1 (FP), located on the basolateral membrane.
- Hephaestin (Hp) facilitates this basolateral transport of Fe^{2+} from the enterocyte to the blood.
- In the plasma, Fe^{2+} is converted back to Fe^{3+} and bound to the iron transport protein transferrin, which can transport the iron to numerous sites in the body, including the bone marrow and liver.
- The cytosolic iron that is stored inside the enterocyte is bound to the protein ferritin and can be subsequently

released in a controlled fashion. These ferritin molecules can aggregate in deposits called hemosiderin, which may collect throughout the body in diseases associated with iron overload.

The absorption of iron is a highly regulated process that is adjusted according to the body's needs.

- Excess iron absorption can lead to iron overload, which occurs in the condition of hemochromatosis.
- To prevent this, absorption is reduced by upregulating ferritin in the enterocyte cytoplasm. This leads to increased formation of iron/ferritin complexes, which are lost in feces when intestinal epithelial cells are sloughed off.
- In addition, the liver produces a peptide hormone called hepcidin, which is a master regulator of iron homeostasis.
  - Hepcidin inhibits iron transport by binding to ferroportin in enterocytes and preventing Fe^{2+} export into the hepatic portal system.
  - Hepcidin also binds the ferroportin on the plasma membrane of reticuloendothelial cells and further inhibits iron release. Consequently, iron absorption is reduced.

The Function of the Exocrine Pancreas

The exocrine pancreas is essentially a factory and a warehouse for the production and storage of digestive enzymes. While its physiology is not as complex as that of the liver—a topic requiring its own chapter—a few details of pancreatic production, storage, and secretory processes are worth mentioning.

- The pancreas possesses a well-developed endoplasmic reticulum and Golgi apparatus for the production of large amounts of protein: the zymogen precursors to digestive enzymes.
- Zymogen-loaded vesicles pinch off from the Golgi to form zymogen granules.
- The zymogen granules cluster near the apical side of the pancreatic acinar cells lining the pancreatic secretory ducts.
    - Neurohormonal signals cause the zymogen granules to be exocytosed (see Ch. 25).
    - The pancreas stores digestive enzymes as inactive zymogens to protect itself from autodigestion.

The pancreas must also secrete fluid to deliver its enzymes to the duodenum.

- No meal: Pancreatic fluid secreted at low rates, chloride is the predominant anion.
- After meal: Pancreatic fluid secreted at high rates during the digestion of a meal, bicarbonate is the predominant anion.
    - This renders the fluid alkaline (pH 7.5–8.0).
    - The alkalinity neutralizes the acidity of chyme coming from the stomach and creates the optimal pH for the functioning of the pancreatic enzymes.

The fate of the pancreatic enzymes (and all other digestive enzymes) subsequent to their digestive action has been a matter of controversy for nearly three decades.

- One theory says that the enzymes, which are made of protein, are themselves digested by proteases (in part by colonic bacteria) and absorbed.
- Another theory suggests that the pancreatic enzymes are absorbed by the intestines and recycled to the pancreas in what would be called an enteropancreatic circulation (See Development Box 24.1, Genetics Box 24.1 and Trauma Box 24.1).

DEVELOPMENT BOX 24.1

The pancreas is formed by the fusion of a ventral and a dorsal anlages that bud from the embryonic foregut. In approximately 10% of people, there is a complete or partial failure of these two buds to fuse, leading to distinct ductal systems. Although most individuals with pancreas divisum are asymptomatic, up to 5% may have episodic abdominal pain and pancreatitis.

GENETICS BOX 24.1

Approximately 10% to 20% of patients with pancreas divisum have a mutation in one or more alleles of the CFTR gene that is the cause of cystic fibrosis.

TRAUMA BOX 24.1

The association between pancreas divisum and pancreatitis is incompletely understood, but some hypothesize that increased pressure in the ductal systems plays a role. This increase in pressure may be caused by narrower papillae for pancreatic secretions to drain into the duodenum. Patients with pancreas divisum are thought to be more susceptible to developing pancreatitis in response to trauma and chemical injury from alcohol and some medications.

PATHOPHYSIOLOGY

Maldigestion occurs when there is a deficiency of digestive enzymes.

A common cause of carbohydrate maldigestion is lactase deficiency in the brush border of the duodenum and jejunum, also known as lactose intolerance:

- Under these circumstances, lactose remains in the lumen unabsorbed and is presented to the lower small intestine and colon.
- The luminal osmotic pressure is increased, which "pulls" water into the lumen. This results in an osmotic diarrhea.
- The undigested lactose is also metabolized by colonic bacteria to lactic acid and CO_2. The gas distends the colon and causes bloating and cramping.

Maldigestion of lipids can occur with a deficiency of pancreatic enzymes. This condition can be present in cases of pancreatic cancer, pancreatitis, and cystic fibrosis.

Malabsorption arises in the context of abnormalities of the alimentary epithelium and may be general to all nutrients, or it may affect specific classes of nutrients, depending on the pathogenesis.

- Inflammation because of autoimmune disease (such as Crohn disease and ulcerative colitis) or infection may decrease the absorptive surface area or render the absorptive surface dysfunctional.
- Surgery may also decrease the absorptive surface area.

There can be nutrient-specific malabsorptive syndromes:

- Scurvy (vitamin C deficiency)
- Rickets (vitamin D deficiency)
- Beriberi (thiamine deficiency)
- Hartnup disease is a rare autosomal recessive disorder in which the carrier system for neutral amino acids is absent.
    - The patient cannot absorb neutral amino acids, such as tryptophan from the lumen of the GI tract (or the renal tubule).
    - However, dipeptides or tripeptides that contain tryptophan can sometimes be absorbed and can be transported to various tissues.

Lipid absorption can be disturbed by several processes.

- Reduced intestinal bile salt concentration can lead to impaired micelle formation. This condition can occur with liver disease because bile salts are produced in the liver.
- It can also occur in the context of conditions affecting the ileum, which interrupt enterohepatic circulation (Fig. 24.22) and thus lead to reduced recycling of bile salts/acids.

The clinical presentation of salt and water malabsorption is diarrhea, which is defined as the excretion of 200 g or more of water in the stools of an adult over 24 hours. Diarrhea can be caused by a variety of mechanisms:

- Hypermotility of the gut leads to diarrhea because of the increased transit rate of chyme through the digestive tract.
    - Water and salts are delivered to the colon faster than the intestinal epithelial cells can absorb them.
    - An increased rate of transit through the intestines also decreases the absorption of nutrients, thereby raising the osmotic pressure of the intestinal lumen. Consequently, water is retained in the lumen.
- Various infectious pathogens may impair the enterocytes' capacity to absorb solutes, leading to high luminal osmotic pressure and retention of water in the lumen.

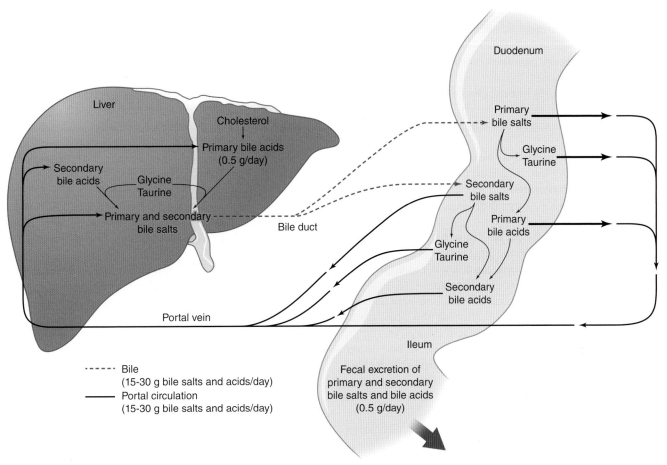

Fig. 24.22 Enterohepatic circulation of bile salts. Bile acids are produced from cholesterol in the liver, where they undergo conjugation with glycine and taurine to form bile salts. Bile salts are secreted into the intestine, where they are modified/deconjugated to form primary and secondary bile acids. In the terminal ileum, the bile acids and bile salts are absorbed and return to the liver via the portal vein. In the liver, the bile acids undergo modification and are resecreted into the intestine.

SUMMARY

- Anabolism is the synthesis of macromolecules from building blocks, a process requiring energy. Catabolism is the degradation of macromolecules into simpler substances, releasing energy. Metabolism is anabolism plus catabolism: the sum total of all chemical reactions in a living being.
- Both energy and building blocks for the construction and maintenance of body tissues come from the digestion (catabolism) and absorption of nutrients taken in by eating.
- The GI tract (alimentary canal) is a tube from the mouth to the anus that digests and absorbs dietary nutrients: carbohydrates, proteins, lipids, nucleic acids, water, vitamins, and minerals.
- Hydrolysis is used in the digestion of all the macronutrients (carbohydrates, proteins, lipids, and nucleic acids). Its general formula is:

$$R'' - R' + H_2O \rightarrow R''OH + R'H$$

- Much of digestion is accounted for by pancreatic enzymes that are released as inactive zymogens into the duodenum through the hepatopancreatic ampulla (the ampulla of Vater).
- Carbohydrates are digested by salivary α-amylase, pancreatic α-amylase, and intestinal disaccharidases, yielding the monosaccharides glucose, fructose, and galactose.
- Glucose and galactose are absorbed by secondary active transport involving an apical Na^+/monosaccharide symporter powered by a basolateral Na^+,K^+-ATPase. Fructose is absorbed by facilitated diffusion.
- Proteins are digested by gastric pepsin, pancreatic proteases, and intestinal peptidases. Pancreatic proteases are secreted as inactive zymogens and activated by intestinal enterokinase. This process yields amino acids, dipeptides, and tripeptides.
- Amino acids are absorbed by secondary active transport involving an apical Na^+/amino acid symporter powered by the basolateral Na^+,K^+-ATPase, as in carbohydrate absorption.

- Lipids are digested via emulsification into droplets by the amphipathic constituents of bile, followed by digestion by pancreatic lipases and cholesterol esterase. This process yields free fatty acids, 2-monoglyceride, free cholesterol, and lysophospholipid.
- Lipids are absorbed by bile salt emulsification of the cleavage products into micelles, which deliver the cleavage products to the intestinal brush border for diffusion into enterocytes.
- Nucleic acids are digested by pancreatic ribonucleases and deoxyribonucleases into individual nucleotides and by pancreatic phosphodiesterases into free bases (purine, pyrimidine) and phosphorylated pentose rings. They are absorbed by active transport.
- A net water uptake of 2 L per day (equal to the amount taken in by drinking) occurs in the large intestine. The Na^+,K^+-ATPase drives Na^+ absorption, causing water to diffuse after it into the enterocytes and the bloodstream.
- Sodium is absorbed in the small intestine and large intestine by active transport. In the small intestine, this active transport is coupled to sugar and amino acid absorption.
- The volume of water and the concentration of Na^+ in the blood (salt and water balance) are not controlled at the level of the GI tract. Rather, the GI tract takes in salt and water in proportion to what is ingested, and the brain and kidney afterward modulate salt and water excretion to keep blood volume and salt concentration within normal limits.
- Chloride is absorbed with sodium because of electrical gradients established by the Na^+,K^+-ATPase pump.
- Bicarbonate (HCO_3^-) is secreted in pancreatic fluid and bile in the duodenum, neutralizing the gastric acidity of chyme. HCO_3^- is absorbed in the jejunum and again secreted in the ileum and colon, where it neutralizes acidic products of bacterial metabolism.
- The fat-soluble vitamins A, D, E, and K are in micelles and are absorbed into the lymph with the other products of lipid digestion. The absorption of most water-soluble vitamins occurs by either facilitated diffusion or sodium-dependent active transport.
- The absorption of vitamin B_{12} (cobalamin) depends on the gastric secretion of IF, which binds vitamin B_{12} and protects it from degradation by pancreatic proteases. Iron is absorbed bound to transferrin.
- Maldigestion results from a digestive enzyme deficiency.
- Malabsorption arises in the context of abnormalities of the alimentary epithelium.

REVIEW QUESTIONS

Directions: Each of the numbered items or incomplete statements in this section is followed by answers or by completions of the statement. Select the one lettered answer or completion that is best in each case.

1. A 65-year-old woman is admitted to the hospital with severe nausea and vomiting and diffuse abdominal pain, including colicky pain in the right upper quadrant. Imaging studies suggest the presence of a gallstone that is occluding the common bile duct and the pancreatic duct. Which of the following would accurately describe the fluid in her duodenum after a meal?
   A. Abnormally high pH
   B. Abnormally low pH
   C. Normal pH
   D. Elevated volume
   E. Infection with *Helicobacter pylori*

2. A 10-year-old child is severely dehydrated after 1 week of copious watery diarrhea with high fever. Oral rehydration therapy could help by:
   A. Slowing intestinal motility
   B. Increasing solute-coupled sodium transport
   C. Increasing the expression of aquaporins
   D. Decreasing the renal excretion of fluid
   E. Improving the digestion of sugars
   F. Healing dysfunctional absorptive cells
   G. Killing bacterial pathogens in the intestine

3. An obese 50-year-old woman undergoes partial gastrectomy to control her appetite. Several months later she is found to be anemic, even though her incisions have healed nicely. The cause could be:
   A. Inadequate vitamin B_{12} in her diet
   B. Inadequate production of intrinsic factor
   C. Poor transcobalamin II production
   D. Inadequate acid production
   E. Bone marrow failure
   F. Inadequate erythropoietin production.

4. Which of the following require micelle formation for intestinal absorption?
   A. Vitamin C
   B. Glucose
   C. Lactose
   D. Leucine
   E. Vitamin D
   F. Bile acids

5. Which of the following must be further digested before it can be absorbed by intestinal cells?
   A. Dipeptides
   B. Tripeptides
   C. Glucose
   D. Alanine
   E. Fructose
   F. Sucrose

ANSWERS TO REVIEW QUESTIONS

1. **The answer is B.** After a meal, pancreatic secretions are alkaline and hence raise the pH of the acidic chyme delivered to the duodenum from the stomach. Obstruction of the pancreatic duct would block these alkaline secretions from reaching the duodenum and would leave the chyme more acidic than usual. The pancreas accounts for 1500 mL of fluid out of the 7 L secreted into the intestines each day. Obstruction of pancreatic secretion would *decrease* the fluid volume of the duodenum rather than increase it. *Helicobacter pylori* infection is associated with peptic ulcer disease, not acute pancreatitis.

2. **The answer is B.** Oral rehydration therapy acts on the glucose/sodium symporter. When intestinal infections compromise the capacity of the Na^+,K^+-ATPase in enterocytes, salt and therefore water absorption are impaired in the intestines. Oral rehydration therapy contains sugar and salt. The diffusion of glucose from the intestinal lumen into the enterocytes across the glucose/sodium symporter results in increased Na^+ and hence water absorption. Oral rehydration therapy does not treat the offending bacteria and does not repair damaged cells. In fact, it relies on the function of the remaining cells with an intact absorptive surface. It does not contain any drugs that distribute into the bloodstream.

3. **The answer is B.** The partial gastrectomy has resulted in decreased production of intrinsic factor owing to a decrease in the number of available parietal cells. Intrinsic factor protects vitamin B_{12} from degradation by pancreatic proteases; if production of intrinsic factor is inadequate, dietary vitamin B_{12} is digested instead of absorbed and cannot conduct its physiologic action of stimulating erythropoiesis (red blood cell production). Transcobalamin II is produced by the liver, which is unaffected by gastrectomy (it assists in the storage of vitamin B_{12} in the liver). The patient's gastric acid production might be below physiologic levels, but this would not affect vitamin B_{12} absorption per se. Bone marrow failure and decreased erythropoietin production (as occurs in renal failure) could also cause anemia in contexts other than the one presented here.

4. **The answer is E.** Fat-soluble vitamins, including vitamin D, E, A, and K, are solubilized in micelles in the intestinal lumen until they can be absorbed by the intestinal epithelial cells. Vitamin C is water-soluble. Bile acids are absorbed by sodium-dependent cotransporters in the ileum.

5. **The answer is F.** Monosaccharides are the only form of carbohydrates that can be absorbed by intestinal epithelial cells. Sucrose is a disaccharide that must be digested before it can be absorbed. Proteins can be absorbed as amino acids, dipeptides, or tripeptides.

25

Control of Gastrointestinal Motility and Secretion

INTRODUCTION

In Chapter 24, we saw that the acquisition of energy and building blocks requires digestion and absorption. We now focus on two other critical gastrointestinal (GI) capabilities, without which digestion and absorption could not occur:

- Motility is the muscular capacity for movement by which the digestive organs agitate food mechanically and propel it through the GI tract.
- Secretion is the process that delivers digestive enzymes, emulsifiers, and fluid at low or high pH into the intestinal lumen to enable digestion and absorption.

Particular sequences of muscular contractions and secretions of specific digestive agents must be orchestrated perfectly in time for digestion and absorption to occur normally. Consequently, motility and secretion are controlled by an elaborate neurohormonal regulatory system.

There are three major components to this regulatory system:
- The central nervous system (CNS), which provides extrinsic innervation and control to the GI tract.
- The enteric nervous system (ENS), sometimes called the "minibrain" of the intestines, which provides intrinsic innervation and control to the GI tract.
- Enteroendocrine cells, which are distributed throughout the GI mucosa.

SYSTEM STRUCTURE

As described in the previous chapter, the entire length of the GI tract shares a similar structural foundation (see Fig. 24.1). Recall that the muscularis has an inner circular and an outer longitudinal sublayer of smooth muscle tissue. The action of these two layers, which constrict the gut in diameter and in length, respectively, provides the basis for peristalsis.

- Between the inner circular and outer longitudinal muscle layers of the muscularis lies the myenteric plexus (Auerbach's plexus), one major component of the ENS (Fig. 25.1).
- The other major component of the ENS is the submucosal plexus (Meissner's plexus), found between the muscularis and the submucosa.

Muscles of the Gastrointestinal Tract

Many muscles and organ systems are involved in chewing and swallowing food.
- Masseter muscle: closes the mandible during biting

- Tongue
- Pharyngeal muscles
- Upper esophageal sphincter: demarcates the transition from the pharynx to the esophagus
- Esophagus
- Lower esophageal sphincter: a tonically contracted zone in the terminal 2 to 4 cm of the esophagus that divides the esophagus from the stomach
- Pyloric sphincter: separates the stomach from the duodenum
- Ileocecal valve: separates the ileum from the large intestine
- Sphincter of Oddi: separates the duodenum and the ampulla of Vater, which carries the bile and pancreatic secretions
- Stomach, small intestine, and large intestine: lined with smooth muscle and myenteric plexus
  - Gap junctions between adjacent smooth muscle cells coordinated contraction and relaxation of the GI tract.
  - The large intestine also possesses three strips of longitudinal muscle called the taenia coli.
- Rectum
- Internal anal sphincter: involuntary smooth muscle
- External anal sphincter: voluntarily controlled striated muscle

Innervation of the Gastrointestinal Tract

As stated earlier, the regulatory system governing GI function includes three components:
- CNS
- ENS
- Enteroendocrine cells

All three are interconnected by nerves, and neurons and enteroendocrine cells both serve as sensors and effectors for the combined CNS/ENS control center. The entire regulatory apparatus is referred to as the brain-gut axis.
- The transmission of information from the GI tract to the brain for processing is via afferent sensory axons, whose cell bodies are located in the submucosal or myenteric plexus.
- Neural commands from the brain and spinal cord—the CNS—are sent in the opposite direction via efferent axons to the computational circuits in the enteric minibrain.

Intrinsic Innervation

The ENS, composed of the submucosal and myenteric plexuses, provides intrinsic innervation of GI tract structures.
- Each plexus is composed of ganglia.
  - The myenteric ganglia form a continuous network from the upper esophagus to the internal anal sphincter.

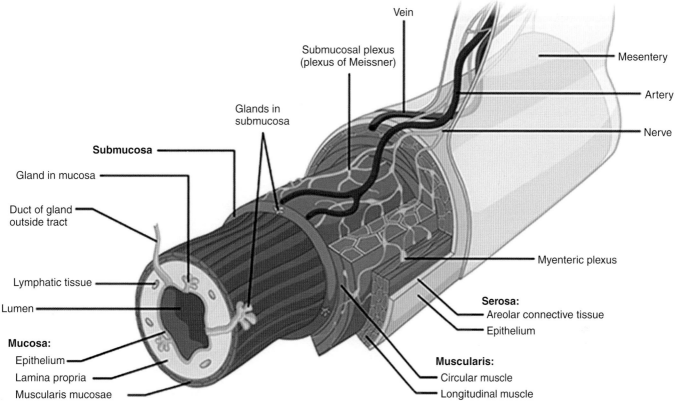

Fig. 25.1 The enteric nervous system (ENS). The myenteric plexus, which controls motility, and the submucosal plexus, which controls secretion and blood flow, make up the ENS. (From Chalazonitis A, Rao M. *Enteric nervous system manifestations of neurodegenerative disease*. Brain Research, Volume 1693, Part B; 2018. Pages 207-213. Fig. 1.)

- The submucosal ganglia are concentrated in the small and large intestine. The ganglia within each layer are connected longitudinally and circumferentially via "highways" of internodal axons.
- The two plexuses are connected via processes akin to bridges traversing the circular muscle layer. These internal highways and bridges are critical for the coordination of activity along the intestinal wall.
- The enteric neurons connect with the intestinal mucosa, secretory cells, blood vessels, smooth muscle cells, sympathetic neurons, parasympathetic neurons, and enteroendocrine cells.

Enteric sensory neurons are responsive to mechanical and chemical stimuli. Interneurons participate in enteric reflexes and are regulated by the hormonal milieu created by surrounding enteroendocrine and neuroendocrine cells.

Extrinsic Innervation

The GI tract is connected extrinsically to the CNS by nerves (Fig. 25.2).
- Above the esophagus, this connection is partly through somatic nerves, which give the CNS partly voluntary control over chewing and swallowing.
- Muscles in the mouth and pharynx are innervated by cranial nerves:
  - V (trigeminal)

- IX (glossopharyngeal)
- X (vagus)
- XII (hypoglossal)
- Taste in the oral cavity is mediated by cranial nerves:
  - VII (facial)
  - IX (glossopharyngeal)
- Afferent and efferent neurons complete a reflex arc through the swallowing center in the brain stem.
- The external anal sphincter is also innervated with a somatic nerve (the pudendal), and therefore the CNS can consciously control either end of the GI tract.

Between the pharynx and the external anal sphincter, the GI tract is extrinsically innervated only by the autonomic nervous system (ANS). The brain thus has little voluntary control over most of the GI tract; it is regulated involuntarily.

The parasympathetic and sympathetic divisions of the ANS regulate the functions of the GI tract, as shown in Fig. 25.3.

The parasympathetic nervous system connects the medulla to the myenteric and submucosal plexuses via the following nerves:
- Vagus nerve innervates the GI tract from the upper esophageal sphincter to the transverse colon.
  - Sensory-motor reflexes carried in the vagus nerve are called vagovagal reflexes (see Fig. 25.3).

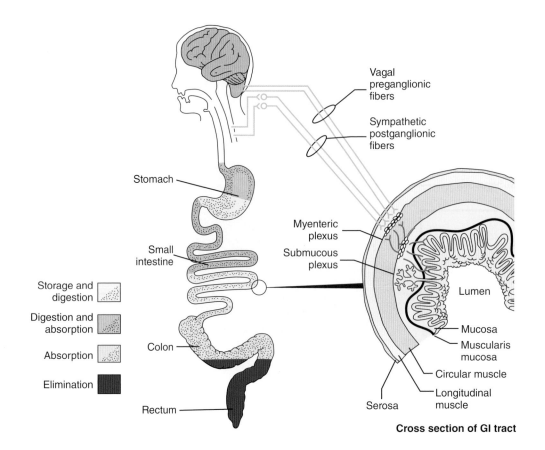

Cross section of GI tract

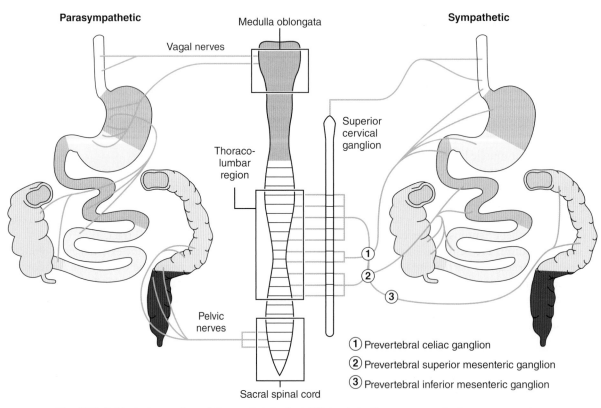

Fig. 25.2 Extrinsic innervation of the gastrointestinal (GI) tract. In the parasympathetic nervous system, nerves project from the medulla oblongata (vagal nerves) and the sacral spinal cord (pelvic nerves). In the sympathetic nervous system, neurons project from the thoracic and first lumbar segments of the spinal cord to form the superior cervical ganglion, as well as the prevertebral ganglion (celiac, superior mesenteric, and inferior mesenteric). (Modified from Wecker L. *Brody's Human Pharmacology*, 6th Ed. Philadelphia: Elsevier, 2018. Fig. 71.1.)

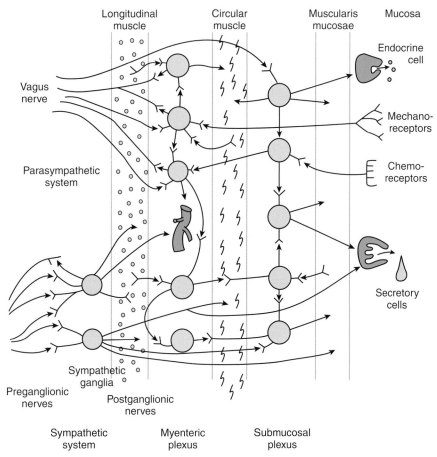

Fig. 25.3 A closer look at the extrinsic innervation of the gastrointestinal tract. The vagovagal reflex receives afferent signals from the mucosa and enteric nervous system (ENS) and delivers efferent signals back to the ENS and mucosa. (From Johnson. *Gastrointestinal Physiology*, 9th Ed. Philadelphia: Mosby Elsevier; 2018. Fig. 2.2.)

- The vagovagal reflex should not be confused with the vasovagal reflex, which parasympathetically drops the heart rate in response to stress-related spikes in blood pressure.
- Pelvic nerves, originating in the sacral spinal cord (S2–S4), innervate the GI tract from the splenic flexure of the colon to the internal anal sphincter.

The sympathetic nervous system innervates the entire GI tract with neurons that arise from the sympathetic chain (located alongside spinal cord levels T5–L2) and travel to the prevertebral ganglia (celiac, superior mesenteric, inferior mesenteric, and hypogastric).

- From the prevertebral ganglia, sympathetic neurons travel along blood vessels to penetrate the intestinal wall.
- Sympathetic fibers synapse with neurons in the enteric plexuses, as well as directly on smooth muscle cells, blood vessels, and the muscularis mucosa.

Overall, parasympathetic stimulation increases smooth muscle contraction, whereas sympathetic stimulation decreases it.

Enteroendocrine Cells

Unlike the endocrine cells of the thyroid or pancreas, which are collected into discrete, isolated glands, GI endocrine cells are distributed over large mucosal areas and are more heterogeneous

in nature. This distribution enables them to respond to a diversity of stimuli over the length of the GI tract with a wide variety of endocrine signals.

GI endocrine cells are derived from the same crypt stem cells that differentiate into enterocytes, as well as goblet cell and Paneth cell lineages.

- They are continuously differentiating from pluripotent intestinal stem cells into specialized cells that secrete one specific agent.
- Like other endocrine cells, they contain many secretory granules full of peptides.
- GI endocrine cells are stimulated at their apical (luminal) surfaces by nutrients, by neural input, or by distention of the GI tract wall.

Gastrointestinal Hormones and Neurotransmitters

GI hormones and neurotransmitters are secreted by enteroendocrine cells and neurons at their axon terminals. They are the final common pathway shared by the nervous and endocrine systems to control the GI system. These factors govern:
- Enzymatic secretion from the stomach
- Enzymatic secretion from the pancreas
- Bile secretion from the liver
- Contraction and relaxation of GI smooth muscle

There are three hormone communication pathways used by GI regulatory substances (Fig. 25.4):

- Endocrine communication occurs when a hormone is released from one tissue into the bloodstream to reach a distant target cell with a receptor for that hormone.
  - Five of the GI peptides—secretin, gastrin, cholecystokinin (CCK), glucose-dependent insulinotropic peptide (GIP), and motilin—are considered endocrine hormones.
- Paracrine communication occurs when an agent is released from endocrine cells into the interstitial fluid to affect neighboring cells with a receptor for that agent.
  - The primary GI paracrine agents are somatostatin and histamine.
- Neurocrine communication occurs when an agent is synthesized and released from neurons in response to an action potential and behaves as a neurotransmitter.
  - The primary neurotransmitters are acetylcholine and norepinephrine.
- Minor neurotransmitters include: gastrin-releasing peptide, nitric oxide (NO), tachykinins (e.g., substance P), enkephalins, and vasoactive intestinal peptide (VIP)

Each regulatory agent exerts its action on the GI tract via binding to a specific receptor on the target cell membrane.

- Hormone receptors in the GI tract belong to a family of G-protein-linked receptors.
- Depending on the receptor, ligand binding activates one of two major intracellular pathways to elicit an immediate response, such as enzyme secretion.
  - The binding of gastrin, CCK, and acetylcholine (ACh) to their respective receptors activates phospholipase C, leading to increased intracellular calcium release.
  - The binding of other substances, including secretin, VIP, and histamine, activates *adenylate cyclase*, which leads to an increased intracellular concentration of cyclic adenosine monophosphate (cAMP).
- Alternatively, hormone binding can elicit a delayed response, such as the activation of gene expression to exert a trophic effect on GI mucosa.

SYSTEM FUNCTION

Table 25.1 shows the motile and secretory events in sequence, along with their neural and endocrine mediators.

Table 25.2 lists the endocrine, paracrine, and neurocrine factors involved in digestion.

Although the regulation of each step of digestion is complex, it is useful to keep a few general principles in mind.

- The parasympathetic nervous system and its end-product, ACh, tend to promote motility and secretion and relax GI tract sphincters.
- The sympathetic nervous system and its end-product, NE, tend to inhibit motility and secretion. The GI tract receives tonic sympathetic output (i.e., a constant, basal level of sympathetic output) so that the default setting of the GI tract is depressed motility, low secretion, and constricted sphincters.

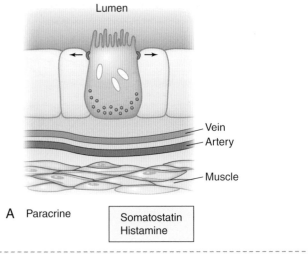

A Paracrine

| Somatostatin |
| Histamine |

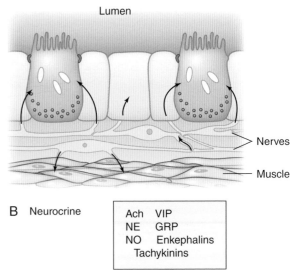

B Neurocrine

Ach	VIP
NE	GRP
NO	Enkephalins
Tachykinins	

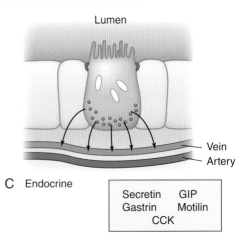

C Endocrine

Secretin	GIP
Gastrin	Motilin
CCK	

Fig. 25.4 Classification of the neurohormonal substances of the gastrointestinal (GI) tract. A, Paracrine substances are released into the interstitium to affect neighbouring cells. B, Neurocrine substances are released directly onto their targets from neuronal axon terminals. C, Endocrine substances are released into the blood stream and circulate to their targets. Not shown are autocrine substances that are released from a given cell and stimulate that same cell. *ACh*, Acetylcholine; *CCK*, cholecystokinin; *GIP*, glucose-dependent insulinotropic polypeptide; *GRP*, gastrin-releasing peptide; *NE*, norepinephrine; *NO*, nitric oxide; *VIP*, vasoactive intestinal peptide.

TABLE 25.1 Motility and Secretion: From Hunger to Defecation

Transit Time	Digestive Event	Regulatory Structure or Mediator Involved
N/A	Perception of hunger	Hypothalamus
	Procurement of food	Cerebral cortex
	Anticipation of eating (cephalic phase of digestion) and preparation of GI tract	Cerebral cortex, cranial nerves, brain stem (dorsal motor nuclei of vagus nerves, salivatory nuclei)
	Tasting of food (oral phase) and preparation of GI tract	Cranial nerves, brain stem (dorsal motor nuclei of vagus nerves, salivatory nuclei)
	Chewing (mastication)	Cerebral cortex, trigeminal nerve (cranial nerve V)
	Initiation of swallowing (deglutition)	Cerebral cortex
1–2 seconds In pharynx, 5–8 seconds in esophagus	Swallowing of food down esophagus into stomach	Vagovagal swallowing reflex, ENS peristalsis
30–45 minutes in stomach	Secretion of acid and pepsinogen (gastric phase)	Vagovagal reflex, gastrin from G cells, histamine from ECL cells
	Mixing and grinding of food in stomach. squirting of chyme into duodenum until stomach is empty	Vagovagal reflex, ENS peristalsis
2–4 hours in small Intestine	Secretion of pancreatic fluid and bile into duodenum (intestinal phase)	Secretin from S cells, CCK from I cells, vagovagal reflex
	Propulsion through small intestine to colon	ENS peristalsis
12–30 hours in colon	Feces formation with water/salt absorption, propulsion toward rectum	ENS peristalsis, mass movement
Seconds to minutes	Defecation	ENS peristalsis, pelvic nerve spinal reflex, cerebral cortex

CCK, cholecystokinin; *ECL*, enterochromaffin-like; *ENS*, enteric nervous system; *MMC*, migrating myoelectrical complex.

TABLE 25.2 Endocrine, Paracrine, and Neurocrine Factors Involved in Digestion

Factor	Secretin	Endocrine Factors
Location	S cells of duodenum and jejunum	
Stimulus	Low pH (<4.5) in duodenum $\rightarrow$ secretin release	
Action	Neutralizes chyme by stimulating pencreatic water and bicarbonate secretion, causes exocytosis of pancreatic enzymes	
Factor	**Gastrin**	
Location	G cells of gastric antrum	
Stimulus	Sight, smell, or taste of food $\rightarrow$ vagal output $\rightarrow$ gastrin release (cephalic phase) Gastric distention and presence of nutrients $\rightarrow$ gastrin secretion (gastric phase) Duodenal distention $\rightarrow$ gastrin secretion from duodenal G cells (intestinal phase)	
Action	Stimulates acid secretion by parietal cells	
Factor	**Cholecystokinin (CCK)**	
Location	I cells and enteric neurons of duodenum and jejunum	
Stimulus	Free fatty acids, triglycerides, peptides, amino acids, and gastric acid in small intestine $\rightarrow$ CCK release	
Action	Causes gallbladder contraction and sphincter of Oddi relaxation, thus allowing bile to enter intestine; causes exocytosis of pancreatic enzymes	
Factor	**Glucose-dependent insulinotropic polypeptide (GIP)[a]**	
Location	Enteroendocrine cells in duodenum and jejunum	
Stimulus	Glucose, triglycerides, or amino acids $\rightarrow$ GIP release	
Action	Stimulates insulin release from endocrine pancreas	
Factor	**Motilin**	
Location	Upper portions of small intestine	
Stimulus	Released in 90-min cycles during fasting state	
Action	Initiates MMC	

TABLE 25.2   Endocrine, Paracrine, and Neurocrine Factors Involved in Digestion—cont'd

Factor	**Somatostatin**	**Paracrine Factors**
Location	D cells in gastric antrum, near gastrin-secreting G cells	
Stimulus	Low pH in stomach → somatostatin (inhibited by parasympathetic input, stimulated by sympathetic input)	
Action	Inhibits acid secretion from parietal cells	
Factor	**Histamine**	
Location	Enteroendocrine cells and mast cells in gastric mucose	
Stimulus	Gastrin	
Action	Stimulates gastric acid secretion via its activation of parietal cells H_2 type receptor	
Factor	**Prostaglandin E$_2$ (PGE$_2$)**	
Location	Stomach	
Stimulus		
Action	Inhibits acid secretion, stimulates mucous production	
Factor	**Acetylcholine (ACh)**	**Neurocrine Factors**
Location	Vagal axon terminals throughout GI tract	
Stimulus	Vagovagal reflexes	
Action	Enhances secretion and motility	
Factor	**Norepinephrine (NE)**	
Location	Sympathetic axon terminals throughout GI tract	
Stimulus	Tonically active	
Action	Inhibits secretion and motility	
Factor	**Gastrin-releasing peptide (GRP)**	
Location	Vagal axon terminals in stomach	
Stimulus	Vagovagal reflex	
Action	Gastrin release from G cells	
Factor	**Vasoactive intestinal peptide (VIP)**	
Location	Vagal axon terminals throughout GI tract	
Stimulus	Vagovagal reflex	
Action	Relaxes sphincters, circular muscle, and dilates blood vessels; stimulates intestinal and pancreatic secretion	
Factor	**Nitric oxide (NO)**	
Location	Vagal axon terminals throughout GI tract	
Stimulus	Vagovagal reflexes	
Action	Relaxes sphincters, circular muscle, and dilates blood vessels	

[a]GIP is also called by its earlier name, gastric inhibitory peptide, but this name does not reflect its behavior at physiologic doses.

CCK, cholecystokinin; *ECL*, enterochromaffin-like; *ENS*, enteric nervous system; *GI*, Gastrointestinal; *MMC*, migrating myoelectrical complex.

Peristalsis is the basic means of propulsion in all parts of the GI tract. In peristalsis, the GI tract wall contracts behind its luminal contents and relaxes in front of them (Fig. 25.5).

- The contraction/relaxation pattern of the musculature then advances along the tract, pushing the luminal contents forward.
- The ENS achieves peristalsis without extrinsic help by sending nervous impulses forward and backward along the GI tract from a site of luminal distention.
  - The backward impulses result in the release of signals to the smooth muscle to contract, such as ACh.
  - The forward impulses result in the release of signals to relax, such as NO.

- Peristalsis is conducted by neurons in the myenteric plexus (as opposed to the submucosal plexus).

The smooth muscle of the GI tract manifests electrical pacemaker activity at all times, like the muscle tissue of the heart.

- Calcium ions are repeatedly flowing into the smooth muscle cells, depolarizing them, and potassium ions are repeatedly being released, repolarizing them.
- These actions lead to rhythmic increases and decreases in wall tension.
- Peristalsis is superimposed upon this underlying pattern of muscular activity.
- The extrinsic influences of the parasympathetic and sympathetic nervous systems are further superimposed on this

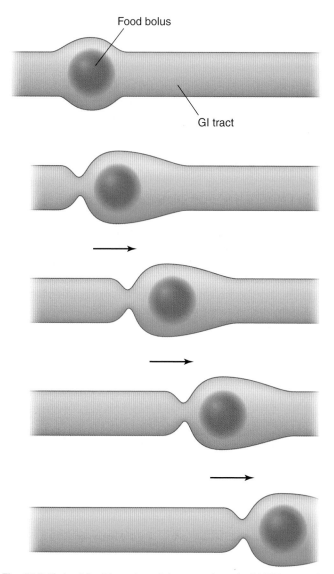

Food bolus

GI tract

Fig. 25.5 Peristalsis. Distention of the gastrointestinal (*GI)* lumen triggers a myenteric reflex that causes circular contraction proximal to the site of distention and dilatation distal to the site of distention. These contractions, termed peristalsis, move the bolus forward, triggering another myenteric reflex, and so on.

basic pattern, with ACh tending to assist in depolarization of the smooth muscle membranes and NE doing the opposite.

Whereas the myenteric system controls GI motility, the submucosal plexus is in perfect position to regulate blood flow and epithelial functions, which mediates secretion.

- Sensory receptors or chemoreceptors in the GI tract are sensitive to mechanical, thermal, osmotic, and chemical stimuli.
- Effector neurons result in motility, electrolyte, and exocrine secretion, and neuroendocrine stimulation.
- A variety of reflexes within the GI system couple the functioning of two or more organs (see Oncology Box 25.1, Development Box 25.1, and Pharmacology Box 25.1).

ONCOLOGY BOX 25.1

Plummer-Vinson syndrome is a risk factor for squamous cell carcinoma of the esophagus and pharynx.

DEVELOPMENT BOX 25.1

Patients with Plummer-Vinson syndrome have a triad of an esophageal web, dysphagia (difficulty swallowing), and iron deficiency anemia. The esophageal web is a thin membrane that can interfere mechanically with the passage of food under peristalsis.

PHARMACOLOGY BOX 25.1

Plummer-Vinson syndrome is treated with iron therapy. This not only addresses the anemia, but often results in resolution of the dysphasia.

Ingestion

Animals acquire nutrients by ingestion (eating), and mouths have been around since the preCambrian beginnings of animal life more than 550 million years ago. It is probably not an exaggeration to say that eating is responsible for the anatomic arrangement of our bodies into segments like those of ancient swimming tunicates and the placement of our organs of sight, audition, olfaction, and gustation in the head, near the mouth.

Anticipation of a Meal

This anticipation of eating, sometimes called the cephalic phase of digestion, is the first stage in the functioning of the GI tract. The brain:

- Signals (via the hypothalamus) the need for food with the subjective sensation of hunger or appetite
- Plans for food procurement (via the cerebral cortex)
- Begins to prepare the digestive tract for action even before eating takes place.

The oral phase of digestion (taste) begins when food reaches the tongue.

- The stimuli of the cephalic and oral phases result in increased parasympathetic output from the dorsal motor nuclei of the vagus nerves and the salivatory nuclei.
- These signals, in turn, increase salivary, gastric, and exocrine pancreas secretion, enhance gallbladder contractility, and relax the smooth muscle of the body of the stomach and the sphincter of Oddi.

Ghrelin is a peptide hormone secreted by epithelial cells of the gastric fundus that also acts to coordinate appetite and energy balance.

- Ghrelin acts on receptors in the anterior pituitary gland to stimulate the release of growth hormone, while its action on receptors in the hypothalamus stimulates appetite.
- Ghrelin also appears to suppress fat utilization in adipose tissue.

Mastication

Mastication, commonly known as chewing, is both a voluntary and an involuntary process involving muscles innervated by cranial nerve V. Like the act of walking, chewing involves certain stereotyped patterns of movement that are partially automatic, although they can be controlled or interrupted with conscious attention.

- To be able to chew, one must have healthy teeth, gums, and mucous membranes.
- Chewing and grinding food enhance digestion by increasing the overall surface area of the food that will be exposed to digestive enzymes.
- Mastication also enhances future gastric emptying (the movement of food onward from the stomach to the duodenum) by decreasing the size of the material that must pass through the small-diameter pyloric sphincter.

Salivation

Salivation, the production of saliva by the salivary glands, is important for many reasons, including:

- Lubrication
- Digestion (secretion of salivary amylase)
- Acid neutralization
- Immunologic function (secretion of immunoglobulin IgA against pathogens)

The salivatory nuclei in the brain stem (which were already stimulated during anticipation of the meal) are further stimulated by the tactile and gustatory sensation of food in the mouth, transmitted to the brain by cranial nerves VII and IX. Efferent sympathetic and parasympathetic fibers in the same nerves also innervate the salivary glands of the mouth, with parasympathetic stimulation increasing salivation.

Deglutition

Deglutition, the physiologic term for swallowing, is the process in which several muscles contract and relax under regulation by the swallowing center in the brain, located in the medulla and lower pons (Fig. 25.6).

- Cranial nerves pass afferent information from the upper GI tract (mouth to esophagus) to the swallowing center.
- Efferent information from the swallowing center returns to the upper GI tract in multiple cranial nerves.
  - Some of these fibers are somatic, arising in the nucleus ambiguus and terminating in striated muscle.
  - Other efferent fibers arise in the dorsal motor nucleus of the vagus nerve and cast parasympathetic axons onto the upper GI smooth muscle.

Deglutition begins voluntarily, as the tongue pushes the food bolus into the posterior oropharynx (Fig. 25.7). This initiates the involuntary swallowing reflex:

Nasopharynx closes→ vocal cords and epiglottis close off the airway to the lungs→pharynx contracts→ upper esophageal sphincter (which is tonically constricted) relaxes→ pharyngeal peristalsis pushes the bolus into the esophagus in less than 2 seconds→ lower esophageal sphincter anticipates passage of the bolus by beginning to relax under parasympathetic influence 1 to 2.5 seconds

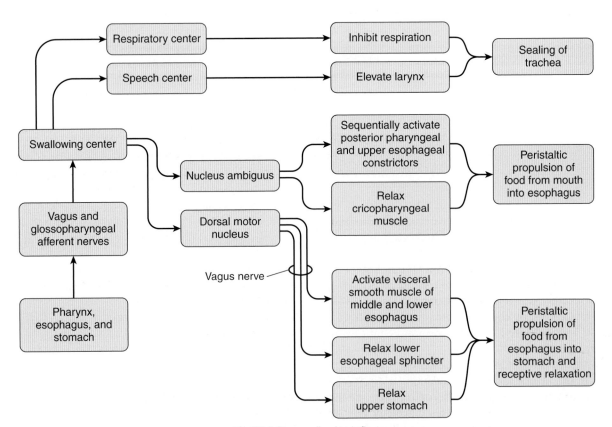

Fig. 25.6 The swallowing reflex.

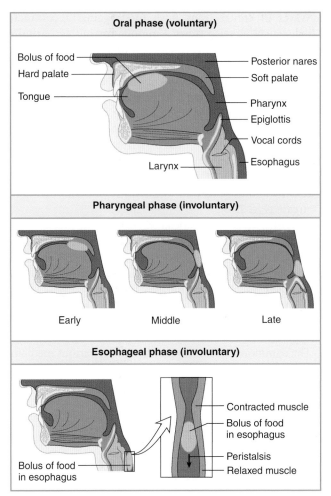

Fig. 25.7 Following chewing (mastication), the tongue pushes food to the back of the mouth, where a reflex response triggered by the trigeminal, glossopharyngeal, and vagus nerves induces swallowing (deglutition). Elevation of the soft palate prevents food from entering the nasal passage. The epiglottis prevents food from entering the trachea. Relaxation of the upper esophageal sphincter allows food to descend into the esophagus. (From Carroll R. *Elsevier's Integrated Physiology*. Philadelphia: Mosby Elsevier; 2007. Fig. 12.3.)

after deglutition→ peristaltic wave traveling down the esophagus pushes the bolus past the lower esophageal sphincter and into the stomach.

If the entire food bolus does not make it through, a secondary peristaltic wave begins at the site of distention and clears the bolus.

The lower esophageal sphincter, like the upper one, is tonically constricted, which is important for preventing acid reflux from the stomach to the esophagus. The sphincter is reinforced by the diaphragm muscle surrounding it and by the positive intraabdominal pressure (as opposed to the negative intrathoracic pressure). (See Clinical Correlation Box 25.1.)

Clinical Correlation Box 25.1

If the upper portion of the stomach slides up into the thorax (hiatal hernia), the low pressure around the lower esophageal sphincter can cause acid reflux into the esophagus.

Finally, the swallowing reflex includes a vagally mediated reduction in the muscle tone of the stomach wall. This "receptive relaxation" allows the stomach to accommodate up to 2 L of fluid without an increase in intragastric pressure (see Clinical Correlation Box 25.2).

Clinical Correlation Box 25.2

What Is Gastroesophageal Reflux Disease?

A 34-year-old man complains to his primary care physician of "burning pain" just below his sternum. The pain has bothered him for almost a year and is aggravated by spicy and fried foods, and especially by caffeine. He has experienced limited relief with over-the-counter treatments like Tums and Pepcid. The patient is instructed to avoid aggravating foods and is prescribed omeprazole (Prilosec). He is also referred to a gastroenterologist for an endoscopy, which shows normal esophageal mucosa. His pain resolves after a month of twice-daily omeprazole, and his dietary changes help in the months following, although he still has pain occasionally.

Reflux (gastroesophageal reflux), the medical term for heartburn, involves the backflow of acid and pepsin from the stomach across the lower esophageal sphincter and into the lower esophagus. Acid and pepsin injure the esophageal mucosa, causing pain because the esophageal mucosa does not share the protections of the gastric mucosa—mucus and bicarbonate production, for example. Gastroesophageal reflux disease (GERD) is chronic reflux; the reflux is present recurrently over a long period of time.

Although gastric secretions do cause the pain, gastric secretion is not elevated in most cases of GERD. Rather, the problem is a failure of the lower esophageal sphincter. Aberrant swallowing may cause the lower esophageal sphincter to open without the appropriate lower esophageal peristalsis afterward. This results in failure to flush refluxed secretions back into the stomach. Postprandial overdistention or irritation of the stomach also increases the likelihood of reflux. Untreated GERD may eventually cause Barrett esophagus, a metaplastic change wherein the esophageal mucosa begins to express features of the gastric mucosa to protect itself from acid. The development of Barrett esophagus carries an increased risk of esophageal cancer.

Several medical treatments for GERD reduce the acidity of gastric secretions, but they do not address the underlying cause of the reflux. Tums (CaCO$_3$) acts as a base and neutralizes the stomach acid so that when it is refluxed, it is not harmful to the esophageal mucosa. H$_2$ blockers, such as ranitidine (Zantac), block the histamine receptor and hence interfere with gastrin's activation of parietal cell acid secretion. Proton pump inhibitors, such as omeprazole (Prilosec), inhibit the parietal cell H$^+$/K$^+$-ATPase. Dietary modification is more successful at eliminating the cause of GERD. The principal surgical treatment for GERD is fundoplication of the lower esophageal sphincter, in which part of the stomach is wrapped around the lower esophageal sphincter to reinforce it. This procedure can now be performed laparoscopically, which makes for an easier recovery than older approaches, but surgery is still reserved for patients in whom medical therapy and dietary modification have failed.

Gastric Motility and Secretion

During fasting, the stomach and small intestine are largely quiescent, aside from the small rhythmic contractions described earlier and what is known as the migrating myoelectric complex (MMC).

- The MMC is a pattern of motility that builds in intensity until it generates one large "housekeeper" contraction, a wave that sweeps from the stomach to the terminal ileum.
- The MMC, which arises every 75 to 90 minutes and lasts for 3 to 6 minutes, pushes any undigested, unabsorbed material

from the stomach and small intestine into the large intestine for excretion.

- It also prevents stasis from occurring within the stomach and small intestine, thereby preventing overgrowth of the small number of bacteria normally present in these organs.
- The MMC is prompted by the neuroendocrine mediator motilin, which is secreted during fasting states by neuroendocrine cells in the proximal small intestine, possibly under the influence of an alkaline duodenal pH (see Clinical Correlation Box 25.3).

Clinical Correlation Box 25.3

The antibiotic erythromycin is a nonpeptide motilin receptor agonist that can be used clinically to stimulate gastrointestinal (GI) motility, but when taken for usual reasons, it can also lead to abdominal discomfort.

When food is delivered to the stomach, stretching the gastric walls, the pattern of motility changes.

- Gastric distention stimulates vagovagal pathways and the ENS, which initiate contractions in the stomach walls.

- Waves of contractions push food against a contracted pyloric sphincter 3 times a minute, mixing and grinding the food and causing small amounts to squirt into the duodenum.

At the same time, gastric distention and the presence of food also stimulate gastric acid secretion from parietal cells through the action of ACh, gastrin, and histamine.

- The vagovagal response to distention deploys ACh to the muscarinic receptors on the parietal cells of the gastric mucosa, directly increasing acid secretion.
- Vagal stimulation of antral G cells and stimulation of the G cells by amino acids lead to gastrin release into the bloodstream (Fig. 25.8).
  - Gastrin reaches the parietal cells through the circulation and acts on the parietal cells directly, increasing H^+ secretion.
  - Gastrin also affects the parietal cells through the intermediary of histamine-containing enteroendocrine cells called enterochromaffin-like (ECL) cells.
  - In response to gastrin, ECL cells secrete histamine, which binds the H_2 receptor on parietal cells and increases H^+ secretion.

The common mechanism by which these various mediators increase H^+ secretion is translocation of H^+/K^+-adenosine

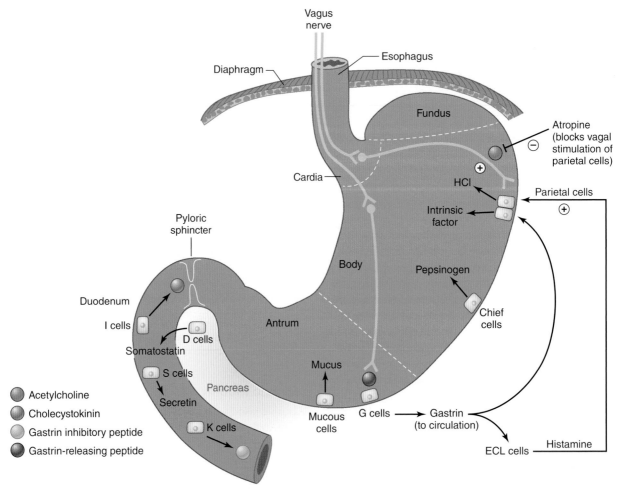

Fig. 25.8 Gastrointestinal (GI) secretory cells. Gastrin in the circulation increases acid secretion primarily through its effects on enterochromaffin-like (*ECL*) cells, which release histamine, rather than through its direct effect on parietal cells. *HCl*, hydrochloric acid.

triphosphatase (ATPase) from intracellular vesicles to the parietal cell membrane.

When the pH drops below 3.0, G cells stop secreting gastrin and D cells secrete the paracrine factor somatostatin, which inhibits gastrin release. Thus the acidification of the gastric contents is self-limiting.

Finally, vagal input and gastrin (as well as other factors) stimulate the gastric chief cells to secrete pepsinogen. Pepsinogen is cleaved by acid pH to form pepsin, an important enzyme in the digestion of proteins.

Duodenal Regulation of Pancreatic and Hepatobiliary Secretion

The entry of food material (called chyme upon leaving the stomach) into the small intestine stimulates three different regulatory pathways that stimulate the pancreas and liver. Two of the signals are hormones secreted by intestinal enteroendocrine cells and one pathway involves the vagus nerve.

- S cells in the mucosa respond to the low pH of chyme by releasing the hormone secretin into the bloodstream. Secretin circulates to acinar cells of the exocrine pancreas and binds basolateral receptors on those cells. This has two main effects:
  - It causes the fusion of zymogen granules with the apical membrane, dumping zymogens (digestive enzyme precursors) into the pancreatic ducts
  - It causes the translocation of H^+-ATPase to the basolateral membrane. This in turn results in increased clearance of H^+ from the cell, enabling the pancreatic cell to make and secrete HCO_3^-, which keeps the pancreatic secretions alkaline and enables neutralization of the acidic chyme.
- I cells in the small intestine respond to luminal proteins, lipids, and their cleavage products by secreting the hormone CCK into the bloodstream.
  - CCK circulates to the pancreas and stimulates pancreatic secretion.
  - CCK also circulates to the smooth muscle of the gallbladder and the sphincter of Oddi. It promotes gallbladder contraction and sphincter relaxation, resulting in the secretion of bile and pancreatic fluid into the duodenum.
  - Pancreatic enzymes and bile acids in the duodenum may have an inhibitory effect on I cells, controlling CCK secretion (and thus pancreatic and hepatobiliary secretion) with negative feedback.
  - CCK has an additional role in signaling satiety to the hypothalamus of the brain.
- Vagovagal reflexes increase pancreatic and gallbladder secretion.
  - Vagal afferents detect intestinal distention and high luminal osmolality, causing vagal efferents to stimulate the pancreas and gallbladder. This is a typical example of a negative feedback loop.
  - CCK acts on the vagal neurons to potentiate these effects.

Ileocecal Regulation of Motility

The terminal ileum regulates not only the passage of chyme into the colon, but also the motility in proximal parts of the small intestine. The ileal brake serves as a feedback system to improve digestion and absorption:
- Lipids in the ileum suggest that chyme moved too fast through the small intestine for proper digestion and absorption to occur.
- Accordingly, the ileal mucosa reacts to lipids in the ileum by sending an inhibitory signal to the ENS of the upper small intestine.

The presence of food in the stomach triggers increased peristalsis in the ileum called the gastroileal reflex.
- This reflex results in the relaxation of the ileocecal sphincter and subsequent flow of chyme (at this point, mostly composed of indigestible matter and water) into the colon.
- The gastroileal reflex is mediated by gastrin and the extrinsic ANS.

Colonic Motility and Defecation

Because the large intestine retains waste material until almost all water can be absorbed, it is a slower-moving portion of the GI tract. The lower-flow conditions allow bacteria to thrive in the colon, unlike in the small intestine.
- Whereas mammals have developed a symbiotic relationship with the intestinal microflora in the colon (see Ch. 27), even symbiotic bacteria are unwanted in the small intestine because they would purloin nutrients from the host and obstruct the absorptive surface.
- For these reasons, the ileocecal sphincter is a one-way valve, and when the cecum is distended by incoming waste matter, a reflex closes the valve.

Wastes pass through the colon by a slower-wave peristalsis.
- In addition, segmental and nonpropulsive contractions occur randomly in the colon that help release water from waste material for absorption
- Intermittently, giant mass movements of fecal material also occur (1–3 times per day), often after the gastroduodenal distention of a meal.
- The gastrocolic reflex occurs when the presence of food in the stomach increases the frequency of mass movements and the motility of the colon. The reflex has a rapid parasympathetic component that is initiated by gastroduodenal stimulation, such as from stomach stretching by food. CCK and gastrin mediate a slower, hormonal component of the gastrocolic reflex.

Either the baseline slow peristalsis of the large intestine or a mass movement can push waste material (at this point termed *feces*) into the rectum.
- Distention of the rectum leads to the defecation reflex when the rectal pressure exceeds 18 mm Hg.
- The reflex includes ENS peristalsis and a spinal parasympathetic reflex (through the pelvic nerve) with relaxation of the internal anal sphincter.
- The internal anal sphincter is otherwise tonically constricted by sympathetic input.

When the involuntary defecation reflex has begun, several voluntary steps are necessary for defecation, the evacuation of feces from the rectum, to occur.
- First, the external anal sphincter must be consciously relaxed.
- Second, the Valsalva maneuver must usually be used to some degree.

- This is the instinctual, but voluntary, event commonly called straining, in which the abdominal wall muscles are contracted against a closed epiglottis to increase intra-abdominal pressure, thereby helping propel the feces through the anal canal.
- The closure of the epiglottis is necessary to sustain the raised intraabdominal pressure. With it open, the raised pressure would move the diaphragm up, forcing air out of the lungs and expanding the abdominal cavity volume at the expense of the thoracic volume.
- With a closed epiglottis, the diaphragm is fixed in place, and abdominal muscle contraction compresses the fixed volume of the abdominal cavity.

PATHOPHYSIOLOGY

Because disorders of motility or secretion lead to disordered digestion and absorption, some of the important derangements of motility and secretion were described in Chapter 24. To that material we will now add the three most common disorders of GI motility, and introduce several less common disorders of motility and secretion that were not touched upon previously.

Common Disorders

Frequent maladies of the digestive tract and often are brief and self-limiting:
- Vomiting
- Diarrhea
- Constipation

Although they account for a significant number of complaints heard by any general practitioner, treatments are less than perfect.

Vomiting

Vomiting, or emesis, serves the functional purpose of expelling potentially harmful luminal contents from the GI tract.
- The vomiting center in the medulla receives signals from both vagal and sympathetic afferents from the stomach and small intestine.
- The stimulus to vomit is often initiated through this pathway by mucosal irritation or overdistention in the GI tract.
- In addition, many metabolic and psychologic stimuli are transduced into signals affecting the medullary vomiting center.
- The anticipation of vomiting is the subjective sensation of nausea.
  Vomiting commences with antiperistalsis, or reverse peristalsis.
- It can bring contents from as far down the tract as the ileum all the way back to the duodenum.
  - The retrograde accumulation of GI contents distends the duodenum until a threshold is reached.
  - The upper GI sphincters relax, and strong contractions of the duodenum, stomach smooth muscle, and abdominal skeletal muscle force the GI contents up the esophagus and out of the mouth.

Diarrhea

Diarrhea is impaired GI water absorption. It results from derangements of the absorptive surface, from abnormalities in the osmotic gradient for small or large intestine water absorption, and from abnormally rapid transit of chyme and feces through the GI tract.

Infections of the GI tract may cause diarrhea by all three of the aforementioned mechanisms.
- Inflammation around mucosal pathogens obstructs the absorptive surface and leaves solutes in the intestinal lumen that would normally be absorbed.
- Solutes in the lumen pose another obstacle for successful water absorption by creating osmotic pressure to retain water in the gut. The resulting distention of the intestine, in combination with inflammatory irritation of the intestinal wall, can provoke ENS and vagovagal reflexes that increase intestinal motility.
- Psychologic factors (anxiety) may also increase parasympathetic input to the GI tract and increase motility.

Constipation

Constipation is impairment or infrequency of defecation, and it is generally caused by two factors, often seen together.
- Decreased water content in the stool, which reduces the lubrication of the stool inside the colon, thereby impeding its forward movement.
- Depressed intestinal motility, which results in a failure to push the feces out toward the rectum and also causes dry stools. Depressed GI motility leads to dry stools because inadequate peristalsis or mass movements slows the transit time of the feces through the colon. With a longer transit time, the feces are exposed to the absorptive surface for a longer period of time, and more water is withdrawn from the stool.

Inadequate dietary intake of fiber and water is the most common cause of constipation.
- With too little water in the diet, too little water is left in the stool.
- Poor fiber content in the chyme delivered to the cecum leads to constipation in two different ways.
  - Less fiber in the diet means less waste matter in the chyme. Consequently, the waste matter delivered to the colon is less bulky. With a smaller mass of waste material, the colon does not experience as much distention, so the luminal contents inspire weaker peristaltic and parasympathetic reflexes.
  - Less undigested fiber means a lower osmolality in the chyme entering the colon. This promotes water absorption, drying out the stool.

Behavioral factors may also contribute to constipation. A daily rhythm of gastrocolic reflexes and mass movements may be established by a regular eating schedule.
- Irregular meals may interfere with this rhythm and reduce mass movements.
- Similarly, irregular opportunities or uncomfortable circumstances for defecation can interfere with regular evacuation of the bowels.
- The longer the feces sit in one place, the more the GI tract's response to distention is attenuated. ENS peristalsis and spinal reflexes are suppressed, and GI motility declines in the distal colon, worsening the problem. Stoppage breeds more stoppage.

Certain populations are at increased risk for constipation.

- The combination of immobility (and hence decreased opportunities for defecation) and decreased fluid intake seen in the geriatric population makes constipation a frequent problem among the elderly or disabled.
- Pregnant women suffer depressed GI motility under the influence of pregnancy hormones, such as relaxin.
- Anxiety-related irritable bowel syndrome may also cause constipation.

- Patients in the hospital are susceptible to constipation owing to infrequent opportunities or uncomfortable circumstances for defecation.

Whatever the cause of the constipation, increased fluid and fiber intake can reverse it or prevent it. Stool softeners and laxatives may provide short-term aid (see Clinical Correlation Box 25.4).

Clinical Correlation Box 25.4

What Is Small Bowel Obstruction?

A 45-year-old man presents to the emergency department with 36 hours of nausea, vomiting, and unrelieved abdominal pain increasing in severity. His last stool was 24 hours ago, and since then he has not passed gas. On examination, his abdomen is distended and bowel sounds are high-pitched and hyperactive. An upright abdominal x-ray shows air-fluid levels; a supine view shows distended bowel proximal to a point in the right lower quadrant and no gas in the colon. Further questioning reveals a history of abdominal surgery, with an appendectomy performed 3 years previously. The patient is diagnosed with complete small bowel obstruction. He receives intravenous normal saline and precautionary antibiotics, a nasogastric (NG) tube is placed, and he is referred for immediate surgery. Laparotomy reveals an adhesion compressing the small bowel in the right lower quadrant. The adhesion is successfully lysed.

Small bowel obstruction (SBO) arises when the bowel is physically (mechanically) compressed. There are two major causes. One cause is adhesions, intraabdominal scar tissue that binds together loops of intestine and can entangle or compress the bowel. Abdominal surgery can lead to adhesions. Another cause of SBO is the condition in which a loop of intestine herniates through the inguinal canal, cutting off luminal flow and blood flow to this portion of the bowel. This condition is called an incarcerated hernia. Whenever a segment of bowel is compressed in two places, as in an incarcerated hernia, the intestine between the compression sites becomes strangulated. Bowel strangulation, a loss of blood supply, can lead to necrosis of the intestine and perforation, or breakdown in the intestinal wall. Perforation introduces bacteria

into the peritoneal cavity, where the bacteria can grow and lead to sepsis. Sepsis is infection of the blood associated with shock, which is widespread vasodilation and consequent hypotension (low blood pressure). Any obstructed intestine becomes inflamed, however, even if it is not strangulated and necrosed, because the obstruction of gastrointestinal (GI) flow leads to bacterial overgrowth inside the GI tract.

Adynamic or paralytic ileus can mimic SBO. This condition arises in the context of gastroenteritis or after surgery. Gastroenteritis and abdominal surgery may acutely stun the myenteric plexus of the small intestine, temporarily abolishing peristalsis. Food fails to move through, causing backup, distention, and antiperistalsis in the upper GI tract. This is why patients are not allowed to eat after abdominal surgery until they recover their bowel motility, as evidenced by bowel sounds (detectable on auscultation of the abdomen).

Bowel sounds are gurgling sounds made by air and fluid passing through the GI tract. A gurgle is called a borborygmus (plural, borborygmi). SBO, by contrast, leads to high-pitched bowel sounds because the distention stretches the intestinal wall taut and raises the frequency of the sound waves it emits during borborygmi. In addition, distention triggers peristaltic and vagovagal reflexes, leading to hyperactive bowel sounds.

SBO is treated with normal saline to replace fluid lost to the intestinal wall, which is undergoing an inflammatory response. The NG tube decompresses the bowel proximal to the obstruction and relieves nausea and vomiting. Antibiotics guard against sepsis. Surgery relieves the causes of mechanical obstruction.

Less Common Disturbances of Gastrointestinal Regulation

Achalasia is a condition resulting from damage to the myenteric plexus in the lower esophagus. A patient with achalasia does not have normal esophageal peristalsis or normal lower esophageal sphincter opening and hence has an abnormal swallowing reflex. Achalasia is a well known complication of chronic Chagas disease, an infection with Trypanosoma cruzi. Injections of botulinum toxin (botox) can relieve the increased lower esophageal sphincter contractility.

This is in contrast to scleroderma, a condition in which excessive fibrosis leads to esophageal dystrophic changes and loss of normal paristalsis (aperistalsis).

Carcinoid tumors of the GI tract are tumors of enteroendocrine cells.

- Well-differentiated carcinoid tumors may secrete hormones in an unregulated fashion.
- For example, Zollinger-Ellison syndrome is a disorder caused by a gastrin-producing tumor (gastrinoma) in the pancreas or duodenum, which leads to gastric acid hypersecretion and severe peptic ulcer disease.

Hirschsprung disease (congenital aganglionic megacolon) is a developmental problem of the GI track that occurs when there is an absence of the colonic ENS. The migration of cells from the neural crest into the large intestine is not complete and therefore the affected part of the colon cannot relax or pass stool, resulting in an obstruction.

SUMMARY

- GI motility (motor activity) and secretion of enzymes and fluid enable digestion and absorption to take place.
- GI tract motility and secretion are controlled by the CNS, the ENS, and the enteroendocrine cells distributed throughout the GI mucosa.
- The ENS is composed of the myenteric plexus, which controls motility, and the submucosal plexus, which controls secretion and blood flow.
- The CNS and ENS communicate via the parasympathetic and sympathetic nervous systems. The parasympathetic nervous system carries afferent and efferent signals between the two in the vagus nerve (a cranial nerve) and the pelvic nerve (a sacral nerve).
- Motility, the propulsion of food, chyme, and feces through the GI tract, is achieved mainly through peristalsis and vagovagal reflexes. Peristalsis is a myenteric reflex in which luminal distention leads to contraction behind and dilatation in front of a bolus of food, driving the bolus forward. Vagovagal reflexes augment peristalsis and coordinate GI contractions with sphincter dilatations and secretions.
- Gastric acid secretion is controlled through enteroendocrine G cells. Vagal input and amino acids on the mucosa stimulate

G cells to release the hormone gastrin, which triggers ECL cells to secrete the paracrine factor histamine. Histamine and vagal input trigger the gastric parietal cells to secrete H^+.
- Enteroendocrine S cells in the duodenal mucosa respond to the low pH of chyme by releasing the hormone secretin into the bloodstream. Secretin stimulates pancreatic secretion.
- Enteroendocrine I cells in the duodenal mucosa respond to luminal proteins, lipids, and their cleavage products by secreting the hormone CCK into the bloodstream. CCK stimulates pancreatic secretion and gallbladder contraction.
- When feces reach the rectum, an autonomic pelvic nerve reflex initiates defecation. Conscious, voluntary compliance with this reflex in the form of external anal sphincter relaxation (and often voluntary straining) is necessary for defecation to be completed.
- Vomiting occurs by antiperistalsis.
- Diarrhea is impaired GI water absorption. Hypermotility plays a role in diarrhea.
- Constipation is impairment or infrequency of defecation. A lack of bulk in the stool (i.e., lack of fiber) reduces colonic motility.

REVIEW QUESTIONS

Directions: Each of the numbered items or incomplete statements in this section is followed by answers or by completions of the statement. Select the one lettered answer or completion that is best in each case.

1. A woman with rectal bleeding is found on examination to have a thrombosed hemorrhoid. Which of the following conditions might predispose her to developing hemorrhoids?
   A. She has had repeated bouts of infectious gastroenteritis in the past year.
   B. She is a vegetarian with a high-fiber diet.
   C. She is in her third trimester of pregnancy.
   D. She has Zollinger-Ellison syndrome.
   E. She abuses laxatives.
2. H2 blockers are sometimes used in the treatment of heartburn symptoms because:
   A. Overproduction of gastric acid is the most common cause of heartburn.
   B. H2 blockers prevent reflux.
   C. H2 blockers improve lower esophageal sphincter tone.
   D. H_2 blockers inhibit the H^+/K^+-ATPase.
   E. H2 blockers can help control heartburn symptoms.
3. A 70-year-old man has suffered several small strokes in his medulla. Since then, he can initiate swallowing but has not

been able to move food all the way from his esophagus to his stomach. The stroke has probably disabled:
   A. The salivatory nucleus
   B. The nucleus ambiguus
   C. The dorsal motor nucleus of the vagus nerve
   D. ENS peristalsis
   E. The myenteric plexus
4. A 39-year-old woman has severe epigastric pain for several days. She has had five peptic ulcers in the past 3 years. Her fasting gastrin level is 800 pg/dL (elevated). What is the most likely diagnosis?
   A. Small bowel obstruction
   B. Food poisoning
   C. Pancreatitis
   D. Zollinger-Ellison syndrome
   E. Celiac disease
5. Which of the following is not considered an endocrine hormone?
   A. Gastrin
   B. Norepinephrine
   C. Secretin
   D. Motilin
   E. Glucose-dependent insulinotropic polypeptide (GIP)

ANSWERS TO REVIEW QUESTIONS

1. **The answer is C.** Pregnancy slows GI motility, leading to constipation, which is the usual cause of hemorrhoids. Constipation causes hemorrhoids by requiring straining with high intraabdominal pressures. Gastroenteritis, a high-fiber diet, and laxative abuse would cause diarrhea. Zollinger-Ellison syndrome would cause peptic ulcer.

2. **The answer is E.** H2 blockers control heartburn symptoms by lowering the acidity of gastric secretions. They do not prevent reflux. They do not reinforce the lower esophageal sphincter as surgical fundoplication does. They do not inhibit the H^+/K^+-ATPase as omeprazole does. They block the histamine receptor and thereby prevent activation of the parietal cell. Overproduction of acid is not the cause of reflux; lower esophageal sphincter incompetence and gastric distention are.

3. **The answer is C.** The dorsal motor nucleus of the vagus nerve sends out signals that open the lower esophageal sphincter. The ENS is not affected by a CNS stroke.

4. **The answer is D.** Hypersecretion of gastrin from a gastrinoma will result in an elevated gastric acid output. The patient also has a history of recurrent peptic ulcers suggesting Zollinger-Ellison syndrome.

5. **The answer is B.** Norepinephrine is released from the sympathetic axon terminals throughout the GI tract and is considered a neurocrine factor.

26

Hepatic Physiology

INTRODUCTION

The kidney modifies the contents of the plasma by filtering its components into the urine, whereas the liver modifies the blood contents by metabolically transforming them. The liver is where drugs, hormones, and toxic waste products, such as ammonia, are metabolized to inactive forms.

The liver also plays an important role in carbohydrate metabolism. Specifically, the liver is involved in:

- Glycogen storage.
- Gluconeogenesis.
- Formation of many biochemical compounds from products of carbohydrate digestion and absorption.
  The liver also synthesizes:
- Cholesterol, phospholipids, and most of the lipoproteins required by the body (see Ch. 24).
- Nonessential amino acids and major plasma proteins, including albumin and clotting factor.
  This brief chapter will focus on the liver's role in detoxification and the synthesis of blood proteins.

SYSTEM STRUCTURE

The liver is situated in the right upper quadrant of the abdomen. It has a dual blood supply from the hepatic artery and the portal vein.

- The hepatic artery, which branches off the celiac trunk, is oxygen-rich but nutrient-poor and provides the liver with 20% to 30% of its blood supply.
- The portal vein, which carries blood from the digestive tract, pancreas, and spleen, is oxygen-poor but nutrient-rich and provides the liver with 70% to 80% of its blood supply.

Both of these vessels enter the liver at the porta hepatis, which is also the site at which the common hepatic bile duct leaves the liver. These three vessels—artery, portal vein, and bile duct—form the portal triad. The three vessels of the portal triad divide and subdivide together through the hepatic parenchyma, separating the liver into functional segments called lobules.

Lobules are hexagonal groups of hepatocytes bounded by portal triads at each corner. In the center of each hexagon is a central vein.

- The arterial and portal venous blood mix as they flow toward the center of the lobule in the spaces between hepatocytes called sinusoids (Fig. 26.1).
- The sinusoids empty into the lobular central vein(s), which join together in collecting veins, which coalesce into hepatic veins.
- Hepatic veins leave the liver and empty into the vena cava.

The plates of hepatocytes in the lobule are one or two cells thick, with sinusoids on either side.

- Bile canaliculi, into which bile is secreted, run between hepatocytes and ferry bile away from the center of the lobule and out to the bile duct at the hexagonal corners (Fig. 26.2).
- The endothelium of hepatocytes lacks a basement membrane, which facilitates the exchange between hepatocytes and the blood.
- Specialized macrophages, called Kupffer cells, line the sinusoidal epithelium on the bloodstream side and are involved in host defense and recycling body iron.

The location in the liver between a hepatocyte and a sinusoid is called the space of Disse or the perisinusoidal space.

- Fenestrations and endothelial discontinuity makes this region highly permeable to the exchange of solutes between the hepatocytes and sinusoidal blood plasma.
- The space of Disse contains hepatic stellate cells, which play an important role in storing fat soluble vitamins, such as vitamin A.
- Inflammation to these cells, such as following liver injury, results in collagen production in the space of Disse, fibrosis, and impaired hepatic function.

The functions of the liver are performed by the various hepatocyte organelles.

- The mitochondria of hepatocytes have enzymes that take part in the urea cycle.
- The smooth endoplasmic reticulum (ER) is the site of glycogen synthesis, the conjugation of bilirubin, and the detoxification of foreign substances.
- The rough ER is the site of the synthesis of plasma proteins, such as albumin, fibrinogen, and prothrombin.
- Lysosomes take part in the receptor-mediated endocytosis of lipoproteins, such as low-density lipoprotein (LDL) and high-density lipoprotein (HDL), as well as chylomicrons.
- Hepatocyte peroxisomes remove peroxide generated by oxidases, and they are the site of long-chain fatty acid oxidation.
- The Golgi apparatus is responsible for the glycosylation and secretion of plasma proteins, such as transferrin, and lipoproteins, such as very-low-density lipoprotein (VLDL).

SYSTEM FUNCTION

As stated earlier, this chapter will focus on just a few of the liver functions that have not been detailed in other chapters. Particular aspects of liver physiology are helpful not only in predicting the consequences of disease, but also in understanding the clinical signs and symptoms by which liver disease is diagnosed.

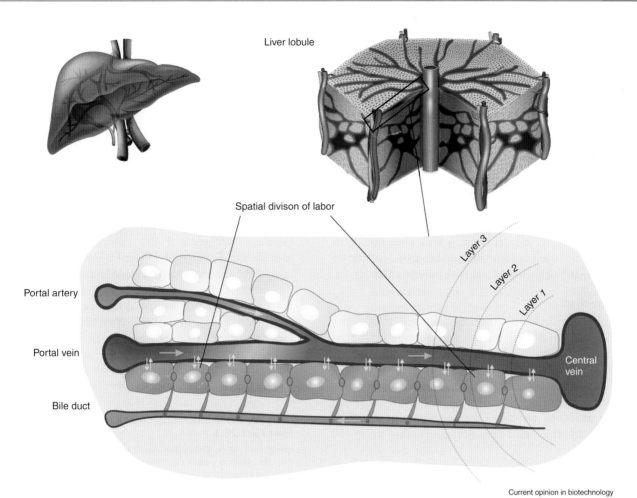

Fig. 26.1 Hepatic microcirculation. The bile canaliculi arise between two cells, and the bile ducts arise within the lobule between two plates of hepatocytes apposed with one another. (From Moor AE, Itzkovitz S. Spatial transcriptomics: paving the way for tissue-level systems biology. *Curr Opin Biotechnol.* 2017;46:126-133. Fig. 2.)

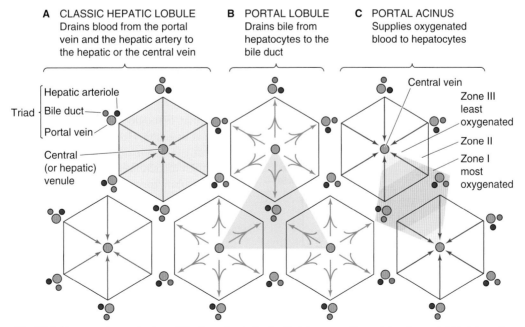

Fig. 26.2 Hexagonal organization of the liver. Central vein; Portal space with contains the portal triad: hepatic artery (*red*), portal vein (*blue*), bile duct (*green*). (From Boron W, Boulpaep E. *Medical Physiology*, 3rd Edition. Elsevier; 2016. Fig. 46.3.)

Detoxifying Actions of the Liver

We will focus on three significant detoxifying mechanisms within the liver:
- Drug metabolism
- Ammonia metabolism
- Metabolism of bilirubin (a breakdown product of heme from red blood cells and the cause of jaundice)

These processes are not hormonally controlled; they are governed by the kinetics of hepatic enzyme-substrate interactions.
- In other words, when more toxic substrate is present in the blood, the rate of enzymatic reactions in the liver increases.
- When the enzymes are saturated, which does not occur under physiologic circumstances, the toxic substrates accumulate in the blood and can have adverse effects.

Drug Metabolism

The liver plays a critical role in the transformation of drugs and xenobiotic compounds into inactive and hydrophilic (water-soluble) substances that are readily eliminated from the body through bile or urine.

Two sets of enzymatic reactions take place in hepatocytes to serve these purposes (Fig. 26.3).
- Phase I reactions are slow, energy-consuming reactions catalyzed by the heme-containing cytochrome P-450 enzymes.
  - These reactions result in oxidation, reduction, or hydrolysis of the parent compound.
  - Three gene superfamilies (I, II, III) encode different cytochrome P-450 enzymes, each with different substrate specificities.
  - Sometimes a phase I reaction alone is adequate to inactivate a drug and prepare it for elimination. Often, however, the phase I product is a toxic intermediate such as a free radical that must be inactivated by a phase II conjugation reaction.

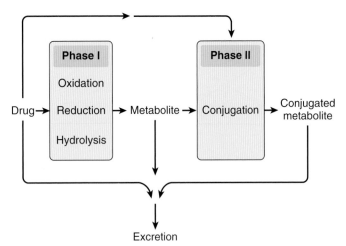

Fig. 26.3 Drug inactivation. Some drugs are excreted without modification, some after phase I, some after phase II. Some drugs undergo phase II conjugation reactions without ever undergoing a phase I reaction by a cytochrome P-450 enzyme.

- Phase II reactions, which are much faster and less energy-dependent than phase I reactions, add bulky polar groups to the metabolites of the phase I reactions, inactivating them and rendering them even more water-soluble.

Most of the enzymes involved in phase I and phase II reactions are located in the smooth ER of hepatocytes, so that toxic metabolites cannot interact with the rest of the cell.

Recall from renal physiology that the clearance of a compound from the blood by an organ is the volume of plasma rid of the substance by that organ per unit time. Drug clearance varies in different contexts.
- Newborns, whose cytochrome P-450 enzymes are poorly developed, clear drugs more slowly, as do older adults.
- Genetic cytochrome P-450 polymorphisms have been identified in members of different ethnic groups, which may contribute to altered metabolism of certain drugs.
- The presence of a second drug in the plasma may also affect the metabolism of the first drug (e.g., by inducing the expression of cytochrome P-450 enzymes, thereby increasing clearance of the first drug).
- Certain foods have also been found to interact with medications as a result of interference with the hepatic and intestinal cytochrome P-450 enzymes (see Fast Fact Box 26.1).

Fast Fact 26.1

Grapefruit and grapefruit juices contain furanocoumarin derivatives that inhibit cytochrome P450 enzymes and subsequently increase the bioavailability of certain drugs.

The Elimination of Bilirubin

Bilirubin is a yellow pigment formed from the hemoglobin of old red blood cells by macrophages.
- Bilirubin gives the yellowish hue to a healing bruise, and the metabolites of bilirubin give the yellow color to urine and the brown color to feces.
- However, before bilirubin gets into either urine or feces, it must be removed from the bloodstream and transformed by the liver.

Recall that hemoglobin contains heme—a porphyrin ring with iron at its center. Heme is metabolized inside macrophages to biliverdin (a green pigment, also seen in healing bruises), which is then metabolized to bilirubin (Fig. 26.4).
- The bilirubin formed in this process is insoluble and is referred to as unconjugated bilirubin, or indirect bilirubin.
- Unconjugated bilirubin is carried in the blood tightly bound to the blood protein albumin and is taken up by hepatocytes.

In the hepatocytes, bilirubin is conjugated in the smooth ER to glucuronic acid by the enzyme glucuronyltransferase.
- After conjugation, it is known as conjugated bilirubin (also bilirubin diglucuronide or direct bilirubin), and it is water-soluble.
- Conjugated bilirubin is secreted into the bile canaliculus and is expelled in bile from the gallbladder to the duodenum.

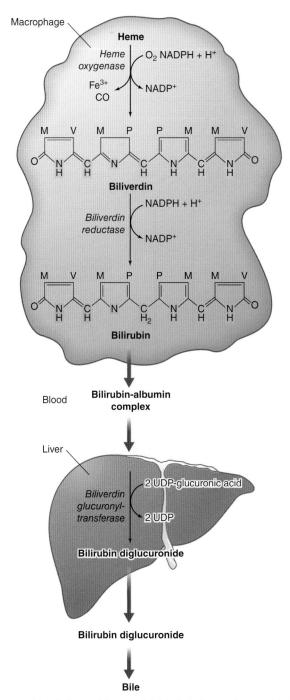

Fig. 26.4 Metabolism of heme. *M*, Methyl; *P*, propionate; *V*, vinyl. The conversion of heme to bilirubin consists of a two-step reaction catalyzed by heme oxygenase, which converts heme to biliverdin, and biliverdin reductase, which converts biliverdin to bilirubin. Note that the drawing is not drawn to scale: the liver is the largest organ in the abdomen, whereas a macrophage is only one cell.

- Conjugated bilirubin is deconjugated and reduced by intestinal bacteria to urobilinogen.
  - Some of the urobilinogen is reabsorbed by the enterocytes. This urobilinogen circulates to the kidney where it is oxidized to urobilin and excreted in the urine (hence urine's yellow color).
  - The urobilinogen remaining in the intestine is oxidized to stercobilin, which colors feces brown (Fig. 26.5).

Jaundice, a yellow pigmenting of the skin, is because of hyperbilirubinemia, high levels of bilirubin in the blood.
- Hyperbilirubinemia may be caused by
  - The increased breakdown of red blood cells (hemolysis).
  - The failed excretion of bilirubin in the bile.
- If the blood contains high levels of indirect (unconjugated) bilirubin, this is most consistent with a hemolytic cause of jaundice.
- If the blood contains high levels of direct (conjugated) bilirubin, it suggests a disorder of the liver itself.
- Severe hyperbilirubinemia in newborns can lead to kernicterus, where bilirubin accumulation in the basal ganglia, hippocampus, or brain stem causes neurologic impairment or death. Different mutations in the gene encoding UDP-glucuronosyltransferase can result in either a relatively mild or a severe form of hyperbilirubinemia. Since these conditions impair conjugation, patients have an indirect hyperbilirubinemia. The mild version is called Gilbert's syndrome, and typically is not clinically significant except that patient may have jaundice if they take certain medications or if they have hemolysis. The severe forms are called Crigler-Najjar syndrome, in which case the indirect hyperbilirubinemia can damage the central nervous system and may even lead to death within months of birth.
- In adults, hyperbilirubinemia can result from a number of conditions including infection with the Chinese liver fluke Chlonorchis sinensis (see Environmental Box 26.1, Oncology Box 26.1, and Pharmacology Box 26.1).

🏠 ENVIRONMENTAL BOX 26.1

Ingestion of raw or undercooked freshwater fish in endemic areas, such as the Far East can lead to infection with *Clonorchis sinensis*, the Chinese liver fluke, and species of the genus *Opisthorchis*. Once ingested, this parasite can enter the bile ducts, mature over the course of 4 weeks, and then reside in small to medium sized bile ducts, the pancreatic duct, or the gallbladder for up to decades. Acutely, patients by asymptomatic or may have right upper quadrant abdominal pain, diarrhea, and fatigue. Chronically, in addition to the acute symptoms, patients can develop gall stones (forming around dead worms), biliary obstruction (from stones or worms), anorexia, and unintentional weight loss

✳ ONCOLOGY BOX 26.1

Patients with a chronic, high burden of liver flukes may develop a malignancy of the biliary system called cholangiocarcinoma. Symptoms of this form of cancer may include abdominal pain and a palpable mass, unintentional weight loss, jaundice, and the accumulation of peritoneal fluid called ascites.

🔖 PHARMACOLOGY BOX 26.1

The antihelminthic agent praziquantel is the drug of choice for eradication of liver flukes. Alternatives include albendazole, mebendazole, and tribendimidine.

The Elimination of Ammonia

Ammonia is formed during the metabolism of amino acids.

If ammonia were not transformed into urea in the liver, it would bind α-ketoglutarate to form glutamate in the brain.
- Depletion of α-ketoglutarate saps the citric acid cycle of an important intermediary and leaves the neurons short on adenosine triphosphate (ATP).

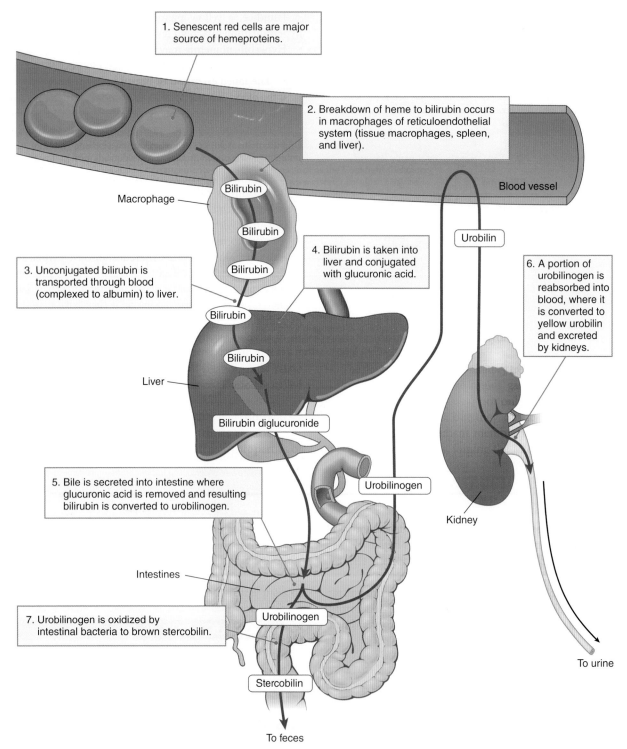

1. Senescent red cells are major source of hemeproteins.

2. Breakdown of heme to bilirubin occurs in macrophages of reticuloendothelial system (tissue macrophages, spleen, and liver).

Blood vessel

Bilirubin

Macrophage

Bilirubin

Urobilin

4. Bilirubin is taken into liver and conjugated with glucuronic acid.

Bilirubin

6. A portion of urobilinogen is reabsorbed into blood, where it is converted to yellow urobilin and excreted by kidneys.

3. Unconjugated bilirubin is transported through blood (complexed to albumin) to liver.

Bilirubin

Bilirubin

Liver

Bilirubin diglucuronide

Urobilinogen

5. Bile is secreted into intestine where glucuronic acid is removed and resulting bilirubin is converted to urobilinogen.

Kidney

Intestines

7. Urobilinogen is oxidized by intestinal bacteria to brown stercobilin.

Urobilinogen

To urine

Stercobilin

To feces

Fig. 26.5 Excretion of heme byproducts. Although it is not shown, some of the reabsorbed urobilinogen is resecreted in bile in addition to being excreted in urine. (Modified from Kumar V, Abbas A, Aster J. Robbins & Cotran. *Pathologic Basis of Disease*, 9th Edition. Elsevier; 2014. Fig. 18.27.)

- In addition, glutamate can pick up another ammonia to form glutamine, decreasing glutamate and its metabolic product, gamma-amino butyric acid (GABA).
- Thus the major neurotransmitters are depleted (glutamate and GABA) while the excess glutamine within brain cells acts osmotically to increase cell water, leading to cerebral edema.

- These metabolic effects can lead to alterations in mental status and ultimately to coma and death.

Hence the hepatic urea cycle is critical for the organism's survival. This cycle is described thoroughly in biochemistry texts, but will not be fully explored within this text (see Fast Fact Box 26.2).

Albumin

Hepatocytes are the site of the synthesis of clotting factors (see Ch. 7) and the synthesis of albumin, the most important blood protein.

Albumin has three critical functions:

- Maintaining intravascular oncotic pressure.
  - Albumin makes up half of the normal intravascular protein content and thus is essential for holding water inside the blood vessels.
  - Albumin is also the main protein found in the interstitium or extravascular space (though it exists here in lower concentrations than in blood).
- Binding and transport of hormones, drugs, and other blood-borne factors.
- Binding free radicals (see Fast Fact Box 26.3).

Because albumin is not stored, it cannot be released "on demand." At any time, 10% to 60% of hepatocytes are actively synthesizing albumin.

- The liver can only increase its albumin production by a factor of 2 to 3, but albumin production is sensitive to changes in the intravascular oncotic pressure.
- When the intravascular oncotic pressure falls, the rate of albumin synthesis increases.
- Albumin synthesis is also influenced by hormones, such as insulin, glucagon, thyroxine, and cortisol.

PATHOPHYSIOLOGY

A number of processes can lead to liver dysfunction. When the dysfunction is severe, it is called liver failure. Causes of liver failure include:

- Viral hepatitis (inflammation of the liver because of viral infection, such as infection with hepatitis B virus).
- Drug toxicity (including alcoholic hepatitis).
- Autoimmune hepatitis.
- Metabolic diseases, such as Wilson disease and hemochromatosis (see Clinical Correlation Box 25.1 and 26.2).

A common endpoint of all chronic liver conditions is scarring of the liver. Irreversible scarring is referred to as cirrhosis. One mechanism of chronic liver inflammation that can lead to cirrhosis is Schistosomiasis, an infection with the blood fluke Schistosoma mansoni (Western hemisphere) or Schistosoma japonicum. As opposed to cirrhosis induced by chronic damage from alcohol (see below), patients with end stage liver disease from Schistosomiasis develop varices that can hemorrhage, but do not develop hepatic encephalopathy.

Other causes of cirrhosis include chronic pancreatitis and non-alcoholic steatohepatitis (NASH).

Inflammation and cirrhosis of the liver have predictable results. Because the liver is the principal site of energy metabolism, liver disease can interfere with these anabolic and catabolic functions.

- Altered carbohydrate metabolism in patients with cirrhosis can result in impaired glucose metabolism manifesting with hyperglycemia or hypoglycemia.
- Altered lipid metabolism can result in hyperlipidemia, which can manifest as subcutaneous accumulations of cholesterol called xanthomas.
- Altered protein synthesis and degradation result in decreased levels of serum albumin and clotting factors, which contribute to the development of edema and coagulopathy (abnormal blood clotting), respectively.
- Reduced levels of albumin and other carrier proteins in the blood can also lead to increased levels of free (unbound) hormones or drugs, leading to unpredictable pharmacokinetics.
- The metabolism of drugs, hormones, and toxic byproducts may be inadequate in liver failure. The consequences are longer drug and hormone half-lives and the accumulation of toxic agents like ammonia, as described earlier above.

In addition to interfering with metabolic liver functions, cirrhosis also interferes with the function of the liver mechanically.

- Scar tissue, which accumulates as a result of increased collagen production by hepatic stellate cells, prevents blood from flowing easily through the liver tissue. This reduces permeability across the space of Disse and the fenestrated sinusoidal endothelium.
- Consequently, low-pressure portal venous blood cannot easily get to the central veins of the liver lobules, and blood backs up in the portal system.

As more portal blood is delivered than can be removed, portal blood pressure rises; this condition is called portal hypertension.

- Portal hypertension may cause fluid to weep from the liver capsule. This fluid is called *ascites*, and it accumulates in the peritoneal cavity, where it poses an infection risk (as low-flow conditions always do by providing bacteria purchase on cell membranes and extracellular proteins).

- In addition, the loss of fluid from the intravascular space decreases the systemic blood pressure, stimulating the kidneys to retain more salt and water. This worsens the portal hypertension, more ascites develops, and more water is retained in a vicious cycle.

Portal hypertension also forces portal blood into collateral paths from the portal system to the inferior vena cava.

- A portosystemic route of communication expands in the gastroesophageal area, leading to dilated veins known as esophageal varices, which are susceptible to bleeding.
- Furthermore, portosystemic routes of venous return to the vena cava represent a shunt past the liver, which bypasses metabolism of toxic substances and thereby worsening the consequences of liver failure.

Finally, disease may also affect the biliary system.

- Inflammation of the gallbladder and bile ducts is called cholecystitis. A common cause of cholecystitis is gallstones (which in turn result from supersaturation of bile with cholesterol among other causes).
- When the biliary ducts (cystic duct, hepatic duct, or common bile duct) are blocked, the condition is described as cholestasis. Cholestasis prevents bile from reaching the intestine where it normally emulsifies fats, leading to maldigestion. When a gallstone blocks the pancreatic duct, it may lead to acute pancreatitis.

The Assessment of Liver Function

Liver dysfunction is reflected in various blood tests. The three best indicators of liver function are as follows.

Prothrombin Time

- Prothrombin is one of the blood clotting factors, and the prothrombin time is the rate at which prothrombin is converted to thrombin in the cascade of activation events that lead to blood clotting.
- When hepatic synthesis of clotting factors is impaired, the prothrombin time is increased.
- Clotting factors produced in the liver, with vitamin K as a cofactor, are factors II (prothrombin), VII, IX, and X.
  - These factors have in common a posttranslational protein modification of glutamic acid residues to œí-carboxyglutamic acid (GLA), which, as a dicarboxylic acid, allows for Ca^{2+} binding.
  - These vitamin K-dependent and calcium-dependent reactions are blocked by the anticoagulant warfarin.

Serum Bilirubin

- Serum bilirubin levels may be elevated in either hepatic or biliary disease, both of which impair the clearance of bilirubin from the blood.
- The retention of bilirubin can lead to jaundice (discussed earlier), and the retention of bile salts can lead to pruritus (itching) because of the deposition of bile salts in the skin.

- Conjugated bilirubin is water-soluble and present in plasma water. Thus it is filtered by the renal glomeruli and appears as a pigment in the urine in the case of hepatic disease.
- In contrast, unconjugated bilirubin is heavily albumin-bound so it is not filtered, nor secreted into the urine when plasma levels are increased.

Serum Albumin

- Although low serum albumin can be a sign of liver disease, hypoalbuminemia takes weeks to develop because of the long half-life of albumin, and it is therefore not a reliable measure of hepatic synthetic function in acute liver disease.

The presence of certain liver-specific enzymes in the blood also serves as an indicator of liver disease:

- Aspartate aminotransferase (AST)
- Alanine aminotransferase (ALT)
  - ALT is more specific than AST for measuring hepatocellular injury, as AST is also found in muscle, kidney, brain, pancreas, and red blood cells.

The leakage of these enzymes into the circulation is a marker for ongoing hepatocellular inflammation. Whereas bilirubin levels may be elevated in cholestasis or intrinsic liver disease, AST and ALT are more specific for intrinsic liver disease (see Fast Fact Box 26.4).

Fast Fact 26.4

An aspartate aminotransferase (AST)/alanine aminotransferase (ALT) ratio greater than 2:1 is found most often in alcoholic liver disease.

Alternatively, an ALT that is greater than the AST is suggestive of viral hepatitis.

Alkaline phosphatase (ALP) is present in the hepatocyte canalicular plasma membrane and the luminal membrane of bile duct epithelium.

- In cholestatic states, the bile acid accumulation stimulates the synthesis and release of ALP. Hence elevated ALP levels are indicative of cholestasis.
  - ALP is also found in a number of other tissues, including bone. The source of an elevated ALP can be confirmed by measuring the levels of 5'-nucleotidase and gamma-glutamyl transpeptidase (GGT).
  - If 5'-nucleotidase and GGT levels are also increased, the elevated ALP is likely from liver and not from bone.
- GGT is often elevated in people who consume three or more alcoholic drinks per day. It is a measure of immoderate intake and can be used to confirm sobriety in alcoholics (see Clinical Correlation Box 26.3).

Clinical Correlation Box 26.3

What Is Alcoholic Hepatitis?

A 60-year-old woman presents with fatigue, nausea, vomiting, and abdominal distention. She noticed that her abdomen has been swelling slowly over the past few weeks. Her past medical history is significant for ovarian cancer, which was treated with chemotherapy without recurrence, and high blood pressure, for which she is taking a β-blocker called atenolol. She consumes, on average, two beers and mixed drinks each day with no concomitant illegal drug use. On physical examination, there is moderate ascites and an enlarged liver and spleen. Her laboratory findings include total bilirubin 1.4 mg/dL (normal 0.1–1.0 mg/dL), alkaline phosphatase 373 U/L (20–70 U/L), aspartate aminotransferase (AST) 79 U/L (8–20 U/L), alanine aminotransferase (ALT) 34 U/L (8–20 U/L), albumin 2.9 g/dL (3.5–5.5 g/dL), and prothrombin time 16.9 seconds (11–15 seconds). Computed tomography scan reveals ascites and an enlarged liver with no masses. A liver biopsy shows hepatocyte injury and necrosis, fatty changes, inflammation, and fibrosis.

This is a classic example of alcoholic hepatitis. Alcohol abuse remains the leading cause of hepatitis and cirrhosis in the United States. The patient has a history of excessive alcohol consumption. She has an AST/ALT ratio of greater than 2:1. The pathologic changes evident on her liver biopsy are consistent with alcoholic hepatitis, which involves "fatty change," or steatosis. Steatosis, the deposition of excess fat in the liver, results from the activity of alcohol dehydrogenase, which yields excess nicotinamide adenine dinucleotide phosphate (NADPH). NADPH stimulates lipid production. The decreased serum albumin concentration and increased prothrombin time together reflect chronic liver disease, with the serum albumin contributing, along with portal hypertension, to the development of ascites. The increase in total bilirubin is consistent with impaired hepatic clearance because of injury and necrosis. The elevated alkaline phosphatase is reflective of the fatty liver changes and fibrosis, which interfere with biliary secretion.

SUMMARY

- The liver modifies the blood contents by metabolically transforming them.
- The liver is a major site of the synthesis of glycogen, glucose, and ketone bodies, thereby playing a fundamental role in energy metabolism.
- The liver governs cholesterol metabolism, mediating its transport to the peripheral tissues and its excretion from the body. The liver also mediates fat absorption by secreting bile (an emulsifier) into the duodenum.
- The liver produces albumin and the clotting factors.
- The liver metabolizes drugs, hormones, and toxic byproducts.
- Hepatic cytochrome P-450 enzymes conduct phase I reactions to detoxify drugs, in which the drug is oxidized, reduced, or hydrolyzed. Phase II reactions are conjugation reactions that inactivate toxic metabolites from phase I. Both phase I and phase II render toxic agents more water-soluble to enhance their elimination in urine or bile.
- Bilirubin, a metabolite of heme from red blood cells, is conjugated in hepatocytes and excreted in bile. Bilirubin is reduced to urobilinogen in the intestine.
- Some urobilinogen is reabsorbed into the blood and oxidized and excreted by the kidney as urobilin. Some urobilinogen remains in the intestine and is oxidized to stercobilin.

- The hepatic urea cycle inactivates free ammonia, a product of protein metabolism.
- Albumin creates oncotic pressure in the blood, helping to hold water inside the blood vessels, and serves as a transport protein for hormones, drugs, electrolytes, and other agents.
- A common endpoint of various types of liver diseases is cirrhosis, the scarring and dysfunction of liver tissue.
- Liver failure reduces albumin production and clotting factor production with predictable results: edema and clotting abnormalities. Cirrhosis and hypoalbuminemia together contribute to the formation of ascites—cirrhosis by creating portal hypertension, hypoalbuminemia by lowering oncotic pressure.
- Cholestasis is obstruction of the biliary ducts.
- Hemolysis, intrinsic liver disease, and cholestasis lead to high levels of bilirubin in the blood and jaundice. Hepatic hyperbilirubinemia leads to high conjugated bilirubin levels; hemolytic hyperbilirubinemia leads to high unconjugated bilirubin levels.
- Levels of AST and ALT are high in intrinsic liver disease. Levels of ALP are high in cholestasis.
- Alcoholism is the most common cause of cirrhosis.

REVIEW QUESTIONS

Directions: Each of the numbered items or incomplete statements in this section is followed by answers or by completions of the statement. Select the one lettered answer or completion that is best in each case.

1. A 48-year-old man with a long history of alcoholism suffers hematemesis and is treated with balloon tamponade. The source of his bleeding is likely to be:
   A. The central veins of the hepatic lobules
   B. The hepatic sinusoids
   C. The left gastroepiploic artery
   D. Esophageal varices
   E. The splenic vein

2. A 43-year-old woman is evaluated for jaundice. She has an elevated total bilirubin level and her direct (conjugated) bilirubin level is 1 mg/dL. AST is 35 U/L, ALT is 41 U/L, and alkaline phosphatase is 197 U/L. Her prothrombin time is 15 seconds and her albumin level is 3.4 g/dL. Sonography shows that her gallbladder diameter is more than 4 cm. The cause of her jaundice is probably:
   A. Alcoholic steatohepatitis
   B. Autoimmune hepatitis
   C. Acute pancreatitis
   D. Hemolytic anemia
   E. Cholestasis

3. Which of the following substances present in urine accounts for its yellow color?
   A. Heme
   B. Bilirubin
   C. Urobilinogen
   D. Urobilin
   E. Stercobilin
4. What cell type in the liver removes intestinal bacteria that enter the portal circulation?
   A. Hepatic stellate cells
   B. Kupffer cells
   C. Hepatocytes
   D. Fenestrated sinusoidal cells
   E. Ito cells
5. A 27-year-old woman is evaluated for cirrhosis. Genetic analysis reveals a mutation in a hepatocyte copper transporting ATPase. Slit lamp examination of the eyes is remarkable for Kayser-Fleischer rings. What is the likely diagnosis?
   A. Hepatic adenoma
   B. Jaundice
   C. Hepatic steatosis
   D. Wilson disease
   E. Alcoholic hepatitis

ANSWERS TO REVIEW QUESTIONS

1. **The answer is D.** Alcoholism is the most common cause of cirrhosis. Chronic cirrhosis leads to portal hypertension, which creates fragile venous collaterals called esophageal varices. Alcoholics with esophageal varices frequently bleed into the upper gastrointestinal tract and vomit blood (hematemesis).
2. **The answer is E.** A distended gallbladder is suggestive of biliary obstruction and cholestasis. The elevated direct bilirubin level rules out hemolysis as the cause of jaundice. Cholestasis can cause pancreatitis, but pancreatitis does not cause jaundice.
3. **The answer is D.** Bilirubin is secreted in bile and reduced to urobilinogen in the intestine. Urobilinogen is absorbed into the bloodstream. Before excreting it, the kidney oxidizes urobilinogen to urobilin, which gives urine its yellow color.
4. **The answer is B.** Kupffer cells are phagocytic cells that destroy bacteria and foreign proteins as part of their role in host defense.
5. **The answer is D.** Kayser-Fleischer rings are a pathognomonic sign of Wilson disease. The disease is also characterized by hemolytic anemia, asterixis, dementia, and basal ganglia degeneration, most of which are the result of copper accumulation throughout the body.

27

The Gastrointestinal Immune System

INTRODUCTION

As described in Chapter 8, the immune system is a complex cellular network that defends the body against danger. To do so, the immune system must distinguish between safe and dangerous substances.

- Safe or nonthreatening substances can be part of the body itself (e.g., normal extracellular molecules, cells, and tissues) or foreign (e.g., foods and commensal bacterial).
- Dangerous materials can be part of the body (e.g., cancer cells) or foreign (e.g., pathogenic bacteria, viruses, and parasites).

With each meal, we ingest an enormous number of nonself molecules, many of which are potential antigens. Thus the enteric immune system is one of the largest tissue-specific immune organs in the body, as it must defend the enormous surface area of the gastrointestinal (GI) tract.

ENTERIC IMMUNE SYSTEM STRUCTURE

The immune system of the GI tract can be divided into "nonimmunologic" and "immunologic" defenses.

- Nonimmunologic defenses
  - Mechanical barriers (epithelial cells, the mucous layer of the GI tract called the glycocalyx)
  - Mechanical actions (the peristaltic movement of the GI tract)
  - Components of GI secretions (gastric hydrochloric acid)
  - Commensal or symbiotic nonpathogenic GI microorganisms (which compete with potential pathogens for space and nutrients)
- Immunologic defenses
  - Immune cells that either reside in or patrol the GI tract
  - Immune system molecules produced by such cells

Gastrointestinal Immune System Tissues
Nonimmune Tissues
The epithelial lining is arguably the most important nonimmune tissue component of the GI defenses.

- In the oral cavity stratified, squamous epithelial lining prevents microorganisms from penetrating into deeper tissues.
- In the stomach, small intestine, and large intestine, epithelial cells held together by tight junctions provide a similar barrier through which antigens cannot pass (Fig. 27.1).

Immune Tissues
The gut-associated lymphoid tissue (GALT) is composed of innate and adaptive immune cells arranged in a pattern similar to that in lymph nodes and the spleen. GALT is located throughout the GI tract in the lamina propria, just beneath the epithelial lining.

- The tonsils are the largest GALT of the oropharynx and can be seen on physical examination.
- Peyer's patches are found throughout the small intestine, although the majority of them are found in the ileum and jejunum. they contain 200 to 400 lymphoid follicles.
- The large intestine does not have Peyer's patches but does have numerous GALT follicles. The appendix especially has large aggregates of such lymphoid tissue.

Mesenteric lymph nodes are typical lymph nodes located in the gut mesentery. Lymphatic channels form the lamina propria of the small intestine (called lacteals) lead to mesenteric lymph nodes.

Gastrointestinal Immune System Cells
Nonimmune cells that contribute to host defense of the GI tract include commensal bacteria and other nonpathogenic microorganisms. Among immune cells, both innate and adaptive immune cells protect the GI tract.

- Some are resident cells stationed among epithelial cells or in the lamina propria.
- Others circulate through the body, exiting the blood at high endothelial venules to patrol the GI mucosa in search of pathogens, and then entering the lymphatic system to return to the blood.

Nonpathogenic Bacteria
The intestinal tract is sterile at birth but is soon colonized in an oral-to-anal direction. The trillions of microorganisms making up the normal enteric flora or "microbiome" is influenced by diet and medications. These microorganisms live symbiotically with the human host, receiving a steady supply of nutrients while producing substances useful to the host (such as vitamin K) and preventing the colonization and penetration of the alimentary tract of pathogens by competing with them for space and resources (see Clinical Correlation Box 27.1).

Fast Fact 27.1

An estimated one-fourth of the cells of the intestinal mucosa are lymphoid cells.

Approximately 70% of the body's antibody-secreting B cells are located in the intestine. About 5×10^{10} immune cells reside in the gastrointestinal tract, equal to the number in the bone marrow.

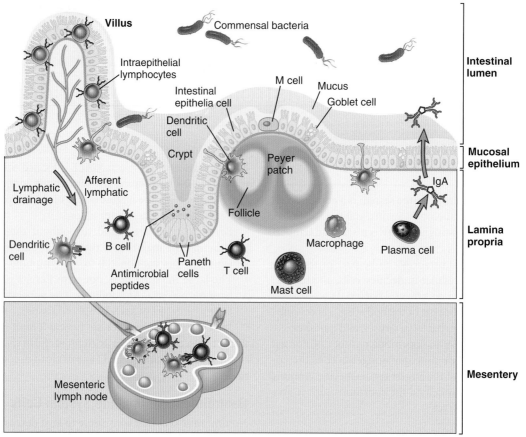

Fig. 27.1 Tissue and cellular components of the gastrointestinal (GI) immune system. Nonimmune defenses, such as the mucus layer and epithelial layer, are present throughout the GI tract. Innate immune cells, such as antigen-presenting cells (macrophages and dendritic cells) and mast cells, are present in the lamina propria. Adaptive immune system T cells, B cells, and plasma cells are found scattered among epithelial cells, in the lamina propria, or in the context of gut-associated lymphoid tissue (GALT), such as lymphoid follicles. Clusters of lymphoid follicles form Peyer's patches. (Modified from Abbas AK, Lichtman AH, Pillai S, et al. *Cellular and Molecular Immunology*, 8th Edition. Philadelphia: Elsevier; 2015.)

Innate Immune Cells

Antigen-presenting cells (APCs) include:
- Macrophages.
- Dendritic cells reside in the lamina propria of the gastric mucosa and can extend portions of their membrane into the gut lumen to sample antigens.
- Mast cells.

The top of each Peyer's patch is covered by a specialized epithelial cell known as a microfold or M cell. M cells sample luminal contents and shuttle these antigens into the Peyer's patches *via* transcytosis (Fig. 27.2).
- M cells do not contain specific receptors to bind antigens.
- Rather, they are located in pits where antigens are likely to deposit, and they are not covered with secretory immunoglobulins (see later) that prevent the binding of antigens.
- Thus M cells sample a large percentage of gut antigens.

Kupffer Cells

As described in Chapter 26, the liver removes damaging chemicals and potentially toxic compounds from the blood. Most intestinal venous blood enters the liver via the portal circulation, carrying the wide array of potentially infectious microbes and other antigenic materials that bypass the GI tract defenses and would enter the circulation. Kupffer cells are fixed (i.e., noncirculating) macrophages located within the

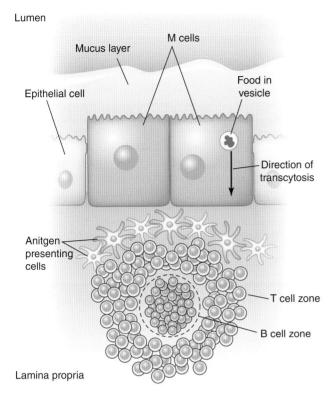

Fig. 27.2 Cellular structure of a Peyer's patch. The luminal "cap" of the patch is composed of M cells that transport luminal contents into the lamina propria via transcytosis. There, antigen-presenting cells, such as dendritic cells and macrophages, digest and present antigen to T cells. The germinal center of a Peyer's patch has a central area of B cells and a surrounding area of T cells.

liver sinusoids. They engulf many soluble antigens from the portal circulation.

Adaptive Immune Cells

The lymphocytes of the adaptive immune system (T cells and B cells) are located in three anatomic areas:

- Among epithelial cells
- Within the loose connective tissue of the lamina propria
- In the lymphoid follicles of the GALT and Peyer's patches. Each follicle is made up of a germinal center (containing mostly B cells) surrounded by collections of T cells and additional B cells, as well as a number of APCs

Many of the mucosal T cells of the GI tract are of the Th17 variety, while many of the B cells (or their plasma cell derivatives) produce immunoglobulin (Ig)A (see later).

Gastrointestinal Immune System Molecules

Both nonimmune and immune molecules are important in the defense of the GI tract.

Nonimmune Molecules

In the oropharynx, saliva contains several nonimmune antibacterial molecules, including:

- Lactoferrin, which binds iron present in food or saliva, depriving bacteria of this needed element.
- Lysozyme (also known as muramidase), which hydrolyzes

constituents of bacterial cell walls, compromising their integrity and thus damaging or destroying susceptible microbes.
- Lactoperoxidase, which, in the presence of hydrogen peroxide (H_2O_2), catalyzes the oxidation of a number of microbial molecules, disrupting their functions in bacterial structure and/or metabolism.

In the stomach, gastric acid prevents invasion by microorganisms. The gastric pH is usually less than 4 on the luminal side, and many microorganisms cannot survive in this acidic environment. (See Clinical Correlation Box 27.2.)

Clinical Correlation Box 27.2

Helicobacter pylori is a bacterial species that can survive in the acidic environment of the stomach. Infection with *H. pylori* is a major cause of gastritis and peptic ulcer disease, and is a risk factor for gastric adenocarcinoma and lymphoma. *H. pylori* cells reside in the mucus layer covering gastric epithelial cells, and possesses the urease enzyme that allows it to produce ammonia that buffers the gastric acid in an envelope around the bacterial cell. A diagnostic urea breath test takes advantage of the activity of the urease enzyme, allowing physicians to diagnose *H. pylori* infection noninvasively. *H. pylori* infection can be treated with conventional antibiotics.

The small intestine contains many digestive secretions that inhibit or destroy microorganisms, including:

- Bile salts.
- Pancreatic enzymes such as trypsin.
- Mucus, a complex mixture of glycoproteins and proteoglycans secreted by goblet cells interspersed among mucosal epithelial cells, forms a layer covering epithelial cells, prohibiting bacterial adherence and thus decreasing the probability that a pathogen will gain entry.

Immune Molecules

Defensins insert into and disrupt bacterial cell walls.
- Alpha-defensins are innate immune proteins produced by small intestine Paneth cells and neutrophils.
- Beta-defensins are produced by large intestine epithelial cells.

IgA is an antibody secreted by plasma cells (see Ch. 8) in the salivary ducts and within the gastric mucosa, the small intestine, and the large intestine.
- IgA coats bacteria preventing them from adhering to epithelial cells.
- In the gut, IgA is usually in a dimeric form with two individual IgA molecules joined by a joining protein called the J chain.
- Because each IgA molecule has two antigen binding sites (Fig. 27.3), the dimeric structure of intestinal IgA gives it four antigen-combining sites and allows it to agglutinate targets.
- In addition to the J chain, IgA in the gut also has a secretory component (SC), a transmembrane protein located at the basolateral surface of intestinal epithelial cells that binds to the dimeric IgA and causes the complex to be taken up by the epithelial cell and transported into the lumen

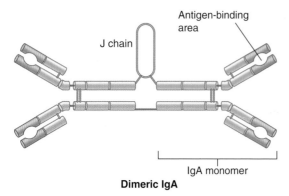

Dimeric IgA

Fig. 27.3 Structure of dimeric immunoglobulin (Ig)A. Dimeric IgA is composed of two IgA monomers linked by a joining or J chain. Because each IgA monomer has two antigen binding sites, dimeric IgA has a total of four such sites.

- The entire complex of dimeric IgA, the J chain, and the SC is referred to as secretory IgA (sIgA).

$\alpha_4\beta_7$ integrin is a molecule expressed on enteric immune system T and B lymphocytes. As these T and B cells circulate in the blood, this integrin allows these cells to exit the vasculature and reenter the GI mucosa by binding to a ligand called MadCAM-1 expressed on the endothelial cells of gut postcapillary venules.

CCR9 and CCR10 are chemokine receptors expressed by enteric immune system T and B cells.

- They bind the chemokines CCL25 and CCL28, respectively.
- These chemokines are expressed by intestinal epithelial cells, and attract the T and B cells out of the circulation and back into the gut mucosa.

SYSTEM FUNCTION

Both nonimmune and immune mechanisms function in an integrative fashion within the GI tract.

Nonimmune Mechanisms

A major nonimmune, macroscopic defense process is peristalsis, which prevents bacteria from remaining in contact with one area for a prolonged period of time.

- This decreases the chance of bacterial adherence and translocation across the epithelium.
- In addition, by mixing the contents of the GI tract and contributing to macroscopic digestion, peristalsis increases the opportunity for contact between small particles and the antigen-sampling cells of the gut.

Immune Mechanisms

The enteric immune system prevents and responds to infection, but must do so in a way that limits inflammation that would cause structural damage to and impair the function of the alimentary tract.

- In many cases, this involves the neutralization of potential pathogens without generating a large inflammatory response.
- In other cases, such as contact between the GI immune system and beneficial proteins derived from foods, the best immune reaction is apparently none, a response called tolerance.

To distinguish between beneficial nonself and potentially harmful nonself, the cells of the enteric immune system sample and analyze the contents of the GI tract, a procedure called antigen processing (see Development Box 27.1 and Environmental Box 27.1).

Antigen Sampling and Processing

Once antigens adhere to the apical surface of M cells, they are taken up via phagocytosis and pinocytosis into the cell and packaged into vesicles, trafficked through the cytosol, and released on the basolateral side where they are delivered to APCs, such as dendritic cells and macrophages in Peyer's patches.

- The APCs process the antigens by digesting them and present them to T cells by inserting antigenic peptides into the clefts of major histocompatibility complex (MHC) II molecules and displaying them on the APC surface.
- T cells may recognize these antigenic peptides in MHC II clefts by means of their cell surface T-cell receptors.

A T cell that recognizes antigen may then respond in a number of ways, depending on the context in which the antigen is presented and the subtype of T cell involved.

- If certain costimulatory signals are present, a T cell will generate signals to initiate inflammation. This may occur if antigens from a pathogenic bacterium or virus are detected and recognized.
- Another T-cell response may instruct B cells in the gut to mature into IgA-secreting plasma cells.
- If the antigen is harmless, however, and costimulatory signals are absent, the T cell may ignore the information or even initiate a program to suppress inflammation in response to

the antigen. This antiinflammatory response is one type of tolerance mechanism, and many GI mucosal T cells are of the Th17 subtype that possess potent antiinflammatory and tolerizing effects.

Intestinal epithelial cells may also take up antigen from the gut lumen and deposit them on the basal side of the epithelial layer where they are processed by APCs.

- Antigens may also pass between intestinal epithelial cells (called the paracellular route) and encounter immune cells in the lamina propria of the small intestine.
- This type of antigen movement is usually prevented by the tight junctions between epithelial cells.
- However, in situations where these junctions are disrupted (such as in infection, ischemia, or inflammation), antigen can pass from the intestinal lumen into the lamina propria.

Hepatic Kupffer cells also engulf antigenic proteins and present them to T cells, thus triggering an immune response. In this way, many antigens and potentially infectious agents that are able to bypass the intestinal immune system are cleared by Kupffer cells in the liver.

Immunoglobin A Production and Function

Once a B cell receives appropriate signals from T cells, it can mature into a plasma cell that secretes antigen-specific IgA.

- Once released from the plasma cell, dimeric IgA binds to the basolateral surface of intestinal epithelial cells by means of a specific receptor and is transported to the apical side of the epithelial cell via transcytosis.

- Once on the apical side, the epithelial cell receptor is enzymatically cleaved, releasing the sIgA.
- That portion of the epithelial cell receptor that remains bound to the dimeric IgA is the SC (Fig. 27.4).

Once released into the lumen, sIgA binds to antigens, such as those on the surface of potential pathogenic microorganisms, preventing them from adhering to the intestinal epithelial cells, entering those cells, and damaging the mucosa. sIgA can also bind to and neutralize potentially harmful products of pathogenic organisms, such as bacterial toxins.

sIgA does not activate inflammatory and cytotoxic immune system responses, such as the complement system. If classical immune responses (including inflammation and cell death) were induced by sIgA, the gut would be in a constant state of inflammation and would no longer be able to carry out its degradative, secretory, and absorptive functions.

Encountering Pathogens

Food may be heavily colonized with potentially pathogenic microorganisms, yet the host is protected from serious infection throughout the processes of digestion, absorption, and elimination.

- In the oropharynx, salivary enzymes such as lactoferrin, lysozyme, and lactoperoxidase impair or damage microorganisms.
- The epithelial barriers of the GI tract prevent access into the lamina propria and blood vessels beneath, and the mucous layer and sIgA prevent adherence to the epithelium.

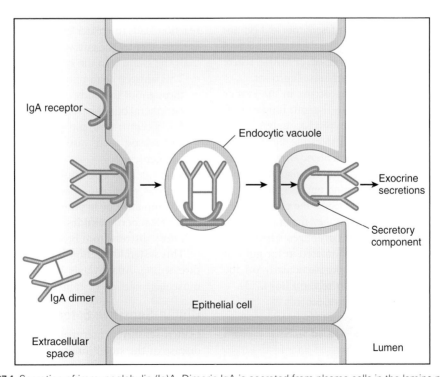

Fig. 27.4 Secretion of immunoglobulin (Ig)A. Dimeric IgA is secreted from plasma cells in the lamina propria. It is bound by a receptor on the basolateral surface of gastrointestinal epithelial cells and endocytosed. By the process of transcytosis, the vesicle carries the IgA to the basolateral surface, where it is released into the lumen. Enzymatic cleavage of the epithelial cell receptor frees the IgA, but part of the receptor remains attached and is called the *secretory component*. (McPherson RA. *Henry's Clinical Diagnosis and Management by Laboratory Methods.* Elsevier; 2017: p. 913–928.e1. Fig. 46.4.)

- After being swallowed, food is subject to peristalsis, which helps prevent adherence.
- In the stomach, gastric acid may damage the microorganisms.
- In the duodenum, bile and pancreatic digestive enzymes may do the same.
- In the jejunum and ileum, antigen is captured and delivered by M cells, and processed by APCs, such as dendritic cells, macrophages, and B cells.
  - Some APCs may present antigen to T cells in mucosal lymphoid tissue, while others may move to mesenteric lymph nodes to do so.
  - T cells and B cells in lymphoid tissues and Peyer's patches, other GALT structures, and mesenteric lymph nodes may respond by proliferating and increasing the output of antigen-specific sIgA to neutralized microorganisms and their toxic products.
  - Those T and B cells that exit lymphoid tissues to enter the circulation home back to the GI mucosa by expressing $\alpha 4\beta 7$ and CCR9 and/or CCR10, allowing them to bind to MadCAM-1 and CCL25 and/or CCL28, respectively.
- In the large intestine, resident normal flora microbes compete with pathogens for nutrients and space.

If a pathogen should gain access despite the safeguards, the APCs, T cells, and B cells of the mucosa can respond by initiating an inflammatory reaction to destroy the invader. If a microorganism succeeds in entering the circulation, hepatic Kupffer cells may intercept it. Finally, the vast majority of ingested microorganisms are excreted in the stool.

The GI immune system does not work in isolation. Because T cells and B cells are mobile, they can encounter antigen in the GI tract and then move to other tissues. In the respiratory and genitourinary tracts, such cells may enter lymphoid tissues similar to GALT (called mucosa-associated lymphoid tissue, or MALT) where they may share information or carry out defensive functions.

- For example, after antigen processing occurs in the Peyer's patches and other lymphoid tissue in the gut, immature B cells are stimulated by T cells to begin producing IgA.
- Many of these B cells exit the small intestine through the lymphatic channels and enter the mesenteric lymph nodes.
- They are then transported into the systemic circulation, where B cells not only return to the small intestine, but also travel to the salivary glands, the eye, the bronchial tissue, the genitourinary tract, and the mammary glands, where they may mature into plasma cells and produce large amounts of antigen-specific IgA.
- Thus protection against antigen encountered in the gut can be conferred on the body as a whole, particularly on the other mucosal tissues (see Clinical Correlation Box 27.3).

Clinical Correlation Box 27.3

Researchers have found higher rates of infection in critically ill patients who are fed via routes other than the alimentary tract, or "parenterally" (e.g., with total parenteral nutrition [TPN], a form of intravenous, liquid nutrition), compared with those who are fed via the gut. One hypothesis suggests that this is because decreased gastrointestinal (GI) exposure to antigen results in poorer immune system education and thus weakened defenses at the skin and mucosal surfaces, such as the respiratory, genitourinary, and GI tracts.

SYSTEM PATHOPHYSIOLOGY

Like the immune system as a whole, the enteric immune system can malfunction in one or more of three ways and result in disease:

- By not defending the body from danger (immunodeficiency).
- By attacking normal, healthy body tissues or cells (autoimmunity).
- By generating an inflammatory response against a benign nonself substance (hypersensitivity).

Food Allergy

Depending on the definition and the stringency of inclusion criteria, an estimated 6% to 8% of children in Western countries and 1% to 4% of the adult population have some type of food allergy, a hypersensitivity reaction directed against one or more food antigens.

The common foods in a Western diet that provoke allergies include eggs, cow's milk, tree nuts, peanuts, wheat, soy, fish, and shellfish.

Reactions occur when food antigen enters the lamina propria and binds to the surface of resident mast cell by means of membrane-bound antigen-specific IgE. Cross-linking of mast cell surface IgE by food antigens induces mast cell activation, with the release of inflammatory mediators such as:

- Histamine
- Prostaglandin D2
- Leukotriene C4

These mediators cause vasodilation and leakage of fluid from the vascular space into the lamina propria causing edema.

A potential positive feedback loop can occur if the initial reaction leads to greater gut barrier breach, allowing more food antigen to enter the gut wall, activate more mast cells, and eventually be swept into the systemic circulation.

- This antigen load and the mast cell mediators are carried throughout the body, activating mast cells at other sites and peripheral blood basophils (which also bear the high affinity IgE receptor and can therefore bind allergen specific IgE and release their vasoactive mediators on encounter with allergen).
- This can lead to diffuse hives, itching, and swelling of the mucous membranes, and in its most extreme form can be accompanied by hypotension from vasodilation (decrease in the total peripheral resistance, see Chs. 9 and 10) and respiratory distress from bronchoconstriction (see Ch. 13).

This systemic reaction is called "anaphylaxis" and can be life threatening. Anaphylaxis is treated with an immediate intramuscular injection of epinephrine.

Gluten-Sensitive Enteropathy

Gluten-sensitive enteropathy, also called celiac disease, is a disease of the small intestine that leads to malabsorption and nutritional deficiencies. It is a hereditary disease and the prevalence varies by geographic location, ranging from 1 in 300 people in areas of Ireland to 1 in 5000 people in North America. It can manifest at any age.

Gluten is a cereal protein found in wheat and rye. Gluten-sensitive enteropathy is linked to a specific component of gluten called the gliadin fraction, which is relatively resistant to digestion. The enteric enzyme tissue transglutaminase (TTG) deamidates and thereby increases the toxicity and immunogenicity of the gliadin molecule. The deamidated gliadin alters gut epithelial cells and leads to their being destroyed by innate immune cells called natural killer (NK) cells.

Some gliadin is engulfed by enteric APCs. Almost all patients with celiac disease express either the human leukocytes antigen (HLA)-DQ8 or HLA-DQ2 genes that code for MHC class II peptide presenting proteins on their APCs. APCs present deamidated gliadin peptide to CD4+ T cells, and those with a T-cell cell receptor that recognizes the gliadin peptide + MHC II complex are activated and release proinflammatory cytokines. The T cells also enteric B cells, which produce a number of antibodies, chief among them being an IgA that binds to the patient's own TTG.

The inflammation and subsequent gut mucosal damage lead to malabsorption, manifested clinically as diarrhea, vitamin deficiencies, weight loss, and anemia.

Celiac disease is diagnosed by a consistent history and by detecting IgA anti-TTG, but definitive diagnosis is by fulfilling these criteria:
- Evidence of malabsorption in the presence of a normal diet.
- An abnormal jejunal biopsy in which blunting of the villi is seen in conjunction with deepening of the crypts.
- Improvement after beginning a gluten-free diet (Table 27.1), which is the treatment (see Clinical Correlation Box 27.4).

Clinical Correlation Box 27.4

Malabsorption can be assessed using a D-xylose absorption test. D-xylose is a pentose sugar that is well absorbed across normal intestinal mucosa but is not absorbed across abnormal mucosa. If the D-xylose is absorbed, it enters the bloodstream and is then excreted in the urine unchanged; if not, it is lost in the stool. Thus measuring urine D-xylose levels or serum D-xylose levels can be an indicator of D-xylose absorption and intestinal absorption in general. To perform the test, the patient fasts for 8 hours and is then given a 25 mg D-xylose load orally. The urine is then collected for 5 hours after the oral load and the total urinary D-xylose measured. If the urinary excretion is less than 15% of the given load, malabsorption is suggested.

Inflammatory Bowel Disease

There are two major types of inflammatory bowel disease, Crohn disease and ulcerative colitis (UC), in which there is inappropriate inflammation that damages the GI tract.

Crohn Disease

- Characterized by patchy inflammatory lesions that often start as aphthous ulcers but then progress to involve the full thickness of the gut wall (Fig. 27.5A). Lesions may occur anywhere from the oropharynx to the anus. Ulcers and fissures may progress to cause perforation and fistulas. Scar formation may lead to obstruction by strictures.
- Symptoms include abdominal pain, diarrhea (often with visible blood in the stool), and weight loss partially because of malabsorption. Numerous other symptoms, including fever, skin rashes, joint disease, and anemia, may be present.
- Evidence suggests that there is an overly exuberant inflammatory response and/or a loss of tolerance to nonpathogenic gut bacteria. Approximately 30% of patients have a defect in NOD2/CARD15, an innate immune receptor for the bacterial cell wall component peptidoglycan.
  - Normal NOD2/CARD15 senses peptidoglycan and leads to the activation of epithelial cells and Th17 cells and increased production of mucus and innate antimicrobial peptides.

TABLE 27.1 Some Gluten-Containing Foods to be Avoided by Patients With Gluten-Sensitive Enteropathy		
Baking soda	Graham flour	Rye
Beer	Gravy cubes	Scotch
Bran	Ground spices	Soy sauce
Bread flour	Malt	Starch
Bulgur	Malt vinegar	Vegetable starch
Caramel color	Mustard powder	Certain vitamins
Couscous	Nuts	Wheat
Dextrins	Pasta	White vinegar

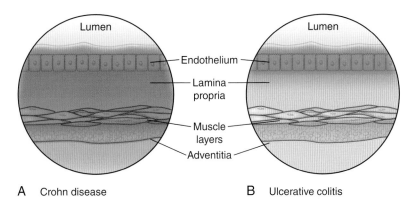

A Crohn disease   **B** Ulcerative colitis

Fig. 27.5 Inflammatory bowel diseases. A, In Crohn disease, patchy inflammation affects the full thickness of the gut wall. Lesions may occur anywhere along the gastrointestinal (GI) tract from oropharynx to anus. B, In ulcerative colitis, there is continuous inflammation affecting the more superficial GI mucosa. Lesions involve the distal large bowel at a minimum and may affect the entire large bowel.

- Mutant NOD2/CARD15 fails to induce these protective responses and leads to epithelial barrier impairment, microbial invasion, epithelial damage, and destructive inflammation in the attempt to defend the GI mucosa.
- The diagnosis is made by a typical history and the gross and histologic patterns of lesions as determined by abdominal radiographic imaging and endoscopy with biopsy.
- Treatments include antiinflammatory and immunosuppressive drugs, and antibiotics are effective in some cases. Often, however, surgical resection of inflamed tissue is necessary, although disease often recurs after surgery.

Ulcerative Colitis

- Inflammation is superficial instead of affecting the entire thickness of the gut wall and is continuous instead of patchy

(see Fig. 27.5B). Although Crohn disease may affect any portion of the GI tract, UC by definition is limited to the colon, although the inflammation may involve as little as the rectum or as much as the entire large intestine.
- Typical symptoms of abdominal pain and bloody diarrhea may be accompanied by fever and extraintestinal symptoms that resemble Crohn disease.
- UC is diagnosed by a history of typical symptoms and visualization of the inflamed colonic epithelium by colonoscopy.
- Medical treatment includes antiinflammatory and occasionally immunosuppressive drugs, but antibiotics do not seem to be efficacious. If severe disease called toxic megacolon or cancer arises, surgical resection of the entire large intestine (total proctocolectomy) is curative.

SUMMARY

- The enteric immune system not only protects the gut from the large antigenic and infectious burden it faces on a daily basis, but also contributes to mucosal immunity of the whole body.
- Potentially dangerous microorganisms and antigens are neutralized in a way that does not cause frequent, severe, or protracted inflammation that would interfere with the digestive and absorptive functions of the GI tract.
- Nonimmune mechanisms include the epithelial barrier, the mucous layer, and peristalsis.
- Immune mechanisms include the organized sampling of antigens by innate APCs and the coordinated responses of adaptive T cells and B cells.
- The epithelial barrier is a critical nonimmune structure that prevents pathogens from entering the body via the GI tract.
- Innate immune cells such as APCs and mast cells and adaptive immune cells (T cells and B cells) are distributed throughout the gut mucosa in three compartments: in the epithelial lining, in the loose connective tissue of the lamina propria, and in the more organized GALT.
- GALT is present throughout the GI tract. In the small intestine, large collections of GALT follicles form the Peyer's patches.

- Nonpathogenic colonic microorganisms (normal flora) benefit the host not only by aiding digestion and producing important metabolic factors such as vitamin K, but also by competing with potential pathogens for nutrients and space.
- Mucus, secreted by cells, such as goblet cells, forms a layer in which potential pathogens are trapped.
- IgA is secreted by plasma cells and transported into the gut lumen via transcytosis. sIgA binds to antigens and neutralizes them, preventing them from adhering to the epithelial lining and gaining access to the lamina propria, but without inducing inflammation.
- M cells overlying Peyer's patches sample luminal contents and transport them into the lamina propria. There, APCs process antigens and present them to T cells.
- Food allergies occur when food antigens cross-link IgE on the surface of GI mast cells.
- Gluten-sensitive enteropathy is an inflammatory disease of the GI tract in which there is an inappropriate reaction to gliadin.
- Inflammatory bowel diseases, Crohn disease and ulcerative colitis, are disorders in which chronic, inappropriate inflammation occurs in the gut.

REVIEW QUESTIONS

Directions: Each of the numbered items or incomplete statements in this section is followed by answers or by completions of the statement. Select the one lettered answer or completion that is best in each case.

1. In the small intestine, which of the following plays an important role in preventing bacterial adherence?
   A. IgE
   B. IgG
   C. Mucus secreted by goblet cells
   D. Nonpathogenic bacteria
   E. Neutrophils

2. What properties of M cells allow them to sample antigen effectively from the small intestinal lumen?
   A. They have a receptor-mediated active transport system for hundreds of antigens.

   B. They are not covered by IgA.
   C. They protrude above the epithelial cells and are thus able to capture antigen as it passes by.
   D. They lack a nucleus, making them more efficient at antigen capture.

3. Gluten-sensitive enteropathy is characterized by which of the following histologic features?
   A. Flattening of intestinal crypts and elongation of intestinal villi
   B. Flattening of intestinal villi and elongation of intestinal crypts
   C. Obstruction of intestinal crypts by mucus impaction and fibrosis
   D. IgE antibodies against gliadin
   E. Bleeding into the muscle layer of the gut wall

4. A 67-year-old man presents to the emergency department with a 1-week history of diarrhea. He had been taking antibiotics for pneumonia when the diarrhea started. Which of the following elements would be the most appropriate part of his diagnostic and treatment plan?
   A. Evaluation of his PT and PTT
   B. Administration of vitamin K
   C. Assay of stool for Clostridium difficile toxins
   D. Abdominal CT
   E. Upper GI endoscopy

5. A 37-year-old, previously healthy patient has been in the intensive care unit for 2 weeks following a high-speed motor vehicle accident that has left him in a coma. He has been unresponsive since admission, and he has been losing weight. The ICU team discusses starting him on total parenteral nutrition (TPN). What concerns are germane when considering this strategy?
   A. He will be at higher risk of developing systemic infections if he is fed parenterally instead of via the GI tract.
   B. Feeding him with TPN will require placement of a central line and all the risks associated with placing that line.
   C. He will not be able to receive sufficient calories through TPN.
   D. The large volume of fluid of TPN will cause heart failure.

6. Inflammatory bowel disease such as Crohn's disease can be treated effectively by any or all of the following EXCEPT:
   A. Surgical resection of severely inflamed, fibrotic, or perforated tissues
   B. Antibiotics
   C. Anti-inflammatory biologic agents
   D. Immunosuppressive agents
   E. Bone marrow transplant

ANSWERS TO REVIEW QUESTIONS

1. **The answer is C.** Both IgA and mucus secreted by goblet cells in the small intestine prevent bacteria from adhering to intestinal epithelial cells. Although IgE and IgG play smaller roles in small intestinal immunity, they are not major factors in preventing bacterial adherence. Nonpathogenic bacteria are normally found in the large intestine, not the small intestine. Neutrophils are normally rare in the lamina propria and do not prevent pathogen adherence.

2. **The answer is B.** M cells reside in pits between epithelial cells and antigen is likely to drop into these pits. M cells are not covered with mucus or IgA and thus are effective at sampling antigen. They do this through pinocytosis and not receptor-mediated active transport. Like most body cells except mature red blood cells, M cells have a nucleus.

3. **The answer is B.** Gluten-sensitive enteropathy is characterized both by a flattening of small intestinal villi and by elongation of intestinal crypts, but not by a flattening of crypts or elongation of villi. While patients may have IgA, IgG, or even IgE antibodies directed against the gliadin fraction of gluten, the presence of such antibodies is a serologic, not a histologic, feature of the disease. Bleeding generally does not occur in the deeper muscle layers of the gut wall in this disease.

4. **The answer is C.** The patient's history of antibiotic use raises the possibility of C. difficile infection. The patient's stool should be sent for C. difficile toxin assay; if the result is positive, he should be treated with an antibiotic such as metronidazole. Neither abdominal CT nor upper GI endoscopy is indicated initially in this case. If the patient had a long history of antibiotic use coupled with malnutrition and the inability to eat, the possibility of vitamin K deficiency coagulopathy would exist and merit evaluation. In this case, however, it seems less likely.

5. **The answer is A.** TPN is used to provide nutritional support to patients who cannot maintain adequate oral intake. It is administered through a peripherally inserted central catheter (PICC line) or a central venous line, so this patient might not need the latter. TPN can provide sufficient calories to patients. However, these patients are often at increased risk of systemic infection owing in part to the fact that their GI tract is no longer seeing the amount of antigen it usually encounters and thus the immune system is stimulated less. In a previously healthy 37-year-old, heart failure from fluid overload is possible but is less likely.

6. **The answer is E.** Crohn's disease can be effectively treated with surgery when necessary, with antibiotics on occasion, with anti-inflammatory biologic agents (such as infliximab), with and immunosuppressive agents (such as corticosteroids). While removal of the colon is curative for patients with ulcerative colitis, Crohn's disease involves the entire GI tract from mouth to anus and thus surgery is a last resort for refractory disease. Bone marrow transplant, while it might theoretically be helpful, is not an accepted treatment for Crohn's disease.

Gastrointestinal Physiology

D.L. is a 9-year-old female who is being seen by her pediatrician for the fifth time this summer. She has been seen for multiple gastrointestinal (GI) complaints including abdominal pain, bloating, and frequent nausea. Her mother is worried because she continues to lose weight despite being given extra servings of food at meals and close monitoring.

PRESENTATION: HISTORY AND PHYSICAL EXAMINATION

D.L. has had multiple visits and inpatient hospitalizations during her life for GI-related complaints. When she was an infant she was had been hospitalized twice for intussusception and underwent surgery. She has always been a small girl but recently she has fallen off her growth curve and is now less then fifth percentile for height and weight. Her mother tells you that D.L. has frequent loose watery stools and complains of abdominal pain frequently. They have tried a number of new dieting strategies, including staying away from rich foods and decreasing dairy products, but this has not helped. D.L. seems fatigued during the visit and she reports not feeling like participating in her usual summer activities or even riding her bike with her friends. She has not traveled at all this summer.

On physical examination D.L. is sitting comfortably on the examination table. She is alert but fatigued, however she can answer questions without difficulty. Her neurologic and cardiovascular examinations are in unremarkable. Her respiratory examination is clear to auscultation and percussion. Her abdominal examination demonstrates diffuse tenderness without peritoneal signs or distention. She has pruritic papules on her knees and buttocks that her mother states have been there for a few weeks. There are two large areas of ecchymosis on her right arm and one on her shin.

DISCUSSION

The differential diagnosis for D.L. includes a number of potential etiologies. The most likely cause of her findings given her history and physical examination would be celiac sprue. Commonly known as celiac disease, it is a gluten induced enteropathy of the small intestine. Patients are unable to absorb multiple nutrients due to an inflammatory response to gluten, a component of wheat, rye, and barley. Undiagnosed, it can lead to a number of nutrient deficiencies with long- and short-term consequences. The differential diagnosis includes lactase deficiency, which largely was ruled out when D.L. removed diary from her diet.

Tropical (as opposed to celiac) sprue is less likely given her history but could be ruled out if a biopsy of the small bowel did not show infiltration of monocytes. Whipple disease, is a rare bacterial infection that could cause a similar presentation and could be tested for by looking for PAS⊕-Macrophage infiltrates on biopsy or a polymerase chain reaction for the bacteria *Tropheryma whippelii*.

The pruritic papular rash found on D.L.'s skin examination is common in celiac disease patients and is referred to as *dermatitis herpetiformis*. It is caused by granular immunoglobulin (Ig) A deposits in the dermal papillae.

PRESENTATION: LABORATORY TESTS AND BIOPSY

Initial laboratory tests included a tissue transglutaminase antibody (tTG)-IgA class, a basic metabolic profile (BMP), a complete blood count (CBC), an erythrocyte sedimentation rate (ESR), vitamin D and B12 and folate to measure vitamin deficiencies, iron, iron binding capacity, and ferritin to detect iron deficiency. The results for D.L. are:

Anti-TTG Antibody, IgA: Positive

BMP: Na 140 mEq/L, K 4.8 mEq/L, Cl 101 mEq/L, HCO_3 24 mEq/L, blood urea nitrogen 16 mg/dL, Cr 0.88 mg/dL, glucose 98 mg/dL, estimated glomerular filtration rate >60 mL/min/1.73 m^2

CBC: White blood cell 12.48 cells/μL, hemoglobin 7.2 g/dL, hematocrit 21.4 %, platelets 132,000/μL

Erythrocyte sedimentation rate: 26 mm/h (elevated)

Vit. D Level: 22 ng/mL (normal range 20–80 ng/mL)

B12: 550 pg/mL (normal range 250–900 pg/mL)

Folate: 11 ng/mL (normal range >5.2 ng/mL)

Iron: 40 mcg/dL (normal range 37–158 mcg/dL)

Iron binding capacity: 200 mcg/dL (normal range 220–460 mcg/dL)

Ferritin: 120 ng/mL (normal range 13–150 ng/mL)

DISCUSSION

Celiac disease is an enteropathy that may lead to multiple vitamin deficiencies. D.L. has some of these deficiencies reflected in her laboratory results. Her hemoglobin demonstrates an unexpected anemia that results from having insufficient iron stores, as iron is a necessary component for hemoglobin synthesis. This type of anemia is known as iron-deficiency anemia and results from immune mediated inflammatory damage to a portion of the small bowel where iron, B12, and folate are absorbed.

Vitamin K deficiency is also a common in celiac disease and is most likely the main contributing factor to the bruises found during physical examination.

COURSE

The signs and symptoms were suspicious for celiac sprue and the tTG assay is highly sensitive and specific for the disease. D.L. was diagnosed with celiac disease and was able to make modifications in her diet even before definitive testing by endoscopy with biopsy could be completed. She saw significant improvements with the avoidance of gluten and the appropriate nutritional supplementation. She began maintaining weight and

her dermatitis herpetiformis was treated with a course of a topical steroid ointment with good effect. She follows closely with her pediatrician and has not required further treatment with glucocorticoids.

DISCUSSION

Further workup for a patient like D.L. could involve the gastroenterology team and the attainment of small bowel biopsies. The classic histologic findings in celiac disease are flattened intestinal villi, lymphocyte infiltration, and hyperplasia and lengthening of intestinal crypts (Fig. 27.1.1)

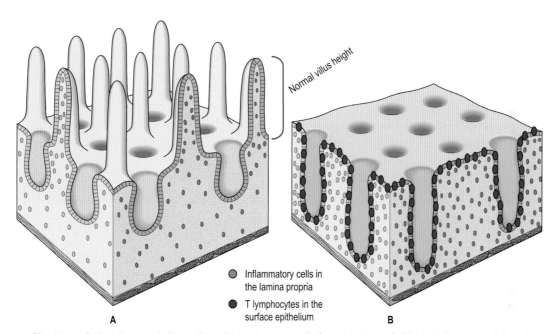

● Inflammatory cells in the lamina propria

● T lymphocytes in the surface epithelium

Normal villus height

A   B

Fig. 27.1.1 Celiac disease. A, Normal small bowel mucosa. B, Complete loss of villi (total villous atrophy) and increased inflammatory cells in the lamina propria in coeliac disease. (From Grabsch, Heike. *Underwood's Pathology.* © 2019; p. 318-355. Fig. 15.13.)

Endocrine Physiology

28

The Endocrine Pancreas: Fed and Fasted Metabolic States

INTRODUCTION

In the 1920s, Frederick Banting and Charles Best isolated insulin and made possible the treatment and survival of millions of diabetics. This helped initiate the era of modern medicine, in which the empiricism of the 18th century and its practice in the 19th century came to fruition in the wondrous cures of the 20th century.

This discovery was made possible by early research into pancreatic function that focused on the difference in hormonal signalling between the acini, the cells that secrete digestive enzymes, and those in the islets of Langerhans.

- Islets have an endocrine function, secreting hormones into the bloodstream to act at distant target sites.
- Acini have an exocrine function, secreting enzymes out of the body and into the lumen of the intestines.

The major pancreatic endocrine hormones, insulin and glucagon, serve to regulate the body's metabolism of carbohydrates, lipids, and proteins.

- By controlling the construction and breakdown of these energy-containing organic molecules, they ensure a constant supply of energy to cells regardless of fluctuations in dietary intake.
- Insulin promotes storage of energy-laden molecules, while glucagon promotes the consumption of energy stores.

SYSTEM STRUCTURE: THE ISLETS OF LANGERHANS

The pancreas lies in the posterior abdomen behind the peritoneum (i.e., retroperitoneal). This organ typically weighs 80 to 100 g in volume; it extends from the curvature of the duodenum to the medial edge of the spleen (Fig. 28.1). (For more detail on the exocrine functions of the pancreas, see Chs. 24–25).

As previously mentioned, the endocrine pancreas is responsible for hormone secretion (Fig. 28.2).

- This organ is organized histologically into islets of Langerhans, which are roughly spherical clusters of cells that account for 1% to 2% of the total weight of the pancreas.
- Islets are buried amid the pancreatic acinar cells (acini), which make up the exocrine pancreas.

The islets of Langerhans consist primarily of beta cells and alpha cells.

- Beta cells synthesize and secrete the peptide hormone insulin.
- Alpha cells make and secrete the peptide hormone glucagon.
- Others cell types include:
  - Delta cells, which synthesize somatostatin
  - PP cells, which make pancreatic polypeptide
  - D1 cells, which secrete vasoactive intestinal peptide (VIP)
  - Enterochromaffin cells, which secrete serotonin

Hormonal Protein Structure

Because the major products of the endocrine pancreas—insulin and glucagon—are peptide hormones, the organelles involved in protein synthesis and secretion play important roles in the islet cells.

- Insulin (Fig. 28.3)
  - The intracellular production of an insulin molecule begins with a large peptide precursor called preproinsulin, which is cleaved into proinsulin and then insulin.
  - The final product of this intracellular processing—the active hormone insulin—consists of two protein chains, known as A and B, which are 21 and 30 amino acids in length, respectively, bridged by a connecting C chain of 31 amino acids.
- Glucagon
  - Synthesized in alpha cells in a precursor form called preproglucagon, which is then processed to proglucagon, which is then processed to form glucagon.
  - The active hormone glucagon is a 29-amino-acid, single-chain polypeptide.

The Insulin and Glucagon Receptors

Although diffusely expressed, insulin receptor is most highly expressed in three organ systems:

1. Liver
2. Muscle
3. Adipose tissue

The insulin receptor is a transmembrane protein complex with four subunits.

Insulin binds to the extracellular domain of the receptor.

- This activates the cytosolic domain, which is a tyrosine kinase.

Glucagon, on the other hand, binds to transmembrane receptors on hepatocyte and triggers the adenylate cyclase/cyclic adenosine monophosphate (cAMP) pathway. (See the online appendix to Ch. 1 on signal transduction for a fuller explanation of tyrosine kinase and cAMP mechanisms.)

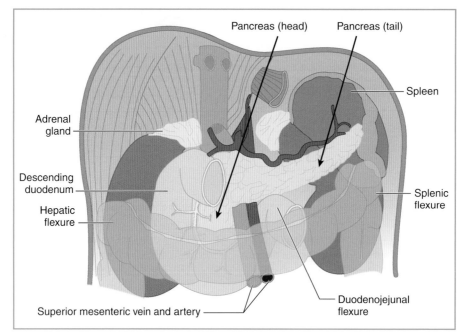

Fig. 28.1 The pancreas. The pancreas is situated in the posterior abdomen. This drawing depicts its blood supply. (Modified from Bogart. *Elsevier's Integrated Anatomy*. Philadelphia: Mosby Elsevier; 2007. Fig. 5.26.)

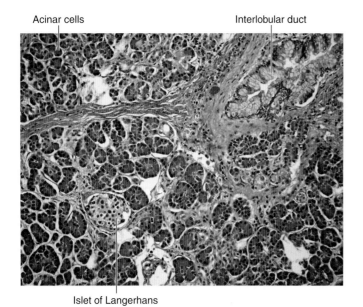

Fig. 28.2 Histology of the pancreas. The islets of Langerhans (endocrine tissue) are surrounded by acinar cells. Within the islet, note the alpha cells at the periphery (large cells with a darker cytoplasm) and the central, lighter beta cells. (From MacLennan G. *Hinman's Atlas of Uro-Surgical Anatomy*, 2nd Edition. Elsevier; 2012. Fig. 6.23.)

SYSTEM FUNCTION: THE REGULATION OF PLASMA GLUCOSE CONCENTRATION

Insulin and glucagon, the major hormones produced by the endocrine pancreas, govern the metabolism, storage, and release of energy-storing molecules. These molecules include:

- Carbohydrates
- Lipids
- Proteins

Energy is stored in their bonds that can be liberated by digestion and chemical breakdown in the body. Most body tissues can use any of these forms of fuel.

Glucose is the predominant molecule regulated by the pancreas, and, as such, the pancreas' regulatory apparatus is tied most closely to the plasma glucose level. This is critical because glucose is the primary fuel source for the brain.

- The brain contains no significant stores of glycogen (the polymerized storage form of glucose).
- The brain is inaccessible to other sources of energy, like fatty acids, because the blood-brain barrier limits neuronal absorption of fatty acids from the bloodstream.
- Thus decreased glucose in the plasma can have severe consequences for neurologic function.

To understand the effects of insulin and glucagon, it is prudent to discuss the differences between fed and fasting states (see Fast Fact 28.1).

Fast Fact Box 28.1

Insulin means money in the bank (i.e., storage and synthesis). Glucagon means money is gone (i.e., broken down and used to sustain vital processes).

- Fed state
  - Postmeal, following digestion of carbohydrates and subsequent absorption of glucose into the bloodstream.

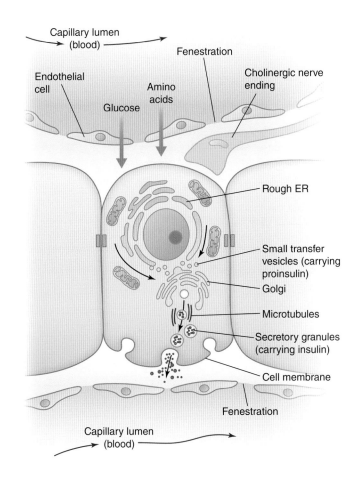

Fig. 28.3 Insulin production in the beta cell. The nucleus transcribes messenger ribonucleic acid (mRNA) that codes for proinsulin. Ribosomes on the rough endoplasmic reticulum (*ER*) translate the mRNA into the proinsulin peptide. Vesicles shuttle the proinsulin to the Golgi apparatus, which secretes granules loaded with proinsulin. Proinsulin is cleaved here, and the granules store the insulin, which is later exocytosed.

- ↑ plasma glucose.
- ↑ insulin production from the beta cells of the pancreas.
- Insulin promotes anabolic ("synthesis and storage") processes (Fig. 28.4).
  Uptake and storage of glucose (glycogenesis).
  Uptake and storage of amino acids and triglycerides.
- Fasting state
  - ↓ plasma glucose.
  - ↑ glucagon production from the alpha cells of the pancreas.
  - Glucagon promotes catabolic ("breakdown") processes to supply the brain with glucose (Fig. 28.5).
    Breakdown of glycogen (glycogenolysis)
    Synthesis of glucose (gluconeogenesis)
    Synthesis of ketone bodies as alternate fuel sources

Although insulin acts fairly independently in the fed state, glucagon is supported by several other hormones in the promotion of fasted-state metabolism.
- Glucocorticoids
- Epinephrine
- Growth hormone
- Human chorionic somatomammotropin (in pregnancy)
  Collectively, these hormones are known as the counterregulatory hormones because of their effect on fasting state metabolism.
- Insulin decreases the plasma glucose level and drives fed metabolism.
- Counterregulatory hormones increase the plasma glucose level and drive fasted metabolism.

Insulin Secretion

The primary trigger for insulin secretion from beta cells is elevated plasma glucose level. Beta cells detect the increased glucose level through the intracellular enzyme glucokinase.
- When the plasma glucose level rises, glucose diffuses down its concentration gradient through the glucose transporter (GLUT)1 and GLUT2 transporters into the beta cells.
- Glucokinase, which is very sensitive to changes in the glucose concentration at physiologic levels, proceeds to phosphorylate the glucose.
- This acts to trap glucose inside the cell so that it may undergo glycolysis.
  After glycolysis, increased concentration of adenosine triphosphate (ATP) inhibits ATP-sensitive K^+ channels on the beta cell.
- This leads to depolarization of the cell.
- Depolarization triggers voltage-sensitive Ca^{2+} channels, leading Ca^{2+} to flood into the cell and further depolarize the beta cell.
- Increased Ca^{2+} concentrations eventually trigger exocytosis of insulin granules (Fig. 28.6).
- The set point at which glucokinase triggers insulin release is a plasma glucose concentration of 5 mmol/L (90 mg/dL).
  By this sensing mechanism, the postprandial ("after meal") spike in plasma glucose stimulates the beta cells of the pancreas and results in a biphasic increase in plasma insulin levels (Fig. 28.7). The constitution of the meal will determine the exact amount of insulin secreted.
- Within 3 to 5 minutes of beta-cell stimulation, the insulin concentration rapidly rises in the bloodstream to as much as 10 times the basal level.
  - This occurs because of immediate release of stored insulin from cytoplasmic granules.
- Over the next 15 to 20 minutes, a second peak in insulin concentration gradually occurs.
- This represents both the further release of stored insulin *and* the release of newly synthesized insulin (see Clinical Correlation Box 28.1).

Clinical Correlation Box 28.1

Diabetic patients will inject differing amounts of insulin before a meal depending on the carbohydrate content (a process known to the diabetic as carbohydrate counting).

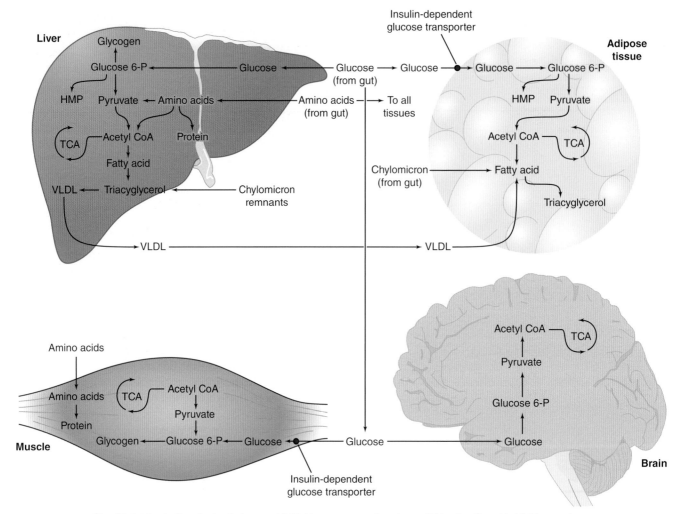

Fig. 28.4 Metabolism in the fed state. *HMP*, Hexose monophosphate; *TCA*, tricyclic acid; *VLDL*, very low-density lipoprotein.

Beyond elevated plasma glucose, other stimuli of insulin secretion include:

- Increased plasma amino acids
- Increased plasma fatty acids
- Acetylcholine (i.e., increased parasympathetic tone)

In addition, endocrine signals from the gut called incretins are also known to promote insulin production and secretion in response to a meal.

- *GIP*, gastroinhibitory polypeptide
- *GLP-1*, glucagon-like polypeptide-1

In contrast, insulin secretion is inhibited by:

- Low plasma glucose
- Norepinephrine and epinephrine (i.e., increased sympathetic tone)

The autonomic nervous system is thought to have separate glucose-sensing capabilities, through which it controls insulin secretion in parallel with the direct effect of glucose on the beta cells. Specifically, glucose-sensing neurons in the hypothalamus detect low blood sugar levels and stimulate the sympathetic nervous system (see Clinical Correlation Box 28.2).

Clinical Correlation Box 28.2

In diabetic patients, increased sympathetic tone produces the warning signals of hypoglycemia, such as sweating, tachycardia, and restlessness. Fortunately, these warning signs occur before the glucose level is low enough to cause changes in consciousness. However, long-term diabetics, even with well-controlled blood sugar levels, may lose their sensitivity to hypoglycemia, and the loss of warning signals may result in episodes of neurologic dysfunction as a first sign of hypoglycemia.

Insulin Action

As insulin mediates metabolism in the fed state, its functions are generally anabolic (i.e., promoting the synthesis and storage of molecules rather than consumption). However, insulin also promotes the use of glucose by stimulating glycolysis, the breakdown of glucose into constituents that may enter into the citric acid cycle or undergo anaerobic energy extraction.

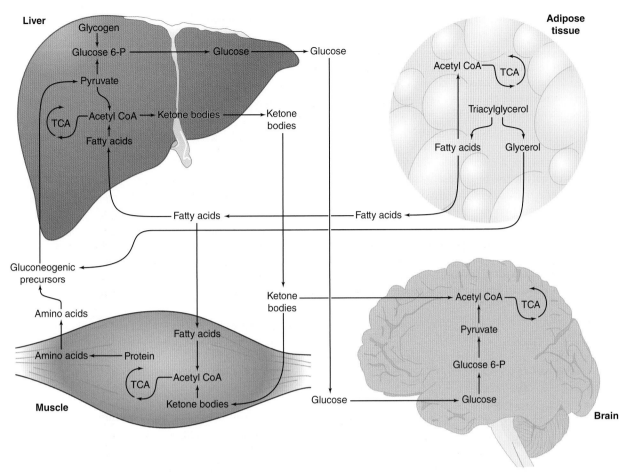

Fig. 28.5 Metabolism in the fasted state. *TCA*, Tricyclic acid.

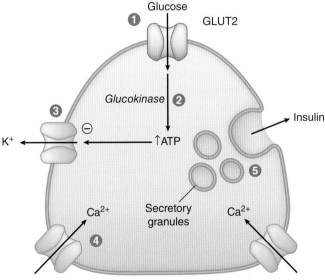

Fig. 28.6 Glucose-sensing mechanism of the pancreatic beta cell. (1) Glucose binds the glucose transporter 2 (*GLUT2*) receptor of the beta cell. (2) In the presence of elevated glucose levels, glucokinase promotes glycolysis and hence oxidative phosphorylation, increasing the level of adenosine triphosphate (*ATP*). (3) ATP inhibits ATP-sensitive K⁺ channels and decreases K⁺ efflux. (4) Decreased K⁺ efflux depolarizes the cell, which triggers voltage-gated Ca²⁺ channels and creates Ca²⁺ influx and further depolarization of the inside of the cell. (5) Ca²⁺ promotes exocytosis of insulin-laden granules.

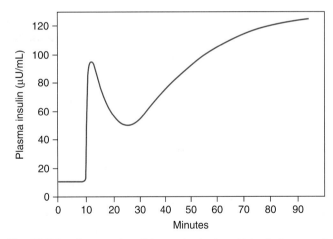

Fig. 28.7 Insulin secretion. This graph charts a biphasic increase in plasma insulin concentration after the ingestion of a bolus of glucose (at time 0).

The Effects of Insulin on Carbohydrate Metabolism

Insulin responds to conditions of elevated plasma glucose via three primary mechanisms:

1. Insulin increases the uptake of glucose into liver, skeletal muscle, and adipose cells.
   - Occurs because of the expression of specific GLUT glucose transporters on these tissues.

GLUT4: Skeletal muscle and adipose tissue.
GLUT2: Liver.

- This allows glucose to be absorbed down its concentration gradient by facilitated diffusion.
- Once inside the cells, elevated levels of glucose can drive glycogen synthesis and glycolysis by a mass effect.

2. Insulin directly enhances glycogen synthesis and glycolysis.
   - Stimulates storage of glucose as glycogen by activating glycogen synthase, an enzyme that links glucose molecules.
   - Stimulates glycolytic use of glucose by increasing the activity of several enzymes in the glycolytic pathway that convert glucose to pyruvate in the production of ATP (Fig. 28.8).

3. Conversely, insulin inhibits glycogen breakdown and gluconeogenesis.
   - Prevents the breakdown of glycogen by inhibiting glycogen phosphorylase, an enzyme that degrades glycogen.

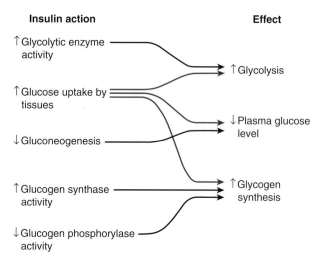

Fig. 28.9 Effects of insulin on carbohydrate metabolism.

- Inhibits gluconeogenesis by decreasing the availability of key substrates for gluconeogenesis, such as free fatty acids (FFAs).

Fig. 28.9 summarizes the effects of insulin on carbohydrate metabolism.

The Effects of Insulin on Lipid Metabolism

Insulin's main role in lipid metabolism is to promote fat storage in adipose tissue during the fed state. Insulin accomplishes this through three primary mechanisms:

1. Insulin inhibits fat breakdown.
   - Hormone-sensitive lipase typically functions to release FFAs.
   - FFAs are a freely diffusible constituent of triglyceride molecules (also known as triacylglycerol), the storage form of fat (Fig. 28.10).
   - By inhibiting lipase, insulin decreases plasma levels of circulating fats (FFAs) and increases the level of stored triglycerides in adipose tissue.
   - Decreased plasma FFA also indirectly stimulates glucose uptake by cells, because FFA normally inhibits glucose uptake by cells.

2. Insulin increases the de novo synthesis of fat (lipogenesis), particularly in liver and adipose cells.
   - Liver
     Excess glucose is first converted to glycogen for storage. After the hepatocyte glycogen concentration exceeds a certain point, feedback inhibition prevents further glycogen synthesis.
     The excess glucose is then converted to fat.
   - Adipose tissue
     Excess glucose is first converted to glycerol, which then forms triglyceride

3. Insulin stimulates lipid uptake into adipose cells.
   - Stimulates the enzyme lipoprotein lipase (LPL).
   - LPL is activated by very low-density lipoprotein (VLDL) and hydrolyzes the triglyceride of VLDL to produce intermediate-density lipoprotein (IDL), fatty acids, and glycerol.
   - This ultimately leads to lipid uptake within the cells.

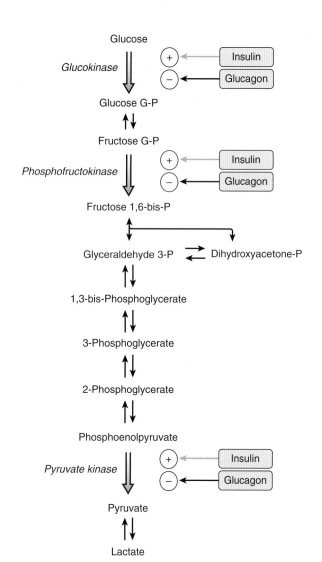

Fig. 28.8 Insulin stimulation of glycolysis. Insulin activates enzymes at several stages along the glycolytic pathway, resulting in an increased utilization of glucose. Glucagon has an inhibitory effect on the same enzymes.

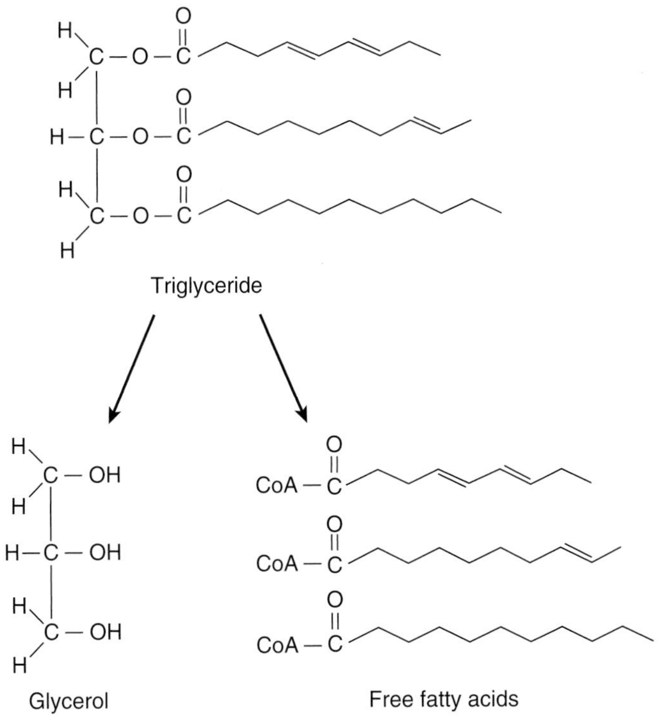

Fig. 28.10 Triglyceride (triacylglycerol), the storage form of fat, and its constituents: glycerol and free-fatty acids (FFAs). Insulin inhibits the breakdown of triglyceride into its components and keeps freely diffusible FFAs out of the bloodstream.

The Effects of Insulin on Protein Metabolism

As mentioned previously, insulin also favors the storage of proteins in tissues in the fed state. Broadly, insulin accomplishes this by:

- Stimulating the transport of free amino acids into liver and muscle cells, thus providing the building blocks for protein formation.
- Inhibiting the catabolism of proteins.

Glucagon Secretion

Glucagon secretion from the alpha cells of the islets of Langerhans is triggered by:

- Low plasma glucose (chief stimulus)
- Norepinephrine and epinephrine
  Conversely, glucagon secretion is inhibited by:
- High plasma glucose
- Insulin
- Fatty acids

Glucagon Action

As the major counterregulatory hormone, glucagon functions to antagonize the actions of insulin. It is the key regulator of metabolism in the fasted state.

- Raises plasma glucose levels via stimulation of glycogenolysis and gluconeogenesis.
- Increases availability of fatty acids via activation of hormone-sensitive lipase in adipose cells.

- Decreases plasma amino acid levels via increased uptake into liver cells.
  - Instead of participating in peptide synthesis, these amino acids are funneled into gluconeogenesis to provide carbon backbones.

During a prolonged fasting state, glucagon action predominates and *ketone bodies* are eventually produced in the following manner:

- Under the influence of glucagon, activation of hormone-sensitive lipase increases the breakdown of adipose tissue triglyceride stores into FFAs.
- Both FFAs and amino acids are oxidized in the liver to acetyl-CoA under the influence of glucagon.
- Buildup of acetyl-CoA that drives the formation of ketone bodies—namely acetoacetate and hydroxybutyrate—by a mass effect (Fig. 28.11).

Ketone bodies serve as fuel substrates in the muscles and elsewhere to preserve any available glucose for use in the brain (see Clinical Correlation Box 28.3).

Clinical Correlation Box 28.3

The state called ketosis, meaning high levels of ketone bodies in the plasma, occurs in starvation and in pathologic conditions, such as diabetes.

Other Pancreatic Hormones

Somatostatin, which is also expressed in the central nervous system and the gastrointestinal tract, is produced in the islets by delta cells.

- Although its exact metabolic role is not completely clear, it likely acts in a paracrine (locally acting from the source of secretion) fashion to inhibit insulin and glucagon secretion.
  Pancreatic polypeptide is synthesized in the PP cells of the islets.
- Secreted in response to protein-containing meals.
- Stimulates the secretion of gastric and intestinal enzymes and inhibits intestinal motility.
  Other substances produced in the islets include:
- VIP, made by D1 cells, which stimulates glycogenolysis.
- Serotonin, made by the enterochromaffin cells, whose pancreatic function is not yet elucidated

In summary, the pancreas regulates metabolism, primarily through the secretion of insulin and glucagon. These hormones integrate activity in the liver, skeletal muscle, and adipose tissue during both fed and fasted states to maintain a constant level of plasma glucose.

PATHOPHYSIOLOGY: DYSREGULATION OF THE PLASMA GLUCOSE LEVEL

An abnormal glucose level may result from three general types of conditions:

- Pathology within the pancreas may cause inadequate or excessive production of pancreatic hormones.

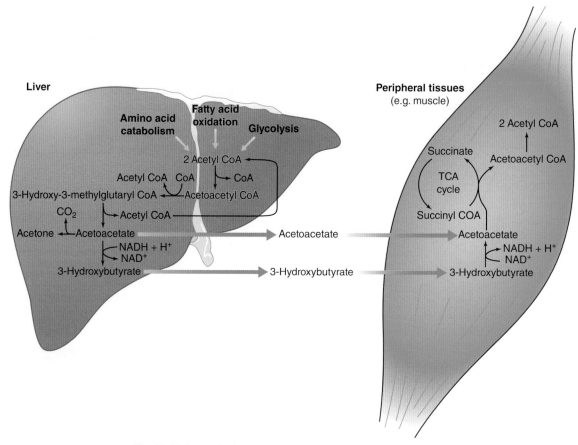

Fig. 28.11 Ketone body production and utilization. *TCA,* Triclyclic acid.

- Target sites of the pancreatic hormones may become insensitive to those hormones.
- There is an excess or deficiency of the extrapancreatic counterregulatory hormones (growth hormone, epinephrine, and glucocorticoids).

Low plasma glucose is called hypoglycemia, whereas high plasma glucose is called hyperglycemia.

- Severe hypoglycemia may lead to confusion, stupor, loss of consciousness, and coma.
- Severe hyperglycemia leads to
  - Short-term
    Polydipsia (excessive thirst, because of increased serum osmolality)
    Polyuria (excess urination, because of osmotic diuresis after the kidney's capacity for glucose reabsorption is overwhelmed)
    Disturbances of mental status and coma
  - Long-term
    Blood vessel injury and ultimately acceleration of atherosclerosis

Islet Cell Tumors

Islet cell tumors involve a proliferation, either benign or malignant, of any of the cell types that normally make up the islet. This may lead to an elevation of the plasma levels of the hormone produced by that cell type.

The most common type is the beta-cell tumor, also called an insulinoma.

- It is associated with high levels of circulating insulin, which leads to hypoglycemia.
- Glucagon, which normally functions to elevate blood sugar, cannot reverse the hypoglycemia because its secretion is inhibited by the high levels of circulating insulin.
- Thus the other counterregulatory hormones then become more important in preserving the plasma glucose level.
  - High levels of epinephrine may result in adrenergic symptoms, such as tachycardia (high heart rate) and jitteriness.

Tumors involving other cells of the islets, such as the alpha cells (glucagonomas) and the delta cells (somatostatinomas), have also been reported but are considerably rarer (See Genetics Box 28.1 and Oncology Box 28.1).

GENETICS BOX 28.1

Pancreatic endocrine tumors like insulinoma, glucagonoma, somatostatinoma, and VIPoma occur at an increased frequency in patients with Multiple Endocrine Neoplasia type 1 (MEN1). Most patients with this rare syndrome have a mutation in the *MEN1* gene on chromosome 11q13. The disease is transmitted in an autosomal dominant manner.

ONCOLOGY BOX 28.1

As the syndrome name implies, patients with *MEN1* can have neoplasms not only of cells of pancreatic islets, but carcinoid tumors, adenomas of the anterior pituitary, and tumors of the adrenal cortex as well. The protein product of the *MEN1* gene, menin, is believed to be a tumor suppressor, and *MEN1* gene mutations inhibit the normal function of menin. According to the "two hit" model of tumour pathobiology, a cell such as a pancreatic neuroendocrine cell undergoes malignant transformation when in addition to the inherited defect in one *MEN1* gene, there is a somatic mutation in the remaining normal *MEN1* gene from the other parent. Such cells therefore entirely lack functional menin tumor suppressor and generate tumors.

Diabetes Mellitus

Diabetes mellitus (DM) is a condition of impaired insulin action that leads to hyperglycemia. As the seventh leading cause of death in the United States today, DM has become an enormous public health issue and merits close attention from aspiring physicians.

The short-term signs and symptoms of DM include
- "The polys"
  - Polydipsia (excess thirst)
  - Polyuria (excess urination)
  - Polyphagia (excess hunger, because of insufficient use of glucose)
- High plasma and urine glucose levels

The longer-term consequences of DM are usually categorized as microvascular complications and macrovascular complications:
- Microvascular complications
  - Retinopathy
  - Peripheral neuropathy
  - Nephropathy, frequently progressing to renal failure
- Macrovascular complications
  - Atherosclerosis, manifesting as
    Coronary artery disease
    Cerebrovascular disease
    Peripheral vascular disease (see Clinical Correlation Box 28.4 and 28.5)

Clinical Correlation Box 28.4

The combination of peripheral neuropathy, which can lead to foot injury owing to impaired sensation, and peripheral vascular disease, which compromises blood flow to the feet, can lead to nonhealing ulcers of the feet and ultimately to amputation.

Clinical Correlation Box 28.5

One mechanism that has been considered important in causation of diabetic neuropathy involves sorbitol. Sorbitol is a 6-carbon polyalcohol that can be formed from glucose by aldose reductase. In the presence of hyperglycemia, glucose can enter the nerve, form sorbitol, and cause osmotic swelling, as sorbitol is trapped inside the cell because of its lack of membrane permeability. This can lead to permanent damage to the nerve. This mechanism is also involved in cataract formation in the setting of diabetes mellitus, because of sorbitol accumulation within the lens.

TABLE 28.1 Distinctions Between Type 1 and Type 2 Diabetes

	Type 1 Diabetes	Type 2 Diabetes
Previous nomenclature	Insulin-dependent diabetes mellitus (IDDM), juvenile-onset diabetes	Noninsulin-dependent diabetes mellitus (NIDDM), adult-onset diabetes
Percent of total diabetes mellitus cases (%)	10–20	80–90
Pathophysiology	Autoimmune destruction of beta cells in pancreatic islets → insufficient production of insulin	Insulin resistance, with eventual insulin deficiency
Typical age range	<30 years	>40 years
Association with obesity	No	Yes
Insulin sensitivity	High	Low
Necessity of insulin therapy	Always	Occasionally

The disorder has been classified into two different types, each with distinct clinical and pathologic features. Table 28.1 summarizes the major distinctions between the two types.

Type 1 Diabetes

In type 1 diabetes, autoimmune attack on the islet beta cells because of islet cell antibodies destroys significant numbers of these cells. Consequently, the pancreas cannot make adequate amounts of insulin, and hyperglycemia follows.

In type 1 diabetes, as in other autoimmune diseases, the immune system falsely recognizes a nonforeign protein as though it were foreign and mobilizes an inflammatory response against cells expressing that protein.
- Autoimmunity likely because of a combination of genetic susceptibility and precipitating environmental trigger.
- Consequently, it may be possible to detect type 1 diabetes early on and thus prevent further disease progression (Fig. 28.12).

Type 2 Diabetes

Type 2 diabetes appears to begin with a syndrome of insulin resistance and progresses toward insulin deficiency. Insulin resistance means that the adipose, skeletal muscle, and hepatic tissues do not respond to insulin as they do under normal physiologic circumstances.
- Because insulin does not have its intended effect in this context, plasma glucose levels remain high.
- Consequently, the pancreas produces higher-than-normal levels of insulin (hyperinsulinemia) in a persistent attempt to lower plasma glucose.
- Thus, insulin resistance can be diagnosed by high levels of insulin relative to a given level of plasma glucose (see Fast Fact Box 28.2).

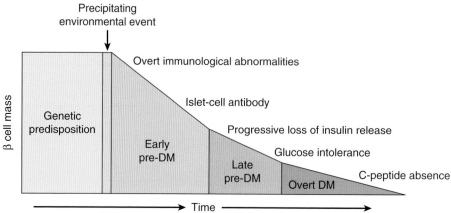

Fig. 28.12 Progression of type 1 diabetes. *DM*, Diabetes mellitus.

Fast Fact Box 28.2

Obesity is strongly correlated with insulin resistance, and it has been proposed that the increased intracellular levels of fatty acids in obese people interfere with insulin signaling. Other factors produced by adipose cells may interfere with insulin function and secretion.

As the disease progresses, however, the capacity of beta cells to secrete insulin declines. The pathophysiology of this phenomenon is a matter of active debate:
- Amyloid, which is normally secreted along with insulin, may deposit in beta cells and interfere with insulin secretion.
- Chronic exposure of beta cells to high glucose levels (and hence to increased glucose metabolism) may also generate increased levels of reactive oxygen species that can injure the genome and impair expression of the genes for proinsulin.

Treatment of Diabetes Mellitus

Because of distinct mechanisms of disease, treatment differs between the two types of DM. However, both rely heavily on patient education.
- Type 1 DM
  - Dietary modification (low-sugar diet)
  - Insulin replacement
    Human insulin mass-produced using recombinant bacteria
    Both short-acting and long-acting preparations available to inject subcutaneously:
      Short-acting: prevent acute hyperglycemia, as may otherwise occur with meals
      Long-acting: maintain insulin level in blood over a longer period of time
    Insulin pumps, which feed insulin continuously into a subcutaneous port, mimic the physiologic basal levels of insulin and more closely mirror normal pancreatic function.

- Type 2 DM
  - Dietary modification (low-sugar diet)
  - Weight loss (reduces insulin resistance)
  - Oral hypoglycemic medications
    Sulfonylureas ($\uparrow$ insulin secretion)
    Metformin ($\uparrow$ insulin sensitivity)
    Thiazolidinediones ($\uparrow$ insulin sensitivity)
    Alpha-glucosidase inhibitors ($\downarrow$ glucose absorption)
    GLP-1 analogs ($\uparrow$ insulin secretion)
    Dipeptidyl peptidase-4 analogs ($\uparrow$ insulin secretion)
  - In progressive cases, may need insulin replacement (see Clinical Correlation Box 28.6)

Clinical Correlation Box 28.6

Diabetic ketoacidosis (DKA) is a life-threatening complication that can arise in patients with diabetes mellitus, most commonly in type 1 diabetics.
- DKA arises from a severe shortage of insulin, causing the body to switch from metabolism of carbohydrates to metabolism of fatty acids.
- This leads to production of ketone bodies, which accumulate in the body.

Symptoms of DKA include:
- Kussmaul respirations (shallow, rapid breathing)
- Nausea/vomiting and abdominal pain
- Delirium
- Fruity breath (because of exhaled acetone)

Laboratory results in DKA will demonstrate:
- Hyperglycemia
- Anion-gap metabolic acidosis ($\uparrow H^+$, $\downarrow HCO_3^-$)
- High blood ketone levels
- Hyperkalemia
  - Note: this actually reflects decreased intracellular K^+, because the absence of insulin causes a transcellular shift of K^+.

Treatment centers around rehydration via intravenous fluids, insulin, K^+, and occasionally glucose if necessary to prevent hypoglycemia.

SUMMARY

- The pancreas consists of both exocrine tissue that secretes enzymes into the gut lumen and endocrine tissue that secretes hormones into the bloodstream. Exocrine structures called *acinar cells* surround the endocrine tissue, called the islets of Langerhans.
- The islets of Langerhans are primarily composed of alpha cells and beta cells. Glucagon is made in alpha cells, and insulin is made in beta cells.
- Glucagon and insulin receptors occur in high concentrations on the cell membranes of adipose, skeletal muscle, and hepatic tissue.
- Glucagon signaling is transduced through a cAMP-mediated pathway, whereas insulin signaling is transduced through a tyrosine kinase-mediated pathway.
- Insulin and glucagon function together regulate the plasma glucose level. Glucagon raises plasma glucose to ensure an adequate supply of glucose to the brain, whereas insulin lowers plasma glucose to promote the storage and use of excess glucose.
- High plasma glucose levels stimulate insulin secretion from beta cells through a glucokinase-mediated sensing mechanism. Glucokinase's effects on glycolysis and hence on intracellular ATP ultimately depolarize the cell and promote the exocytosis of granules of stored insulin.
- During fed states, insulin leads to storage and macromolecule production.
  - Promotes glycogen production and glycolysis.
  - Promotes binding of free fatty acids to glycerol to form triglyceride.
  - Promotes protein synthesis.
  - In addition, inhibits the degradation of these same macromolecules and inhibits glucagon secretion.
- During fasting states, glucagon leads to macromolecule breakdown.
  - Promotes glycogenolysis and gluconeogenesis.

- Promotes degradation of triglycerides into fatty acids and glycerol to feed gluconeogenesis.
- Promotes hepatic uptake of amino acids to feed gluconeogenesis.
- Counterregulatory hormones that also raise plasma glucose and counter insulin's actions are growth hormone, glucocorticoid, and epinephrine.
- When glucagon levels are chronically high, acetyl-CoA accumulates from the degradation of triglyceride and protein that can lead to formation of ketone bodies. These serve as alternate fuel sources for the body so that the brain can use any available glucose.
- Other hormones produced by the islet of Langerhans include somatostatin, pancreatic polypeptide, VIP, and serotonin.
- Low plasma glucose is called hypoglycemia, whereas high plasma glucose is called hyperglycemia.
- Islet cell tumors lead to increased levels of pancreatic hormones. The most common type is the beta-cell tumor, also called an insulinoma, which leads to hypoglycemia.
- Diabetes mellitus is a condition of impaired insulin action that leads to hyperglycemia. The short-term signs and symptoms include polydipsia, polyuria, polyphagia, and high plasma and urine glucose levels. The longer-term sequelae are injuries to large and small blood vessels.
- In type 1 diabetes, autoantibodies against beta cells reduce beta-cell mass and hence reduce insulin secretion. Chronic lack of insulin-mediated glucagon inhibition can put the body into a fasted-state metabolism, worsening the hyperglycemia and leading to ketosis. The mainstay of therapy is subcutaneous injection of insulin.
- Type 2 diabetes begins with insulin resistance in adipose, liver, and muscle tissue. Insulin resistance is correlated with obesity. As the disease progresses, insulin secretion also declines. Treatment options include weight loss, oral hypoglycemic medication, and administration of exogenous insulin.

REVIEW QUESTIONS

Directions: Each of the numbered items or incomplete statements in this section is followed by answers or by completions of the statement. Select the one lettered answer or completion that is best in each case.

1. A 73-year-old woman comes to the emergency room with worsening disorientation and stupor. The workup reveals pronounced hypoglycemia, hyperinsulinemia, and a pancreatic mass. Which of the following explains the woman's failure to compensate for her hypoglycemia?
   A. Glycogen deficiency
   B. Excess free fatty acids
   C. Decreased alpha-cell mass
   D. Glucagon inhibition
   E. Adrenal suppression

2. A 13-year-old girl is admitted to a psychiatric ward for treatment for an eating disorder. She is severely malnourished and underweight. It is likely that:
   A. Her glucagon levels are low

   B. Her plasma glucose level is low
   C. Her tissues are insulin-resistant
   D. Her tissue glycogen stores are depleted
   E. Her gluconeogenesis enzymes are depleted

3. An obese 50-year-old man notices a significant increase in his thirst and appetite over the past few months and complains of frequent urination. He has a long family history of type 2 diabetes but has never had any symptoms of it before now. The mechanism behind his hyperglycemia is likely to involve:
   A. An impaired glucokinase-mediated signaling pathway
   B. An impaired tyrosine kinase-mediated signaling pathway
   C. Decreased beta-cell mass
   D. Impaired glucagon action
   E. Impaired insulin secretion

ANSWERS TO REVIEW QUESTIONS

1. **The answer is D.** The woman has an insulinoma. The consequent high levels of insulin cause the hypoglycemia and also inhibit glucagon secretion, preventing counterregulatory compensation for the low plasma glucose level. Glycogen deficiency could interfere with the counterregulatory response to the low plasma glucose level because the counterregulatory hormones derive glucose from glycogenolysis; however, hyperinsulinemia *increases* glycogen stores rather than decreases them. Hyperinsulinemia decreases levels of free fatty acids, binding them into triglycerides by inhibition of hormone-sensitive lipase. Decreased alpha-cell mass would interfere with the compensation for hypoglycemia by limiting the amount of glucagon that can be produced. However, hyperinsulinemia does not reduce glucagon secretion by decreasing alpha-cell mass; rather, it inhibits secretion from alpha cells. Adrenal suppression would also interfere with the response to hypoglycemia because the adrenal glands produce glucocorticoid, a counterregulatory hormone. Hyperinsulinemia does not, however, suppress the secretion of any of the counterregulatory hormones besides glucagon.

2. **The answer is D.** The girl's metabolism is in a fasted state. Decreased consumption of carbohydrates initially lowers the plasma glucose level, and glucagon secretion increases. Glucagon levels would therefore be elevated, not low. Glucagon promotes glycogenolysis to increase the glucose level at the expense of glycogen stores, so glycogen stores would be depleted. The plasma glucose level may not be low because of successful counterregulatory compensation for the decreased dietary supply of glucose. Insulin resistance is associated with obesity, not malnourishment. Although her liver would be conducting more gluconeogenesis to provide glucose to the bloodstream to feed the brain, increased metabolic activity is not associated with a decrease in enzyme levels.

3. **The answer is B.** The man has type 2 diabetes with insulin resistance. Because the insulin receptor in insulin's target tissues (liver, muscle, and fat) is a tyrosine kinase, peripheral insulin resistance is likely to involve this signaling pathway. The glucokinase signaling pathway mediates glucose sensing and insulin secretion in beta cells. Early in the progression of type 2 diabetes, insulin secretion and beta-cell mass are normal. There is no glucagon impairment in type 2 diabetes. Furthermore, impaired glucagon action would lead to hypoglycemia, not hyperglycemia.

29

The Pituitary Gland

INTRODUCTION

The hypothalamus and pituitary gland constitute an elegant center of hormonal control known as the hypothalamic-pituitary axis (HPA).
- Each hormone controlled by the pituitary is regulated separately along its own pathway, or "axis."
- The HPA integrates information from the body's internal and external environments with higher cortical input.
- The HPA then orchestrates changes in the multiple physiologic systems controlled by the pituitary hormone axes, allowing for coordinated hormonal responses to stimuli.
  - Necessary for daily activities (i.e., eating, sleeping), but also for efficient response to illness and other physiologic stress.

Pituitary hormones act on both endocrine and nonendocrine sites, including the kidneys, adrenal glands, thyroid, ovaries, testes, breast, uterus, and vascular smooth muscle. These hormones are essential to metabolic and autonomic nervous system function and also support changes that occur throughout life.

SYSTEM STRUCTURE

The pituitary gland (or hypophysis, meaning "undergrowth") is a small endocrine gland (0.5–0.9 g). The pituitary gland is located below the hypothalamus, attached to it by the pituitary infundibulum, or neural stalk (Fig. 29.1).
- The pituitary rests in the sella turcica (Latin for "Turkish saddle") of the sphenoid bone.
- It is separated from the brain and its surrounding arachnoid membranes and cerebrospinal fluid by a reflection of the dura mater called the diaphragmatic sellae.
- The pituitary is inferior and slightly posterior to the optic chiasm.
- It lies posterior to the air-filled sphenoid sinus and adjacent to the venous cavernous *sinuses* through which travel cranial nerves III, IV, and VI and the internal carotid artery.
- Any of these anatomic structures may be compressed and disturbed by pituitary tumors (see Clinical Correlation Box 29.1).

Clinical Correlation Box 29.1

Surgeons often reach the pituitary through a transnasal approach via the sphenoid sinus. Surgical equipment is inserted up the nasal cavity and through the sphenoid bone, giving access to the cranium.

Gross Anatomy

The pituitary has three divisions, the most important of which are the anterior and posterior lobes (Fig. 29.2):
- Anterior lobe (adenohypophysis)
  - Synthesizes and secretes six hormones (Table 29.1)
    Adrenocorticotropic hormone (ACTH)
    Thyroid-stimulating hormone (TSH)
    Growth hormone (GH)
    Follicle-stimulating hormone (FSH)
    Luteinizing hormone (LH)
    Prolactin
- Posterior lobe (neurohypophysis)
  - Stores and releases two hormones (see Table 29.1):
    Antidiuretic hormone (ADH)
    Oxytocin
- Infundibulum
  - Stalk-like structure that connects the pituitary to the hypothalamus.
  - Consists of the more proximal median eminence and the distal stalk.
  - Contains vasculature carrying hypothalamic hormones to the anterior pituitary and neural tracts that project from the hypothalamus to the posterior lobe.

Histology of the Anterior Lobe

The anterior lobe consists of cords of secretory cells, fibroblasts, and capillary endothelial cells. The secretory cells are named according to the staining properties of their granules:
- Chromophils
  - Acidophils
  - Basophils
- Chromophobes
  - Few or no secretory granules.
  - May represent undifferentiated chromophils, or chromophils that have released their granules.

The acidophils and basophils are further classified on the basis of the hormones they produce (Table 29.2):
- Acidophils
  - Somatotrophs (GH)
  - Lactotrophs (Prolactin)
- Basophils
  - Corticotrophs (ACTH)
  - Thyrotrophs (TSH)
  - Gonadotrophs (FSH, LH)

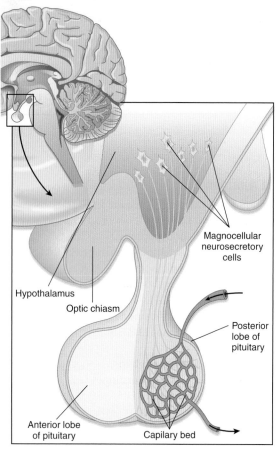

Fig. 29.1 Midsagittal cross-section of the hypothalamus. The infundibulum connects the pituitary with the hypothalamus. (Modified from Larsen PR et al, eds. *Williams Textbook of Endocrinology*, 10th Edition. Philadelphia: Saunders; 2003.)

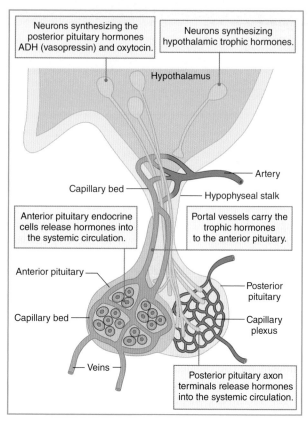

Fig. 29.2 Anterior and posterior pituitary. The posterior pituitary comprises axonal projections from cell bodies in the hypothalamic nuclei. Both anterior and posterior pituitary cells secrete hormones into a capillary plexus supplied by the hypophyseal arteries and the pituitary portal circulation, bringing blood from the hypothalamus. (Modified from Carroll R. *Elsevier's Integrated Physiology*. Philadelphia: Mosby Elsevier; 2007. Fig. 13.4.)

TABLE 29.1	**Pituitary Hormones**		
Compound	**Size (kDa)**	**Structure**	**End Organ**
Anterior Pituitary			
ACTH	MW 4500	39 aa[a]	Adrenal cortex
TSH	Glycoprotein MW 28,000	alpha subunit[b]: 89 aa beta subunit: 112 aa	Thyroid
GH	MW 21,500	191 aa polypeptide	IGF-1 production; growth and metabolic effects
FSH	Glycoprotein MW 29,000	alpha subunit[b]: 89 aa beta subunit: 115 aa	Ovaries Testes
LH	Glycoprotein MW 29,000	alpha subunit[b]: 89 aa beta subunit: 115 aa	Ovaries Testes
Prolactin	MW 22,000	198 aa polypeptide	Breast
Posterior Pituitary			
ADH		Nonapeptide (9 aa)	Vascular smooth muscle; distal tubule of kidney
Oxytocin		Nonapeptide (9 aa)	Mammary gland smooth muscle; uterus

ACTH, Adrenocorticotropic hormone; *ADH*, antidiuretic hormone; *FSH*, follicle-stimulating hormone; *GH*, growth hormone; *IGF-1*, insulin-like growth factor-1; *LH*, luteinizing hormone; *MW*, molecular weight; *TSH*, thyroid-stimulating hormone.
[a]aa, amino acid.
[b]The alpha subunits of TSH, FSH, and LH, as well as hCG (human chorionic gonadotropin, a compound released by the placenta), are identical; the beta subunits are distinct and give each its identity and function.

TABLE 29.2   Anterior Lobe Cell Types

Cell Type (% of Anterior Lobe Cells)	Staining Properties	Secretory Granules (nm)	Hormone Product(s)
Somatotroph (50)	Acidophilic	300–400	GH (somatotropin)
Lactotroph (mammotroph) (10–25)	Acidophilic	200 (600 in pregnant or lactating women)	Prolactin
Corticotroph (15–20)	Basophilic	400–550	ACTH[a] (corticotropin)
Thyrotroph (<10)	Basophilic	120–200	TSH (thyrotropin)
Gonadotroph (10–15)	Basophilic	250–400	FSH, LH

[a]Corticotrophs synthesize and releases multiple peptides; see text.
ACTH, Adrenocorticotropic hormone; *FSH*, follicle-stimulating hormone; *GH*, growth hormone; *LH*, luteinizing hormone.

The anterior pituitary depends on stimulating factors from the parvocellular (small-diameter) neurons of the hypothalamus.

- The axons of these neurons release substances into the fenestrated capillaries of the median eminence.
- These capillaries coalesce into hypophyseal portal vessels that travel down the infundibulum, form another capillary bed, and release substances to the anterior pituitary.
- This is known as the pituitary portal circulation (see Clinical Correlation Box 29.2).

Clinical Correlation Box 29.2

Portal Circulations

In the systemic circulation, the vascular sequence is arteries → capillaries → veins. In a portal circulation, such as in the pituitary or the liver, there is an additional set of veins and capillaries, yielding the sequence arteries → capillaries → veins → capillaries (or venules) → veins. A portal system is used to transport substances in a focused, undiluted fashion to a site for a specific purpose, such as detoxification (liver) or hormonal signaling (pituitary).

Histology of the Posterior Lobe

The posterior lobe contains the unmyelinated axons of hypothalamic neurosecretory cells, pituicytes (specialized glial cells), and capillary endothelial cells.

- No hormone synthesis occurs in the posterior lobe.
  Magnocellular (large-diameter) hypothalamic neurons originate in the paraventricular and supraoptic nuclei.
- Their axons carry hormones down the infundibulum into the posterior lobe, where they are stored.
- The axon terminals are adjacent to fenestrated capillaries and release hormones directly to the systemic circulation without making use of the pituitary portal circulation.

SYSTEM FUNCTION

As previously mentioned, each pituitary hormone is controlled by a corresponding HPA. Each axis has several factors modulating its activity, including:

- Primary regulatory agents (major)
- Regulatory agents of other HPAs
  - In other words, pathology in one axis can readily disrupt others.
- Changes in body metabolism or electrolyte balance
- Higher cortical input
  The primary control mechanisms include (Fig. 29.3):
- Hypothalamic releasing factors
  - A positive releasing factor stimulates the release of a compound, whereas a negative factor inhibits its release.
  - All the hypothalamic regulatory hormones are peptides, except dopamine, which is a biogenic amine.
  - Most hypothalamic and pituitary hormones are secreted in bursts, known as pulsatility.
- Feedback loops
  - Definition: the end-product of a chain of events feeds back to an earlier step.
    If the effect is inhibitory, this is called negative feedback.
    If the effect is stimulatory, this is called positive feedback.
  - Negative feedback is more common because it prevents the overproduction of a compound; when a sufficient amount of a hormone has been produced, it shuts off its own releasing process.
  - Example: Hypothalamic thyrotropin-releasing hormone (TRH) prompts TSH from the pituitary gland, which leads to thyroid hormone release from the thyroid; this subsequently inhibits both TRH and TSH.

The pituitary gland also provides the basis for adaptations at various life-cycle stages or during a chronic illness.

- In these settings, significant changes in pituitary hormones and the systems they regulate are made possible by changes in gland size.
- During pregnancy, for example, lactotroph hyperplasia occurs to provide a needed increase in prolactin.

The Anterior Pituitary

The six hormones synthesized in the anterior pituitary (ACTH, TSH, GH, FSH, LH, and prolactin) individually affect the activity of one or more target organs (Fig. 29.4). They are under the influence of several hypothalamic regulatory factors:

- Corticotropin-releasing hormone (CRH)
- TRH
- Growth hormone-releasing hormone (GHRH)
- Gonadotropin-releasing hormone (GnRH)
- Hypothalamic inhibitory factors
- Somatostatin
- Prolactin-inhibiting factor (PIF)

The roles of these regulatory factors are summarized in Table 29.3.

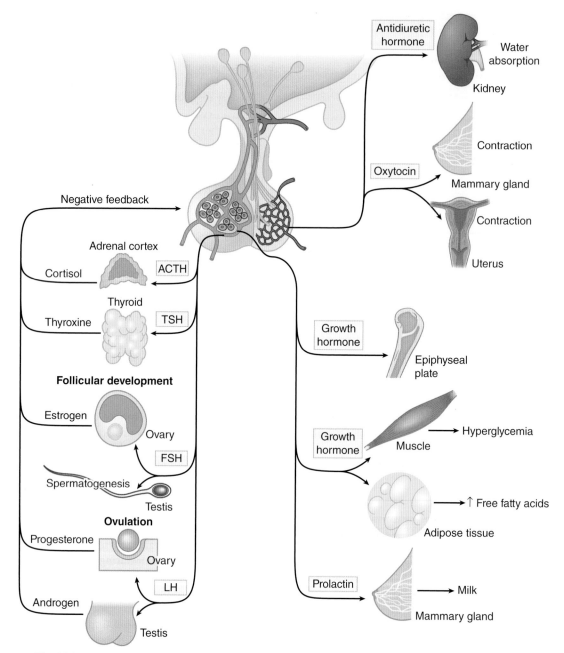

Fig. 29.3 Actions of pituitary hormones on target tissues. *ACTH*, Adrenocorticotropic hormone; *FSH*, follicle-stimulating hormone; *LH*, luteinizing hormone; *TSH*, thyroid-stimulating hormone

Corticotrophs

Corticotrophs produce the hormone ACTH, which is initially synthesized as proopiomelanocortin (POMC), a 28,000-molecular-weight prohormone whose primary breakdown product is ACTH.

- Function
  - ACTH causes the release of glucocorticoids (and, to a lesser extent, mineralocorticoids and adrenal androgens) from the adrenal cortex (see Ch. 31).
  - Over time, ACTH also promotes the growth of the adrenal cortex; in its absence, the gland atrophies.
  - The role of ACTH in adrenal gland function and corticosteroid synthesis is described more fully in Chapter 31.

- Regulation (see Fig. 29.4)
  - (+)
    Pulsatile release of CRH from the hypothalamus stimulates a diurnal pattern of ACTH release, characterized by an early morning peak and an evening nadir.
    ADH is a less-potent stimulator of ACTH release and acts predominantly through the potentiation of CRH activity.
  - (−)
    Cortisol feedback inhibits the release of CRH and ACTH.
    ACTH inhibits CRH release via a short feedback loop (Fig. 29.5).

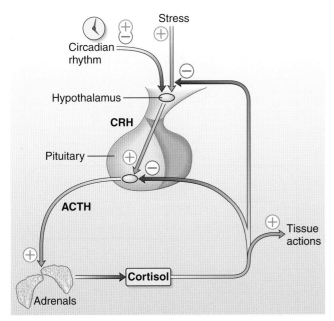

Fig. 29.4 Hypothalamic-pituitary-adrenal axis. Plus signs represent stimulation; minus signs represent inhibition. *ACTH*, Adrenocorticotropic hormone; *CRH*, corticotropin-releasing hormone. (From *Kumar & Clark's Cases in Clinical Medicine.* Elsevier; 2013: p. 411-460; Fig. 14.5.)

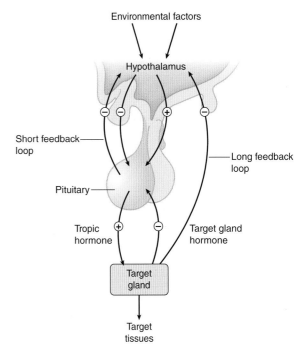

Fig. 29.5 Feedback loops. The short and long feedback loops are depicted as having a negative (inhibitory) feedback effect, but they may also have a positive (stimulatory) feedback effect.

TABLE 29.3	Hypothalamic Regulatory Hormones	
Hypothalamic Hormone	**Structure**	**Function[a]**
Thyrotropin-releasing hormone (TRH)	Tripeptide (3 aa[b])	Stimulates TSH release by thyrotroph; stimulates prolactin release by lactotroph
Corticotropin-releasing hormone (CRH)	41 aa polypeptide	Stimulates ACTH release by corticotroph
Gonadotropin-releasing hormone (GnRH)	Decapeptide (10 aa)	Stimulates FSH and LH release by gonadotroph
Growth hormone-releasing hormone (GHRH)	44 aa polypeptide	Stimulates GHRH release by somatotroph
Somatostatin	14 aa peptide	Inhibits GH release by somatotroph; inhibits TSH release by thyrotroph
Prolactin-inhibiting factor (PIF)	Dopamine[c]	Inhibits prolactin release from lactotroph

[a]Primary function. Almost all hypothalamic hormones have some effects on each of the anterior pituitary cell types.
[b]aa, amino acid.
[c]Evidence indicates that there may be additional PIFs. However, dopamine appears to be the primary PIF.
ACTH, Adrenocorticotropic hormone; *FSH*, follicle-stimulating hormone; *GH*, growth hormone; *LH*, luteinizing hormone; *TSH*, thyroid-stimulating hormone.

Both psychologic and physical stressors, such as trauma and illness, increase ACTH levels to promote cortisol synthesis via a variety of mechanisms.
- Fever is associated with cytokine-mediated release of CRH.
- Catecholamines and opioids can stimulate ACTH release.

Thyrotrophs
Thyrotrophs produce the hormone TSH.
- Function
  - TSH regulates the synthesis and secretion of thyroid hormones (see Ch. 30).
  - TSH also promotes thyroid growth.
- Regulation (Fig. 29.6)
  - (+)
    Hypothalamic secretion of TRH causes TSH synthesis, posttranslational glycosylation, and release.
    There is a pulsatile, circadian pattern of TSH release that peaks in the early morning and reaches its nadir in the late afternoon.
  - (−)
    Somatostatin inhibits TSH release from the pituitary.
    The thyroid hormones thyroxine (T4) and triiodothyronine (T3)— primarily the more physiologically active T3— inhibit TSH and TRH release via long feedback loops.
    TSH inhibits TRH release via a short negative-feedback loop.
  Starvation, stress, exercise, and illness all decrease TSH secretion via many mechanisms, including increased cortisol (i.e., stress response).
- Cortisol decreases TSH by decreasing the sensitivity of the pituitary to TRH.
- During starvation, the lowering of TSH decreases the overall basal metabolic rate and preserves scarce energy sources.

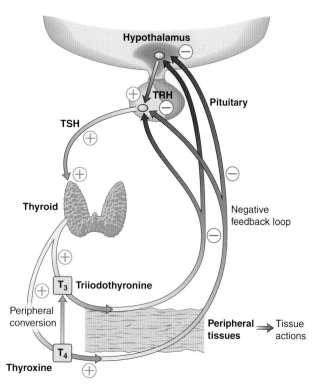

Fig. 29.6 Hypothalamic-pituitary-thyroid axis. *Plus signs* represent stimulation; *minus signs* represent inhibition. *TRH,* thyrotropin-releasing hormone; *TSH,* thyroid-stimulating hormone. (From *Kumar and Clark's Clinical Medicine.* Elsevier; 2017: p. 1175-1240; Fig. 26.2.)

Somatotrophs

Somatotrophs produce the hormone GH.

- Unlike other anterior pituitary hormones, GH does not prompt the release of another hormone from a specific endocrine gland.
- In addition, GH indirectly promotes the release and actions of insulin-like growth factor-1 (IGF-1), also known as somatomedin-C.
  - The liver secretes IGF-1 into the systemic circulation, whereas other tissues respond to GH by secreting IGF-1 locally as a paracrine factor.

Because GH and IGF-1 are intimately related, it is useful to explore them together by organ system:

- Function
  - Musculoskeletal

    Both promote long-bone growth at the epiphysis (growth plate) via a process known as endochondral ossification.

    Chondrocytes (cartilage-producing cells) multiply, grow, and lay down cartilage that then undergoes calcification.

    GH binds to receptors on epiphyseal prechondrocytes → promotes differentiation into chondrocytes, which secrete IGF-1 → chondrocyte proliferation → long-bone growth.
  - Renal

    IGF-1 as well as insulin increases distal nephron collecting dust epithelial Na$^+$ channel function, leading to increase Na$^+$ reabsorption. Some patients who have overproduction of IGF-1 or an increase in circulating insulin may therefore develop edema.

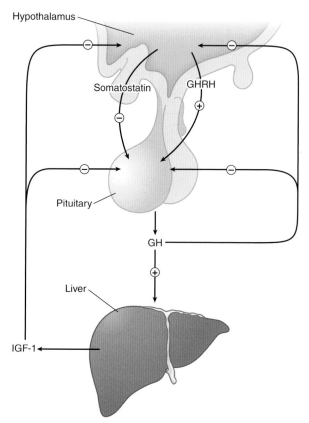

Fig. 29.7 Growth hormone secretion. *Plus signs* represent stimulation; minus signs represent inhibition. *GH,* Growth hormone; *GHRH,* growth hormone releasing hormone; *IGF,* insulin-like growth factor.

- Metabolic
  - GH produces anabolic effects on protein metabolism and catabolic effects on carbohydrate/lipid metabolism.

    Protein: increases synthesis directly

    Carbohydrate: inhibits insulin action in the liver ("diabetogenic") but preserves glycogen stores in liver ("glycostatic")

    Lipid: increases activity of hormone-sensitive lipase
  - IGF-1 has a synergistic effect on protein metabolism but opposes GH action on carbohydrate/lipid metabolism.

    Protein: inhibits breakdown

    Carbohydrate: Binding IGF-1 receptors on skeletal muscle (not adipocytes or hepatocytes) result in glucose uptake and utilization; inhibits GH's effects on glucose metabolism.

    Lipids: Short-term antilipolytic, long-term lipolytic by unknown mechanisms.
- Regulation (Fig. 29.7)
  - (+)

    GH secretion is mediated by GHRH from the hypothalamus.

    GH release mediated by higher-order central nervous system centers, including the hippocampus and amygdala, and occurs mostly during sleep (70%).

    GH levels peak during adolescence and decrease with age, linking metabolic changes and growth induction such that the body ensures that it will have the metabolic substrate necessary for growth.

- (−)

  GH secretion is inhibited by somatostatin from the hypothalamus.

  IGF-2 provides feedback inhibition at the hypothalamus and pituitary.

  In addition, GH inhibits GHRH release via short-loop feedback inhibition.

GH secretion changes in response to virtually any stress or change in endocrine function or metabolism.

- Hypoglycemia is a potent stimulus to GH release.
- Strong evidence indicates that emotional deprivation can impair GH secretion and even lead to growth failure. For example, institutional abuse and profound neglect have been found to produce dwarfism.

Of note, the GH axis interacts with almost every other pituitary axis.

- Cortisol increases GH release; the linking of these two counterregulatory hormones facilitates a more effective response to hypoglycemia.
- Thyroid hormone T3 potentiates the pituitary response to GHRH, increasing GH levels (see Clinical Correlation Box 29.3).

Clinical Correlation Box 29.3

Consequently, in hypothyroidism, the growth hormone response to growth hormone-releasing hormone is blunted, so hypothyroidism typically retards growth in children. Again, the pituitary coordinates events: when the body's thyroid function is low, as in illness, it is an inopportune time for growth.

Gonadotrophs

Gonadotrophs produce two hormones, LH and FSH, also known as the gonadotropins. These hormones act on the ovaries and testes, although both their function and regulation is complex and merits further exploration in Chapters 34 and 36.

- Function
  - Their effects include both gametogenesis and the production of sex steroids.
- Regulation (Fig. 29.8)
  - Context-dependent (+ or −)

    Hypothalamic GnRH governs the secretion of LH and FSH.

    If pulsatile → (+) regulation

    If nonpulsatile → (−) regulation

    Estrogen

      Typically (−) caused by inhibition of GnRH

      During follicular phase of the menstrual cycle, (+) feedback stimulates LH secretion from the pituitary and creates mid-cycle LH "surge"

  - (−)

    Women

      Progesterone decreases GnRH secretion.

      LH/FSH decrease GnRH secretion.

      Inhibin, made in the ovarian granulosa cells, blocks FSH secretion in the late follicular phase of the menstrual cycle.

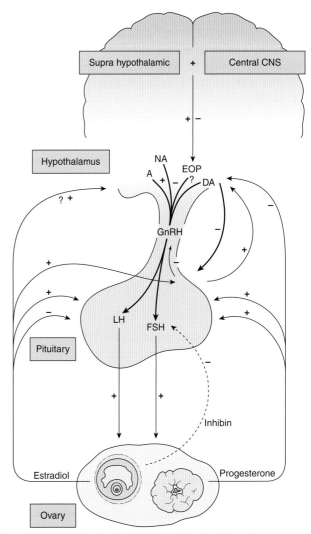

Fig. 29.8 Hypothalamic-pituitary-gonadal axis. *Plus signs* represent stimulation; *minus signs* represent inhibition. *A,* Adrenaline; *DA,* dopamine; *CNS,* central nervous system; *EOP,* endogenous opioids; *FSH,* follicle-stimulating hormone; *GnRH,* gonadotrophin-releasing hormone; *LH,* luteinizing hormone; *NA,* noradrenaline; *PRL,* prolactin. (From Shaw RW. *Gynaecology,* 4th Edition. Elsevier; 2011: p. 197-211; Fig. 15.15.)

Men

  Testosterone and dihydrotestosterone from testicular Leydig cells suppress LH (but not FSH) via the suppression of GnRH.

  Inhibin, made in the testicular Sertoli cells, inhibits FSH release (see Clinical Correlation Box 29.4).

Clinical Correlation Box 29.4

Pulsatility is necessary for gonadal activity. Continuously elevated gonadotropin-releasing hormone (GnRH) leads to the suppression of luteinizing hormone (LH) and follicle-stimulating hormone (FSH), perhaps because of the downregulation of GnRH receptors. This phenomenon is used in the therapy of hyper-LH/FSH states, such as central precocious puberty by treating patients with a long acting depot GnRH analogue. A depot medication is a long term storage form of the agent that slowly diffuses into it volume of distribution. Such long acting GnRH analogues are used to treat some gonadal malignancies such as testicular cancer and can decrease blood flow to the gonads.

As with other hormonal systems, stress and other environmental changes (including the usual course of development) modulate the activity of this system.

- In anorexia nervosa, the levels of GnRH, gonadotropins, and the sex steroids decrease leading to amenorrhea, preventing a possible pregnancy in the setting of "starvation."
- In early childhood, there is central inhibition of GnRH secretion and the pituitary is exquisitely sensitive to negative feedback by gonadal steroids.
- In puberty, central inhibition is lifted and the sensitivity of the pituitary to negative feedback declines, leading to a transition to adult pattern of pulsatile GnRH (and thus gonadotropin) secretion.
- At menopause, with the lack of circulating sex steroids from the ovaries, levels of LH and FSH rise.

Lactotrophs

Lactotrophs produce the hormone prolactin, which acts primarily at the mammary gland.
- Function
  - Promotes breast development and lactation.
  - Inhibits spermatogenesis and ovulation.
  - Like other anterior pituitary hormones, prolactin is secreted in a pulsatile fashion with peak levels occurring at the end of the night.
- Regulation (Fig. 29.9)
  - (+)
    TRH acts at the level of the pituitary to stimulate prolactin release.
    Decrease in dopaminergic inhibition.
    Estrogen causes increased synthesis and release of prolactin, in anticipation of need for postpartum prolactin.
  - (−)
    Unlike other anterior pituitary hormones, prolactin regulation is predominantly through hypothalamic inhibition.
    The major inhibitory factor is dopamine, which tonically inhibits prolactin release.
    Through a short feedback loop, prolactin promotes hypothalamic dopamine release and thus "tunes down" its own release (see Genetics Box 29.1 and Development Box 29.1).

> ### 🧬 GENETICS BOX 29.1
>
> Patients with combined pituitary hormone deficiency (CPHD) have insufficient production of one or more hormones because of a defect in pituitary cell differentiation. The most common genetic abnormalities are mutations in the PROP-1 gene that encodes a transcription factors in cells that normally differentiate into various components of the pituitary. Without the PROP-1 transcription factor, pituitary development is impaired.

> ### 🧬 DEVELOPMENT BOX 29.1
>
> Combined pituitary hormone deficiency (CPHD) manifests in young children as decreased stature and impaired growth, as most patients have a deficiency in growth hormone. Some patients have hypothyroidism as well, because of a lack of thyroid-stimulating hormone. There is variable impairment in the development of other pituitary cells. In adulthood, some patients develop adrenal insufficiency (lack of adrenocorticotropic hormone) or impaired fertility (low follicle-stimulating hormone and luteinizing hormone).

The Posterior Pituitary

The hypothalamic hormones released by the posterior lobe of the pituitary are two peptide hormones, ADH (also known as vasopressin) and oxytocin.
- Their structures are quite similar, differing by only two amino acids.
- Recall that these compounds are synthesized in neuronal cell bodies in the hypothalamus but stored in neuronal axons in the posterior pituitary.

Antidiuretic Hormone

- Function
  - The primary role of ADH is to promote water retention at the level of the renal distal tubule.
    Binds V_2 receptor → causes the fusion of aquaporin-containing vesicles with the luminal membrane of the distal tubules → increases water permeability and thereby allowing water reabsorption.
  - Stimulates thirst.
  - Mediates vasoconstriction.
    Binds V_1 receptor
- Regulation
  - Plasma osmolarity over 280 mOsm/kg H_2O
    Osmoreceptors in anterior hypothalamus → triggers supraoptic and paraventricular nuclei → release of ADH.
    This system is very sensitive: a small increase in osmolarity causes rapid ADH release, water retention, and the restoration of normal osmolarity.
  - Decreased blood volume
    Baroreceptors in left atrium and aortic arch/carotid arteries → stimulation of CNIX and CX → hypothalmic activation → ADH release.
    This system is less sensitive than the osmolarity system, and thus significant changes in blood pressure or volume are required to causes ADH release.

Oxytocin

- Function
  - Oxytocin is responsible for stimulating lactation by leading to the contraction of myoepithelial cells in the breasts, causing milk flow.
  - Oxytocin also maintains labor by causing uterine smooth muscle contraction. Myometrial cells express a large number of oxytocin receptors during pregnancy.
    Oxytocin is frequently used at pharmacologic doses to induce labor by promoting uterine contraction, and it is also used to promote postpartum uterine contraction.
  - Oxytocin's function in men is unclear, but it may in increase motility in seminiferous tubules and seminal vesicles.
- Regulation
  - (+)
    Suckling induces the release of oxytocin. Interestingly, visual or psychologic stimuli suggestive of suckling can also provoke this response.
  - (−)
    Both beta-agonists and opioids appear to have an inhibitory effect on oxytocin secretion.

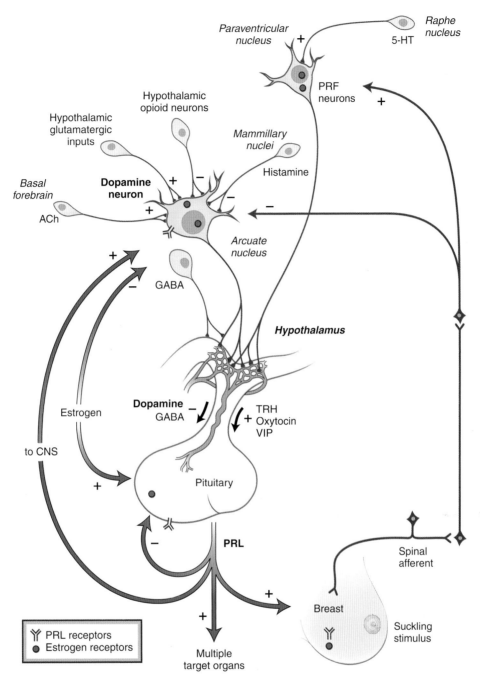

Fig. 29.9 Prolactin secretion. *Plus signs* represent stimulation; *minus signs* represent inhibition. *CNS,* Central nervous system; *GABA,* γ-aminobutyric acid; *PRF,* prolactin releasing factor; *PRL, prolactin* (From Melmed S. *Williams Textbook of Endocrinology,* 14th Edition. Elsevier; 2019. Fig. 7.27.)

During pregnancy, the increased endogenous opioids in response to stress have the effect of preserving oxytocin stores for parturition and uterine contraction.

PATHOPHYSIOLOGY

Pituitary pathology is broadly caused by three categories of problems:

1. Insufficient pituitary hormone secretion
2. Excessive pituitary hormone secretion
3. Mass effects of enlarging pituitary tumors

Typically, the disruption of one HPA also alters the others. Pituitary pathology thus leads to a gross disruption of the endocrine and metabolic processes that the pituitary carefully regulates.

Anterior Pituitary Lobe Pathology

The entire anterior pituitary lobe can be destroyed in certain clinical scenarios:

- Infarction because of hemorrhage (i.e., after massive hemorrhage during childbirth, referred to as Sheehan syndrome)

- Head trauma (i.e., a car accident that leads to a sudden halting of motion of the head can shear the infundibulum)

In this case, all the pituitary hormones will be decreased or absent. This is known as panhypopituitarism.

More commonly, through injury or developmental anomaly, a single cell type will be deficient or absent. The effects of deficiencies of the various anterior pituitary hormones follow logically from their function.

- GH deficiency in children leads to short stature.
- FSH/LH deficiency causes hypogonadism.
- ACTH deficiency leads to adrenal insufficiency.
- TSH deficiency causes central hypothyroidism, which is much rarer than primary hypothyroidism, caused by disease of the thyroid gland itself.

In the anterior pituitary, the most common type of overgrowth pathology is a pituitary adenoma, a tumor of one of the chromophil or chromophobe cells. It may be:

- Large (macroadenoma) or small (microadenoma)
- Functioning (hormone-secreting) or nonfunctioning

A functioning pituitary adenoma causes abnormal elevation of the hormone it produces, but can also lead to hypofunction of other cell types by taking up necessary space and nutrients.

- The most common of these is a prolactin-secreting tumor, or prolactinoma.
  - Prolactinomas lead to hypogonadism and galactorrhea (milky discharge from the breasts).
- GH excess during childhood causes gigantism, whereas during adulthood it leads to acromegaly (see Clinical Correlation Box 29.5).

Clinical Correlation Box 29.5

Acromegaly results from the excess production of growth hormone (GH), usually because of a tumor of the pituitary.

- Acromegaly typically arises in middle age, when the epiphyseal plates at the ends of the long bones have already sealed—thus, there is no change in height.
- However, soft tissues and bones of the face remain responsive to this excess GH and grow. This results in visceromegaly, brow and jaw protrusion, lengthening of the vocal cords resulting in deepening of the voice, and hyperpigmentation of the skin.

By contrast, gigantism results from an excess production of GH during childhood when the epiphyseal plates of the long bones have not yet sealed, resulting in excess height.

- Robert Wadlow, the tallest man known to have lived and a known patient with gigantism, grew to 8 feet 11 inches tall.

Posterior Pituitary Pathology

The most clinically significant disease involving the posterior lobe of the pituitary is a deficiency of ADH, a condition known as central diabetes insipidus (DI).

- Because of lack of ADH, patients are unable to retain water and excrete large amounts of dilute urine, leading to increased plasma osmolarity.
- Central DI is common after trauma or neurosurgical resection of tumors near the pituitary.
  - It may be transient (secondary to postoperative swelling) or permanent.

Because central DI is a deficiency of ADH, it can be treated with a synthetic form of ADH, DDAVP (desmopressin acetate) (see Fast Fact Box 29.1).

Fast Fact Box 29.1

Antidiuretic hormone (ADH) deficiency refers to central diabetes insipidus (DI), not to be confused with nephrogenic DI, which occurs when ADH is present but the kidney cannot respond properly.

Mass Effects From Pituitary Tumors

The classical presentation of a patient with an enlarging pituitary tumor is a bitemporal hemianopsia (bilateral loss of lateral vision fields) resulting from compression of the optic chiasm (Fig. 29.10).

- Compression of the central optic nerve fibers that innervate the nasal retinae and supply the lateral visual fields causes a loss of peripheral vision.

However, tumors may also invade the nearby cavernous sinus, compromising the integrity of the internal carotid artery or of cranial nerves II, IV, or VI, which travel through it.

- This can lead to diplopia or other vision changes.

Because pituitary tumors exert dual effects—(1) hormonal overproduction and (2) mass effect on the optic nerves—visual changes with evidence of hormonal dysfunction should arouse clinical suspicion of a pituitary tumor. (See Clinical Correlation Box 29.6, Clinical Correlation Box 29.7 and Clinical Correlation Box 29.8).

Clinical Correlation Box 29.6

Craniopharyngiomas are slow-growing brain tumors that develop from embryonic tissue precursors to the pituitary gland, particularly from cells that for the pituitary stalk. These cells are known as odontogenic cells, meaning that they typically differentiate to form teeth. As such, craniopharyngiomas are often calcified and visible on x-ray (Fig. 29.11). As with other tumors in the pituitary region, craniopharyngiomas can cause growth failure, pituitary insufficiency, and bitemporal hemianopsia because of impingement on the optic chiasm.

Clinical Correlation Box 29.7

A 51-year-old man is referred to his endocrinologist with decreased libido and impotence. He also reports worsening headaches over the past several months, and says that he was involved in a motor vehicle accident where he did not see an incoming car at a four-way stop sign. On exam, he has decreased peripheral vision. Laboratory testing demonstrates decreased serum testosterone, luteinizing hormone (LH), and follicle-stimulating hormone (FSH) in addition to elevated serum prolactin. Magnetic resonance imaging demonstrates a large pituitary mass encroaching on the optic chiasm.

Prolactinomas are the most common type of functional pituitary tumors, representing a hyperplasia of pituitary lactotrophs and subsequent overproduction of prolactin (see Fig. 29.11A and B):

- High prolactin suppresses both LH and FSH, leading to hypogonadal symptoms.
- The size of the tumor compresses the optic chiasm, leading to bitemporal hemianopsia.
- Treatment revolves around both medical and surgical therapies.
  - Medical: Dopamine agonists, that is, bromocriptine, to suppress prolactin secretion.
  - Surgical: Resection of the tumor via the sphenoid sinus.

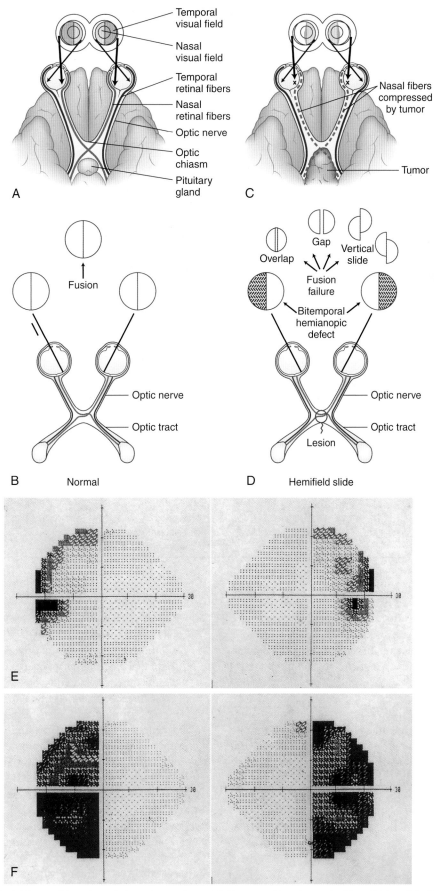

Fig. 29.10 The world as viewed through a patient with bitemporal hemianopsia. (From Melmed S. *Williams Textbook of Endocrinology*, 14th Edition. Elsevier; 2019. Fig. 9.6.)

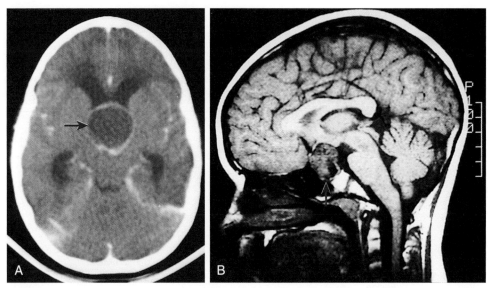

Fig. 29.11 A, Craniopharyngioma on computed tomography scan (red arrow). Calcification is very visible. **B,** Magnetic resonance imaging (the red arrow shows the craniopharyngioma). A, Courtesy Michael Painter, MD, Children's Hospital of Pittsburgh, Pittsburgh, PA. B, Courtesy Department of Neuroradiology, University Health Center of Pittsburgh, Pittsburgh, PA. (From *Zitelli and Davis' Atlas of Pediatric Physical Diagnosis*, 7th Edition. Fig. 16.45.)

Clinical Correlation Box 29.8

Magnetic resonance imaging (MRI) relies on the spinning properties of the protons in the nuclei of hydrogen atoms. The spin of individual protons lends them a magnetic polarity that makes them sensitive to magnetic fields.

- If the spin aligns with the field → low-energy state
- If the spin is in opposition with the field → high-energy state
  If the proton shifts in orientation from high to low-energy state, energy is released; in the opposite scenario, energy is absorbed.
- When energy is produced in the form of radio waves, the resonance of this energy between protons and the MRI spectrometer creates a measurable signal.
- This is tested in full 360 degrees.

As human tissue is mainly water, hydrogen is the most abundant tissue in the body.

- Differing amounts of hydrogen content allow us to distinguish fat, bone, muscle, and other tissues from one another.
- MRI may also be used to detect tumors, such as pituitary adenomas.
  MRI does not pose a carcinogenic risk as x-rays do, as radio waves are lower-energy and do not break chemical bonds in the same fashion. However. . .
- Radio waves can heat body tissues if the machine malfunctions.
- The powerful magnets used can cause metal objects to fly through the air! Everything that enters an MRI room, including medical equipment, must be deemed "MRI-safe" before entry.

■ SUMMARY

- The pituitary is divided into anterior and posterior lobes. The anterior lobe, also known as the adenohypophysis, is an extension of the ectodermal tissue of the hypothalamus. The posterior lobe, also known as the neurohypophysis, is an extension of the neuroectodermal tissue of the hypothalamus.
- The anterior pituitary hormones are part of a hypothalamic-pituitary (HP) axis. The hypothalamus secretes a hormone that stimulates the pituitary to secrete a hormone, and the pituitary hormone in turn stimulates a target organ to secrete its hormone.
- The HP axes are governed by releasing factors and feedback loops.
- The six axes of the anterior pituitary and their major function are as follows:
  - Hypothalamic-pituitary-adrenal axis: secretion of cortisol and response to stress.
  - Hypothalamic-pituitary-thyroid axis: secretion of thyroxine.

- Growth hormone axis: release of insulin-like growth factor-1 (IGF-1, long bone growth, promotion of protein synthesis and carbohydrate/lipid breakdown.
- Hypothalamic-pituitary-gonadal axis: promote the gonadal production of sex steroids.
- Prolactin axis: promotes breast development and lactation.
- The posterior pituitary secretes antidiuretic hormone (ADH) and oxytocin. ADH is primarily important in the regulation of serum osmolality. Oxytocin promotes milk secretion and may promote the uterine contractions of labor.
- Pituitary pathology causes three broad problems: (1) insufficient pituitary hormone secretion; (2) excessive pituitary hormone secretion; or (3) mass effects of enlarging pituitary tumors.
- The most common form of pituitary pathology is the pituitary adenoma, and the most common functional pituitary adenoma is the prolactinoma.
- Mass effects of pituitary tumors may include visual field deficits, hemorrhage because of invasion of the cavernous sinus, and cranial nerve palsies.

REVIEW QUESTIONS

Directions: Each of the numbered items or incomplete statements in this section is followed by answers or by completions of the statement. Select the one lettered answer or completion that is best in each case.

1. A 60-year-old man is diagnosed with a prolactin-secreting pituitary microadenoma after a thorough workup for impotence. He is given medication that suppresses prolactin secretion. This medication is likely to mimic the effects of which hypothalamic product?
   A. GnRH
   B. GHRH
   C. CRH
   D. TRH
   E. Dopamine
   F. Bromocriptine
   G. ACTH
   H. FSH
   I. LH
   J. Thyroxin

2. A 41-year-old man is diagnosed with acromegaly after a progressive enlargement of the hands and feet and prognathism. Which of the following lab abnormalities is likely to be observed?
   A. Hypocalcemia
   B. Hypoalbuminemia
   C. Hypoosmolality
   D. Hyperglycemia
   E. Hypernatremia

3. A 28-year-old woman presents with amenorrhea, galactorrhea, and bitemporal hemianopsia. The most likely cause is:
   A. Gonadal failure
   B. Panhypopituitarism
   C. Pituitary adenoma
   D. Gigantism
   E. Acromegaly

ANSWERS TO REVIEW QUESTIONS

1. **The answer is E.** Hypothalamic dopamine inhibits the secretion of prolactin from pituitary lactotrophs. GnRH, GHRH, CRH, and TRH are all hypothalamic hormones with stimulatory, not inhibitory, effects on pituitary tissues other than the lactotrophs. Bromocriptine is not a hypothalamic product; rather, bromocriptine is the medication that mimics dopamine action on the lactotrophs. ACTH, FSH, and LH are produced in the pituitary, not the hypothalamus. Thyroxine is produced in the thyroid gland.

2. **The answer is D.** GH, levels of which are elevated in acromegaly, is a counterregulatory hormone that mimics glucagon action in its effects on carbohydrate metabolism. It promotes gluconeogenesis and increases the plasma glucose level. High levels of GH also increase IGF-1 levels, which mimics the effect of insulin, not glucagon, thus driving down the serum glucose level. Clinically, it is more common to observe an increase in the counterregulatory effects and hyperglycemia.

3. **The answer is C.** The symptoms of hyperprolactinemia and cranial mass effects are indicative of a prolactin-secreting pituitary adenoma. Pituitary adenomas can lead to gigantism or acromegaly, but these produce a different clinical picture. Gonadal steroid production is suppressed in hyperprolactinemia, but gonadal failure alone would not explain galactorrhea (milk production) or cranial mass effects.

30

The Thyroid Gland

INTRODUCTION

The thyroid—named from the Greek *thureoeides*, meaning "shield-shaped"—bears two essential responsibilities in the endocrine system:
- Maintains metabolic rate necessary for heat generation in warm-blooded species.
- Promotes normal growth and development from fetal life into childhood.

Roughly 5% of the U.S. population has a diagnosed thyroid disorder, and perhaps another 5% has undiagnosed thyroid disease, according to the American Association of Clinical Endocrinologists. In developing countries where dietary iodine is lacking, thyroid disease is even more widespread. Because of the prevalence of thyroid disease and its accessibility to treatment, an understanding of thyroid physiology is of great clinical importance.

SYSTEM STRUCTURE

The thyroid gland is located in the neck anterior to the trachea and inferior to the larynx and cricoid cartilage (Fig. 30.1). It consists of right and left lobes connected by an isthmus and weighs around 15 to 20 g (see Clinical Correlation Box 30.1).

Clinical Correlate Box 30.1

Under pathologic conditions, the neuroendocrine signals may demand more thyroid hormone for a sustained period of time, resulting in the hypertrophy of the gland to many times its normal size, causing it to protrude visibly from the neck.

The follicles represent the functional units of the thyroid gland (Fig. 30.2), and are spherical structures less than 0.5 mm in diameter.
- Follicles are filled with thyroglobulin, the glycoprotein precursor to thyroid hormone. The pool of thyroglobulin molecules is referred to collectively as a substance called colloid.
- Each colloid-filled follicle is encapsulated by a capillary-laden basement membrane and lined on the inside by a one-cell-thick cuboidal epithelium.
- The follicles are bundled into lobules by connective tissue, and along the planes of connective tissue travel nerves (parasympathetic and sympathetic), blood vessels, and lymphatics.

The epithelial cells, sometimes called thyrocytes, have different surface proteins on their apical surface, the luminal or colloid-facing side, than they do on their basal surface, the capillary-facing side.
- Accordingly, the apical and basal membranes perform different functions in the biosynthesis and transport of thyroid hormones (see Fast Fact Box 30.1).

Fast Fact Box 30.1

Recall a similar segregation of surface proteins, and similar terminology, from renal physiology, where the inner membranes of the renal tubular cells are called *apical* and the outer membranes called *basolateral*.

Parafollicular cells are scattered among the follicles (see Pharmacology Box 30.1, Pharmacology Box 30.1 and Genetic Box 30.1).

✳ ONCOLOGY BOX 30.1

Malignancies arising from thyroid epithelial cells (thyrocytes) may be well or poorly differentiated. The well-differentiated cancers include follicular and papillary (each with variants or subtypes), while the poorly differentiated include anaplastic and medullary. Of these, papillary is most common. Thyroid cancer often manifests as a mass found by the patient or detected on physical examination. Thyroid examination is best done with a glass of water – the patient drinks while the clinician examines the thyroid as the patient swallows.

💊 PHARMACOLOGY BOX 30.1

Although surgical resection is the primary mode of treatment for thyroid cancer, radioactive iodine is used in some patients as well. Patients who undergo thyroidectomy (i.e., complete removal of the thyroid) require thyroid hormone replacement.

⚛ GENETICS BOX 30.1

Well-differentiated thyroid cancers, like many other malignancies (e.g., lung, hematopoietic) may harbor mutations in the human telomerase reverse transcriptase (hTERT), the gene encoding the enzymatic component of human telomerase. The telomerase ribonucleoprotein polymerase adds repeated TTAGGG sequences to the temini of telomeres, the structures on the ends of chromosomes that progressively shorten with repeated mitosis. In normal cells, telomere shortening eventually leads to programmed cell death (apoptosis), but in cells with hTERT mutations, the addition of sequences to telomeres prevents this, thus contributing to the malignancy. hTERT mutations are associated with persistent and more lethal differentiated thyroid cancers.

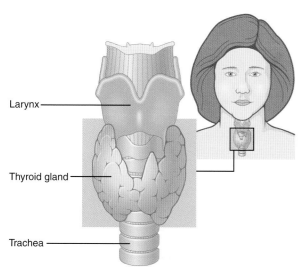

Fig. 30.1 Anatomy of the thyroid gland. A normal variant of thyroid anatomy includes a pyramidal lobe extending upward from the isthmus. (Modified From Guyton AC, Hall JE. *Guyton and Hall Textbook of Medical Physiology*, 13th Edition. Elsevier; 2015. Fig. 77.1.)

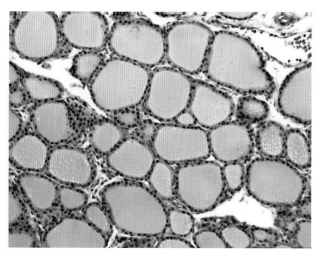

Fig. 30.2 Thyroid follicles. The follicles are filled with colloid (thyroglobulin). Thyroglobulin is iodinated, and iodotyrosyls are coupled in the follicle lumina.

Tyrosine

MIT (3-moniodotyrosine)

DIT (3,5-diiodotyrosine)

Thyroxine, T_4 (3,5,3',5'-tetraiodothyronine)

T_3 (3,5,3'-triiodothyronine)

Reverse T_3 (3,3',5'-triiodothyronine)

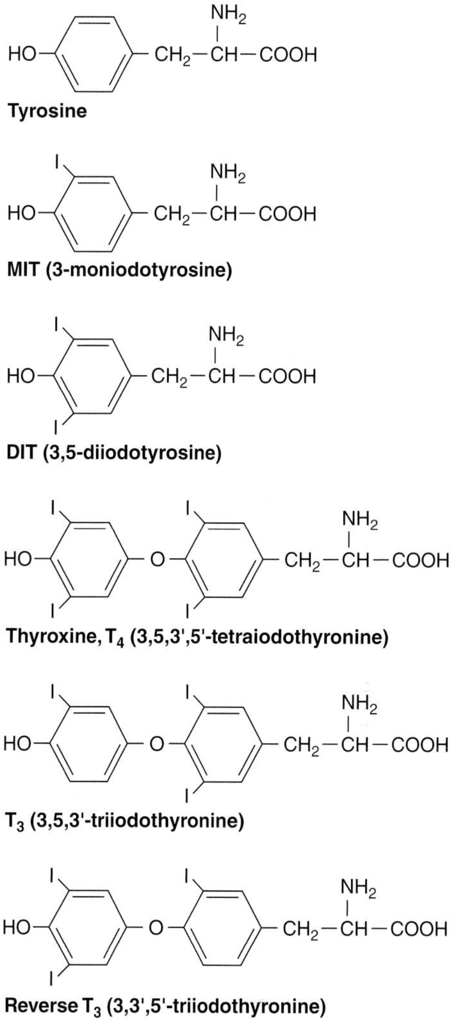

Fig. 30.3 Structure of tyrosine, MIT, DIT, T_4, T_3, and Reverse T_3 (rT_3). The iodinated carbons on the inner benzene ring are labeled 3 and 5. The carbons on the outer benzene ring are labeled 3' and 5'. T_3 has no iodine moiety at the 5' carbon. Thus it is a 5' deiodinase that converts T_4 to T_3. rT_3 has no iodine moiety at the 5 carbon. Thus it is a 5 deiodinase that converts T_4 to rT_3, thereby inactivating it.

- They produce calcitonin, a hormone that aids in the regulation of plasma calcium concentration via:
  - Inhibition of calcium absorption by the intestines
  - Inhibition of osteoclast activity
  - Inhibition of reabsorption of calcium in the kidney

The Biosynthesis of Thyroid Hormones

There are two primary types of thyroid hormone (Fig. 30.3), which are identical except for their number of iodine moieties:
- Thyroxine (T_4): four iodine moieties
- Triiodothyronine (T_3): three iodine moieties

Thyroid hormone, like epinephrine and norepinephrine, is a modified molecule of the amino acid tyrosine.
- Whereas tyrosine has one benzene ring (a hydroxyl-bearing phenol group), thyroid hormone incorporates a second benzene ring in its side chain.

- Thyroid hormone also has iodine moieties on both of its benzene rings.
  - In T_4, there are two atoms of iodine on each ring
  - In T_3, there are two atoms of iodine on one ring and one atom of iodine on the other

When T_3 is synthesized, either the phenol ring or the inner ring may receive two atoms of iodine. If the outer phenol ring bears two atoms of iodine, the molecule is inactive and is called reverse T_3 (rT_3).

Ingredients for Thyroid Hormone: Thyroglobulin, I^-, and H_2O_2

Under enzymatic control, tyrosine is combined with iodine to form T_4 and T_3 in the follicle lumen (Fig. 30.4).
- Thyroglobulin
  - A glycosylated protein scaffold, thyroglobulin, is constructed in the endoplasmic reticulum with multiple tyrosine groups (tyrosyls) along its length.

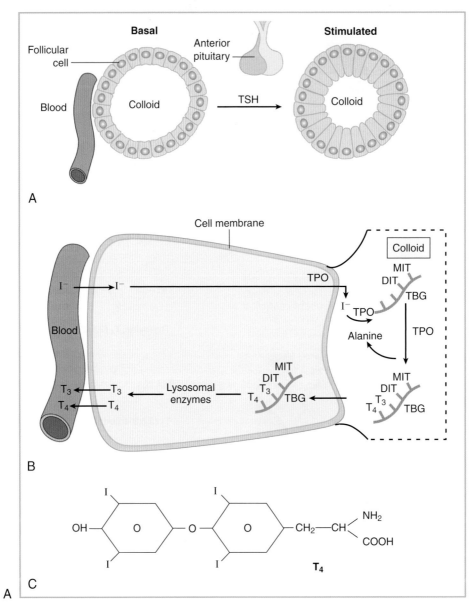

Fig. 30.4 A and B, Biosynthesis of thyroid hormone. *DIT,* Diiodotyrosine; *MIT,* monoiodotyrosine; *T₃,* triiodothyronine; *T₄,* thyroxine; *TBG,* thyroxine-binding globulin; *TPO,* thyroid-peroxidase, *TSH,* thyroid-stimulating hormone. (A, from Kester M, Karpa K, Vrana K. *Elsevier's Integrated Review: Pharmacology,* 2nd Edition. Elsevier; 2011. Fig. 12.5.)

- The thyroglobulin molecules are then exocytosed into the follicle lumen.
- Iodine (I^-)
  - Dietary iodine diffuses from the follicular capillaries across the basal Na^+/I^- symporter (NIS) and into the thyrocyte cytoplasm.
  - The energy driving this I^- uptake comes from the Na^+,K^+-ATPase, which has suppressed the intracellular Na^+ concentration.
    Extracellular Na^+ flows down its concentration gradient across the NIS and into the cell.
    Because NIS couples Na^+ movement to I^- movement, the influx of Na^+ drives an influx of I^-. This is an example of secondary active transport.

- When I^- accumulates inside the cell, it forms a concentration gradient across the apical membrane that permits flow through the I^-/Cl^- transporter (pendrin) and into the follicular lumen.
- Hydrogen peroxide (H_2O_2)
  - H_2O_2 is produced in the lumen by nicotinamide adenine dinucleotide phosphate oxidase associated with the apical membrane.

Iodination

Once thyroglobulin, I^-, and H_2O_2 have been congregated in the follicle lumen near the apical membrane, thyroid peroxidase (TPO) catalyzes the oxidation of I^- to an intermediate species.

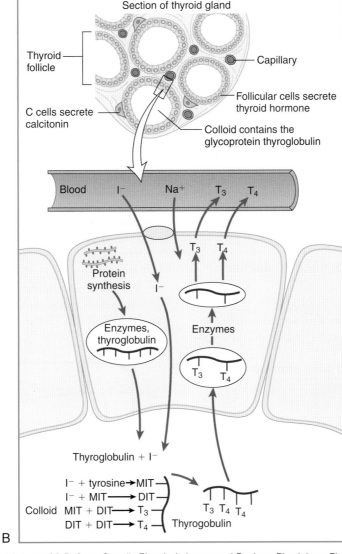

Section of thyroid gland

Thyroid follicle

Capillary

C cells secrete calcitonin

Follicular cells secrete thyroid hormone

Colloid contains the glycoprotein thyroglobulin

Blood · I⁻ · Na⁺ · T₃ · T₄

Protein synthesis

I⁻

Enzymes, thyroglobulin

Enzymes

T₃ · T₄

T₃ · T₄

Thyroglobulin + I⁻

I⁻ + tyrosine → MIT
I⁻ + MIT → DIT
Colloid MIT + DIT → T₃
DIT + DIT → T₄

T₃ T₄ T₄
Thyrogobulin

B

Fig. 30.4 cont'd B, from Carroll. *Elsevier's Integrated Review: Physiology.* Fig. 13.6.)

- H_2O_2 serves as the electron acceptor for this reaction.
- The oxidized iodine intermediate then binds the benzene rings of the tyrosyl groups, which are sitting on the thyroglobulin backbone.
- This is termed iodination of thyroglobulin (or organification of iodine).
  - If the tyrosyl binds one iodine atom, the group is called monoiodotyrosine (MIT).
  - If the tyrosyl binds two iodine atoms, the group is called diiodotyrosine (DIT).

The Formation of T₄ and T₃

At this stage, thyroid peroxidase catalyzes a second oxidation-reduction reaction.

- One tyrosine hydroxyl group loses its hydrogen and binds an adjacent tyrosine benzene ring, linking two iodinated rings together.
  - Two DIT moieties join to form T₄ on the thyroglobulin scaffold.

- Alternatively, a DIT and an MIT bind together to make T₃.
- The mature thyroglobulin, loaded with T₄ and T₃, as well as uncoupled DIT and MIT, is finally released from the apical epithelial surface into the large pool of mature thyroglobulin (colloid).

When signals from the brain mandate the secretion of thyroid hormone, mature thyroglobulin is endocytosed and transported into lysosomes.

- Here, T₄, T₃, DIT, and MIT are cleaved from the thyroglobulin backbone and the backbone is digested.
- The biologically inactive DIT and MIT are metabolized, and their iodine is recovered for another round of iodination.
- T₄ and T₃ are conducted to the basal membrane and transported into the capillary blood.

Almost all the thyroid hormone released by the thyroid is in the form of T₄. Roughly 80 to 100 mcg of T₄ is secreted per day, versus a daily output of around 4 mcg of T₃ and 2 mcg of rT₃.

SYSTEM FUNCTION

The thyroid gland is under control of the hypothalamus-pituitary-thyroid axis, a cascade of signals originating in the brain that controls the secretion of hormone from the thyroid gland (Fig. 30.5).

- The hypothalamus first secretes thyrotropin-releasing hormone (TRH).
- This leads the pituitary gland to release thyroid-stimulating hormone (TSH)—also called thyrotropin.
- TSH triggers the production of thyroid hormone and also promotes its secretion from the thyroid gland.

The hypothalamic-pituitary-thyroid (HPT) axis features classic negative feedback control.

- The axis end-product, thyroid hormone, circulates back to the hypothalamus and the pituitary in the bloodstream and inhibits the release of its own control signals, TRH and TSH.
- Thyroid hormone thereby delimits its own production and secretion.

The Regulation of Thyroid Hormone Production and Secretion

Thyrotropin-Releasing Hormone

TRH is produced from cleavage from a prohormone by *prohormone convertases* in the paraventricular nucleus of the hypothalamus.

- From here, TRH is transported along neuronal axons into the hypothalamic median eminence.

- Finally, TRH is secreted into the portal blood vessels that connect the hypothalamus to the anterior pituitary.

TRH production and secretion is fairly constant, leading to a relatively constant plasma level of thyroid hormones.

- This is in keeping with a fundamental task of thyroid hormone to ensure a constant supply of body heat under any circumstances.
- Negative feedback from thyroid hormone is the chief regulator of TRH output.

When TRH reaches the pituitary in the portal blood, it acts on the thyrotroph cells (TSH-secreting cells) of the anterior pituitary. It accomplishes this via TRH receptors on the cell membranes of pituitary thyrotrophs (Fig. 30.6).

- The TRH receptor is a G-protein-linked seven-transmembrane receptor that stimulates TSH gene expression through a Ca^{2+}-mediated signaling pathway.
- TRH stimulation of the receptor $\rightarrow$ production of TSH.
- TRH also influences the bioactivity of TSH produced.
  - Promotes posttranslational modification of the oligosaccharide chains on TSH.
  - This facilitates TSH secretion and prolongs its half-life.

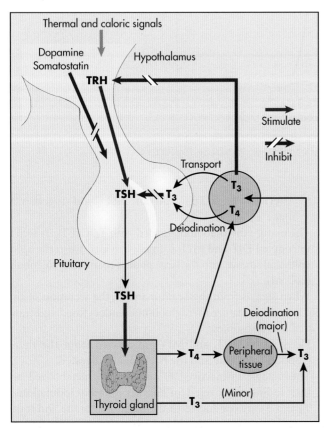

Fig. 30.5 The hypothalamic-pituitary-thyroid axis. *Plus signs* represent stimulation; *minus signs* represent inhibition. T_3, Triiodothyronine; T_4, thyroxine; *TRH*, thyrotropin-releasing hormone; *TSH*, thyroid-stimulating hormone. (From Berne and Levy *Principles of Physiology*. Fig. 46.4.)

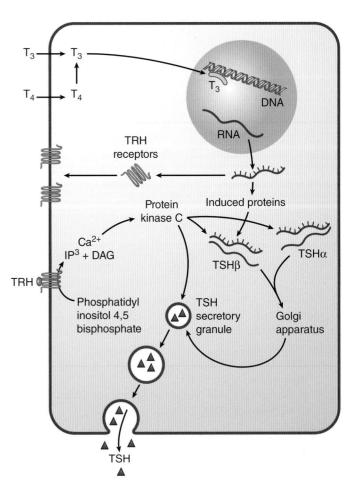

Fig. 30.6 Signaling mechanisms by which thyrotropin-releasing hormone (*TRH*) acts on pituitary thyrotroph cells. *DAG*, Diacylglycerol; *DNA*, deoxyribonucleic acid; *IP3*, inositol triphosphate; *RNA*, ribonucleic acid; T_3, Triiodothyronine; T_4, thyroxine; *TSH*, thyroid-stimulating hormone.

Thyroid-Stimulating Hormone

TSH is a glycoprotein hormone that, like TRH, binds to a G protein-linked receptor (Fig. 30.7).

- The TSH receptor is located on the basal membrane of the thyroid follicle cells and triggers increased intracellular cyclic adenosine monophosphate (cAMP).
- The cAMP-mediated signaling cascade promotes increased thyroid hormone biosynthesis and secretion.
- A phospholipase C-mediated signaling pathway also participates.

Ultimately, TSH acts in numerous ways to aid in the production and circulation of thyroid hormone:

- Gene expression of proteins involved in thyroid hormone biosynthesis and secretion.
- Phosphorylation and activation of proteins involved in the same.
- Growth and cell division of the thyrocytes.
- Blood flow to the thyroid follicles.
  Improves iodine and oxygen delivery to the thyroid.
  Improves circulation of secreted thyroid hormone to the body.

TSH secretion is controlled by TRH, as described earlier, and it is also subject to the same negative feedback effects that act upon the TRH-secreting cells.

- Increased levels of T_4 and T_3 dampen the pituitary response to TRH and hence suppress TSH production and secretion.
- Conversely, decreased levels of thyroid hormone disinhibit TSH secretion, and the plasma TSH level goes up, driving the thyroid gland to replenish the blood levels of thyroid hormone.

Clinically, the TSH level is the single most important indicator of thyroid function.

- If the thyroid is making a normal amount of thyroxine, the TSH level will be in the normal range.
- If the thyroid is underperforming (e.g., owing to the destruction of thyroid tissue), the TSH will be high.
- If the thyroid is overperforming (e.g., owing to unregulated hormone production), the TSH will be low (see Clinical Correlation Box 30.3).

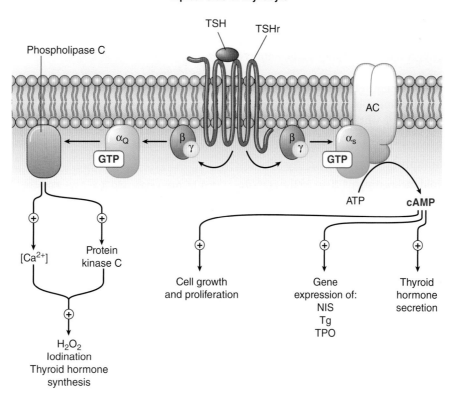

Fig. 30.7 Signaling mechanisms by which thyroid stimulating hormone (*TSH*) acts on thyroid cells. *AC*, Adenylate cyclase; *ATP*, adenosine triphosphate; *cAMP*, cyclic adenosine monophosphate; *GTP*, guanosine triphosphate; *H₂O₂*, hydrogen peroxidase; *NIS*, Na⁺/I⁻ symporter; *Tg*, thyroglobulin; *TPO*, thyroid peroxidase; *TSHr*, TSH receptor.

Clinical Correlation Box 30.3

Lack of functional thyroid hormone will lead to a dearth of feedback inhibition of the secretion of thyroid-stimulating hormone (TSH), which will promote thyroid hypertrophy (goiter). As such, people who are deficient in iodine can develop thyroid hypertrophy because of decreased production of functional thyroid hormone, despite the fact that their thyrotropin-releasing hormone (TRH)-TSH axis is intact. This condition is corrected by thyroid supplementation, and is rarely seen today because of the use of iodized salt, which supplies sufficient amounts of iodine in meals.

Other Controls: Thyroglobulin and Iodine Levels

In addition to TRH/TSH-mediated control of thyroid hormone and negative feedback effects, at least two lesser factors affect the regulation of thyroid hormone production and secretion.

- Thyroglobulin
  - Mediates a negative feedback effect via autocrine action on the follicle containing it.
    Accumulation of thyroglobulin in follicle $\rightarrow$ suppression of gene expression for proteins involved in thyroid hormone biosynthesis
- Iodine
  - Low availability $\rightarrow$ limitation of thyroid hormone production
    Thyroid hormone cannot be produced in adequate amounts
  - Excessive amounts $\rightarrow$ negative feedback
    Excess iodine monopolizes binding sites on follicular thyroid peroxidase
    This leads to inefficient iodination of thyroglobulin.
- Amount of T_3 versus rT_3
  - Plasma levels of T_3 are known to drop and levels of rT_3 known to rise during prolonged fasting or in nonthyroidal illnesses.
  - The mechanism is not completely understood, but the effect is probably to slow metabolism and conserve energy when food is scarce or when energy is needed for healing.

Thyroid Hormone Transport

As stated earlier, the thyroid makes roughly 20 to 25 times more T_4 than T_3 each day. However, T_4 is the major circulating form of thyroid hormone. Why?

- While the liver converts some of the T_4 to T_3, T_3 is also absorbed by tissues and metabolized more quickly than T_4.
- The end result is that total T_4 concentrations in the plasma average somewhere around 100 nmol/L, while the total T_3 concentrations are somewhere around 2 nmol/L.

Like many other hormones, thyroid hormone binds to carrier proteins found in the blood. In fact, once T_4 and T_3 enter the bloodstream, nearly all of these hormones are taken up by the plasma proteins that transport them (Fig. 30.8).

- Whatever T_4 and T_3 remains unbound in the plasma is referred to as free T_4 and free T_3.
- The association reaction of thyroid hormone and carrier protein is reversible and is governed by an equilibrium constant.

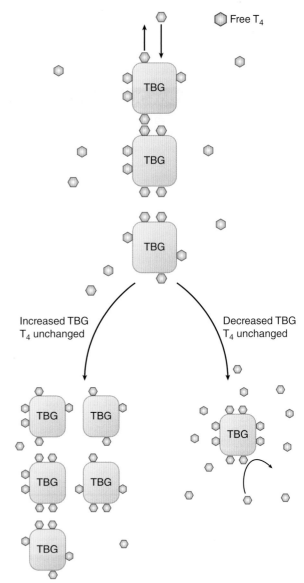

Fig. 30.8 Thyroxine (T_4) binding to thyroxine-binding globulin (*TBG*). If the amount of TBG is increased without a change in T_4, more T_4 is bound. In normal physiology, this situation is transient, as the decreased free T_4 will result in increased TSH. This, in turn, will increase the free T_4 level until the TBG is loaded with T_4 and the free T_4 is back in the normal range, and it is how increased TBG levels yield increased total T_4 levels, as in pregnancy.

- Free T_4 + carrier protein $\leftrightarrow$ Bound T_4
- Free T_3 + carrier protein $\leftrightarrow$ Bound T_3
- To enter cells and alter their functioning, T_4 and T_3 must be unbound from their carrier proteins.
  - As such, bound T_3 and T_4 can be thought of as a reserve pool of thyroid hormone that is functionally inactive.

When the transport proteins pass by the cells in the periphery, they unload the T_4 and T_3.

- Unloading occurs because of the cellular uptake of T_4 and T_3 from the extracellular fluid.
- This action drops the plasma concentration of free T_4 and T_3.
- This in turn shifts the equilibrium between protein and thyroid hormone toward dissociation (see Fast Fact Box 30.2).

Three proteins bind T_4 in the blood:
1. Albumin
2. Transthyretin (TTR)
3. Thyroxine-binding globulin (TBG)

TBG, not to be confused with thyroglobulin (the thyroid hormone precursor), carries the vast majority of T_4 in plasma. It thus serves as an extrathyroidal reservoir of T_4, protecting the T_4 supply from fluctuations in thyroidal output.

- If T_4 production falls in the thyroid (e.g., because of low dietary iodine intake), the TBG reservoir of T_4 can buffer the peripheral tissues against T4 shortage until adequate T_4 production is resumed.
- However, if T_4 underproduction is sustained—as in chronic autoimmune thyroiditis, for instance—the TBG buffer supply will eventually be exhausted and the level of free T_4 will fall.
- Under physiologic conditions, the plasma protein reservoir also prevents losses of T_4 and T_3 to the urine because the large carrier proteins are not filtered at the glomerulus (see Clinical Correlation Box 30.4 and 30.5).

Clinical Correlation Box 30.4

In pregnancy, placental estrogen increases hepatic production and decreases hepatic clearance of thyroxine-binding globulin (TBG), thus increasing the size of the TBG reservoir. This increases the **total** thyroxine (T_4) (bound T_4 + unbound T_4) in the mother without increasing the free T4 concentration. This enables the mother to supply the fetus with thyroid hormone without compromising her own supply.

Clinical Correlation Box 30.5

The free thyroxine index (FTI) estimates the level of free thyroxine (T_4). In the test, thyroxine-binding globulin (TBG) is exposed to a form of T_3 bearing a radioisotope of iodine. Radio-triiodothyronine (T_3) binds any available binding sites on the TBG; any remaining radio-T_3 is bound by a special resin.
- Low resin binding → more available TBG sites for radio-T_3 → implies low T_4
The FTI is calculated by multiplying the total T_4 by the percentage of radio-T_3 bound by resin.

The Actions of Thyroid Hormone

Although T_4 is the major circulating form of thyroid hormone, T_3 is the active form of thyroid hormone inside cells.

- As the majority of the thyroid hormone supply is in the form of T_4, the majority of thyroid hormone in the plasma must be converted to T_3 to act upon cells.
- The deiodinases are the enzymes responsible for converting T_4 to active T_3, and they are present throughout the body.

Activation and Inactivation by Deiodinases

Deiodinases in the liver create T_3 that circulates to sites of action in the tissues, whereas deiodinases in the peripheral tissues also create T_3 that acts locally.

- Circulating T_3, which is less well bound to the plasma proteins, diffuses quickly into the cells and stimulates the intracellular T_3 receptor.
- Type I and type II 5′ deiodinases then convert T_4 to T_3.
- The type I 5′ deiodinase in the liver is chiefly responsible for manufacturing circulating T_3 (see Clinical Correlation Box 30.6).

Clinical Correlation Box 30.6

An example of local triiodothyronine (T_3) activation is found in the pituitary gland. For thyroid hormone to have its negative-feedback effect on thyroid-stimulating hormone (TSH) secretion, thyroxine (T_4) must enter the thyrotroph and be deiodinated to T_3. The T_3 then acts inside the thyrotroph to suppress TSH production and secretion.

The 5 deiodinase (as opposed to 5' deiodinase) in the tissues inactivates both T_4 and T_3.
- Inactivates T_4 by conversion to rT_3.
- Inactivates T_3 by conversion to T_2 (diiodothyronine)

The Thyroid Hormone Receptor

Thyroid hormone binds intracellular thyroid hormone receptors (TRs) that complex with thyroid hormone response elements (TREs) and bind nuclear deoxyribonucleic acid (DNA), thereby influencing gene expression.

- TRs have a much higher affinity for T_3 than they do for T_4, which accounts for the importance of T_3 as the active form of thyroid hormone.
- TRs are present in most body tissues, but particular TR subtypes or isoforms may predominate in one tissue or another.
  - Different isoforms may complex differently with TREs to produce distinctive thyroid hormone effects in a tissue-dependent manner.

In addition to actions mediated by the well-known TR, research has begun to illuminate other pathways of thyroid hormone action.

- Faster, nongenomic activity
  - Receptors for T_4 and T_3 at the cell surface may mediate these actions instead of the slower mechanism of altered gene expression.
  - Signaling mechanisms include the activation of various protein kinases and alterations in solute transport.
- Mitochondrial effect
  - Thyroid hormone appears to act directly on transcription factors associated with the *mitochondrial genome*.

Metabolic and Thermogenic Actions

The predominant means by which thyroid hormone ramps up metabolism is via stimulation of oxidative phosphorylation and thus mitochondrial O_2 consumption.

- Stimulation by T_3 increases the rate of adenosine triphosphate (ATP) synthesis and consumption.

- The increased churning of the oxidative phosphorylation machine results in more molecular motion, and hence more thermogenesis.

T_3 increases mitochondrial O_2 consumption and the heat dissipation associated with it by a number of different direct mechanisms:

- Enhances expression of mitochondrial proteins that enhance oxidative phosphorylation.
- Promotes mitochondriogenesis.
- Increases permeability for protons in the mitochondrial membrane.
  - Recall that during oxidative phosphorylation, the electron transport chain concentrates protons in the intermembrane space of the mitochondrion.
  - The proton gradient then causes protons to flow through the ATP synthetase, making ATP from adenosine diphosphate (Fig. 30.9).
  - By increasing the membrane's proton permeability, the process of making ATP becomes more inefficient. Thus more energy is wasted as heat.

In addition, T_3 increases mitochondrial O_2 consumption through several indirect mechanisms:

- Increases expression of Na^+,K^+-ATPase.

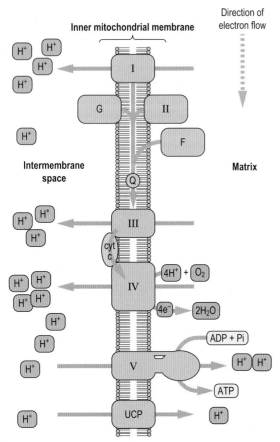

Fig. 30.9 Adenosine triphosphate (*ATP*) synthesis in oxidative phosphorylation. A proton gradient from the intermembrane space to the mitochondrial matrix drives ATP synthesis. Complex V is ATP synthetase. *ADP*, Adenosine diphosphate; *UCP*, uncoupling protein. (From Baynes J, Dominiczak M. *Medical Biochemistry*, 5th Edition. Elsevier; 2018. Fig 8.5.)

- Promotes early increase in lipogenesis, followed by lipolysis. This provides fatty acids as substrate to the citric acid cycle and thus stimulates more energy release.
- Increases cardiac contractility and heart rate, which increases oxygen delivery to the tissues and consumes large amounts of energy in cardiac muscle cells.
  - Increases expression of myosin isoform with greater ATPase activity $\rightarrow$ increased force and speed of contraction.
  - Increases expression and activity of the sarcoplasmic Ca^{2+} ATPase $\rightarrow$ increased force and speed of contraction.
  - Increased venous return to the heart by venoconstriction $\rightarrow$ increases contractility by increasing preload.
  - Potentiates sympathetic effects on the heart by increasing the expression of adrenergic beta receptors.

Influences on Growth and Development

Although the mechanisms are not completely understood, it is clear that thyroid hormone plays a major role in growth and development.

- Deficiencies in thyroid hormone in fetal life or in infancy can retard neurologic development.
- Thyroid hormone promotes growth hormone synthesis in the pituitary.
- Normal levels of thyroid hormone are important for both male and female fertility.

Summary of Thyroid Function and Regulation:

Under the influence of TRH, TSH is released from the anterior pituitary. The stimulation increases iodine uptake via anion exchange into the thyroid gland for organification. Patients with high TSH will increase T4 release from the pituitary, while patients with low TSH will decrease release due to a feedback loop for T3. Though 80% of the total thyroid hormone produced by the thyroid gland is T4, the tri-iodinated T3 is the active hormone supporting hypermetabolism, body temperature, and growth. T4, bound to thyroid-binding globulin (TBG), is taken up by peripheral cells, especially the liver, kidney, and brain, where it can be de-iodinated to T3 by de-iodinase enzyme, or to reverse T3 (rT3), an inactive form of iodinated hormone. The T3 secreted into the extracellular space by these organs is available for negative feedback on TRH and TSH. The direction of change (i.e., T4 converted to either T3 or rT3) is regulated as a way to decrease T3 in situations like starvation, where a high metabolic rate would be pathogenic.

PATHOPHYSIOLOGY: THYROID HORMONE EXCESS AND DEFICIENCY

The main categories of thyroid disease are:

- Hyperthyroidism (excessive thyroid hormone)
- Hypothyroidism (deficient thyroid hormone)

The consequences of each dysfunction follow logically from knowledge of thyroid function and its effect on energy metabolism.

Hyperthyroidism

The core symptoms of hyperthyroidism are caused by increased energy metabolism:

- Weight loss despite increased appetite

- Palpitations
- Heat intolerance and sweating
- Diarrhea
- Anxiety (see Clinical Correlation Box 30.7)

Clinical Correlation Box 30.7

Certain inflammatory conditions of the thyroid, such as Hashimoto thyroiditis (discussed in detail later), can lead to damage of the integrity of thyroid follicles, resulting in the release of stored thyroid hormone and subsequent thyrotoxicosis.

Symptomatic hyperthyroidism is called thyrotoxicosis. Infrequently, severe thyrotoxicosis leads to the sudden onset of thyroid storm, a life-threatening condition marked by very high fever.

Hyperthyroidism is most commonly caused by an autoimmune condition called Graves disease (Fig. 30.10), and less frequently a thyroxine-secreting tumor of the thyroid gland.

- In Graves disease, antibodies to the TSH receptor stimulate the receptor in the same way that TSH itself does.
- This leads to an unregulated and constant overactivity of the thyroid gland.
- Signs/symptoms:
  - Under the influence of TSH-like stimulation, the thyroid gland hypertrophies, forming a *protruding goiter*.
  - Because proteins in the extraocular muscles resemble the TSH receptor, the anti-TSH receptor antibodies also cause inflammation in the eye sockets, causing the eyes to protrude—a condition called exophthalmos.

When the thyroid escapes pituitary control and secretes too much T_4, the pituitary thyrotrophs are suppressed and secrete less TSH.

- Hyperthyroidism is thus associated with a low TSH in the majority of cases.
- In the case of a TSH-secreting pituitary tumor, hyperthyroidism is accompanied by a high TSH level, and treatment would involve resection of the pituitary tumor.

The treatment of hyperthyroidism revolves around pharmacologic, radiation, and surgical therapies:

- Pharmacologic

- Antithyroid
  Propylthiouracil (PTU) and methylmercaptoimidazole, also called methimazole, inhibit thyroid peroxidase. PTU also inhibits peripheral activation of T_4.
- Symptomatic
  Beta-adrenergic receptor blockers, such as propranolol, can help control symptoms, especially palpitations and tachycardia.
- Radiation
  - Administration of radioactive iodine to ablate the malfunctioning thyroid tissue.
- Surgical
  - Removal of the thyroid gland.

Hypothyroidism

The core symptoms of hypothyroidism result from reduced energy metabolism:
- Weight gain despite low appetite
- Constipation
- Intolerance to cold
- Fatigue
- Depression
- Dry skin and hair
- Heavy menstrual periods

In severe hypothyroidism, proteins and sugars may accumulate in the skin owing to sluggish metabolism, promoting a form of superficial edema called myxedema.

Hypothyroidism is most commonly caused by an autoimmune condition called autoimmune thyroiditis, also known as Hashimoto thyroiditis.

- In this condition, antibodies to thyroglobulin or thyroid peroxidase interfere with thyroid hormone synthesis.
- Thyroid hormone levels in the blood are low whereas the TSH level is high.
- Chronic stimulation of the thyroid tissue by TSH may lead to goiter. However, inflammation may also fibrose the thyroid, keeping it small.

Iodine deficiency, other forms of thyroiditis (e.g., viral), and drug side effects (lithium, amiodarone) may also cause hypothyroidism.

Hypothyroidism is treated with exogenous thyroxine, administered in the form of a daily pill.

- Dosages increase for hypothyroid mothers during pregnancy by 25% to 50%.
- However, whether the patient is pregnant or not, dosage is always titrated to normalize the plasma TSH level.
- As previously stated, the TSH is the most important lab test in the diagnosis and treatment of thyroid disease (see Clinical Correlation Box 30.8).

Clinical Correlation Box 30.8

Postpartum thyroiditis is a medical phenomenon that follows birth in about 5% of women. It may involve hyperthyroidism, hypothyroidism or both. Typically, hyperthyroidism arises first, followed either by a return to normal or hypothyroidism, which may become permanent.

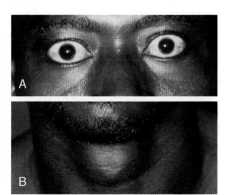

Fig. 30.10 Graves disease is a common cause of hyperthyroidism, an overproduction of thyroid hormone, which causes enlargement of the thyroid and other symptoms, such as exophthalmos, heat intolerance, and anxiety. (From Stern T, Fava M, Wilens T, Rosenbaum J. *Massachusetts General Hospital Comprehensive Clinical Psychiatry*, 2nd Edition. Elsevier; 2010. Fig. 21.19.)

Postpartum thyroiditis is likely caused by changes in the immune system during pregnancy, resulting in antibodies targeting the thyroid, leading to subacute lymphocytic thyroiditis.

SUMMARY

- Thyroid hormone causes increased energy metabolism and thermogenesis, in addition to promoting normal growth and development from fetal life through childhood.
- Thyroxine (T_4) is the major circulating form of thyroid hormone, but triiodothyronine (T_3) is the active form.
- T_4 is made in thyroid follicles from tyrosine-containing thyroglobulin, I^-, H_2O_2, and thyroid peroxidase.
- T_4 is produced and secreted by the thyroid gland under the control of hypothalamic TRH and pituitary TSH as part of the HPT axis. The HPT axis is governed by negative-feedback effects of T_4 on TRH and TSH-secreting cells.
- T_4 is transported in the blood bound to TBG. It is activated by conversion to T_3 by deiodinases in the liver and in the tissues themselves.
- T_3 binds an intracellular TR that binds TREs. The TR-TRE complex binds nuclear DNA and alters its transcription.

- T_3 primarily acts to stimulate mitochondrial oxidative phosphorylation, which concomitantly increases heat dissipation. It also leads to increased expression of the Na^+,K^+-ATPase, increased lipogenesis and lipolysis, and increased cardiac contractility and heart rate.
- Hyperthyroidism is defined by thyroid hormone excess, whereas hypothyroidism is defined by thyroid hormone deficiency.
- Graves disease and autoimmune thyroiditis are two common autoimmune conditions that cause hyperthyroidism and hypothyroidism, respectively.
- Hyperthyroidism is treated with medical and surgical methods of reducing thyroid activity, whereas hypothyroidism is treated with exogenous thyroxine.
- Measurement of the serum TSH level is the critical test for diagnosis of thyroid disorders.

REVIEW QUESTIONS

Directions: Each of the numbered items or incomplete statements in this section is followed by answers or by completions of the statement. Select the one lettered answer or completion that is best in each case.

1. A woman has been taking 100 mcg qd of levothyroxine for autoimmune thyroiditis for the past 4 years. During that time, her TSH has remained below 2.0 mU/L. She is now pregnant, and in the 11th week of pregnancy, she has an elevated TSH level of 7.5 mU/L (normal, 0.4–5.0 mU/L). A possible cause of her elevated TSH is the fact that:
   A. Antibodies are stimulating her TSH receptors.
   B. Her levothyroxine dose is too high.
   C. Her thyroxine-binding globulin (TBG) levels are increased.
   D. High human chorionic gonadotropin (hCG) levels are mimicking TSH action.
   E. The placenta is producing TSH.
   F. The fetus's pituitary gland is producing TSH.
   G. The fetus's thyroid gland is producing T_4.
   H. She has a toxic thyroid adenoma.

2. A 10-year-old child with congenital hypothyroidism might be expected to exhibit which of the following signs?
   A. Tall stature, cachexia, and low IQ
   B. Short stature, a potbelly, and low IQ
   C. Tall stature, cachexia, and high IQ
   D. Tall stature, a potbelly, and low IQ
   E. Short stature, cachexia, and low IQ

3. Propylthiouracil interferes with more than one process essential to normal thyroid function, but methimazole interferes with just one. Which is it?
   A. Thyroid hormone synthesis
   B. Thyroid hormone transport
   C. Conversion of T_4 to T_3
   D. Binding of T_3 to thyroid receptor
   E. T_3 stimulation of mitochondrial O_2 consumption

ANSWERS TO REVIEW QUESTIONS

1. **The answer is C.** TBG levels increase in pregnancy because placental estrogen stimulates hepatic TBG production and decreased hepatic clearance of TBG. TBG soaks up T_4, transiently decreasing the level of free T_4, lifting negative feedback on the pituitary, and yielding increased TSH secretion. Because the woman cannot increase her endogenous T_4 production in response to the high TSH level, her TSH level remains elevated. All the other possible causes listed, aside from (E) and (F), are states of high T_4 and hence low TSH. TSH receptor-stimulating antibodies are found in autoimmune thyroid disease, but they are present in Graves disease, not autoimmune thyroiditis, and Graves antibodies cause high T_4 and low TSH levels. Serum human chorionic

gonadotropin is thought to mimic TSH action during pregnancy, but again this would increase T_4 and depress TSH. (E) and (F) are not true causes of high maternal TSH.

2. **The answer is B.** Sustained thyroid deficiency from birth impairs growth hormone secretion (short stature), lipolysis in adipose tissues (leading to fat accumulation and potbelly), and neurologic development (low IQ).

3. **The answer is A.** Both propylthiouracil and methimazole inhibit thyroid peroxidase inside thyroid follicles, preventing normal iodination and coupling of thyroid hormone precursors. Propylthiouracil also interferes with deiodination of T_4 to T_3.

31

The Adrenal Gland

INTRODUCTION

The adrenal gland plays a pivotal role in human endocrine physiology. It is subdivided into two sections, which function separately and originate from different embryonic tissues.

The outermost shell of the adrenal gland, the adrenal cortex, is divided into three layers:
1. Zona glomerulosa
2. Zona fasciculata
3. Zona reticularis

Together, these layers produce three kinds of steroid hormones:
1. Aldosterone, a mineralocorticoid, modulates electrolyte and fluid balance by stimulating sodium retention in the kidney's collecting ducts.
2. Cortisol, a glucocorticoid, plays a crucial role in the body's stress response, in the regulation of protein, glucose, and fat metabolism, in the maintenance of vascular tone, and in the modulation of inflammation.
3. Androgens are critically important during fetal life as a substrate for placental estrogen production, but they only play a minor role during adult life.

The adrenal medulla is the inner core of the adrenal gland. It produces the catecholamines epinephrine and norepinephrine (NE), which are also important components of the stress response.

Adrenalectomy will lead to cardiovascular failure and death within a few days from a lack of cortisol, which maintains blood vessel tone and blood pressure.

SYSTEM STRUCTURE: ADRENAL ANATOMY AND EMBRYOLOGY

The adrenals are triangular retroperitoneal organs located at the superior poles of the kidneys, lateral to the 11th thoracic and first lumbar vertebrae. They are supplied by three separate arteries (Fig. 31.1):
1. Superior adrenal artery, a branch of the inferior phrenic.
2. Middle adrenal artery, a branch of the aorta.
3. Inferior adrenal artery, a branch of the renal artery (see Clinical Correlation Box 31.1).

Clinical Correlation Box 31.1

Because of the rich blood supply from multiple locations, the adrenals are a frequent site of metastases from distant primary cancers. This rich blood supply, however, is crucial to the function of the adrenals, as they ensure that the adrenals have ample access to the bloodstream to facilitate efficient hormonal secretion.

The adrenal arteries anastomose into a subcapsular plexus, which in turn branches into arteries that flow inward. These arteries form capillary networks in both the cortex and the medulla of the adrenal gland (Fig. 31.2).

The venous drainage of the adrenal glands differs depending on the side:
- The left adrenal vein drains into the left renal vein.
- The right adrenal vein drains directly into the inferior vena cava (IVC) (see Fast Fact Box 31.1).

Fast Fact Box 31.1

This drainage is analogous to the testicular and ovarian veins. The left testicular/ovarian vein drains into the left renal vein, while the right testicular/ovarian drains right into the inferior vena cava.

In addition to structure and function, the medulla and cortex of the adrenal glands differ in embryologic origin.
- The cortex arises from the mesoderm, whereas the medulla derives from the ectoderm.
- The mesodermal gonadal ridge gives rise to the steroidogenic cells of the ovaries and testes, as well as the adrenal cortex precursor cells, which migrate to the retroperitoneum.
- These mesodermal cortical cells are invaded by migrating ectodermal neural crest cells, which will become the medulla.
- By week 8 of fetal life, these two subdivisions have unified as one organ.

SYSTEM FUNCTION: THE ADRENAL CORTEX

The adrenal cortex makes up 80% to 90% of the adrenal gland by volume and comprises three histologically and functionally distinct zones, each of which makes a different steroid (Fig. 31.3). Starting from the outermost, these layers are:
1. The zona glomerulosa, which produces aldosterone;
2. The zona fasciculata, which produces cortisol; and
3. The zona reticularis, which produces adrenal androgens, primarily dehydroepiandrosterone (DHEA) and androstenedione.

The Role of Corticotropin-Releasing Hormone and Adrenocorticotropic Hormone

Production of the steroids in the adrenal cortex is regulated by the hypothalamic-pituitary-adrenal (HPA) axis (Fig. 31.4).
- The hypothalamus first releases corticotropin-releasing hormone (CRH).

- This stimulates the anterior pituitary to release proopiomel-anocortin (POMC), a precursor molecule that is cleaved into four main products:
  - Melanocyte-stimulating hormone
  - Beta-lipotropins
  - Beta-endorphins

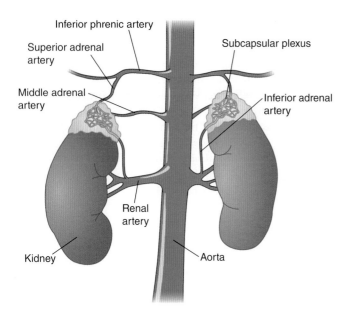

Fig. 31.1 Arterial supply to the adrenal glands. The adrenal arteries are not drawn to scale, nor drawn in their exact anatomic locations.

- Adrenocorticotropic hormone (ACTH), also known as corticotropin
- ACTH is released into the bloodstream and acts in the cortex, stimulating the synthesis and release of steroid products including cortisol, the adrenal androgens, and aldosterone. The HPA axis features classic negative feedback control.
- The axis end-product, cortisol directly inhibits both CRH and ACTH production.
- This regulates all adrenal cortical hormone production, with the exception of aldosterone.
  The cortex responds dramatically to stimulation from ACTH, leading to elevated steroid production within minutes (Fig. 31.5).
- ACTH activates a receptor on the adrenal cell membranes that is linked to a G-protein-mediated pathway that increases intracellular levels of cyclic adenosine monophosphate (cAMP).
- This ultimately leads to phosphorylation and hence activation of the enzyme cholesteryl ester hydrolase (CEH).
  - This promotes the conversion of cholesteryl esters into free cholesterol.
  - The free cholesterol then supplies the steroid synthesis pathways, as described later (see Fast Fact Box 31.2).

Fast Fact Box 31.2

Chronic stimulation with excessive adrenocorticotropic hormone (ACTH) causes bilateral adrenal hypertrophy, whereas removal or destruction of the pituitary, which is responsible for producing ACTH, conversely leads to adrenal atrophy.

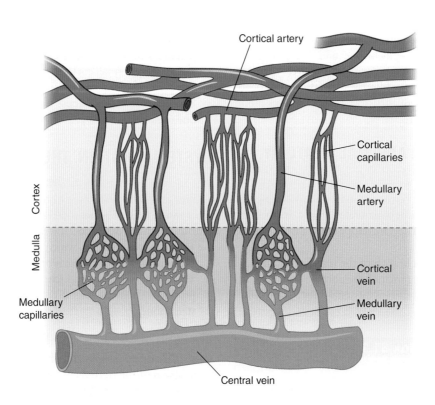

Fig. 31.2 Vasculature inside the adrenal glands. The subcapsular plexus gives rise to arteries that form medullary capillary beds and to arteries that form cortical capillary beds.

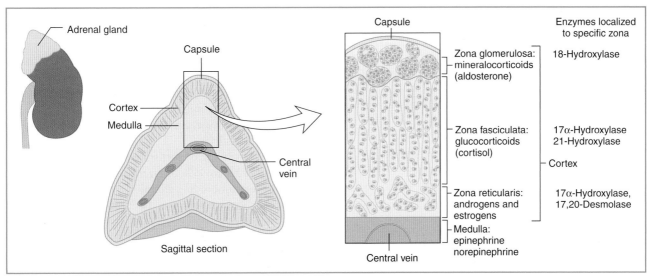

Fig. 31.3 Adrenal zonation. (From Carroll R. *Elsevier's Integrated Physiology.* Philadelphia: Mosby Elsevier; 2007. Fig. 13.9A.)

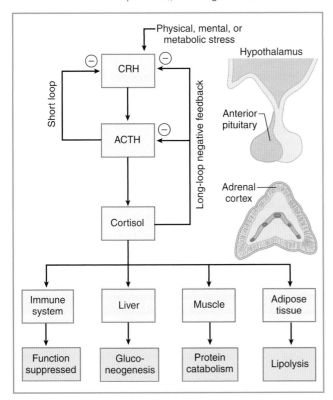

Fig. 31.4 Hypothalamic-pituitary-adrenal axis. Stress, circadian rhythms, and negative feedback from cortisol all influence the paraventricular nucleus of the hypothalamus and modulate corticotropin-releasing hormone (*CRH*) output. Stressors may be organic in nature (such as hypoglycemia or infection) or psychologic. *ACTH,* Adrenocorticotropic hormone. (From Carroll R. *Elsevier's Integrated Physiology.* Philadelphia: Mosby Elsevier; 2007. Fig. 13.11.)

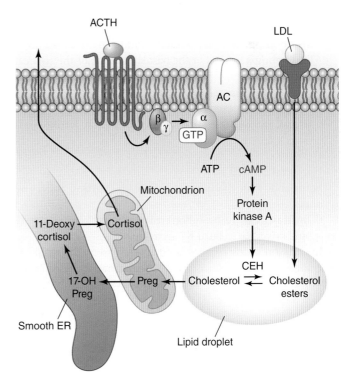

Fig. 31.5 Action of adrenocorticotropic hormone (*ACTH*) on the adrenal cortex. *AC,* Adenylyl cyclase; *ATP,* adenosine triphosphate; *cAMP,* cyclic adenosine monophosphate; *CEH,* cholesteryl ester hydrolase; *G,* G protein (linking the receptor to the adenylyl cyclase); *GTP,* guanosine triphosphate; *LDL,* low-density lipoprotein; *Preg,* pregnenolone (cortisol precursor); *R,* ACTH receptor; *Smooth ER,* smooth endoplasmic reticulum.

Cortical Hormones: Their Actions and Regulation

As steroids, the cortical hormones all share certain functional features:

- Secreted into the adrenal blood vessels and circulate from the adrenal veins to target tissues all over the body.
- Pass readily into lipid membranes of target tissues and into the intracellular cytosol.

- Bind cytosolic receptor proteins, which in turn bind to particular deoxyribonucleic acid (DNA) sequences in the nucleus to initiate the transcription of messenger ribonucleic acid (mRNA), ultimately resulting in the synthesis of new proteins.

Table 31.1 summarizes the actions of the cortical steroids.

TABLE 31.1 Actions of the Cortical Steroids

Adrenal Hormone	Main Actions
• Aldosterone	• Increases salt and water reabsorption from kidney tubules • Increases K$^+$ secretion in kidneys
• Cortisol	• Counterregulatory effects: increases blood sugar, increases catabolism of triglyceride and protein • Antiinflammatory/immunosuppressant effects
• Androgens	• Maintains blood vessel tone and hence blood pressure • Help determine male sex characteristics during fetal development and puberty

Aldosterone Action

Aldosterone plays a key role in the regulation of fluid balance by enhancing the ability of kidney tubules to absorb salt and water. It accomplishes this in two ways:

- Directly stimulates the production and activity of Na$^+$,K$^+$-ATPase pumps located in the basolateral side of the cortical collecting ducts.
  - This leads to increased sodium reabsorption in exchange for potassium excretion.
  - Recall that increased reabsorption of sodium leads to passive water reabsorption and increased extracellular fluid volume.
- Upregulates apical Na$^+$ channels, directly increasing sodium permeability on the luminal side of the cortical collecting ducts.
  - Increased Na$^+$ reabsorption creates tubular electronegativity and drives paracellular K$^+$ secretion.

In addition, aldosterone acts on H$^+$-ATPase in the renal tubule and has other effects on acid-base balance. As aldosterone acts on the levels of these inorganic (mineral) electrolytes, it is termed a mineralocorticoid.

Aldosterone Regulation

Aldosterone is the only adrenal cortical hormone that is secreted largely independently of ACTH.

A small amount of ACTH from the pituitary is required for aldosterone release, but aldosterone is regulated mainly by two other control mechanisms:

1. Serum potassium level
   a. Elevated K$^+$ triggers aldosterone secretion → stimulates renal K$^+$ excretion via the Na$^+$/K$^+$ pump.
2. Renin-angiotensin-aldosterone system (RAAS)
   a. Low blood pressure triggers aldosterone secretion via the RAAS pathway → increases salt (and thus water)–reabsorption → raises the extracellular fluid volume and blood pressure.

Cortisol Action

Cortisol has a multitude of actions, and derivatives of this hormone are used frequently in a variety of medical therapies.

Cortisol is consequently one of the most challenging adrenal hormones to understand and at the same time one of the most clinically relevant.

- Cortisol is produced mostly by the zona fasciculata, with some production in the zona reticularis.
- It mainly serves as a glucocorticoid (explained later), but also exerts a weak mineralocorticoid effect.
- Cortisol's precursor, corticosterone, also exhibits some glucocorticoid activity.

About 20 to 30 mg of cortisol is secreted per day by the adrenals, with 90% to 95% of circulating cortisol bound in the plasma to cortisol-binding globulin.

Glucocorticoid action can be thought of mainly in two broad categories:

- Metabolic
- Antiinflammatory

Although the myriad metabolic actions of cortisol can be daunting, it is useful to remember that cortisol acts to prepare the body for stress.

- During stress, the body requires rapidly usable energy for the brain in the form of glucose.
- To accomplish this, glucocorticoids act through several mechanisms:
  - Increases all gluconeogenic enzymes to raise hepatic gluconeogenesis 6-fold.
  - Blood sugar levels climb, while peripheral uptake and use of glucose decrease.
  - Increase release of fatty acids and amino acids from lipid and muscle breakdown, respectively, to fuel gluconeogenesis.
  - Synthesis of protein and fat is halted.
- In other words, glucocorticoids are counterregulatory hormones, alongside glucagon, epinephrine, and growth hormone.
  - Glucocorticoids oppose insulin action. However, unlike glucagon, glucocorticoids do not promote glycogen breakdown. This phenomenon is known as glucocorticoid's glycostatic effect (see Clinical Correlation Box 31.2).

Clinical Correlation Box 31.2

The stress response induced by cortisol is intended to be temporary. If exposure to cortisol is prolonged, the body will suffer deleterious effects because of a disruption of the normal balance between insulin and cortisol. This leads to a prolonged state of catabolism, leading to striae, skin thinning, and muscle weakness.

Causes include:
- Cushing disease (excess adrenocorticotropic hormone production)
- Long-term treatment with prednisone

Cortisol also has powerful effects on the immune system, which accounts for the widespread use of glucocorticoids as antiinflammatories and as immunosuppressants. Cortisol reduces the inflammatory response by both blocking the early stages of inflammation and speeding the resolution of inflammation. Inflammation is decreased in a number of specific ways:

- Stabilization of white cell granules, which release proteolytic enzymes during inflammation.
- Decreased capillary permeability (leading to decreases edema).

- Decreased production of prostaglandins and leukotrienes, both of which are powerful stimuli of inflammation.
- Decreased leukocyte migration.
- Decreased interleukin-1 (IL-1) and IL-6 release, which are proinflammatory cytokines.
- Direct suppression of T cells.
- Decreased production of lymphocytes and antibodies (see Fast Fact Box 31.3).

Fast Fact Box 31.3

Because of the powerful immunosuppressant effects of cortisol, patients taking glucocorticoids for prolonged periods can become immunocompromised and have an increased risk for infections.

Cortisol is also a powerful modulator of the allergic response, acting to:
- Decrease eosinophil production.
- Increase eosinophil apoptosis.
- Limit the inflammation that can be deadly in anaphylaxis.

Finally, cortisol acts to maintain blood pressure by potentiating catecholamines and by directly supporting blood vessel tone.

Importantly, cortisol can bind to the mineralocorticoid receptor (MR) in the collecting duct of the kidney at equal affinity as aldosterone. To prevent cortisol from causing hyypertension, potassium loss, and metabolic alkalosis, cortisol is converted to cortisone, which is inactive at MR. This is achieved by 11-beta-hydroxysteroid dehydrogenase type 2. In the adrenal gland, the opposite occurs via 11-beta hydroxysteroid dehydrogenase which converts cortisone (often given therapeutically) to the active form of cortisol. This enzyme can be blocked by glycyrrhizic acid in licorice, so that someone who consumes licorice may develop the syndrome of hyperaldosteronism due to the patient's cortisol binding to MR.

Cortisol Regulation

The median eminence of the hypothalamus is responsible for the production of CRH.
- CRH is produced in response to a variety of stressful stimuli, such as trauma, infection, catecholamines, or surgery.
- CRH is released in a circadian cycle, leading to a diurnal variation with cortisol levels peaking in the early morning. CRH triggers ACTH release from the anterior pituitary. ACTH is also modulated by antidiuretic hormone (ADH), which acts synergistically with CRH to stimulate ACTH release.

Cortisol is almost exclusively regulated by ACTH, which activates CEH.
- This ultimately increases the production of pregnenolone, a cortisol precursor.
- Cortisol inhibits CRH and ACTH in a classic negative-feedback loop.

The Androgens

The adrenal androgens, like the gonadal androgens, are male sex hormones—that is, they help determine and maintain male sex characteristics. The principal adrenal androgens are:
- Androstenedione

- DHEA
- DHEA-S (a sulfated form of DHEA)

These hormones have only a minor effect on adult physiology compared with the gonadally produced hormones (such as testosterone), which account for the majority of sex hormone effects. In fact, the adrenal androgens are about one-fifth as potent as testosterone.

However, androstenedione can be converted to testosterone, which is in turn converted to dihydrotestosterone (DHT) and estradiol in extraadrenal tissues. These androgens are most important during fetal development and puberty.
- In the fetus, the adrenal glands are much larger proportionally than in the adult.
- In addition, they possess a layer known as the provisional or fetal cortex exists, which is analogous to the adult zona reticularis.
- This layer produces DHEA-S, which is converted by the placenta into androgens and estrogens.

Adrenal androgens are also important during adolescence, when they stimulate the development of pubic and axillary hair in women.
- This increase in adrenal androgen secretion is known as adrenarche.
- Adrenarche and puberty normally coincide, but they are actually two physiologically separate events.
- Androgen production continues into adulthood and declines with age.

Steroid Biosynthesis

All the products of the adrenal cortex are steroid hormones, which have a standard four-ring structure and are produced by a similar biosynthetic pathway (Fig. 31.6).

Cholesterol provides the basic four-ring steroid framework.
- Although the adrenals can synthesize cholesterol de novo from acetyl CoA, 80% of the cholesterol used in adrenal hormone synthesis comes from dietary cholesterol packaged as cholesteryl ester in circulating low-density lipoprotein (LDL) particles.
- CEH converts the esters to free cholesterol in response to ACTH.
- The rate-limiting step in hormone biosynthesis is the transfer of cholesterol to the inner mitochondrial membrane of adrenal cells via the steroidogenic acute regulatory protein.
- Finally, cholesterol is converted to pregnenolone, catalyzed by the enzyme desmolase.

Once pregnenolone is made from cholesterol, it flows downhill through each zone of the cortex, undergoing successive modifications to the basic steroid ring.
- These modifications result in a distribution of various steroid products throughout the adrenal cortex (Fig. 31.7).
- The steroids are released immediately after synthesis; very little of the cortical hormones are stored.
- This is in contrast to the medulla, which packages and stores its products for release under stimulus at a later time.

Some enzymes in the steroid biosynthetic pathways are common to all three zones, while others are unique to a specific adrenal zone.

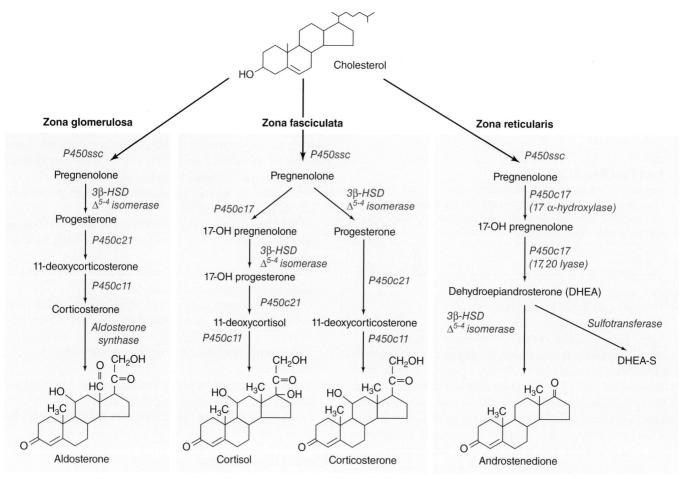

Fig. 31.6 Steroid hormone biosynthetic pathways along with location of synthesis in the adrenal cortex. *DHEA,* Dehydroepiandrosterone. (From Ortsäter H, Sjöholm Å, Rafacho A. Regulation of glucocorticoid receptor signaling and the diabetogenic effects of glucocorticoid excess. *Open Access Peer-Reviewed Chapter.* DOI: 10.5772/51759.)

Pregnenolone flows across zones and also undergoes progressive transformation along each zone's unique enzymatic pathway unless an enzyme deficiency in one pathway acts as a roadblock.

- Such a condition prevents further modification of the steroid product, leading to an excess of premodification substrate

that leads to shunting of production into the remaining intact routes of hormone synthesis.

- An example of this hormonal roadblock is found in the pathologic condition congenital adrenal hyperplasia (CAH) (see Clinical Correlation Box 31.3).

Clinical Correlation Box 31.3

A newborn girl in the nursery is found to have an abnormal genital examination. She has an enlarged clitoris and a single urogenital sinus instead of separate openings for the vagina and urethra. She also is found to have low blood pressure and a high plasma K+ level. With a putative diagnosis of congenital adrenal hyperplasia (CAH), the infant receives hydrocortisone and fludrocortisone (a medical mineralocorticoid), as well as daily salt supplements, as well as a surgical consultation.

Patients with CAH are deficient in *21-hydroxylase,* an enzyme that converts:

- Progesterone to corticosterone in the zona glomerulosa; and
- 17-hydroxyprogesterone to cortisol in the zona fasciculata.

This deficiency causes the precursors to accumulate, causing them to overflow into the androgen biosynthetic pathway. They are then converted by 17,20-lyase into dehydroepiandrosterone (DHEA) and androstenedione. With the lack of cortisol to provide negative feedback, the hypothalamus and pituitary continue to churn out corticotropin-releasing hormone and adrenocorticotropic hormone (ACTH) to attempt to produce more cortisol, leading to adrenal hypertrophy and further shunt to the androgenic pathway.

Thus the broad pathophysiology of the disease lies in:

- Deficiency of aldosterone and cortisol
  - Aldosterone deficiency → salt-wasting crisis with profound hyponatremia, hyperkalemia, hypotension, and nonanion gap metabolic acidosis
  - Cortisol deficiency → aberrant carbohydrate metabolism and dangerous hypotension
- Excess of androgenizing hormones
  - Large amounts of DHEA can lead to clinically significant levels of testosterone, virilizing external genitalia in female fetuses to produce *ambiguous genitalia.*
  - Male newborns with CAH may go unnoticed.

Administration of glucocorticoids can correct these defects and suppress ACTH, thus decreasing androgen production. In addition, administration of mineralocorticoids and salt tablets can counteract salt wasting. Surgical management to correct virilized genitalia may also be pursued, although this has become a controversial topic in the past several decades.

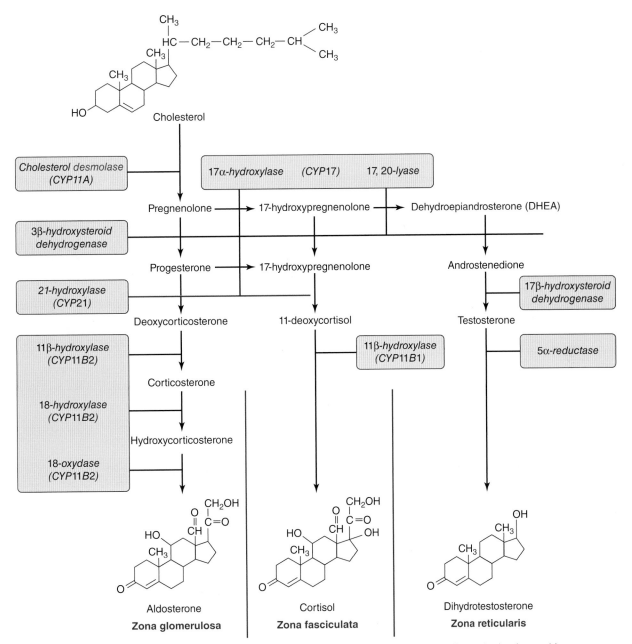

Fig. 31.7 Steroid biosynthesis. The line next to 21-hydroxylase is highlighted to indicate the barrier to aldosterone and cortisol synthesis posed by 21-hydroxylase deficiency. Such a barrier causes progesterone and 17-hydroxyprogesterone to build up, which decreases the rate of conversion of pregnenolone to progesterone and of 17-hydroxypregnenolone to 17-hydroxyprogesterone. In turn, pregnenolone and 17-hydroxypregnenolone build up and drive increased dehydroepiandrosterone (DHEA) formation.

PATHOPHYSIOLOGY: DISEASES OF CORTICAL OVER- AND UNDERPRODUCTION

Levels of cortisol and aldosterone normally vary in response to changing conditions in the body. For example, during stress, cortisol levels rise; in hypotension, aldosterone levels rise.

Pathologic conditions, however, may interfere with the adrenal cortex's normal response to stimuli. These conditions are classified as follows:

- Overproduction of adrenal hormone(s)
- Underproduction of adrenal hormone(s)

Note that these conditions may coexist for different hormones, as with CAH discussed earlier.

Diseases of Overproduction

Diseases of overproduction may be either be:
- Primary, that is, originating in the adrenal gland itself; or
  - CAH
  - Adrenal carcinomas or adenomas
- Secondary, that is, originating outside the adrenal gland
  - ACTH overproduction in the pituitary → overproduction of cortisol

- Chronic stimulation of the RAAS pathway because of renal disease → overproduction of aldosterone

Hypercortisolism

Excess glucocorticoid exposure, called hypercortisolism, can lead to a variety of disease manifestations and is one of the most serious adrenal derangements. Excess glucocorticoids may be the result of endogenous overproduction or exogenous administration of glucocorticoid drugs in higher-than normal amounts.

Endogenous cortisol overproduction can be classified into two categories:
- ACTH-dependent
  - Accounts for 85% of endogenous hypercortisolism.
  - Includes Cushing disease (pituitary adenoma producing ACTH), ectopic ACTH or CRH production.
- ACTH-independent
  - Accounts for 15% of endogenous hypercortisolism.
  - They include primary causes intrinsic to the adrenal gland, such as adrenal adenoma and adrenocortical carcinoma.

Exogenous glucocorticoids—drug preparations like prednisone or large quantities of steroid inhalers—can also lead to hypercortisolism (see Pharmacology Box 31.1).

> ### 💊 PHARMACOLOGY BOX 31.1
>
> Iatrogenic Cushing syndrome is generally the result of the use of pharmacologic glucocorticoids at supraphysiologic doses, and rarely from the administration of adrenocorticotropic hormone. Although oral drugs like prednisone are the most common cause, injected (for arthritis), inhaled (for asthma), and even topical steroid medications may be culpable. Progestins with cortisol-like effects may lead to Cushing disease. Nonsteroid drugs that impair hepatic metabolism of steroids (e.g., the human immunodeficiency virus drug ritonavir) can increase the risk of Cushing disease among patients using inhaled steroids.

Hypercortisolism resulting from any cause yields a constellation of clinical findings known as Cushing syndrome. The signs and symptoms of cortisol excess, first described by Harvey Cushing in 1932, include:
- Truncal obesity
- Round and full face ("moon facies")
- A "buffalo hump" of fat on the posterior neck
- Pigmented skin striae and thinned skin with easy bruising
- Muscle weakness and osteoporosis
- Hypertension, and hyperglycemia (Fig. 31.8) (see Fast Fact Box 31.4)

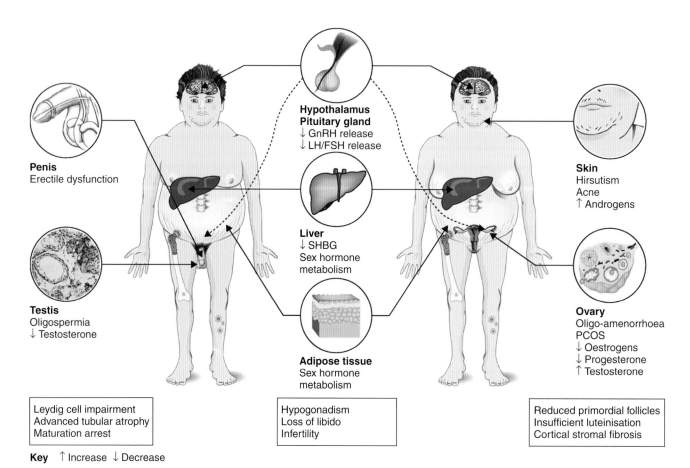

Key ↑ Increase ↓ Decrease

Fig. 31.8 Cushing syndrome signs and symptoms. *GnRH*, Gonadotropin-releasing hormone; *FSH*, follicle-stimulating hormone; *LH*, luteinizing hormone; *PCOS*, polycystic ovary syndrome; *SHBG*, sex hormone-binding globulin. (From: Pivonello R, Isidori AM, De Martino MC, et al. Complications of Cushing's syndrome: state of the art. *Lancet Diabetes Endocrinol.* 2016;4(7):611-629; Fig. 6 ©.)

These signs and symptoms emerge from a variety of pathophysiologic mechanisms related to the normal action of cortisol:

- The catabolic effects of cortisol cause muscle weakness, osteoporosis, striae, bruising, and hyperglycemia.
- The abnormal fat distribution is believed to be caused by increased lipolysis, which affects the extremities more than the trunk.
- Virilizing symptoms of hirsutism and acne can accompany ACTH-dependent hypercortisolism as a result of androgen overproduction from excessive ACTH.
- Hyperpigmentation is also seen with elevated ACTH levels and is believed to be caused by ACTH cross-reacting with melanocyte-stimulating hormone receptors on melanin-producing cells (see Clinical Correlation Box 31.4).

Clinical Correlation Box 31.4

Several tests are available to diagnose Cushing syndrome, each with varying degrees of sensitivity and specificity.
- Plasma cortisol level
  - Performed at night
  - Normally, circadian rhythms cause a drop in cortisol secretion at night; thus elevated levels imply Cushing syndrome
- 24-hour urine-free cortisol
  - Cushing syndrome leads to increased renal cortisol filtration and excretion
- Dexamethasone-suppression test
  - Administer dexamethasone, a powerful glucocorticoid that normally suppresses adrenocorticotropic hormone (ACTH) production just as cortisol does
  - ACTH-dependent processes (such as pituitary adenomas) will not respond to this negative feedback
  - Thus failure to suppress ACTH with dexamethasone indicates an ACTH-dependent cause of hypercortisolism

Hyperaldosteronism

As with hypercortisolism, hyperaldosteronism can be classified into two categories:

- Primary
  - Conn syndrome (aldosterone-producing adrenal adenoma)
- Secondary (extraadrenal)
  - Activation of the RAAS pathway because of overproduction of renin or a primary renal disorder involving decreased renal perfusion (i.e., renal artery stenosis).

Signs and symptoms of hyperaldosteronism include:

- Hypokalemia
- Hypernatremia
- Diastolic hypertension
- Polyuria
- Muscle weakness

Diagnosis is made by demonstrating a failure to suppress aldosterone production after intravenous saline loading. It may also be characterized by low plasma renin levels owing to the negative feedback from elevated aldosterone levels.

The hypertension seen in primary hyperaldosteronism is typically mild, caused in part by the phenomenon of aldosterone escape (also called mineralocorticoid escape). This occurs because the kidney can compensate through modification of other methods of volume control.

- The unregulated aldosterone secretion increases salt reabsorption in the distal tubule, leading to increased water reabsorption and increased fluid volume.
- However, other renal mechanisms respond to the increase in circulatory volume and pressure by reducing salt reabsorption and promoting diuresis.
- Decreased expression of distal NaCl cotransporters may also contribute to aldosterone escape.

Diseases of Underproduction

Like hyperaldosteronism, adrenal insufficiency can be categorized as:

- Primary
  - Addison disease
- Secondary
  - ACTH deficiency because of pituitary trauma, or suppression of ACTH release by exogenous glucocorticoids

Primary adrenal insufficiency, or Addison disease, is characterized typically by both aldosterone and cortisol deficiency.

- It is most often caused by adrenal cortex destruction.
  - Most common cause is autoimmune.
  - Other causes of cortex destruction include adrenal hemorrhage, tuberculosis, cytomegalovirus infection, certain medications, metastases, human immunodeficiency virus infection, and rare familial disorders, such as adrenal leukodystrophy.
- Another cause of primary adrenal insufficiency is caused by genetic deficiency of synthetic enzymes, most commonly 21-hydroxylase as seen in CAH.

Because of destruction of the entire adrenal cortex, glucocorticoid, mineralocorticoid, and androgen production can all be affected at once.

- Cortisol deficiency → fatigue, weakness, anorexia, weight loss, hypotension, and hypoglycemia.
- Aldosterone deficiency → deficient, hyperkalemia and salt craving may be present as well.
- Androgen deficiency → decreased hair growth in women (limited because of minor effect of androgens in adults).

The lack of cortisol feedback on the pituitary leads to increased ACTH production, which can be detected serologically or upon dermatologic examination, which reveals ACTH-related hyperpigmentation. This hyperpigmentation is caused by excess ACTH binding to melanocortin receptors, leading to several downstream effects including increased pigmentation (Fig. 31.9). Cortrosyn, an ACTH analog, can also be used to challenge the adrenals and test for primary adrenal insufficiency.

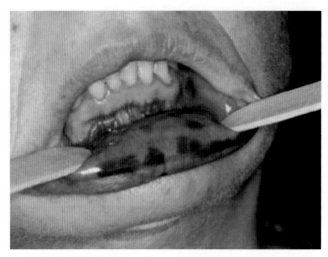

Fig. 31.9 Hyperpigmentation from Addison disease showing darkening around the gums. (From Farag AM. Head and neck manifestations of endocrine disorders. *Atlas Oral Maxillofac Surg Clin North Am.* 2017;25(2):197-207; Fig. 5.)

Primary adrenal insufficiency may present initially as an acute Addisonian crisis.

- This occurs when a patient with underlying undiagnosed adrenal disease encounters a stressor, such as surgery or infection, and cannot mount an appropriate cortisol response.
- The crisis is characterized by anorexia, nausea, vomiting, abdominal pain, hyponatremia, and hyperkalemia.
- Addisonian crises can be fatal if not rapidly treated with cortisol replacement, fluids, and glucose.

Secondary adrenal insufficiency arises from pituitary ACTH deficiency, and usually results only in cortisol deficiency as aldosterone production does not rely on ACTH.

- When a patient is treated with steroids, it can take some time for the pituitary to recover fully after the steroids have been stopped. Patients on high-dose or chronic steroids should always be tapered off the drugs to allow for adequate recovery of pituitary function.
- Similarly, patients taking glucocorticoids chronically, which causes suppression of their HPA axes, may often require "stress-dose steroids"—an increased amount of exogenous corticosteroids when undergoing surgery, trauma, or major illness—to mimic the physiologic response to stress.

SYSTEM FUNCTION: THE ADRENAL MEDULLA

At the core of the adrenal glands are the adrenal medullae, which are part of the sympathetic nervous system and are responsible for the production of catecholamines, epinephrine and NE. Catecholamines are essential modulators of the rapid response to stress, triggering a variety of fight-or-flight responses:

- Increased heart rate
- Elevated cardiac output
- Increased blood glucose levels

The parenchymal cells of the medulla, known as chromaffin cells, are derived from neural crest cells.

- Like postganglionic sympathetic neurons, the medulla is innervated by cholinergic preganglionic sympathetic neurons.

- Chromaffin cells are widely distributed throughout the body during fetal life, but the majority degenerate after birth, leaving the adrenal medulla as the main locus of chromaffin cells.

In contrast to adrenal cortical cells, medullary cells are full of secretory granules, which are storehouses for catecholamines, adenosine triphosphate (ATP), opiate-like enkephalins, and proteins called chromogranins, which bind to catecholamines. These cells are split into two types:

- Epinephrine-producing (80% of output)
- NE-producing (20% of output)

The Synthesis, Storage, and Release of Catecholamines

Catecholamines, which are all amines with a phenyl ring, include (Fig. 31.10):

- Dopamine
- NE
- Epinephrine

Just as cholesterol is the common precursor of adrenal cortical hormones, *tyrosine* is the precursor for catechol synthesis.

- Tyrosine comes from the diet, or it can be synthesized from phenylalanine.
- Tyrosine hydroxylase is the rate-limiting enzyme and catalyzes the production of dihydroxyphenylalanine (DOPA) from tyrosine.
  - Stimulated by acetylcholine (ACh), a preganglionic sympathetic neurotransmitter.
- DOPA is converted to dopamine and then to NE.
  - NE is then taken up into granules by an ATP-driven monoamine transport, or
  - NE may also be converted to epinephrine in the cytosol by phenylethanolamine-*N*-methyltransferase and packaged into secretory granules.
- Both NE and epinephrine are stored in granules until release is triggered.

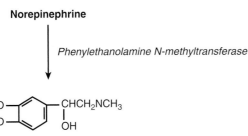

Fig. 31.10 Catecholamine biosynthesis. Catecholamines are produced from a tyrosine precursor in the adrenal medulla. This pathway is stimulated by input from the sympathetic nerves.

The adrenal medulla is the main producer of epinephrine in the body, whereas adrenergic axons make mostly NE.

The release of secretory granules occurs by exocytosis of the entire granule contents directly into the extracellular space and circulatory system.

- ACh stimulates voltage-gated calcium channels to open, causing an influx of calcium, which triggers process of exocytosis.
- Blood flow to the medulla increases significantly during the secretion of catecholamines, likely as a means of expediting

the distribution of the catecholamines to the rest of the body.
- Once in the bloodstream, NE and epinephrine are active for 10 to 30 seconds, then exert weaker activity for up to several minutes.

Catecholamines are metabolized by two systems, monoamine oxides, found in nerve endings, and catechol-O-methyltransferase, which is present in many tissues throughout the body. The main product of epinephrine degradation is vanillylmandelic acid (VMA).

Catecholamine Actions and Regulation

Like cortisol, the catecholamines have a wide variety of effects in a great many tissues. As they are not steroids, however, they bind to receptors on the surface of target tissues.

Catecholamine Actions

Catecholamines have effects on two main systems:
- Hemodynamic
  - Lead to increased heart rate, cardiac output, blood vessel tone, and extracellular fluid volume.
  - Collectively causes increased blood pressure.
- Metabolic
  - Act as counterregulatory hormones to oppose insulin action and mimic glucagon.
  - Epinephrine is up to 10 times more metabolically active than NE and acts to increase the metabolic rate and stimulate glycogenolysis.
  - Both NE and epinephrine elevate plasma glucose levels by suppressing glucose utilization, increasing glucagon levels, and decreasing insulin production.

NE and epinephrine both act at adrenergic receptors, of which there are two types, alpha receptors and beta receptors.
- NE has greater alpha activity, whereas epinephrine has an equal effect on alpha and beta receptors.
- Alpha1-receptor stimulation mediates:
  - Blood vessel constriction, which elevates total peripheral resistance and arterial blood pressure.
  - Stimulates the kidneys to secrete renin, initiating the RAA cascade and leading to tubular salt reabsorption and extracellular fluid volume expansion.
- Beta1-receptor mediates:
  - Increased cardiac activity.

Regulation of the Adrenal Medulla

Both the postganglionic sympathetic nerve endings and the adrenal medulla release catecholamines in response to signals from the nervous system.
- The brain registers stress or hypotension and discharges impulses along the sympathetic nerves.
- When the sympathetic nerves that innervate the adrenal gland are stimulated, the adrenal medulla releases NE and epinephrine, a sympathetic stimulus that affects the body globally by traveling in the bloodstream.

Recall that NE and epinephrine have a short half-life. Thus they do not regulate their own medullary release by negative feedback as cortisol does.

PATHOPHYSIOLOGY: MEDULLARY DYSFUNCTION

As in the adrenal cortex, medullary pathology can be classified as two processes:
- Overproduction of catecholamines
- Underproduction of catecholamines

Catecholamine Overproduction

Pheochromocytomas are catecholamine-producing tumors of chromaffin cells, the majority of which arise from the adrenal gland (90% of cases) but may also arise from extraadrenal chromaffin islands that persist after fetal life. They are rare and are perhaps most remarkable for their overrepresentation as a favorite "zebra" on medical boards.

Pheochromocytomas usually produce both NE and epinephrine and are characterized by paroxysmal symptoms indicating intermittent catecholamine release:
- Headache
- Pallor
- Palpitations
- Diaphoresis (sweating)
- Hypertension

Diagnosis is made by collecting a 24-hour urine sample and testing for catecholamines, metanephrines, and VMA.

Catecholamine Underproduction

Isolated adrenal underproduction of catecholamines usually does not lead to any sequelae, as the rest of the sympathetic nervous system can adequately perform the same functions. However, autonomic dysfunction that involves the sympathetic nerves can occur.
- Autonomic dysfunction may be idiopathic or secondary to diabetes, autoimmune disorders, or central nervous system infections.

- This dysfunction typically leads to postural hypotension (see Clinical Correlation Box 31.5).

Clinical Correlation Box 31.5

Waterhouse–Friderichsen syndrome can be caused by fulminant infection from *Neisseria meningitidis*, which leads to hemorrhagic necrosis of the adrenal glands, leading to adrenal failure (Fig. 31.11). Infection with Neisseria can also lead to septic shock, organ failure and hemorrhage, and disseminated intravascular coagulation.

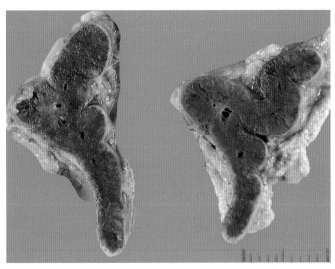

Fig. 31.11 Extensive hemorrhage of the adrenal glands because of Waterhouse-Friderichsen syndrome. (From Connolly AJ, Finkbeiner WE, Ursell PC, et al. Atlas of gross autopsy pathology. In: *Autopsy Pathology: A Manual and Atlas.* Elsevier; 2016: p. 186-319. Fig. 16-256.)

▌ SUMMARY

- The two portions of the adrenal gland are the cortex and the medulla.
- The three layers of the cortex from outermost to innermost are the zona glomerulosa, which secretes the mineralocorticoid aldosterone; the zona fasciculata, which secretes the glucocorticoid cortisol; and the zona reticularis, which secretes adrenal androgens, DHEA, and androstenedione.
- The adrenal glands have excellent arterial supply with superb vasodilatory capacity, which facilitates hormonal secretion.
- The HPA axis regulates adrenal secretion from the cortex. The hypothalamus releases CRH, which stimulates the anterior pituitary to release ACTH.
- ACTH triggers increased CEH conversion of cholesteryl ester to cholesterol, thereby increasing intracellular cholesterol levels. Steroid production from cholesterol, in particular

cortisol, increases. Cortisol inhibits the secretion of CRH and ACTH in a classic negative-feedback loop.
- Aldosterone increases salt and water reabsorption in the kidney and K^+ secretion in the kidney. Its secretion is regulated primarily by the RAA system (which responds to blood pressure) and the plasma K^+ level.
- Cortisol affects metabolism, as well as the immune and cardiovascular systems.
- The adrenal androgens are physiologically important during fetal development and puberty but are less important and less potent than the gonadal androgens (such as testosterone) during the other periods of life.
- All steroids are derived from cholesterol and pregnenolone, a modified form of cholesterol. Cholesteryl esters are delivered to the adrenal by LDLs in the blood and converted to cholesterol by CEH.

- In the disease congenital adrenal hyperplasia, 21-hydroxylase deficiency causes decreased production of cortisol and aldosterone, an overflow of precursors into the androgen pathways, and excess production of adrenal androgens.
- Hypercortisolism, an overproduction of cortisol, leads to Cushing syndrome. Hypercortisolism may have ACTH-dependent causes, such as pituitary adenoma and ectopic ACTH-secreting tumors, or ACTH-independent causes, such as adrenal tumors or exogenous glucocorticoid administration.
- Hyperaldosteronism may arise from adrenal tumors or kidney disease.
- Destruction of the adrenal glands owing to various causes leads to primary adrenal insufficiency (Addison disease). Secondary adrenal insufficiency results from decreased

ACTH production, whether because of pituitary pathology or the suppression of ACTH by the administration of exogenous glucocorticoids.
- The catecholamines epinephrine and norepinephrine mediate the fight-or-flight response, which includes increased heart rate, elevated cardiac output, and increased blood glucose levels.
- Catecholamines are made from the common amino acid precursor tyrosine.
- Many central nervous system-processed signals, including stress and hypotension, cause increased sympathetic nervous output, thereby driving the release of adrenal catecholamines.
- Pheochromocytomas are extremely rare catecholamine-secreting tumors of the adrenal medulla.

REVIEW QUESTIONS

Directions: Each of the numbered items or incomplete statements in this section is followed by answers or by completions of the statement. Select the one lettered answer or completion that is best in each case.

1. A newborn girl is observed to have ambiguous genitalia, low blood pressure, and hyperkalemia and is diagnosed with congenital adrenal hyperplasia. Her 21-hydroxylase deficiency has caused which of the following patterns of adrenal hormone derangement?
   A. Decreased cortisol, decreased aldosterone, increased adrenal androgens
   B. Decreased cortisol, increased aldosterone, increased adrenal androgens
   C. Increased cortisol, decreased aldosterone, decreased adrenal androgens
   D. Increased cortisol, increased aldosterone, decreased adrenal androgens
   E. Increased cortisol, decreased aldosterone, increased adrenal androgens

2. A 27-year-old man is treated with oral prednisone (a glucocorticoid) to control a severe asthma exacerbation. After 2 weeks on the medication, his wheezing resolves and he decides to stop taking the prednisone without tapering his doses as prescribed. Two days later, he comes to the emergency room with symptoms of fatigue, weakness, and anorexia. He

is hypotensive and hypoglycemic. He probably has adrenal insufficiency because:
   A. His adrenal cortex is unresponsive to ACTH.
   B. His ACTH secretion is low because of pituitary dysfunction.
   C. His ACTH secretion has been suppressed by exogenous glucocorticoids.
   D. His adrenal glands have been destroyed by lymphocytic infiltration.
   E. He has an ACTH-secreting pituitary adenoma.
   F. He has an adrenal adenoma.
   G. He has an adrenal pheochromocytoma.
   H. Exogenous glucocorticoids have injured his adrenal glands.

3. A 25-year-old woman with type I diabetes is hospitalized with a severe case of double pneumonia. During her hospital stay, she requires higher-than-usual doses of insulin. This is because:
   A. Elevated glucagon secretion has increased her plasma glucose level.
   B. Alveolar inflammation has liberated glucose into the blood.
   C. Her intake of carbohydrates has increased dramatically.
   D. Elevated cortisol secretion has increased her plasma glucose level.
   E. Her adrenal function has been suppressed.

ANSWERS TO REVIEW QUESTIONS

1. **The answer is A.** The 21-hydroxylase deficiency in CAH results in a failure to convert progesterone into deoxycorticosterone in the aldosterone pathway and a failure to convert 17-hydroxyprogesterone into 11-deoxycortisol in the cortisol pathway. Pregnenolone levels consequently rise and drive conversion to 17-hydroxypregnenolone and then DHEA, an androgen. CAH therefore decreases cortisol and aldosterone output, while it increases the secretion of androgens, leading to the development of ambiguous genitalia in female infants.

2. **The answer is C.** Administration of an exogenous glucocorticoid (prednisone) has suppressed ACTH production from

his pituitary. When the prednisone is abruptly withdrawn, his pituitary cannot immediately generate enough ACTH to stimulate the adrenals to make normal amounts of cortisol. The patient has a form of secondary adrenal insufficiency. Exogenous glucocorticoids are always prescribed on a taper (i.e., with progressively decreasing doses of the glucocorticoid) to relieve ACTH suppression gradually. Destruction of the adrenals causes primary adrenal insufficiency, which also leads to low cortisol levels, but there is no indication of primary adrenal pathology in this case. A functioning pituitary or adrenal adenoma causes hypercortisolism, not adrenal insufficiency. A pheochromocytoma is a rare tumor of the adrenal medulla that does not cause adrenal insufficiency, but rather increased catecholamine secretion.

3. **The answer is D.** The stress of infection has driven the patient's hypothalamus to increase CRH secretion, which in turn elevates the level of ACTH and then cortisol in the bloodstream. Cortisol's insulin-opposing, counterregulatory effect elevates the plasma glucose level. The insulin dose must therefore be increased to cover the higher level of glucose. Other causes of hyperglycemia would also require an increased insulin dose, but we know that infection has engaged her CRH response to stress. Her adrenal function is fine, as it is mounting an effective response to stress.

32

Calcium Regulation: Parathyroid Physiology

INTRODUCTION

Calcium plays a fundamental role in the physiology of all living organisms.
- At the macroscopic level, calcium is essential to maintaining the structural integrity of the skeleton.
- At the molecular level, calcium is central to several physiologic processes, including neurotransmitter release, signal transduction, and blood coagulation.

Parathyroid hormone (PTH), the main product of the parathyroid glands, and vitamin D together regulate the serum calcium level.

SYSTEM STRUCTURE: THE PARATHYROID GLANDS AND THE DISTRIBUTION OF CALCIUM AND PHOSPHORUS

The parathyroid gland synthesizes and secretes PTH. Typically, there are four parathyroid glands, with pairs located at the superior and inferior margins of the thyroid capsule (Fig. 32.1).
- Each parathyroid gland is small, averaging $6 \times 4 \times 2$ mm in size and weighing 40 mg.
- The parathyroid develops at 5 to 14 weeks of gestation from the third and fourth branchial pouches.

There are two types of cells in the parathyroid:
1. Chief cells
   a. Critical for synthesis and secretion of PTH.
2. Oxyphil cells
   a. Unknown function, but have been shown to produce parathyroid-relevant genes, as well as certain autocrine and paracrine factors.

Extracellular and Intracellular Pools of Calcium

The extracellular pool of calcium (the concentration of calcium in the plasma) is tightly regulated and remains remarkably constant, varying from 8.8 to 10.4 mg/dL (2.2–2.6 mM). This extracellular pool consists of three fractions:
1. Free, ionized calcium (50%)
2. Protein-bound calcium (40%)
3. Calcium complexes with anions, such as citrate and phosphate (10%)

The free, ionized calcium fraction is physiologically active and under close regulation by PTH.

The equilibrium between free, protein-bound, and complexed fractions may change under certain conditions.
- Acidosis increases the proportion of free calcium, while alkalosis decreases it.
- Increases in citrate and phosphate concentration can also decrease ionized calcium levels.
  - Examples: Blood transfusion (contains citrate for preservation), crush injury (releases phosphate).

On an intracellular level, the concentration of free calcium is only 0.1 µM, or 1/10,000th of the extracellular concentration.
- The magnitude of this gradient allows for rapid flow of calcium into the cell when calcium channels are opened, transiently increasing the intracellular concentration 10-fold to 100-fold.
- Calcium pumps and exchangers actively restore and maintain this large gradient.
- The endoplasmic reticulum, microsome, and mitochondria store calcium in bound form where it is available for rapid intracellular release when signaled.

Inputs and Outputs of Calcium

For calcium levels to remain stable, the daily amount of calcium absorption must equal the amount of excretion (Fig. 32.2).
- Dietary intake
  - The dietary intake of calcium of an American adult averages 0.4 to 1.5 g of calcium per day.
  - For reference, a quart of milk contains about 1.0 g of calcium.
- Gastrointestinal absorption
  - Around 50% dietary intake is absorbed by the gastrointestinal tract, which is regulated by vitamin D (discussed later).
  - In addition, the body secretes calcium into the lumen of the gastrointestinal tract in digestive juices.
  - Incomplete absorption of dietary and secreted calcium results in an average of 0.35 to 1.0 g of calcium lost in the stool every day.
  - This balances out to a net gut absorption of 0.15 to 0.4 g of calcium per day (see Fast Fact Box 32.1).

Fast Fact Box 32.1

During periods of growth, pregnancy, and lactation, vitamin D increases the absorption of calcium.

- Renal absorption
  - Net inputs from the gut are matched by losses from the urinary tract.

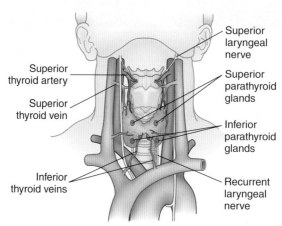

Fig. 32.1 Anatomy of the parathyroid glands. The four small parathyroid glands are found in the capsule of the posterior thyroid or embedded in the thyroid tissue. They share the thyroid's blood supply. (From Miller FR, Netterville JL. Surgical management of thyroid and parathyroid disorders. *Med Clin North Am.* 1999;83(1):247; Fig. 1.)

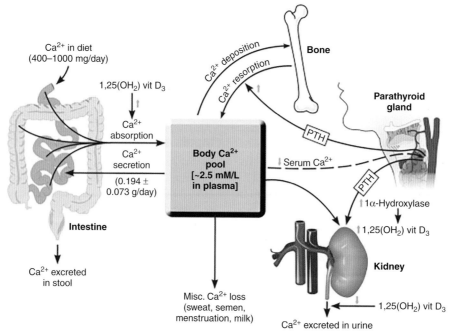

Fig. 32.2 The dietary intake of calcium of an American adult. (From Kiela PR, Ghishan FK. Molecular mechanisms of intestinal transport of calcium, phosphate, and magnesium. In: *Physiology of the Gastrointestinal Tract*, 6th Edition. Elsevier; 2018: p. 1405-1449; Fig. 59.1.)

- The kidney filters 10.0 g of calcium per day.
- It reabsorbs 98% of the calcium, excreting only 0.15 to 0.3 g in the urine.

The skeleton serves as both a reservoir and a destination for calcium, depending on the hormonal milieu. There is a dynamic balance between the pool of calcium in the skeleton and in the extracellular fluid (ECF).

- Skeleton versus ECF
  - About 98% of the body's 1- to 2-kg total store of calcium is found in the skeleton as calcium hydroxyapatite $[Ca_{10}(PO_4)_4(OH)_2]$.
  - The ECF described earlier contains a small fraction—only 0.9 g.

- Remodeling
  - During the course of normal day-to-day bone remodeling, 0.25 to 0.5 g of calcium enters and leaves the ECF from the skeleton, for a net skeletal balance of 0.
  - In times of duress, the skeleton can rapidly mobilize its pool of calcium and replenish the calcium in the critical ECF pool in a matter of hours.

This skeletal reservoir is sufficient to prevent hypocalcemia for months to years.

  - However, mobilization of these skeletal reservoirs, as might be expected, can lead to fractures as the bone is depleted of calcium (see Clinical Correlation Box 32.1).

In light of the effects of aging on bone mass, it is recommended to increase dietary intake of calcium with age.
- By increasing dietary calcium levels, the body relies less on the skeletal calcium reservoir for maintaining appropriate levels of calcium in the body.
- The skeletal reservoir is thus protected and the integrity of the skeletal system preserved.

Phosphorus

The hormones that regulate calcium homeostasis are also responsible for regulating phosphorus homeostasis. Phosphorus has numerous roles throughout the body, including:
- Component of calcium hydroxyapatite that forms bone, phosphorus.
- Covalently modifies enzymes and substrates during signal transduction (in the form of phosphate).
- Participates in energy transactions (e.g., adenosine triphosphate [ATP], creatine phosphate).

The distribution of phosphorus is roughly similar to calcium. The adult human body contains roughly 600 g of phosphorus, distributed as follows:
- Some 85% is stored in crystalline form in the skeleton.
- Around 100 g is found in the soft tissues as phosphate esters.
- Around 550 mg is found in the extracellular pool, which is in equilibrium with soft tissues and bone.
  - Phosphorus, generally in the form of inorganic phosphate (HPO_4^{2-} and $H_2PO_4^-$), circulates at concentrations of 2.8 to 4 mg/dL (0.9–1.3 mM) (see Fast Fact Box 32.2).

The gastrointestinal tract absorbs phosphorus considerably more efficiently than calcium, which is more than sufficient for daily requirements.

The regulation of phosphate levels takes place primarily at the level of the kidney by PTH, but vitamin D also plays a role.
- Increased PTH levels lead to lower plasma phosphate levels by enhancing urinary phosphate excretion.
- Vitamin D defends against hypophosphatemia by inhibiting the production of PTH.

Overall, the regulation of calcium balance is much tighter than the regulation of phosphate.

SYSTEM FUNCTION: PARATHYROID HORMONE AND VITAMIN D

Two principal hormones regulate plasma levels of calcium in response to rapid, daily fluxes of calcium inputs and outputs:
- PTH
- Vitamin D
  - 1,25-dihydroxyvitamin D ($1,25(OH)_2D$) is the active metabolite of vitamin D.

Specifically, PTH and vitamin D work in concert to raise calcium levels.
- PTH regulates calcium minute to minute.
- Vitamin D, on the other hand, acts on a longer time frame and facilitates the effects of PTH.

PTH increases calcium levels by three mechanisms:
1. Increasing bone resorption.
2. Increasing the renal reabsorption of calcium at the proximal tubule.
3. Increasing the synthesis of active vitamin D by the kidney.

Vitamin D increases calcium levels by two mechanisms:
1. Increasing the intestinal absorption of calcium.
2. Increasing bone resorption.

Fig. 32.3 summarizes the actions of and interactions between PTH and vitamin D in response to a hypocalcemic challenge.

Calcitonin, a peptide hormone secreted by C cells in the thyroid, also plays a role in calcium homeostasis by lowering plasma calcium levels. However, the participation of calcitonin in calcium regulation is much smaller than PTH and vitamin D and will be discussed later.

Parathyroid Hormone

As the most significant mediator of calcium homeostasis, PTH warrants a detailed discussion.

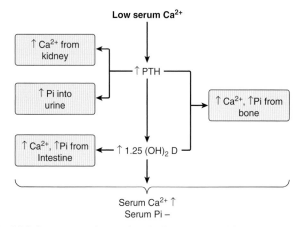

Fig. 32.3 Response to hypocalcemia. Low serum calcium levels lead to an increased release of parathyroid hormone (*PTH*) and increased synthesis of $1,25(OH)_2D$, the active metabolite of vitamin D. The increase in PTH stimulates bone resorption (thereby increasing the flux of calcium from the skeleton to the extracellular fluid), the renal reabsorption of calcium, and the synthesis of vitamin D by the kidney. The increase in vitamin D in turn increases the intestinal absorption of calcium and increases bone resorption. PTH promotes the wasting of phosphate (*Pi*) in the kidney, while vitamin D increases its absorption in the intestine.

Parathyroid Hormone Synthesis

The regulation of PTH synthesis occurs via negative feedback loops.
- Vitamin D and high levels of calcium suppress transcription of the *PTH* gene.
- Conversely, hypocalcemia stimulates the synthesis of PTH.

Parathyroid Hormone Secretion and Calcium Levels

The secretion of PTH is exquisitely sensitive to circulating free, ionized calcium levels (recall that this is the physiologically active pool).
- Decreases in calcium levels increase PTH secretion.
- Fig. 32.4 illustrates the steep, inverse sigmoidal relationship between calcium and PTH secretion.
  - The steep portion of the curve corresponds to the normal range of calcium, reflecting the sensitivity of the parathyroid to minor changes in calcium levels.
  - Small decreases in calcium concentrations dramatically increase PTH secretion.

The parathyroid detects calcium levels through the calcium-sensing receptor, an extracellular, 120-kDa G protein-linked receptor.
- Calcium ions serve as the ligand for this receptor.
- Stimulation of this receptor depresses PTH secretion through the activation of Gq, which is coupled to phospholipase C.
  - This initiates the inositol trisphosphate and diacylglycerol signaling pathway common to many other cell types.
- The same calcium-sensing receptor is also present in renal tubule cells and in the thyroid C cells, which secrete calcitonin (see Clinical Correlation Box 32.2).

Clinical Correlation Box 32.2

Mutations that inactivate the calcium-sensing receptor affect calcium homeostasis. One example is familial hypocalciuric hypercalcemia (FHH), an autosomal dominant, benign condition.
- Key finding: hypocalciuria in the presence of parathyroid hormone (PTH)-mediated hypercalcemia.
- In FHH, the mutation alters the set point for calcium in the parathyroid, leading to inappropriate PTH release and thus hypercalcemia.
- Simultaneously, the same abnormal receptor in the kidney inhibits the renal excretion of calcium, exacerbating the hypercalcemia.

Other Modulators of the Parathyroid Hormone Level

Other factors that influence PTH secretion include magnesium, lithium, and aluminum.
- Magnesium
  - As with calcium, low serum levels of magnesium stimulate PTH secretion, and high levels suppress it.
  - However, paradoxically, chronic, severe hypomagnesemia (1.0 mg/dL, 0.4 mM) suppresses PTH secretion because of depletion of intracellular magnesium levels.
- Lithium
  - Lithium stimulates PTH secretion by changing the set point for PTH secretion (see Fast Fact Box 32.3).

Fast Fact Box 32.3

Hypercalcemia may be seen in patients who receive lithium for manic depression.

- Aluminum
  - High levels of aluminum inhibit PTH secretion.
  - May be seen in patients with renal failure who are dialyzed against solutions containing aluminum, or who are being treated with aluminum-containing phosphate binders for the hyperphosphatemia observed in renal failure.

Table 32.1 summarizes the regulation of PTH synthesis and secretion.

Parathyroid Hormone Structure

PTH, which is derived from the precursor hormone pre-pro-PTH, is a small protein composed of 84 amino acids with a molecular weight of 9300 Da.

Once PTH is processed and secreted, the circulating intact PTH is rapidly metabolized by the liver and kidney.
- PTH has a half-life of only 2 to 4 minutes.
- The rapid breakdown of PTH thus allows the body to respond quickly to changing calcium levels.

The metabolism of PTH becomes clinically relevant when determining the levels of PTH (see Clinical Correlation Box 32.3)

Clinical Correlation Box 32.3

Newer assays for parathyroid hormone (PTH) quantify intact PTH and avoid the pitfalls of earlier approaches, which tended to detect only the carboxyl terminal fragments produced during the breakdown of intact PTH. These carboxyl terminal fragments are cleared by the kidney and accumulate in renal failure, and thus may potentially skew the measurements of earlier assays toward higher PTH values.

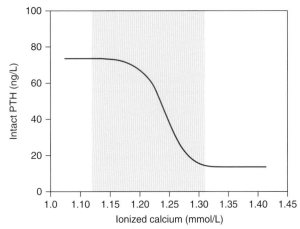

Fig. 32.4 The inverse sigmoidal relationship between serum ionized calcium levels and parathyroid hormone (*PTH*). Parathyroid sensitivity is maximal within the normal range, indicated by the *shaded area*.

TABLE 32.1 The Regulation of Parathyroid Hormone Secretion

↑ Secretion	↓ Secretion
↓ [Ca^{2+}]	↑ [Ca^{2+}] negative feedback
↓ [Mg^{2+}]	↑ [Mg^{2+}]
	Vitamin D (negative feedback via synthesis inhibition)

PTH, Parathyroid hormone.

TABLE 32.2 The Actions of Parathyroid Hormone

↑ Osteoclast activity and number (via osteoclasts)
↑ Calcium reabsorption at distal tubule
↑ Synthesis of 1,25(OH)$_2$D
↓ Activity of vitamin D-24-hydroxylase (deactivator of vitamin D metabolites)
↑ Urinary phosphate excretion

PTH, Parathyroid hormone.

The Actions of Parathyroid Hormone

For a quick overview, see Table 32.2. PTH has direct effects on two organ systems where calcium flux occurs:
- Skeletal system
- Renal system

Recall that the skeletal system is not a static system but a dynamic one. Bone is continuously resorbed and reformed; 5% to 10% of the skeleton turns over annually. There are three types of cells in bone:

1. Osteoblasts synthesize the collagen matrix, or osteoid, where mineralization takes place.
   a. As long as calcium and phosphate are present in the appropriate concentrations, mineralization occurs spontaneously on the collagen scaffolding laid down by osteoblasts.
2. Osteocytes are osteoblasts that are embedded in cortical bone during remodeling. Their physiologic role is not as clear.
3. Osteoclasts are multinucleated giant cells that resorb bone and in the process release calcium and phosphate.
   a. Osteoblasts and osteoclasts coordinate their activities, with osteoblasts generally issuing most of the orders to osteoclasts through cytokines.

In bone, PTH acts via osteoblasts to increase the activity and number of osteoclasts.
- All PTH receptors are found on osteoblasts.
- Osteoblasts mediate the signal from PTH by releasing cytokines, which increase osteoclast activity (Fig. 32.5).
- PTH also recruits more osteoclasts by accelerating the maturation of osteoclast precursors.

Therefore PTH increases the magnitude of bone resorption and therefore the efflux of calcium and phosphate from bone into the circulation.
- Chronic elevations in PTH inhibit osteoblast activity; thus unless the calcium is replaced, the increased osteoclast-mediated bone resorption will be at the expense of skeletal mass and integrity (see Clinical Correlation Box 32.4, Genetics Box 32.1, Development Box 32.1, and Trauma Box 32.1).

Clinical Correlation Box 32.4

Because osteoblasts possess parathyroid hormone (PTH) receptors, intermittent PTH administration paradoxically leads to clinically significant osteoblast activity and enhanced bone formation.

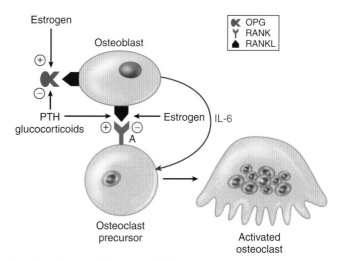

Fig. 32.5 Parathyroid hormone (*PTH*)'s activation of osteoclasts via osteoblasts. Osteoblasts, but not osteoclasts (OC), possess receptors for PTH. When activated by *PTH*, osteoblasts release cytokines, such as interleukin-6 (IL-6) that directly and indirectly stimulate osteoclasts, leading to increased bone resorption and increased release of calcium into the circulation. Receptor activator of nuclear factor-kB ligand (*RANKL*) from the osteoblast in both membrane bounded and soluble forms stimulates osteoclast precursors through receptor activator of nuclear factor-kB (*RANK*), whereas osteoprotegrin (*OPG*) antagonizes RANKL binding to RANK. (Modified from Unnanuntana A, Gladnick BP, Lane JM. Osteoporosis and the aging spine: diagnosis and treatment. In: *The Comprehensive Treatment of the Aging Spine*. Elsevier; 2011: p. 68-73; Fig. 12.1.)

GENETICS BOX 32.1

Patients with autosomal recessive osteopetrosis have impaired function of osteoclasts. Consequently, they have hyperdense bones that, counterintuitively, are more likely to fracture than normal bones. In many patients, this is caused by a mutation in the TCIRG1 gene that encodes the a3 subunit of the vacuolar H$^+$ adenosine triphosphatase (ATPase). This ATPase normally allows osteoclasts to acidify the space between their membrane and the surrounding bone matrix, a critical step in bone catabolism and remodeling. TCIRG1 mutations impair this function. Other affected individuals have a mutation in the CA2 gene that codes for a carbonic anhydrase enzyme isoform critical to both osteoclast development and renal tubular function.

DEVELOPMENT BOX 32.1

Autosomal recessive osteopetrosis presents with short stature and impaired growth, but as bones progressively thicken, patients may develop cranial neuropathies (resulting in blindness of optic nerve dysfunction or hearing impairment from cranial nerve VIII disease) as there is mechanical impingement on cranial nerves from bony overgrowth. This atypical bone growth can also constrict the marrow space and lead to insufficient red blood cell, white blood cell, and platelet production, leading to anemia, leukopenia, and thrombocytopenia, respectively.

TRAUMA BOX 32.1

Ironically, patients with the abnormally thick and dense bones of osteopetrosis are more likely to sustain a fracture with even minor trauma than patients with normal bone structure. With loss of bone marrow function, patients may also have trauma associated hemorrhages because of thrombocytopenia.

In the kidney, on the other hand, PTH performs two functions for calcium homeostasis:

1. Stimulation of calcium reabsorption
2. Increased synthesis of the active metabolite of vitamin D, $1,25(OH)_2D$

PTH raises calcium levels faster and in greater magnitude through the kidney than through bone resorption.

- As mentioned earlier, the kidney filters 10 g of calcium per day, returning 98% of it to the body.
- About 90% of this calcium reabsorption takes place in the proximal convoluted tubule, and this process is not regulated by PTH.
- The fate of the remaining 10% is modulated by PTH at the distal tubule; the presence of PTH increases calcium reabsorption at the distal tubule.

Furthermore, PTH activates 25-hydroxyvitamin D-1α-hydroxylase, the enzyme responsible for converting vitamin D to its most active metabolite, $1,25(OH)_2D$. This enzyme is found in the mitochondria of the proximal tubule.

Phosphate balance is also regulated by PTH. The kidney is the principal site for phosphate regulation, and PTH determines the set point for serum phosphate levels.

- PTH inhibits phosphate reabsorption at the proximal and distal tubule.
- The phosphaturia produced by PTH compensates for (and overshoots) the release of phosphate from bone because of PTH.
- Hence, PTH overall decreases serum phosphate levels.

Through these coordinated effects, the body can increase the levels of calcium without excessively increasing phosphate levels. This avoids the risk of precipitating calcium phosphate crystals in the bloodstream.

- Fig. 32.6 summarizes the actions of PTH on its target organs to raise serum calcium levels and decrease serum phosphate levels.

- Fig. 32.7 illustrates the changes in calcium and phosphate levels when PTH is administered pharmacologically.

The Parathyroid Hormone Receptor

The PTH receptor is found in bone and the kidney. It has a molecular weight of 80,000 Da and is a member of the G-protein receptor superfamily with a seven-transmembrane domain.

- This receptor is coupled to two receptor-associated G proteins, Gs and Gq.
  - The Gs pathway is linked to adenylyl cyclase and increases cyclic adenosine monophosphate.
  - The Gq receptor is coupled to phospholipase C and the inositol trisphosphate and diacylglycerol signaling pathway n increases Ca^{++}.

Parathyroid Hormone-Related Protein

Parathyroid hormone-related protein (PTHrP) is a protein secreted in certain malignancies that mimics the calcium-raising effects of PTH.

- Binding of the PTH receptor requires only the first 34 residues of PTH (intact PTH has 84 residues), and activation of the receptor requires only the first six residues.
- PTHrP is homologous with PTH only at the amino terminus, where they share eight of the first 13 amino acid residues.

This homology becomes clinically important because the secretion of PTHrP by certain malignancies can activate the PTH receptor and cause hypercalcemia. Examples include:

- Renal cell carcinoma
- Squamous cell carcinoma
- Breast cancer

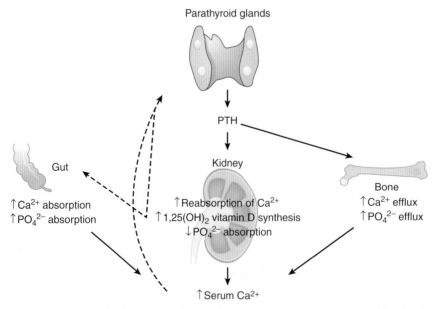

Fig. 32.6 The actions of parathyroid hormone (*PTH*) on its target organs to raise serum calcium levels and decrease serum phosphate levels. (From Bone and mineral disorders in chronic kidney disease. In: Gilbert and Weiner, Eds. *National Kidney Foundation Primer on Kidney Diseases*, 7th edition. Elsevier; 2018: p. 493-505.e1. Fig. 54.1.)

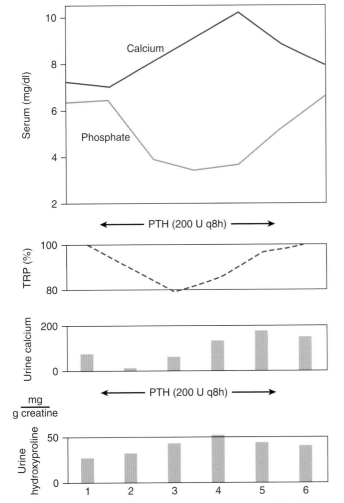

Fig. 32.7 Effect of parathyroid hormone (*PTH*) on a PTH-deficient patient with low plasma calcium and high plasma phosphate levels. PTH increases serum levels of calcium and decreases serum levels of phosphate. Tubular resorption of phosphate (*TRP*) decreases with PTH administration, and hence the urinary excretion of phosphate increases. Urinary calcium levels initially decrease owing to increased calcium reabsorption mediated by PTH. However, urinary calcium levels eventually increase because the filtered load of calcium increases with rising serum calcium concentrations. Rising urinary hydroxyproline levels reflect PTH-mediated bone resorption.

In addition to its relationship to malignancy, PTHrP also has a physiologic role that is currently being determined.
- May aid in breast differentiation.
- May relax smooth muscle, particularly uterine and gastric smooth muscle.

Vitamin D

As mentioned earlier, vitamin D is another key player in calcium homeostasis. Vitamin D increases calcium levels by two principal mechanisms:
1. Increasing the intestinal absorption of dietary calcium.
2. Stimulating the maturation of bone-resorbing osteoclasts.

Vitamin D is a sterol prohormone that needs to be converted (through a sequence of reactions) to its active metabolite,

$1,25(OH)_2D$, before it can participate in calcium regulation. These conversions take place in three locations:
1. Skin
2. Liver
3. Kidney

There are two forms of dietary vitamin D:
1. Vitamin D_3 (cholecalciferol), which is found in animal sources (such as cod liver oil).
2. Vitamin D2 (ergocalciferol), which is found in plant sources.

Both are metabolically equivalent, with the same actions and potency in the body.

Vitamin D Synthesis

The first step of vitamin D synthesis occurs in the skin (Fig. 32.8).
- The starting substrate is 7-dehydrocholesterol (7-DHC) or provitamin D, the immediate precursor of cholesterol.
- In the epidermis, ultraviolet (UV) light from 290 to 310 nm transforms 7-DHC to previtamin D.
- Thermal energy then converts previtamin D to vitamin D over the course of several days.
- This allows for a steady supply of vitamin D after brief UV radiation exposure.

Several factors modulate the production of vitamin D, including:
- Competition for UV energy
  - Melanin pigmentation
  - Exogenous factors, such as sunscreen
- Amount of 7-DHC
  - Decreases with advancing age
  - A 70-year-old person produces only 30% of the amount of vitamin D a young adult produces when exposed to similar amounts of UV light.
- Inactivation of previtamin D and vitamin D
  - Excessive UV radiation

Once vitamin D is synthesized, circulating vitamin D-binding protein draws vitamin D from the skin into the bloodstream.
- Vitamin D-binding protein has a 1000-fold higher affinity for vitamin D compared with previtamin D.

Once in the circulation, vitamin D is transported to the liver where the second step in vitamin D activation occurs.
- Vitamin D is hydroxylated by mitochondrial cytochrome P_{450} vitamin D-25-hydroxylase to create 25(OH)D (Fig. 32.9).
- 25(OH)D is the major circulating form of vitamin D and is also its major storage form in adipose and muscle.
- Vitamin D-25-hydroxylase in the liver is loosely regulated by a negative-feedback mechanism by 25(OH)D.

However, 25(OH)D is not biologically active at its physiologic levels. Thus it is finally transported to the kidney, where the final step of vitamin D activation occurs.
- A second hydroxylation takes place by the mitochondrial cytochrome P_{450} 25(OH)D-1 α-hydroxylase to $1,25(OH)_2D$.
- The $1,25(OH)_2D$ is the most biologically potent form of vitamin D.
  - It is 100 to 1000 times more potent than its precursor!

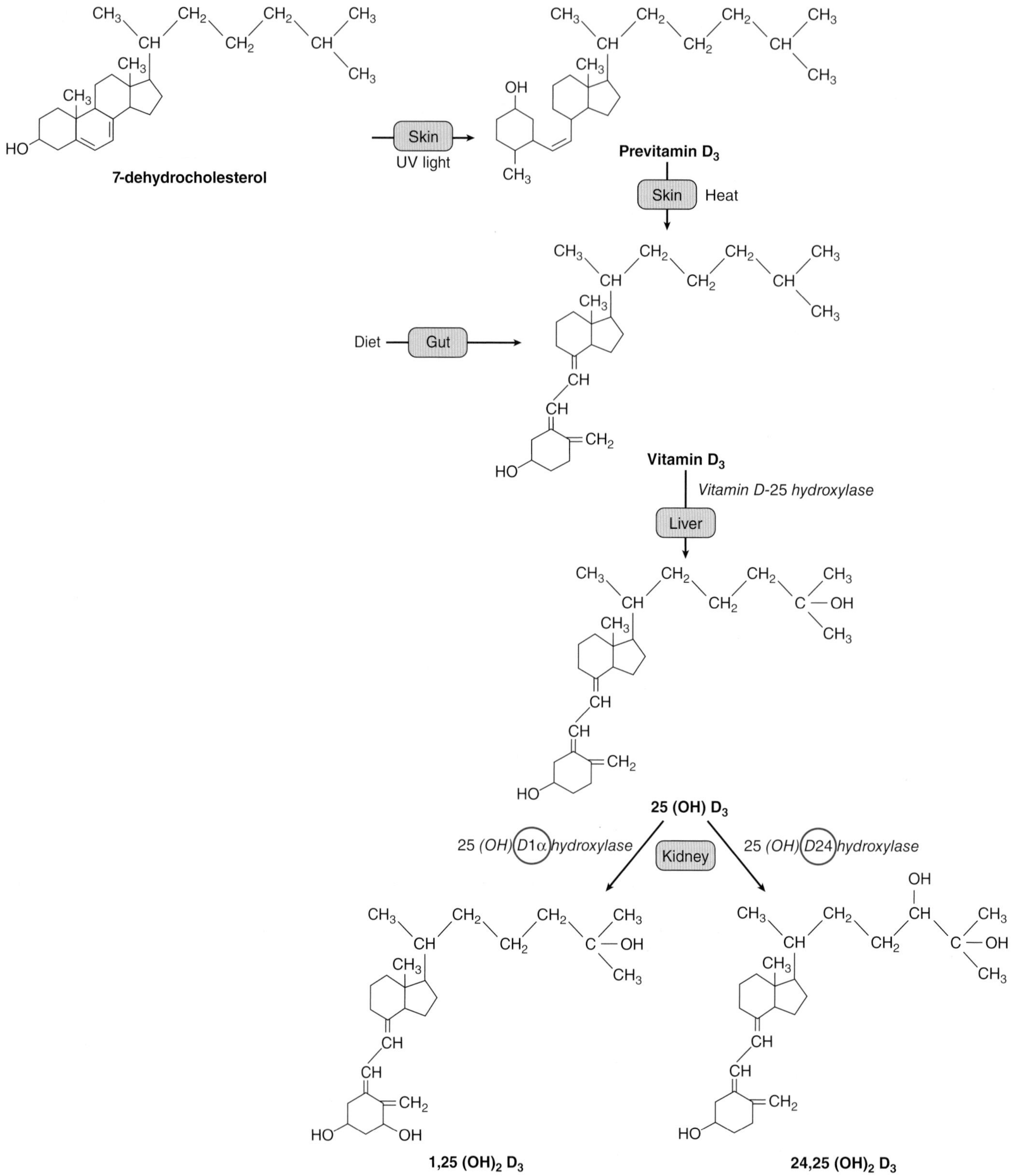

Fig. 32.8 Photochemical, thermal, and metabolic pathways for the synthesis of vitamin D. Vitamin D is synthesized in the skin through the actions of ultraviolet and thermal energy. Vitamin D then undergoes a series of hydroxylations in the liver and in the kidney to become its most active form, 1,25(OH)$_2$D. Vitamin D3 (cholecalciferol) is found in animal sources, while vitamin D2 (ergocalciferol) is found in plant sources. Vitamin D2 closely resembles vitamin D3, except that it bears an extra methyl group.

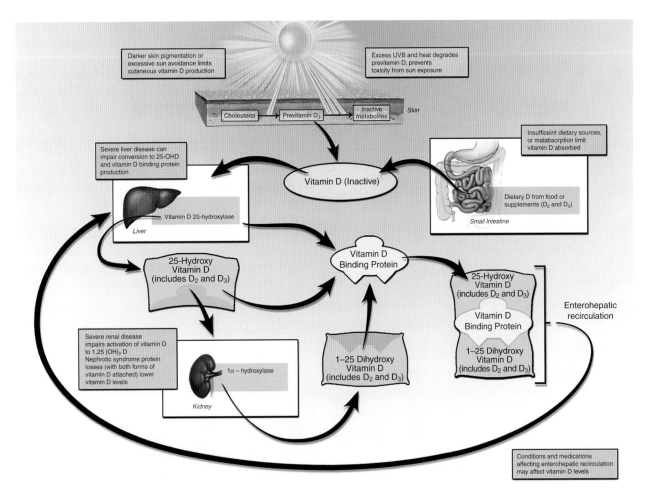

Fig. 32.9 Circulating vitamin D-binding protein draws vitamin D from the skin into the bloodstream. (From Hines SL, Jorn HKS, Thompson KM, et al. Breast cancer survivors and vitamin D: A review. *Nutrition.* 2010;26(3):255-262; Fig. 1.)

- Specifically, this hydroxylation occurs in the proximal convoluted tubule, where 25(OH)D is filtered, reabsorbed, then transformed into 1,25(OH)$_2$D.

This is the rate-limiting step in the metabolism of vitamin D and is the enzymatic step that is under the tightest regulation.

The Regulation of 1,25(OH)$_2$D Production

There are several regulators of 1,25(OH)$_2$D synthesis.
- Positive
  - PTH is the principal determinant.
  - Increases in PTH increase the conversion of 25(OH)D to 1,25(OH)$_2$D by increasing the synthesis of 25(OH)D-1 α-hydroxylase.
  - Hypocalcemia and hypophosphatemia increase 1,25(OH)$_2$D production.
  - Hormonal influences, such as estrogen, prolactin, and growth hormone, also stimulate 25(OH)D-1α-hydroxylase activity, thereby increasing levels of calcium during pregnancy, lactation, and growth.
- Negative
  - Hypercalcemia and hyperphosphatemia inhibit 25(OH)$_2$D production.

TABLE 32.3 The Regulation of 25(OH)D-1α-Hydroxylase	
↑ **Activity**	↓ **Activity**
PTH	1,25(OH)$_2$D (negative feedback)
↓ [Ca^{2+}]	↑ [Ca^{2+}]
↓ [Pi]	↑ [Pi]
Estrogen	
Prolactin	
Growth hormone	

Pi, Phosphate; *PTH,* parathyroid hormone.

- 1,25(OH)$_2$D participates in negative-feedback regulation by inhibiting the transcription of the 25(OH)D-1α-hydroxylase gene.

Table 32.3 summarizes the regulation of 25(OH)D-1α-hydroxylase.

The Mechanism of Vitamin D Action

The mechanism of action of vitamin D is similar to other steroid hormones, such as estrogen and glucocorticoids (Fig. 32.10).

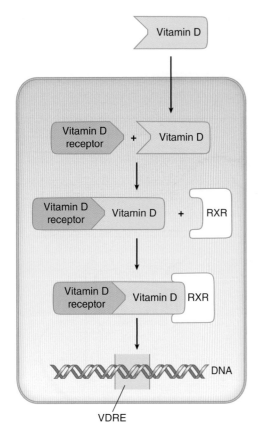

Fig. 32.10 A proposed general mechanism of action of vitamin D (1,25(OH)$_2$D). Free vitamin D enters the cell and binds to the vitamin D receptor (*VDR*). The vitamin D-VDR complex then interacts with the retinoic acid X receptor (*RXR*) to form a heterodimer, which in turn binds to vitamin D response elements (*VDREs*). This binding enhances or inhibits the transcription of the target genes of vitamin D.

- Vitamin D diffuses across cell membranes of its target tissues and forms complexes with specific intracellular receptors.
- The 1,25(OH)$_2$D first binds to the vitamin D receptor (VDR), a member of the nuclear hormone receptor superfamily.
- The 1,25(OH)$_2$D-VDR complex then interacts with the retinoic acid X receptor (RXR) to form a heterodimeric complex, which acts as a transcription factor on specific deoxyribonucleic acid (DNA) sequences.
- These DNA sequences are known as vitamin D response elements (VDREs).
- The interactions between the VDR complex and DNA's VDREs enhances or inhibits the transcription of various genes.

Actions of Vitamin D

In the intestinal tract, vitamin D plays a crucial role by increasing the absorption of calcium and phosphate (Fig. 32.11). Despite its array of effects on bone, the primary role of vitamin D in skeletal physiology is to maintain appropriate concentrations of calcium and phosphate through its effects on intestinal absorption.

- Calcium
  - Most of the active absorption of calcium takes place in the duodenum, while passive transport occurs throughout the rest of the small intestine.
  - Vitamin D increases the efficiency of calcium absorption from 10% to 70%.

Stimulates transcription of multiple proteins, including calbindin and calcium pumps. This occurs over a period of hours.

Directly opens calcium channels in the cell membrane, a phenomenon known as transcaltachia. This occurs over a period of seconds to minutes.
- Phosphorus
  - Active absorption of phosphate occurs primarily in the jejunum.

In bone, vitamin D enhances mobilization of skeletal calcium stores through its effects on osteoblasts and ultimately osteoclasts.
- Osteoblasts
  - Principal target of 1,25(OH)$_2$D.
  - Stimulated to produce cytokines that accelerate maturation of osteoclasts from their precursor and enhance activity.
  - Upregulates a variety of proteins involved in matrix formation, including alkaline phosphatase, osteocalcin, and osteopontin.
- Osteoclasts
  - Increase serum calcium.
  - Facilitate the bone remodeling process.

In the parathyroid gland, vitamin D inhibits the transcription of PTH, completing the feedback loop between PTH and vitamin D. This effect is mediated through a VDRE in the parathyroid chief cells.

Table 32.4 summarizes the actions of vitamin D.

The Biodegradation of Vitamin D

When calcium levels are sufficient, there is no longer a need for 1,25(OH)$_2$D. In response, 25(OH)D may be diverted away from 1,25(OH)$_2$D production in the kidney and metabolized by a series of steps into the water-soluble product calcitroic acid.
- 25(OH)D is deactivated to 24,25(OH)$_2$D through a 24-hydroxylation in the kidney by 25(OH)D-24-hydroxylase.
- 25(OH)D-24-hydroxylase is regulated by 1,25(OH)$_2$D and PTH.
  - 1,25(OH)$_2$D stimulates this enzyme (negative feedback loop).
  - PTH inhibits 25(OH)D-24-hydroxylase.

Other Actions of Vitamin D

Vitamin D has several functions unrelated to its role in calcium homeostasis, with receptors in many "nonclassical" organs that mediate unknown effects. These include:
- Dermatologic
  - Inhibits the proliferation of keratinocytes and fibroblasts.
  - Inhibits the differentiation of keratinocytes.
- Immunologic
  - Inhibits the production of IL-2 by activated T lymphocytes (see Clinical Correlation Box 32.5)

Clinical Correlation Box 32.5

The antiproliferative effects of vitamin D can be used to treat psoriasis, a disorder where there is hyperproliferation of keratinocytes. Calcipotriene, an analog of vitamin D, is used for this purpose.

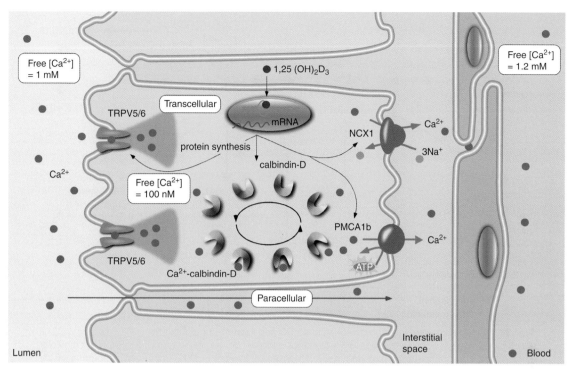

Fig. 32.11 A proposed mechanism of action of vitamin D (1,25(OH)₂D) on the intestine. Vitamin D, through a series of interactions with the vitamin D receptor (VDR), drives the transcription of a variety of genes, including calbindin. Calbindin is a calcium-binding protein believed to transport calcium through the cell. The model depicted here has been proposed to operate in both intestinal and renal epithelial cells. *ATP*, Adenosine triphosphate; *mRNA*, messenger ribonucleic acid; *NCX1*, sodium/calcium exchanger 1; *PMCA*, plasma membrane calcium ATPase; *TRPV*, transient receptor potential vanilloid. (From Dempster D, Marcus R, Cauley J, Feldman D. *Osteoporosis*, 4th Edition. Elsevier; 2013. Fig. 13.7.)

TABLE 32.4 Action of 1,25(OH)₂D (Active Vitamin D)
↑ Intestinal absorption of calcium
↑ Intestinal absorption of phosphate
↑ Osteoclast maturation (via osteoblasts)
↓ PTH synthesis (feedback inhibition)
↑ Synthesis of vitamin D-24-hydroxylase (deactivator of vitamin D metabolites) (feedback inhibition

PTH, Parathyroid hormone.

Nutritional Requirements for Vitamin D

The exact recommended daily allowance for vitamin D depends on age and physiology:

- Adults: 200 IU (international units).
- Infants, children, and pregnant and lactating women: 400 IU.

In general, these demands are met by endogenous synthesis from casual exposure to UV radiation. For example, a whole-body dose of sunlight that produces minimal erythema in Caucasians generates an equivalent oral dose of 10,000 to 25,000 IU. However, the generation of vitamin D depends on a range of factors that affect the intensity of UV radiation, including:

- Environmental: Altitude, geographic location, time of day.
- Individual: Amount of skin exposed, skin pigmentation, age (see Fast Fact Box 32.4).

Fast Fact Box 32.4

In higher latitudes, such as Boston (42°N), there is insufficient ultraviolet radiation to synthesize vitamin D between the months of November and February. During the spring, summer, and fall months in Boston, 5 to 15 minutes of sunlight exposure is all that is necessary to meet daily requirements.

It is not possible to overdose on vitamin D via sun exposure because precholecalciferol is photolyzed into the biologically inert isomer lumisterol (Fig. 32.12).

Dietary fortification of vitamin D also helps prevent against vitamin D deficiency. In the United States, milk has been fortified with vitamin D since the 1930s and contains roughly 400 IU per quart.

Calcitonin

Calcitonin is a 32-amino-acid peptide that reduces serum calcium and phosphate concentrations.

- Calcitonin is secreted by the parafollicular C cells, neural crest derivatives that make up 0.1% of the mass of the thyroid.
- The C cell shares the same calcium-sensing receptor as the parathyroid.
- Increasing calcium levels stimulates secretion of calcitonin by C cells.

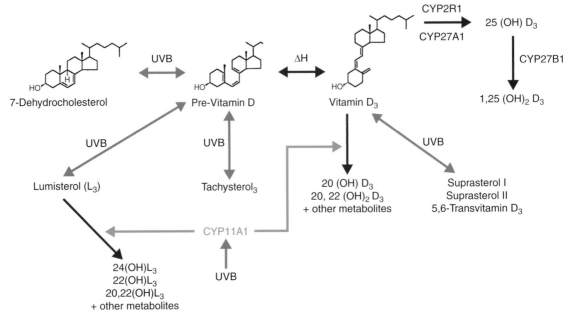

Fig. 32.12 Production and metabolism of vitamin D3 and related compounds in skin. Previtamin D3 is synthesized when the B-ring of 7-dehydrocholesterol is broken on the absorption of a photon of ultraviolet B (*UVB*). At body temperature, previtamin D3 is converted to vitamin D3 . Continued absorption of UV photons by previtamin D or vitamin D3 results in conversion to overirradiation products, such as lumisterol3, tachysterol3, or suprasterols, or 5, 6transvitamin D3. Vitamin D3 is converted in skin to 25-hydroxyvitamin D3 by CYP2R1 (or possibly CYP27A1) and then to 1, 25-dihydroxyvitamin D3 by CYP27B1. The cholesterol side chain cleavage enzyme CYP11A1 is also expressed in skin and upregulated by UV. It can convert vitamin D3 into 20-hydroxyvitamin D3 and at least 10 other products. CYP11A1 can also convert lumisterol3 into 24-hydroxylumisterol3 and several other lumisterol derivatives. (From Feldman D. *Vitamin D*, 4th Edition. *Volume 2: Health, Disease and Therapeutics*. Academic Press; 2018. Fig. 110.3.)

The effects of calcitonin on calcium and phosphate are mediated by osteoclasts and by proximal renal tubule cells, both of which express receptors for calcitonin.

- Inhibits osteoclasts, causing them to shrink and withdraw their bone-resorbing processes.
- Promotes the excretion of calcium, phosphate, sodium, potassium, and magnesium (see Clinical Correlation Box 32.6).

Clinical Correlation Box 32.6

Clinically, calcitonin is important as a marker for medullary thyroid cancer and as a therapeutic agent.
- Increased calcitonin secretion in medullary thyroid cancer can be provoked with calcium or pentagastrin infusions.
- Calcitonin is useful for treating metabolic bone conditions, such as Paget disease and osteoporosis, and also for treating hypercalcemia secondary to malignancy.

However, the physiologic role of calcitonin in humans is not completely clear given the following observations:

- Calcitonin deficiency secondary to thyroidectomy (and hence removal of the C cells) has no effect on calcium or bone metabolism.
- Excess levels of calcitonin, as in medullary thyroid carcinoma, have little if any effect on calcium homeostasis.

PATHOPHYSIOLOGY

Typically, PTH and vitamin D maintain serum calcium levels within normal limits. However, derangements in these regulatory systems can lead to hypercalcemic (excessive calcium) or hypocalcemic (insufficient calcium) states.

Hypercalcemia

The vast majority of cases of hypercalcemia are caused by hyperparathyroidism or malignancy. The mechanisms of hypercalcemia reflect pathology in the body's inputs and outputs of calcium:

- Increased bone resorption (most common mechanism)
- Increased gastrointestinal absorption
- Decreased renal excretion

Symptoms of Hypercalcemia

Normally, calcium and phosphate circulate at concentrations close to their saturation point.

- Above 10.0 mg/dL: Signs and symptoms of hypercalcemia begin to appear.
- Above 13 mg/dL: Calcifications begin to develop at multiple sites.
- Above 15 mg/dL: Medical emergency; coma and cardiac arrest may occur.

Recall that calcium concentrations are tightly maintained inside the cell to generate a steep gradient from out to in (extracellular concentrations are in millimolar quantities, intracellular in nanomolar), so that it has a significant depolarizing potential when it enters. Paradoxically, hypercalcemia actually leads to systemic depression (weakness, reduced muscle reflexes, and fatigue) rather than hyperexcitability.

- Excessive extracellular calcium → inhibition of voltage-gated calcium channels → diminished calcium entry → reduced intracellular calcium → hyperpolarization.

Hypercalcemia negatively affects several different organ systems:

- Cardiovascular
  - Positive inotropic effect
  - Altered conduction
    Shortened QT interval
    Widened T waves
  - Hypertension caused by systemic vasoconstriction
- Musculoskeletal
  - Bony pain (if cause of hypercalcemia is increased bony resorption)
- Neurologic
  - Fatigue
  - Depression
  - Confusion
- Gastrointestinal (inhibitory effect of calcium on smooth muscle contraction)
  - Nausea
  - Vomiting
  - Constipation
- Urologic
  - Polyuria (interferes with antidiuretic hormone on distal convoluted tubule)
  - Kidney stones (excessive calcium precipitation) (see Fast Fact Box 32.5)

Fast Fact Box 32.5

The mnemonic "stones, bones, groans, and moans" reviews the symptoms of hypercalcemia. "Stones" refers to kidney stones; "bones" to signs and symptoms of bone resorption seen in hyperparathyroidism, "groans" to a wide variety of gastrointestinal complaints and maladies, and "moans" to an array of mental symptoms, from lethargy to behavioral changes.

Causes of Hypercalcemia

Causes of hypercalcemia include:

- Primary hyperparathyroidism
- Malignancy
- Sarcoidosis

Primary hyperparathyroidism (PHP) occurs when there is excessive secretion of PTH. Of note, it is now often diagnosed in early stages because of the routine assessment of serum calcium levels in the clinical setting.

- Epidemiology
  - 80% of cases: PHP is caused by a single parathyroid adenoma, or focal expansion from a single abnormal cell.
  - 15% of cases: Primary hyperplasia of the whole parathyroid gland.
  - 1% to 2% of cases: Parathyroid carcinoma.
- Presentation
  - Some 80% of cases: Asymptomatic or minimally symptomatic because of early diagnosis.
  - Some 20% of cases: Signs and symptoms of hypercalcemia and hypercalciuria (as earlier).
    Less than 10% of cases: Skeletal manifestations, such as *osteitis fibrosa cystica*.
    PTH increases number and activity of osteoclasts.
    Characteristic subperiosteal resorption of cortical bone, bone cysts, and a "salt-and-pepper" appearance of the skull.
- Treatment
  - Surgical, with resection of the tumor or some of the enlarged parathyroid glands.
  - Curative in over 90% of cases (see Clinical Correlation Box 32.7).

Clinical Correlation Box 32.7

In a minority of cases or primary hyperparathyroidism, the underlying cause is resulting from multiple endocrine neoplasia (MEN) syndrome. The types of MEN syndrome that can lead to parathyroid tumors include:

- MEN type 1 (caused by a mutation in the gene *MEN1*)
- MEN type 2a (caused by a mutation in the gene *RET*)

In addition to causing tumors in the parathyroid glands, leading to overproduction and secretion of parathyroid hormone (PTH), these syndromes can result in tumors of the pituitary gland and pancreas in MEN type I, and medullary thyroid carcinoma and pheochromocytoma in MEN type 2a.

Malignancy is the most common cause of hypercalcemia in hospitalized patients, with an incidence of 15 in 100,000 per year.

- Lung cancer, breast cancer, and multiple myeloma account for over 50% of these cases.
- Mechanisms of hypercalcemia of malignancy include:
  - Secretion of PTHrP
  - Direct bone resorption by lytic metastases
  - Release of other tumor factors that predispose to hypercalcemia

Sarcoidosis is a rare but intriguing disorder characterized by chronic, multisystem granuloma formation. Hypercalcemia is seen in 10% of cases of sarcoidosis.

- This is caused by the presence of $25(OH)D\text{-}1\alpha$-hydroxylase activity in macrophages from sarcoid tissue.
- The same mechanism can give rise to hypercalcemia in other granulomatous disorders, including tuberculosis, berylliosis, coccidioidomycosis, histoplasmosis, and leprosy.

Hypocalcemia

Conversely, hypocalcemia generally occurs when the decrease in calcium levels overwhelms the body's homeostatic mechanisms. This is rare because the bone serves as a large reserve of calcium that can readily be liberated into the blood when needed. However, under certain circumstances, PTH and/or $1,25(OH)_2D$ fail to boost the calcium level adequately in the

face of low plasma calcium. The mechanisms of hypocalcemia reflect this:
- Failure of PTH or vitamin D production.
- Resistance to the actions of PTH or vitamin D.
- Precipitous drop in calcium levels.
    - May occur if phosphate levels rise (e.g., in a crush injury), causing precipitation of calcium phosphate.

Symptoms

As with hypercalcemia, there is a paradoxical effect on cellular excitability in the presence of hypocalcemia.
- Low extracellular calcium levels → disinhibition of voltage-gated calcium channels → increased calcium entry → increased intracellular calcium → depolarization.

Accordingly, most of the signs and symptoms of hypocalcemia revolve around increased neuromuscular excitability or irritability.
- Hyperreflexia
- Numbness and tingling around the fingertips, toes, and circumoral region
- Tetany
    - Carpopedal spasm (*main d'acchoucheur*) (Fig. 32.13)
    Flexion of the wrist and metacarpophalangeal joints, extension of the interphalangeal joints, and adduction of the thumb.
    - Laryngospasm (may be life-threatening because of airway obstruction)
- Seizures

Chvostek's and Trousseau's signs are classic indicators of hypocalcemia that reflect increased neuromuscular excitability.
- Chvostek's sign can be elicited by tapping the facial nerve just anterior to the ear and looking for facial muscle contractions (Fig. 32.14).
    - About 10% of people have a positive Chvostek's sign but are otherwise normocalcemic.

- Trousseau's sign is positive when there is carpopedal spasm following the inflation of a blood pressure cuff to 20 mm Hg above systolic pressure for 3 minutes (Fig. 32.15).
    - Ischemia unmasks the heightened excitability of the nerves.
    - Trousseau's sign is more specific than Chvostek's sign, with only 1% to 4% of normal subjects having a positive Trousseau's sign.

In addition, electrocardiogram will show prolonged QT interval because of delayed repolarization.

Causes

Hypocalcemia is associated with several key disorders that may be distinguished based on laboratory results, including:
- Hypoparathyroidism
- Pseudohypoparathyrodism
- Vitamin D deficiency

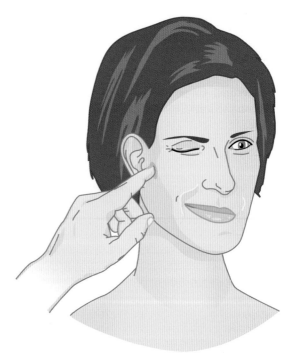

Fig. 32.14 Eliciting Chvostek's sign with a finger tap to the facial nerve, anterior to the ear. (From Carlson K. *AACN Advanced Critical Care* Nursing. Philadelphia, PA: Elsevier; 2009: p. 841-864; Fig. 1.)

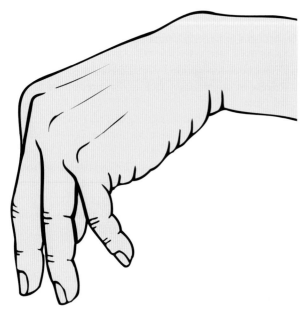

Fig. 32.13 The main d'accoucheur posture of the hand. This posture is seen in the carpal spasm caused by hypocalcemia. (From Murphy M, Srivastava R, Deans K. *Clinical Biochemistry: An Illustrated Colour Text*, 6th Edition. Elsevier; 2019: p. 70-71; Fig. 35.5.)

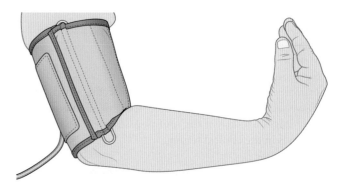

Fig. 32.15 Eliciting Trousseau's sign with an inflation of a blood pressure cuff. (From Innes JA, Dover AR, Fairhurst K. *Macleod's Clinical Examination*. Elsevier; 2018: p. 193-209; Fig. 10.7.)

Hypoparathyroidism is most often caused by inadvertent excision of the parathyroid glands during neck surgery. More rarely, it may be caused by autoimmune disease or congenital absence of the thymus and parathyroid glands (DiGeorge syndrome).
- Insufficient release of PTH
- Characteristic findings include:
  - Hypocalcemia
  - Hyperphosphatemia
  - Normal magnesium level
  - Normal renal function

Pseudohypoparathyroidism is a genetic condition leading to resistance to PTH signaling, rather than absence of PTH release. There are two types of pseudohypoparathyroidism.
- Type 1B is a disorder characterized by resistance only to PTH.
  - Hypocalcemia
  - Hyperphosphatemia
  - Secondary hyperparathyroidism (increased PTH secondary to PTH resistance)
- Type IA features the symptoms found in IB, as well as a distinct phenotype known as Albright hereditary osteodystrophy.
  - Short stature and neck
  - Round face
  - Brachydactyly (especially in the fourth and fifth metacarpal bones)
  - Subcutaneous ossifications
  - Reproductive abnormalities secondary to hypothyroidism

Vitamin D deficiency results in two well-known conditions, osteomalacia and rickets.
- Osteomalacia is a defect in mineralization of the bone matrix or osteoid deposited during normal bone remodeling.
- Rickets is characterized by osteomalacia and inadequate mineralization of the epiphyseal cartilage or growth plate in growing skeleton. Therefore rickets by definition occurs only in children (see Fast Fact Box 32.6).

Fact Fact Box 32.6

In osteoporosis, there is a loss of bone mass overall with a normal mineral-to-collagen ratio, while in osteomalacia, there is a decreased mineral-to-collagen ratio from poor bone mineralization.

Vitamin D deficiency has a variety of etiologies, including:
- Nutritional deficiency (rare in the United States because of dietary fortification).
- Inadequate endogenous production of vitamin D.
- Increased catabolism of vitamin D (as may occur with stimulation of hepatic enzymes by anticonvulsants),

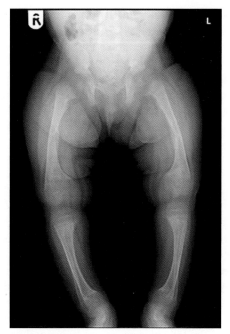

Fig. 32.16 An x-ray of a 2-year-old child with rickets showing the characteristic bowing of the long bones of the leg. (From Jacobs B. Toe walking, flat feet and bow legs, in-toeing and out-toeing. *Paediatr Child Health.* 2010;20(5):221-224.)

- Malabsorption of vitamin D (as in gastrointestinal disorders).
- Defective activation of vitamin D (as in renal disease).
- Resistance to vitamin D (as in genetic disorders).

In both osteomalacia and rickets, insufficient vitamin D levels result in decreased intestinal absorption of calcium and phosphate. Although severe hypocalcemia develops only late in the course of vitamin D deficiency, a suboptimal supply of calcium and phosphate hinders proper bone mineralization. In fact, increases in PTH compensate for deficient calcium absorption by increasing bone resorption with consequent phosphaturia and phosphate losses.

Rickets produces multiple characteristic skeletal findings, reflecting its effects on an active growth plate (Fig. 32.16). These findings include:
- Growth failure
- Pigeon-breast deformity of the sternum
- Bowing of the long bones
- Increased frequency of fractures and diffuse bone pain

Osteomalacia, on the other hand, does not result in prominent skeletal findings; rather, osteomalacia may present as:
- Diffuse skeletal pain
- Bony tenderness
- Proximal muscle weakness
- Fractures from minimal trauma

SUMMARY

- The skeleton is the primary reservoir of calcium in the body.
- PTH and vitamin D are the primary hormones involved in calcium regulation.
- PTH raises calcium levels by: (1) increasing bone resorption, (2) increasing renal reabsorption of calcium at the distal tubule, and (3) increased renal conversion of 25(OH)D to its active metabolite, 1,25(OH)$_2$D.
- Vitamin D raises calcium levels by increasing the intestinal absorption of calcium and increasing the production of osteoclasts.

- Phosphate levels are regulated primarily at the kidney by PTH, wherein increasing PTH decreases plasma phosphate concentrations by promoting phosphate wasting in the urine.
- The net effect of PTH is to restore calcium levels without excessively increasing phosphate levels, which would lead to precipitation of calcium phosphate.
- Vitamin D plays a central role in restoring phosphate levels in extracellular fluid. Hypophosphatemia stimulates renal production of $1,25(OH)_2D$, which in turn increases intestinal absorption of phosphate. Moreover, $1,25(OH)_2D$ inhibits the synthesis of PTH, thereby reducing the renal phosphate excretion mediated by PTH.
- Hypercalcemia (excessive calcium) is most often caused by primary hyperparathyroidism, malignancy, sarcoidosis, and other granulomatous disorders.
- Hypocalcemia (insufficient calcium) is most often caused by primary hypoparathyroidism, pseudohypoparathyroidism, and vitamin D deficiency.

REVIEW QUESTIONS

Directions: Each of the numbered items or incomplete statements in this section is followed by answers or by completions of the statement. Select the one lettered answer or completion that is best in each case.

1. An 11-year-old boy with a history of epilepsy, short stature, and bone deformities is discovered to have low levels of vitamin D as a chronic side effect of his seizure medication. Which of the following responses to hypocalcemia is most significantly impaired in this child?
   A. Increased bone resorption
   B. Increased hydroxylation of inactive vitamin D by the kidney
   C. Increased reabsorption of Ca^{2+} by the proximal tubule in the kidney
   D. Increased secretion of PTH
   E. Increased intestinal absorption of dietary Ca^{2+}

2. A 55-year-old man is diagnosed with sarcoidosis and hypercalcemia. If macrophages are secreting vitamin D-25-hydroxylase, thereby increasing the conversion of vitamin D to its major circulating (and still inactive) form, the macrophages are mimicking a physiologic function of which other tissue?
   A. Skin
   B. Liver
   C. Kidney
   D. Bone
   E. Parathyroid
   F. Intestine

3. After suffering from a kidney stone, a man is diagnosed with hypercalcemia because of primary hyperparathyroidism, which has increased the levels of PTH in his plasma. The PTH is creating hypercalcemia by acting at receptors on which cells?
   A. Chief cells in the parathyroid gland
   B. Osteoclasts in bone
   C. Osteoblasts in bone
   D. Duodenal cells in the gut
   E. Parafollicular C cells in the thyroid gland

ANSWERS TO REVIEW QUESTIONS

1. **The answer is E.** Vitamin D alone promotes increased intestinal absorption of Ca^{2+}, so a deficiency in vitamin D is likely to impair intestinal absorption. Although vitamin D does also promote bone resorption to liberate Ca^{2+} from bone, PTH is the more significant mediator of bone resorption, so bone resorption would not be affected to the same extent as intestinal absorption. The ability of the parathyroid to secrete PTH is normal in this child and so are PTH actions, including bone resorption, increased renal hydroxylation (and activation) of inactive vitamin D, and increased renal Ca^{2+} reabsorption.

2. **The answer is B.** Inactive vitamin D is newly synthesized in the skin or absorbed in the intestine, converted to its major circulating form by vitamin D-25-hydroxylase in the liver, and converted to its active form in the kidney.

3. **The answer is C.** PTH promotes the liberation of Ca^{2+} from bone by acting on the PTH receptor in osteoblasts, which in turn augment the activity of osteoclasts through cytokines. The osteoclasts promote bone resorption and the release of Ca^{2+}. The chief cells of the parathyroid produce PTH. Although negative feedback loops do affect the chief cells, the negative feedback is mediated through vitamin D influence on the cells and not PTH directly. Vitamin D, not PTH, acts on the duodenal cells of the intestine to promote Ca^{2+} absorption. The parafollicular C cells in the thyroid produce calcitonin in response to high levels of serum Ca^{2+}.

33

Calcium Regulation: Bone Physiology

INTRODUCTION

The word skeleton comes from the Greek skellein, meaning to dry up; a dried-up body (skeleton soma) is one with only the bones remaining. Thus etymologically, but also in our cultural imagination, our bones refer to death. However, the skeleton is, like any other organ system, a system dedicated entirely to the functions of life.

The human skeleton is made not only of minerals, but also of blood, proteins, and living cells. The skeletal system's diverse functions include:
- Mineral homeostasis
- Hematopoiesis
- Mechanical support for movement
- Protection
- Determination of body size and shape
    In this chapter, we will explore how the skeleton as an organ interacts with the body, focusing on:
- Anatomy and composition of bones
- Bone resorption and deposition
- Types of fractures and healing process
- Diseases affecting the skeletal system

SYSTEM STRUCTURE

Like many organs, bone is composed of living cells and an acellular matrix. Bone is dominated by its extracellular matrix, with cells making up just a tiny percentage of the total weight. Like most extracellular matrices, the acellular matrix of bone contains polysaccharide chains called glycosaminoglycans.
- These anionic chains bind water and repel one another, creating a viscous but fluid ground substance.
- Bone is also a unique tissue in that its ground substance contains not only protein, but also a heavy proportion of inorganic minerals (Fig. 33.1).

The Acellular Elements
Collagen and Hydroxyapatite
The acellular portion of bone is primarily composed of collagen fibers and calcium phosphate crystals. In some ways, this can be compared with reinforced concrete: the collagen is analogous to the steel rods, and the calcium phosphate crystals are compared with the cement.

The calcium phosphate crystals found on and within the collagen fibers are called hydroxyapatite.
- The chemical formula for hydroxyapatite is $Ca_{10}(PO_4)_6(OH)_2$.
- These crystals are oriented preferentially along the long axis of the collagen fibers.

The collagen fibers in the bone matrix are composed of subunits called tropocollagen.
- Each tropocollagen is a triple-helical supercoil of three polypeptide chains.
- The tropocollagens are cross-linked to one another within the collagen fiber at hydroxylysine and lysine residues (Fig. 33.2).
    - These cross links stabilize the fiber, increase its resistance to deformation, and render it completely insoluble.
    About 85% to 90% of the total protein found in bone consists of collagen. Most of the collagen in bone is type 1 collagen. Other types of collagen are infrequent contributors to bone.

Noncollagen Proteins
Noncollagen proteins (NCP) make up the majority of the remaining bone protein content. These proteins are largely serum-derived and bind to the mineral component of bone. They can be classified into four groups that are somewhat overlapping:
1. Proteoglycans
2. Cell attachment proteins
3. γ-carboxylated proteins
4. Growth factors
    When glycosaminoglycans are rooted to a protein backbone, as is the case in bone matrix, they are called proteoglycans.
- Primarily function to fix hydroxyapatite crystal to the collagen fibers.
- Poorly defined role in promoting and inhibiting mineralization.
    - Intact proteoglycans in high concentrations may inhibit calcification.
    - Partially degraded or sparse proteoglycans may allow calcification to proceed.
    Cell attachment proteins anchor osteoblasts and other bone cells to the bone matrix. Four proteins are recognized as having an integral role in cell attachment:
- Fibronectin
- Thrombospondin
- Osteopontin
- Bone sialoprotein
    The exact physiologic role of the γ-carboxylated proteins is unclear, but measurements of one, called osteocalcin, have proven valuable as markers of bone turnover. Growth factors will be discussed later.

Suspended in the bone matrix, the polypeptide growth factors influence the growth, development, and repair of bone. These factors have various effects on bone and cartilage growth in the fetus and during postnatal life, stimulating the proliferation of osteoblasts and chondroblasts and the proliferation and

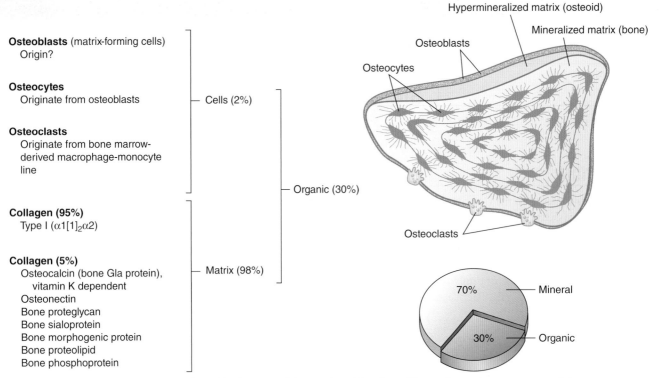

Fig. 33.1 Bone is dominated by its extracellular matrix, with cells making up just a tiny percentage of the total weight.

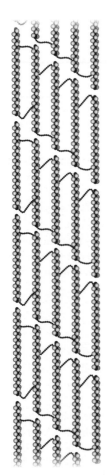

Fig. 33.2 The structure of a collagen fiber.

differentiation of progenitor cells in bone and cartilage cell lines. All of the following factors are produced by osteoblasts and elsewhere in the body and are found in the serum:

- Bone morphogenetic proteins (BMP)
  - Important in early skeletal formation in the embryo.
- Platelet-derived growth factor (PDGF)
  - Promotes chemotaxis in osteoblasts.
- Insulin-like growth factor (IGF)
  - Important in long bone growth.
- Fibroblast growth factor (FGF)
  - May be particularly important in repairing bone injuries.
- Transforming growth factor β (TGF-β)
  - Regulates bone remodeling and enhances osteoblast activity.

Cartilage Versus Bone

Cartilage is another form of extracellular matrix found in the body, composed of proteoglycans and either collagen or elastin.

- Covers the ends of bones inside joints, and is found in the trachea, the tip of the nose, and many other areas of the human body.
- Serves a precursor to bone in the context of fetal development and bone growth before adulthood.
- When cartilage is mineralized (laden with hydroxyapatite) and converted to bone, it has undergone ossification (from the Latin os, meaning bone).

The Cellular Elements

Although bone is mostly mineral, it is anything but fixed and static. Even after an individual has reached maturity, bone remains dynamic, as it is constantly remodeled (destroyed and rebuilt) by cells within the matrix. There are three primary cell types:

1. Osteoblasts
2. Osteocytes
3. Osteoclasts

In addition, the ends of many bones have a cartilage cap, produced by cells called chondroblasts.

Osteoblasts are present at sites of bone formation called remodeling sites. They function to actively produce the protein component of the acellular matrix and regulate bone growth and degradation.

- Extensive rough endoplasmic reticulum and Golgi apparatus equip osteoblasts for abundant protein production.
- Embryologically, they are derived from condensing mesenchyme.

Osteocytes are quiescent osteoblasts suspended in the bone matrix. Approximately 15% of osteoblasts become osteocytes.

- When an osteoblast becomes totally encased in the calcified matrix, its metabolic activity decreases considerably.
- Gas and nutrients are in limited supply, arriving via very small channels called canaliculi.
  - Canaliculi are formed around cytoplasmic processes that extend from the osteoblast during mineralization.
- The processes of many osteocytes are linked via gap junctions, allowing communication and material transfer between cells.
- The osteocytes are eventually phagocytized by osteoclasts during bone resorption.

Osteoclasts are unique and highly specialized cells, present on all bone surfaces and especially at sites of actively remodeling bone. These large, multinucleated cells (10–20 nuclei each) have many primary lysosomes and numerous mitochondria.

- Osteoclasts arise from the hematopoietic cell line in bone marrow.
- Their mononuclear precursors leave the marrow and circulate in the blood. At endosteal (i.e., inner bone) surfaces, they marginate, proliferate, and fuse, forming a ruffled border for bone resorption.
- This border is in fact an extracellular lysosome, sealed off by integrins that bind the osteoclast to the bone surface.

Patterns of Bone Composition

Osteoblasts deposit bone in two distinct patterns, lamellar and woven.

- Woven bone is formed when the osteoblasts deposit the collagen fibers randomly, "weaving" the collagen in a loosely organized pattern.
  - Woven bone is normally present in the fetal skeleton and growth plates.
  - It is produced quickly and has excellent strength in all directions.
  - In an adult its presence always signifies pathology. It is formed at fracture sites, areas of infection, and tumors.
- Lamellar bone, which is deposited more slowly and is stronger, typically replaces woven bone in normal development.
  - Lamellar bone forms the characteristic Haversian systems, with concentric lamellae surrounding a central vascular bundle (Fig. 33.3).

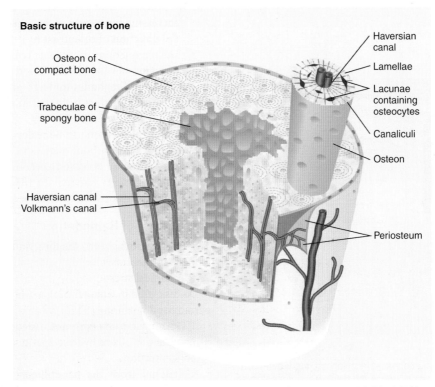

Basic structure of bone

Osteon of compact bone

Trabeculae of spongy bone

Haversian canal
Volkmann's canal

Haversian canal
Lamellae
Lacunae containing osteocytes
Canaliculi
Osteon
Periosteum

Fig. 33.3 Lamellar bone showing the Haversian system. (From Bayliss L, Mahoney DJ, Monk P. Normal bone physiology, remodelling and its hormonal regulation. *Surgery*. 2012;30(2):47-53. © 2011. Elsevier. Fig. 1.)

Lamellar bone may be further subdivided into two types:
- Cortical bone, the tissue at the outer periphery of bones
  - Also called compact bone.
  - 20× more dense than trabecular bone.
- Trabecular bone, the tissue inside of bones
  - Also called spongy bone or cancellous bone.
  - Composed of a porous network of bony arches called trabeculae (the word is Latin for "little beams").
  - Trabeculae are filled with bone marrow.
  The fibrous periosteum is the outer covering of bone.

The Anatomy of Bones

At the gross level, the skeleton is composed of two anatomically distinct types of bones:
- The flat bones of the skull, scapula, mandible, and pelvis.
- The long bones, such as the tibia, femur, and humerus.
  These two bone types are formed by two different kinds of ossification.
- Flat bones are created in the fetus by intramembranous ossification, in which membranes of mesenchymal connective tissue are ossified.
- Long bones result from endochondral ossification during fetal life, the ossification of mesenchyme that has first differentiated into discrete cartilaginous forms.
  Although short bones are more variable in shape, long bones have a characteristic structure (Fig. 33.4).
- The widened end of the bone is called the epiphysis.
  - Increased surface area distributes pressure and reduces stress exerted per area of bone by adjacent, articulating bone.

- Contain a larger proportion of trabecular bone, which makes epiphyses more malleable and better able to absorb stress.
- The long and thin shaft is called the diaphysis.
- The end of the shaft just before the epiphysis is called the metaphysis.
- In growing children, a cartilaginous growth plate divides the epiphysis from the metaphysis, sometimes referred to as the epiphyseal plate (Fig. 33.5).
  - This is an active site of bone deposition.
  - Once the epiphyseal plate is sealed, no more linear growth can occur.
- Arteries enter the bone through holes in the periosteum.
  The epiphyses of bones are capped with cartilage, which enables the formation of two distinct joint types:
- In cartilaginous joints, such as the costochondral joints that connect ribs to the sternum, the cartilage connects one epiphysis directly to another.
- In synovial joints, such as the knee, the cartilage forms a smooth surface for the articulation of two epiphyses.
  - In synovial joints, the space in which the two bones articulate is sealed in a fibrous capsule filled with lubricating synovial fluid.
  Muscles that attach to bones on either side of a joint can flex or extend the joint. Both muscles and ligaments stabilize joints.

SYSTEM FUNCTION

During adulthood, bone is always in a state of balance between simultaneous resorptive processes and depositional ones.
- Osteoclasts digest lacunae in bone and osteoblasts follow behind and fill them in with new bone.
- This process is called remodeling, or bone turnover.
  - Increasing bone mass means that remodeling is tipped in the direction of osteoblast function and bone deposition.
  - Decreasing bone means that remodeling has tipped in the direction of osteoclast function and resorption.
  Before adult life, bones undergo growth—a special form of bone deposition distinct from that in remodeling and driven in part by growth hormone.
- When osteoblasts conduct bone deposition as part of remodeling, they secrete the bone matrix directly onto preexisting bone.
- During growth, however, osteoblast activity is preceded by chondroblast activity. Cartilage is formed and then mineralized or ossified to become bone.

The Control of Remodeling

Two main factors govern the direction that remodeling favors:
1. Ca^{2+} homeostasis
2. Mechanical stress
   As discussed in Chapter 32, Ca^{2+} homeostasis is mediated by parathyroid hormone (PTH), vitamin D, and calcitonin.
- PTH and vitamin D promote osteoclastic bone resorption to liberate Ca^{2+} from hydroxyapatite and raise the serum Ca^{2+} concentration.
- Calcitonin from the parafollicular C cells of the thyroid inhibits bone resorption to suppress the serum Ca^{2+} concentration (see Fast Fact Box 33.1).

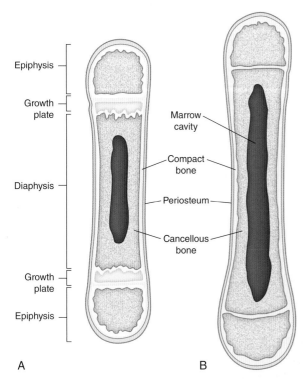

Fig. 33.4 The structure of long bones. A, In childhood, the growth plate consists of a cartilaginous band between the diaphysis and the epiphysis. B, When long bone growth is complete, the growth plate becomes completely ossified. This is sometimes called closure of the epiphyses.

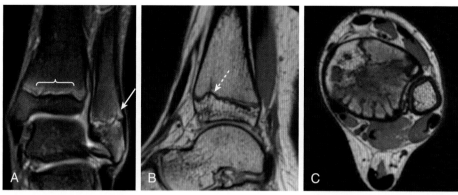

Fig. 33.5 A 12-year-old ballet dancer with normal distal tibial and fibular physis. Coronal proton density (PD) with fat suppression (A), sagittal PD (B), and axial PD (C) demonstrate the development of normal spiculations within the trilaminar physis indicating impending fusion (*curly braces*). Notice the normal laterally undulating distal fibular physis (*solid arrow*). Kump's bump (*dashed arrow*) anteriorly in the tibia reflects the location of earliest physiologic fusion. Axial image at the level of the fusing physis (C) reveals spoke wheel low signal spiculations radiating from the periphery. The physis has a heterogeneous signal intensity when viewed axially owing to its undulating orientation in the longitudinal axis. (From Ma CMY, Ecklund K. MR imaging of the pediatric foot and ankle: what does normal look like? *MRI Clin North Am.* 2017;25(1):27-43. © 2016. Fig. 3.)

Fast Fact 33.1

Several other endocrine axes have minor effects on bone remodeling as well. Glucocorticoids and thyroid hormone appear to promote resorption, while estrogen receptors in bone appear to mediate the inhibition of osteoclast activity.

By mechanisms that remain unclear, mechanical stress also governs the balance in bone remodeling between resorption and deposition (Fig. 33.6).

- Mechanical stress inhibits bone resorption and promotes bone deposition.

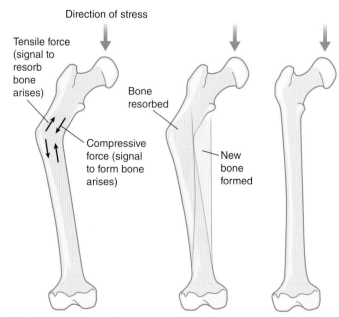

Fig. 33.6 Wolff's law. Bone is remodeled in accordance with planes of stress.

- The skeleton's outward appearance closely reflects the forces imposed upon it.
  - When bones chronically bear weight or muscles chronically exert force upon them, the bones' trabeculae become dense and prominent.
  - Bones protected from stress lose mass.
- Julius Wolff first proposed this attribute of the bones in 1892 and the orthopedic notion that "form follows function" is sometimes called Wolff's law (see Physiology Integration Box 33.1).

Physiology Integration Box 33.1

Recently, investigators have suggested that bones possess a "mechanostat" that can detect strain, compare it with a set point, and influence osteoblasts and osteoclasts in accordance with this afferent information. The specific character and location of such a mechanostat remain to be discovered, but Harold Frost speculates that signals associated with stress could include electric potentials or "fluid shear over cell membranes."

Because of Wolff's law, chronic bed rest or lack of exercise with muscle weakness can put elderly people at risk of osteopenia (decreased bone mass) and fractures. Similarly, astronauts who spend extended periods of time in space are threatened with osteopenia because the low gravity reduces the levels of mechanical stress on their bones and resorption becomes more active than deposition (see Clinical Correlation Box 33.1).

Clinical Correlation Box 33.1

Astronauts who stay weightless in orbit for extended periods of time will actually lose an average of 1% to 2% of their bone mass each month, as compared with a loss of 1% to 1.5% of bone loss in the elderly per year. This characteristic bone loss during spaceflight is known as spaceflight osteopenia. Current regimens attempting to combat spaceflight osteopenia include load bearing exercise regimens, as well as an increased dietary supplementation of vitamin D and calcium.

Finally, it should be noted that bone remodeling is to some extent a self-regulating phenomenon. As mentioned earlier, serum-derived growth factors are embedded in bone during deposition. When this bone is later resorbed, growth factors such as IGF-1, TGF-β, FGF, and PDGF are released. All these factors promote osteoblastic activity.

Bone Deposition in Remodeling

During remodeling, osteoblasts commence bone deposition by secreting a thick seam of type 1 collagen called the osteoid. Over the next 5 to 15 days, mineralization of the collagen fibers follows, also under the regulation of osteoblasts.

- The crystals formed are needle-like and lie alongside or penetrate the collagen fibers.
- The exact process whereby the osteoblasts control the precipitation of crystals is unclear. Under physiologic conditions, the extracellular fluid is supersaturated with hydroxyapatite, which should lead to uncontrolled crystal growth; however, the process is somehow well controlled by the osteoblasts

Bone Resorption in Remodeling

Osteoclasts are not activated directly, but rather indirectly via osteoblasts.

- Recall that only osteoblasts bear the receptor for PTH.
- Under PTH stimulation, osteoblasts signal to osteoclast precursors to stimulate their fusion, differentiation, and activation.

In addition to cytokines, such as interleukin (IL)-6, a receptor in the tumor necrosis factor receptor family, known as receptor activator of nuclear factor kappa B, or NF-κB (RANK), has been shown to be involved in the activation of osteoclasts and consequently bone resorption (see Fig. 32.5).

- RANK is expressed by preosteoclasts.
- RANK-ligand (RANKL) is expressed by osetoblasts and the lining cells of the bone under stimulation by PTH.

- The binding of RANKL to the osteoclast receptor RANK activates osteoclast differentiation and bone resorption.
- A free-floating decoy receptor known as osteoprotegerin (OPG) is also produced by osteoblasts and competes for RANKL, thus modulating bone resorption.
  - Estrogen increases OPG production and may prevent bone resorption by this mechanism.

Once encouraged by the osteoblasts, the osteoclasts resorb bone at the endosteal surfaces by forming extracellular lysosomes with integrin seals.

- Carbonic anhydrase generates protons, which are then extruded across the ruffled border via a variety of pumps, antiporters, and channels.
- Proteolytic enzymes are targeted to the area via mannose-6-phosphate receptors and are released via exocytosis.
- Osteoclastic resorption forms a small pit or lacuna in the bone, sometimes called Howship's lacuna.
- The osteoclast then moves on to a new area on the endosteal surface to start over.
- Meanwhile, bone resorption has released growth factors from the matrix that stimulate the osteoblasts.
- Once the osteoclasts vacate the lacuna, activated osteoblasts move in and begin to lay down osteoid to make new bone.

Together, these events constantly renew the bone matrix and are referred to as the activation-resorption-formation sequence (Fig. 33.7) (see Clinical Correlation Box 33.2).

Clinical Correlation Box 33.2

Paget disease is a disorder of bone remodeling, characterized by an increase in osteoclast-mediated bone resorption and a compensatory increase in new bone formation. This increase in both osteoclast and osteoblast activity results in a disordered mosaic of woven and lamellar bone. This bone is larger, less dense, has increased vascularity, and is more malleable and susceptible to fracture.

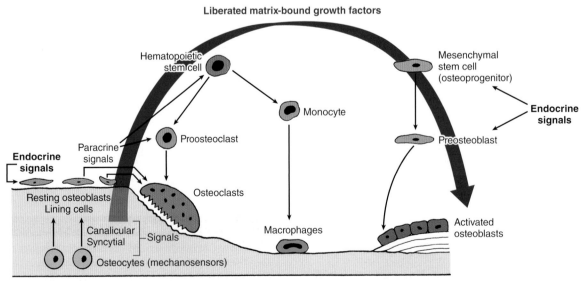

Fig. 33.7 The activation-resorption-formation sequence. Osteoblasts are activated by mechanical or hormonal signals to trigger osteoclastogenesis. Osteoclastic resorption liberates growth factors from the matrix, which stimulate osteoblastic deposition. (Modified from Levy MN, Koeppen BM, Stanton BA. *Berne and Levy Principles of Physiology*, 4th edition. Philadelphia: Elsevier; 2007. Fig. 44.1.)

Bone Deposition in Growth

As mentioned earlier, flat bones are created in the fetus by intramembranous ossification, whereas long bones are the product of endochondral ossification. In endochondral ossification, the bone is modeled in cartilage before ossification occurs (see Fact Fact Box 33.2).

Fast Fact 33.2

Muscular stress on bones may be important to the development of bones in utero as the fetus applies stress to immature bones by kicking and pushing against the uterine walls.

During childhood and adolescence, growth takes place in the long bones along the growth plate between the epiphysis and the metaphysis (see Fig. 33.4).
- The growth plate contains functional zones distributed from the epiphysis to the metaphysis.
  - The epiphysis contains quiescent chondrocytes.
  - The metaphysis contain active chondroblasts that are proliferating and laying down cartilage.
- Osteoblasts then mineralize this cartilage matrix, ossifying it and forming new trabeculae in the metaphysis.
- Orderly cartilage formation is necessary for orderly bone formation.

Growth hormone regulates the growth of bones indirectly by increasing the expression of IGF-1 by cells in the growth plate. IGF-1 then promotes chondroblast and osteoblast proliferation and enhances deposition of the bone matrix by osteoblasts. The exact mechanism of control over chondrocyte growth and differentiation is not completely clear.
- The fibroblast growth factor receptor 3 (FGFR3) appears to stop or slow the growth of chondrocytes in the proliferative zone of the plate.
- A second receptor active in the growth plate is the parathyroid hormone-related peptide (PTHrP) receptor. PTHrP receptors also appear to slow the rate of chondrocyte growth within the plate

PATHOPHYSIOLOGY

Any defect in the regulation or mechanism of bone remodeling may lead to abnormalities in the quality and quantity of bone tissue. This, in turn, may lead to deformities and fractures. Among the causes of skeletal deformity and injury are:
- Abnormal Ca^{2+} homeostasis
- Fracture because of trauma
- Osteoblast or osteoclast dysfunction

Abnormal Calcium Homeostasis

In vitamin D deficiency, poor intestinal Ca^{2+} absorption and hypocalcemia occur. The parathyroid glands secrete PTH to release Ca^{2+} from bone and raise the serum Ca^{2+} (which is critical for normal neuromuscular function).
- PTH activates osteoclasts, and bone resorption prevails over deposition.

- The increased osteoclastic activity results in demineralized and malleable bones.
- Histologically, there is excess unmineralized matrix and wide osteoid seams.

In growing children, the disease is called rickets, and the result is a weak skeleton and bones that deform under the strain of gravity or muscle tension. In adults, vitamin D deficiency with demineralization is called osteomalacia. Causes include malnourishment, inadequate sunlight exposure, and malabsorption.

Hyperparathyroidism is caused by the loss of normal negative-feedback control by high serum calcium.
- This leads to demineralization of bone as osteoclasts increase their activity.
- Although resorption occurs in excess as it does in osteomalacia, in hyperparathyroidism, the serum Ca^{2+} is elevated rather than depressed, leading to a different pattern of bone destruction.

Fractures

Three forces cause fractures (bone breakage):
1. Tension
2. Compression
3. Torsion

Tension stretches bone; compression compacts bone. Bending a bone causes the cortex on one side of the bone to experience tension, the other to be compressed, leading to breakage. Torsion causes part of a bone to rotate about its axis.

Fractures are classified by the bone involved, the anatomic location, and the pattern of the fracture fragments. Fracture patterns are sometimes classified as follows:
- Closed versus open. In an open fracture, the bony fragment penetrates the skin.
- Simple versus comminuted. A simple fracture has a single fracture line. In a comminuted fracture, more than two fragments are created.
- Extraarticular versus intraarticular. In an intraarticular fracture, the fracture line enters the joint cavity.
- Transverse, oblique, or spiral
  - If the fracture line is perpendicular to the long axis of the bone, the fracture is transverse. A direct blow to a bone frequently causes a transverse fracture.
  - If the fracture line is tilted up or down from the perpendicular line, it is called oblique.
  - Twisting or wrenching (torsion) of bone causes a spiral fracture, in which the break occurs along more than one plane. This is commonly seen in skiing injuries.
- Pathologic. A fracture is called pathologic if it occurs in bone that is weakened from an underlying disease.

Bone is unique in its ability to completely reconstitute itself by reactivating processes that normally occur only in embryogenesis—the construction of a cartilage precursor followed by woven bone.

The four stages of bone healing are:
1. Inflammation
2. Soft callus

3. Hard callus
4. Remodeling

The inflammatory phase begins immediately after injury and last for 7 days. During this time, a hematoma (blood clot) forms, filling gaps in the disrupted bone.

- The hematoma contains a fibrin meshwork that seals the site and forms a framework for incoming cells.
- Degranulating platelets at the site release PDGF, TGF-β, and FGF, which activates bone growth.
- The hematoma anchors the bone for healing purposes but provides no significant structural stability.

The proliferation of chondroblasts and the elaboration of cartilage marks the soft callus phase.

- Capillary buds invade, enabling more chondroblasts, osteoclasts, and osteoblasts to populate the callus.
- The callus can only bridge the fracture site under conditions of mechanical stability; that is, if the fractured bone is too mobile at the fracture site, a successful callus cannot form.
- This is the reason for splinting and casting fractures. In some cases, grafting of bone may be necessary to enable a callus to bridge the gap.

Once a soft callus is successfully formed, the callus is gradually calcified and infiltrated by woven bone and is called a hard callus. Finally, the woven bone is remodeled to lamellar bone.

Osteoblast and Osteoclast Dysfunction

The most common disorder occurring at the level of osteoblast and osteoclast function is osteoporosis, a reduction in overall bone mass (osteopenia) that occurs with aging. Because androgens and estrogens dampen osteoclastic activity, the postmenopausal reduction estrogen production puts postmenopausal women at particularly high risk for osteoporosis.

- In the absence of premenopausal estrogen levels, osteoblasts secrete more RANKL, IL-6, and other cytokines that stimulate osteoclastogenesis, leading to increased bone resorption and more brittle bones.
- Although the entire skeleton is involved, disease in the femoral neck and vertebrae tends to pose the most clinical problems.
- Osteopenia in these locations predisposes sufferers of osteoporosis to hip fractures and spinal compression fractures even without significant trauma.

Exercise, bisphosphonate therapy, and calcium supplementation are treatments for osteoporosis.

- Bisphosphonates (pyrophosphate analogues such as alendronate or risedronate) bind to hydroxyapatite in bone and inhibit osteoclast activity or increase osteoclast cell death, helping restore the balance between resorption and deposition.
- Other effective treatments have been developed for patients with severe osteoporosis. Denosumab, a human monoclonal antibody, binds to and inhibits osteoblast-produced RANKL, reducing the binding between RANKL and osteoclast receptor RANK and decreasing osteoclast-mediated bone resorption and turnover.
- Other treatments include teriparatide, a parathyroid hormone analogue, and abaloparatide, a parathyroid hormone-related protein analogue.
- Romosozumab inhibits sclerostin, a glycoprotein that inhibits bone formation.
- Deposition occurs normally on top of the bisphosphonates, which become embedded and inactive in the matrix (see Clinical Correlation Box 33.1).

Clinical Correlation Box 33.3

Whereas most people do not commonly think of cancer as arising out of bone tissue, some particularly malignant cancers do in fact result from processes in bone development that have gone awry. One such tumor of bone is osteosarcoma, an aggressive cancer that arises from transformed cells of mesenchymal origin. Osteosarcoma is a common childhood cancer but can also arise in the elderly, often in the background of other bone pathology, such as Paget disease. Treatment of osteosarcoma is typically a radical surgical resection—unfortunately, this can leave patients as amputees.

Tumor Induced Osteomalacia and FGF23:

Tumor induced osteomalacia, an entity previously called oncogenic osteomalacia, had been associated with tumors that are often benign. Patients suffer from severe hypophosphatemia, with large amounts of phosphorus-wasting in the urine that could not be attributed to elevated parathyroid hormone. This syndrome is now known to be due to a decrease in proximal tubule sodium phosphate reabsorption mediated by increased fibroblast growth factor 23 (FGF23). Further work on the FGF23 syndrome showed that it derives from the bone with receptors in the intestine and the kidney. Its main effects are the phosphaturia as well as suppression production of 1,25 $(OH)_2$ vitamin D.

Hungry bone syndrome:

Hungry bone syndrome is the effect of removing the parathyroid gland or glands due to elevation of PTH. The elevation of PTH may be from a single adenoma within a single gland (primary hyperparathyroidism) or from all glands due to hyperplasia (secondary hyperparathyroidism, which is usually caused by low vitamin D and hypocalcemia). With surgery, there is a decrease in PTH, and subsequently a loss of a stimulus for osteoclast formation and the resorption of calcium that supports the blood calcium. Consequently, unopposed osteoblastic function is responsible for the uptake of calcium into bone and hypocalcemia with tetany. For that reason such patients must be treated, beginning preoperatively, with vitamin D and calcium supplements to prevent hypocalcemia.

SUMMARY

- Bone is composed of cellular and acellular elements. The acellular element, or bone matrix, is made of collagen adorned with hydroxyapatite (calcium phosphate crystals).
- Woven bone is found in the fetus and in pathologic states. Lamellar bone, arrayed in a concentric circle around a blood vessel, is the usual pattern of bone deposition in postnatal life.
- Flat bones are the skull, pelvis, scapula, and so on. Long bones are the humerus, femur, and so on.
- Long bones have a diaphysis, metaphysis, and epiphysis. In growing children and adolescents, a growth plate divides the metaphysis and epiphysis.
- The inside of trabecular bone consists of porous network of bony arches called trabeculae. The pores are filled with bone marrow, where blood cells are made. More compact cortical bone surrounds and contains the trabecular bone.
- Osteoblasts deposit bone. Osteoclasts resorb bone. Osteoblasts control osteoclast proliferation with cytokines, such as IL-6 and RANKL.

- In adults, deposition and resorption occur at all times and remain in equilibrium. Thus they preserve a relatively stable bone mass. This process is called remodeling.
- Calcium homeostasis can shift bone turnover toward deposition or resorption to liberate Ca^{2+} from bone. Mechanical stress shifts remodeling toward deposition along planes of stress, and lack of stress shifts it toward resorption. This is Wolff's law: form follows function.
- During remodeling, osteoblasts deposit new bone (collagen and hydroxyapatite) directly on top of old.
- During fetal growth, bones are modeled in cartilage and then mineralized or ossified with woven bone.
- In childhood and adolescence, cartilage grows at the growth plate and is then ossified with lamellar bone.
- When bone is fractured, it grows a cartilaginous callus, which is then ossified with woven bone. The woven bone is later remodeled into lamellar bone.

REVIEW QUESTIONS

Directions: Each of the numbered items or incomplete statements in this section is followed by answers or by completions of the statement. Select the one lettered answer or completion that is best in each case.

1. Estrogen receptors are expressed on many different cells found in the bone matrix. Estrogen's inhibitory effect on osteoclastogenesis is probably mediated by estrogen receptors on which bone cell?
   A. Osteoclasts
   B. Osteocytes
   C. Chondrocytes
   D. Osteoblasts
   E. Chondroblasts
2. A 96-year-old woman suffers a painful hip fracture with minimal trauma. If bone mineral density testing later shows that she has osteoporosis, her fracture could be described as:
   A. Comminuted
   B. Pathologic

   C. Transverse
   D. Articular
   E. Open
3. An 81-year-old man complaining of back pain is diagnosed with prostate cancer after a transrectal biopsy. His bone scan shows dark areas at several lumbar and thoracic vertebrae, suggesting probable metastases. The dark areas reflect:
   A. Increased bone resorption
   B. Increased bone deposition
   C. Increased bone resorption and deposition
   D. Cancellous bone
   E. Low radionuclide concentration

ANSWERS

1. **The answer is D.** Stimulation of the estrogen receptor on osteoblasts causes inhibition of osteoclastic activity. Osteoblasts control osteoclastogenesis through cytokines, such as IL-6. Estrogen likely acts on the osteoblast, just as PTH acts on the osteoblast to upregulate osteoclastic activity.
2. **The answer is B.** The patient has a pathologic fracture. A pathologic fracture is one that occurs in the context of underlying abnormalities in the bone. In this case, the abnormality is low bone mass owing to osteoporosis. She may also have a

comminuted, transverse, articular, or (less likely) open fracture, but there is not enough information given to diagnose her with anything except a pathologic fracture.
3. **The answer is C.** The dark areas on the bone scan reflect increased bone remodeling, meaning increased resorption and deposition. The cancer promotes the resorption, and the osteoblasts respond to the increased resorption with increased deposition. The dark areas are highly concentrated with radionuclide, not the reverse.

The Female Reproductive System

34

INTRODUCTION

The menstrual cycle defines the reproductive years of a woman's life. It begins with menarche (the onset of menstruation) at about age 8 to 13 years and ends with menopause, which begins at about age 50 years. Evolutionarily, the purpose of each menstrual cycle is to create the opportunity for pregnancy.

Preparation for potential pregnancy is achieved through two concurrent cycles, which together make up the menstrual cycle:
1. The ovarian cycle
2. The uterine cycle

If pregnancy is not achieved on a given month, the nutritive uterine lining is shed in menstruation and a cycle begins anew. If pregnancy is achieved, a transient organ called the placenta creates a new and unique hormonal milieu to support the growth of a fetus. When the baby is delivered and the placenta passed from the body, the menstrual cycle resumes.

SYSTEM STRUCTURE

Gross Anatomy

The Reproductive Tract

The ovaries are the gonads of the human female.
- Approximately 2 to 3 cm each, they are located in the pelvis with one ovary on either side of the uterus within the broad ligaments (Fig. 34.1).
- The ovarian ligaments contain the ovarian artery and vein, which enter and leave the ovary at its hilum.

The fallopian tubes, or oviducts, are hollow structures on either side of the uterus.
- The space inside each tube is continuous at the distal end with the peritoneal cavity and at the proximal end with the cavity of the uterus.
- Each tube is subdivided into a distal infundibulum with tentacle-like projections called fimbriae, an ampulla, and a proximal isthmus (Fig. 34.2).
- Fertilization of the ovum by the sperm occurs in the fallopian tube.
- The fallopian tube conducts the egg from the ovary into the tube and the fertilized egg from the tube into the uterus (Genetics Box 34.1. Pharmacology Box 34.1, and Oncology Box 34.1).

The uterus, or womb, is the chamber in which the fertilized egg will implant and subsequently grow into a fetus.
- It is a muscular organ located in the pelvis posterior to the bladder, anterior to the rectum, and superior to the vagina.

- The components of the uterus include:
  - The fundus, or most superior portion
  - The corpus (body), the upper, pear-shaped portion of the uterus
  - The cervix, the lower, cylindrical portion of the uterus. The ends of the cervix are the internal and the external cervical os.

The vagina, or birth canal, is the passageway leading from the internal female reproductive tract to the external genitalia.

The mons pubis, the labia majora, the labia minora, the clitoris, the hymen, and the greater vestibular (or Bartholin's) glands make up the female external genitalia.

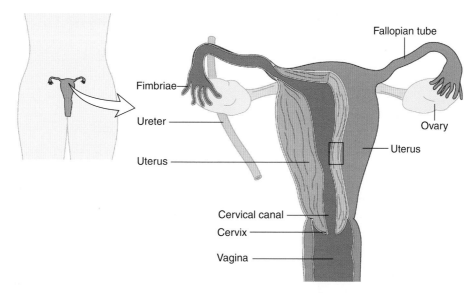

Fig. 34.1 Anatomy of the ovaries. (Modified from Carroll R. *Elsevier's Integrated Physiology.* Philadelphia: Mosby Elsevier; 2007. Fig. 14.3.)

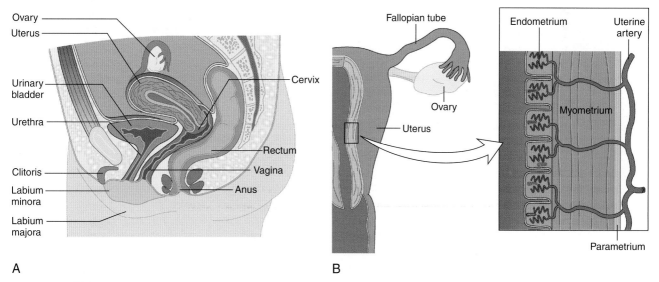

A

B

Fig. 34.2 A, Anatomy of the uterus and B, fallopian tubes. (Modified from Carroll R. *Elsevier's Integrated Physiology.* Philadelphia: Mosby Elsevier; 2007. Fig. 14.3.)

The Central Nervous System

The generation of an egg, the establishment and maintenance of an appropriate environment for fertilization and development, the process of birth, and the nourishment of an infant all require precise functioning of a number of hormone-producing organs in the brain.

- The hypothalamus is located in the diencephalon, the part of the brain that lies above the brain stem and between the two cerebral hemispheres.
- The pituitary gland is a bilobed structure in the sella turcica, in the midline of the brain, just inferior to the hypothalamus (see Ch. 29 for more information).
- As described in Chapter 29, the pituitary gland consists of the anterior pituitary (adenohypophysis) and the posterior pituitary (neurohypophysis).

Histology

Each ovary has two distinct zones (Fig. 34.3):

- The inner medulla contains the ovarian blood vessels.
- The outer cortex that contains the follicles, the functional components of the ovary.

  A follicle is composed of three different cell types:

1. Oocytes
2. Granulosa cells
3. Theca cells

   Each follicle contains a single oocyte, or central egg. The cells closest to the oocyte are granulosa cells, which are surrounded by a basal lamina or basement membrane. Outside this basal lamina are the theca cells.

- When an oocyte leaves the follicle in the process of ovulation, the remaining parts of the follicular tissue—granulosa

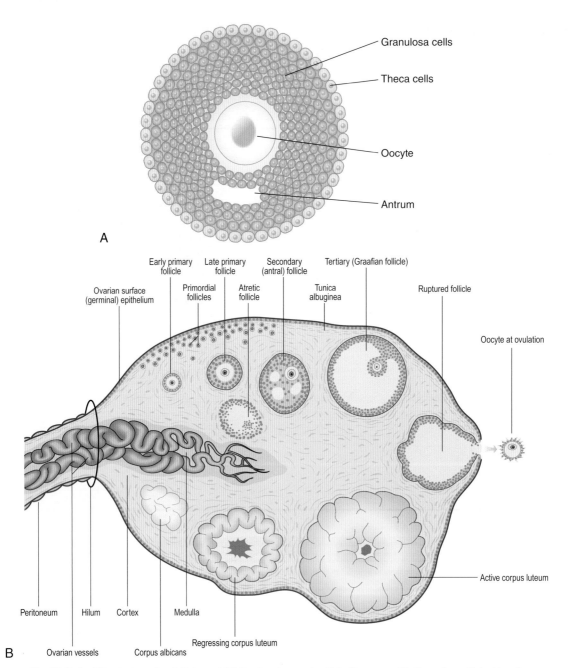

Fig. 34.3 An (A) antral ovarian follicle and (B) its development within the ovary. (Bottom, from Satndring S. *Gray's Anatomy*, 41st Ed. Philadelphia: Elsevier, 2015. p. 1288–1313. Fig. 77.32.)

cells, theca cells, and ovarian fibroblasts—change organization and function and are called the corpus luteum.

- When the corpus luteum degenerates, it turns into a scar-like structure called the corpus albicans.

Smooth muscle and ciliated cells line the inside of the fallopian tubes and help to create a "current" that brushes the fertilized egg toward the uterus.

The walls of the uterus are composed of three layers (see Fig. 34.2):

1. Outer serosa (mesothelium)
2. Thick smooth muscle layer (myometrium)
3. Inner mucosal layer (endometrium)

Likewise, the endometrium is composed of several different tissues:

- The superficial layer of the endometrium, the stratum functionalis, is composed of porous connective tissue (called the stroma) invested with secretory glands.
  - The functionalis grows up to a centimeter thick and then is sloughed during menstruation.
- A deeper layer, the stratum basalis, proliferates to create a new functionalis.
- Arcuate arteries run through the myometrium parallel to the mucosal surface. Two sets of vessels branch off of the arcuates perpendicularly to supply the endometrium.

- The straight arteries, which supply the basalis.
- The coiled or spiral arteries, which supply the functionalis (see Clinical Correlation Box 34.1).

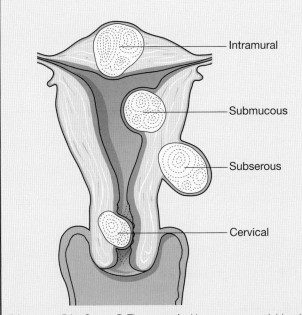
The hypothalamic nuclei (groups of neurons) relevant to the female reproductive system are:

- The arcuate nucleus in the medial basal hypothalamus.
- The paraventricular and supraoptic nuclei, which contain the magnocellular cells.

The anterior pituitary cells most relevant to the female reproductive system are:

- Gonadotrophs (follicle-stimulating hormone [FSH]- or luteinizing hormone [LH]-producing)
- Lactotrophs (prolactin-producing)

The Reproductive Hormones

Steroid Hormones

Many of the hormones required for the proper functioning of the female reproductive system are members of the steroid family, which are derivatives of cholesterol. The steroids germane to female reproduction ("sex steroids") are:

- Pregnenolone
- Progesterone
- Dehydroepiandrosterone (DHEA)
- Androstenedione
- Testosterone
- Estrogens (estrone, estradiol, estriol)

The estrogens constitute a steroid subfamily, each with subtle structural differences.

- Estrone has one OH group, estradiol has two such groups, and estriol has three.
- Estradiol, with two OH groups, is the most abundant and physiologically important of the three.

Like all other steroid hormones, each of the sex steroids must bind to intracellular receptors to exert its influence.

- The distribution of the receptors determines the distribution of the effects of the steroid hormones.
- Progesterone and estrogen receptors are located throughout the body, but principally in the uterus, breast, hypothalamus, and pituitary gland.

Sex steroids are produced by the cells of the ovaries, the maternal and fetal adrenal glands, and the placenta, but many other tissues (e.g., the liver and fat tissues) are also involved in the synthesis, metabolism, and catabolism of these molecules (Fig. 34.4). Estrogen and progesterone are transported in the blood bound to proteins called sex hormone-binding globulins.

Protein Hormones

Gonadotropin-releasing hormone (GnRH) is a protein hormone produced by the arcuate nucleus of the hypothalamus. The gonadotrophs of the anterior pituitary possess GnRH receptors.

The anterior pituitary produces and secretes two protein hormones critical for the proper functioning of the female reproductive system. These hormones are called gonadotropins because they are intimately involved in the function of, and have an affinity (or tropism) for, the gonads. The pituitary gonadotropins are:

1. LH
2. FSH

LH and FSH are both glycoproteins composed of alpha and beta subunits.

- The alpha subunit is common to both hormones and is the same as that of thyroid-stimulating hormone (TSH) and human chorionic gonadotropin (hCG).
- The beta subunit is unique to each hormone and determines the specific action at the target organ or tissue.

Ovarian granulosa cells possess LH and FSH receptors, whereas theca cells have LH receptors but no FSH receptors.

In addition, the ovary produces three glycoprotein hormones that are members of the transforming growth factor beta (TGF-β) superfamily.

1. Activin
   - Acts in a paracrine fashion on sites near to its release.

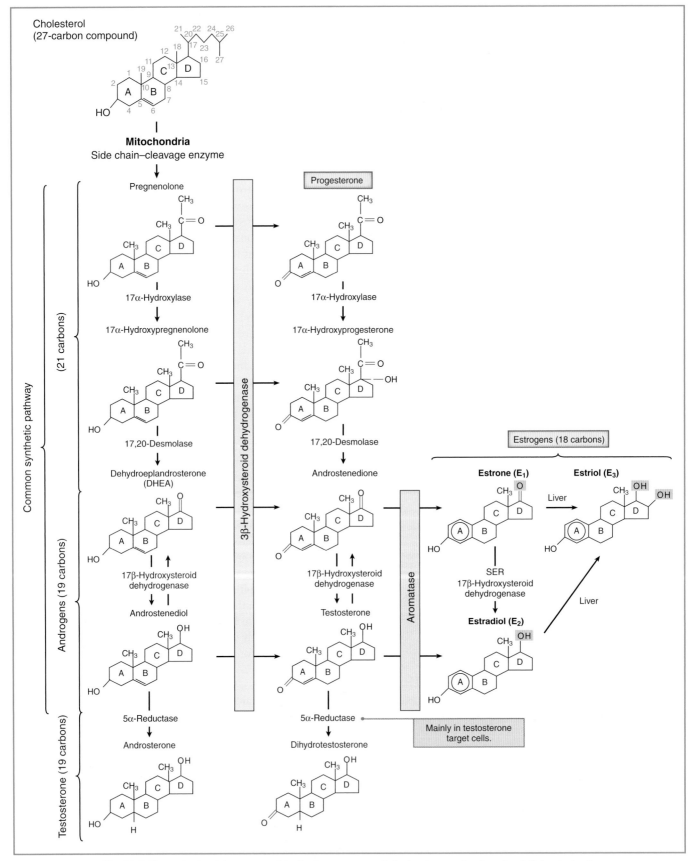

Fig. 34.4 Biosynthesis of the sex steroids. Androgens are made in the theca cells of ovarian follicles, but only the granulosa cells contain aromatase. Therefore androgens must pass from theca to granulosa to be converted to estrogens. (From Carroll R. *Elsevier's Integrated Physiology.* Philadelphia: Mosby Elsevier; 2007. Fig. 14.5.)

- Its role is not yet well understood, although it has been shown to promote and to suppress follicular development in the ovary.
2. Follistatin
   - Binds to and inhibits activin.
3. Inhibin
   - Circulates in the blood from the ovarian follicles to the pituitary, where it binds to receptors on the FSH-secreting gonadotrophs to attenuate FSH secretion.

Fig. 34.5 illustrates the structure of the hormonal system and a simplified schematic of its feedback mechanism, collectively known as the hypothalamic-pituitary-gonadal (HPG) axis. Briefly:

- Pulsatile GnRH promotes the secretion of FSH and LH, whereas constant GnRH inhibits the secretion of FSH and LH.
- FSH and LH stimulate ovarian responses, including secretion of estrogen and progesterone.
- Estrogen and progesterone promote reversible (and at puberty some irreversible) developments of the reproductive tract and feedback negatively on FSH and LH secretion.
- Ovarian-released inhibin inhibits FSH secretion.

Although this abbreviated description may suggest that the HPG axis operates much like the other neuroendocrine axes,

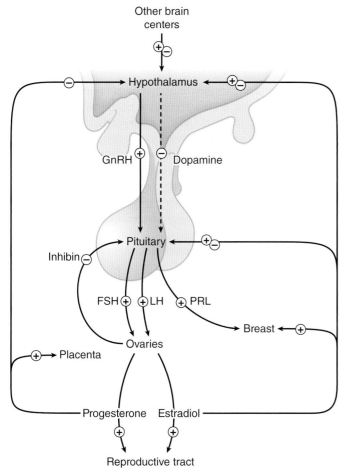

Fig. 34.5 Hypothalamic-pituitary-gonadal axis: an overview. *FSH*, Follicle-stimulating hormone; *GnRH*, gonadotropin-releasing hormone; *LH*, luteinizing hormone; *PRL*, prolactin. *Plus signs* represent stimulation; *minus signs* represent inhibition.

the reproductive axis is actually more complex than the other axes. The function of this system will be explored in detail later.

SYSTEM FUNCTION

Unlike the other organ systems, the reproductive system does not need to be operational at birth, with full functionality only attained with biologic maturity. Reproductive function therefore changes over the lifespan of an individual.

- These changes over time are even more pronounced in the female than in the male.
- One function in particular (oogenesis, the production of eggs) begins in the first weeks of fetal life and is not completed for many years.

Because of the reproductive system's evolving character, we will survey the development of female reproductive function across ages.

Fetal Life

A genetically distinct individual comes into being the moment that a sperm and egg fuse—the moment of fertilization, or conception.

- Each sperm and egg cell contains 23 unpaired chromosomes and is called haploid (having half a set of chromosomes).
- When the cells merge at fertilization, they form a zygote with 23 pairs of chromosomes for a full diploid set of 46.

Twenty two of these pairs are called autosomes; the remaining pair is the sex chromosomes. There are two types of sex chromosomes: an X and a Y.

- If the zygote has two X chromosomes, the resulting fetus is genetically female.
- If the zygote has one X and one Y chromosome, it is genetically male.

Initially, the developmental paths of the male and female gonads and genital systems are identical. The reproductive structures begin to take shape in the fifth week of gestation, when germ cells migrate from the yolk sac into the coelom (body cavity) inside the tiny embryo (Fig. 34.6):

- The germ cells undergo mitotic division during their journey and settle into the inner surface of the embryo's dorsal body wall.
- The germ cells signal the coelomic epithelium to grow and differentiate into two genital ridges lateral to the developing vertebral column.
- The genital ridges are the primordial gonads, and at this time they are still gender-indifferent (neither male nor female).

By the sixth week, two pairs of genital ducts also have developed in every fetus lateral to the genital ridge:

1. The Wolffian ducts, or mesonephric ducts, are the male genital precursors.
2. The Müllerian ducts, or paramesonephric ducts, are the female genital precursors.

If a normal Y chromosome is present (i.e., if the fetus is genetically male), a gene on the Y encodes a zinc finger deoxyribonucleic acid (DNA)-binding protein called testis determining factor (TDF). TDF will initiate a male developmental program for the gonads and genitals of the fetus, preserving

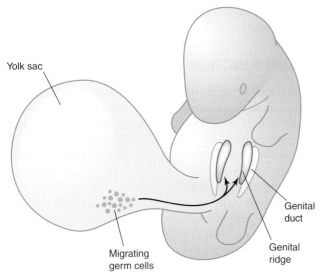

Fig. 34.6 Primordial genitals around the fifth week of life. At this early stage of development, male and female genital structures are undifferentiated.

the Wolffian ducts and causing regression of the Müllerian ducts.

However, the "default" program of the human fetus is to form a female reproductive tract, which occurs as follows:
- After the sixth week of gestation, regression of the gonadal medulla and growth of the cortex occurs.
  - Multiplying germ cells differentiate into oogonia (egg-producing cells).
  - Coelomic epithelial tissue surrounding the oogonia becomes granulosa cells.
  - Mesenchymal stromal cells become theca cells.
  - The Mullerian duct remains while the Wolffian duct regresses.
- By the 9th to 10th week of gestation, the genital structures begin to take shape.
  - The upper Müllerian ducts form the fallopian tubes.
  - The lower Müllerian ducts fuse to produce the uterus, cervix, and upper vagina. The genital tubercle transforms into the clitoris.
  - The urethral folds transform into the labia minora.
  - The genital swellings transform into the labia majora.
  - The urogenital sinus transforms into the lower vagina.
- After the 12th week of gestation, millions of oogonia exist within the fetal ovaries.
  - Oogonia begin meiosis.
  - However, they are inhibited by signaling from the granulosa cells, preventing them from completing meiosis.
  - Delays complete egg development until puberty.

In all fetal body cells outside the ovarian germ cells, one or the other of the two X chromosomes is selected at random to be inactivated and thereafter condenses to form the Barr body. This is called X inactivation.
- Once a given cell has selected either the paternally derived or the maternally derived X chromosome for inactivation, all of its subsequent daughter cells will have the same X chromosome inactivated (see Fast Fact Box 34.1).

Fast Fact Box 34.1

An animal correlate is the calico cat, where random X inactivation of one of the two X chromosomes (each carrying a gene with a different color allele) leads to the different "patches" of color on the calico cat.

Mitosis, Meiosis, and Oogenesis

By the third trimester of fetal life, all or most oogonia have entered meiotic division. This is the beginning of oogenesis—the production of eggs or ova.

Recall that mitosis produces two daughter cells, each with the same 46 chromosomes as the parent cell, whereas meiosis produces two cells with only 23 chromosomes each.

Recall from cell biology that mitosis is divided into six phases (Fig. 34.7):
1. Interphase: This is the nondividing phase in which human cells spend most of their time. At the end of interphase, internal and external signals prompt DNA replication to occur. Interphase is sometimes divided into G_1 phase (quiescent), S phase (DNA replication), and G_2 phase (precell division).
2. Prophase: Chromosomes condense. Owing to replication, every one of the 46 chromosomes has an identical sister called a chromatid. The cell has gone from the usual amount of genetic material, called *2n* (diploid), to 4n.
3. Metaphase: Chromosomes attach to a spindle of microtubules and line up in the midline of the cell, an area designated the metaphase plate.
4. Anaphase: Identical sister chromatids are pulled away from each other along the microtubule spindle with the help of adenosine triphosphate (ATP)-requiring dynein motor proteins.
5. Telophase: Two sets of 46 chromosomes decondense and nucleate on each side of the mother cell.
6. Cytokinesis: The mother cell's cytoplasm splits, and two diploid daughter cells are formed.

Meiosis is divided into two subphases, meiosis I and meiosis II, each with five analogous steps (see Fig. 34.7).
- Meiosis I consists of prophase I, metaphase I, anaphase I, telophase I, and cytokinesis I.
- Meiosis II consists of prophase II, metaphase II, anaphase II, telophase II, and cytokinesis II.

During metaphase I in meiosis I, homologous chromosomes pair up and these 23 *pairs* line up on the metaphase I plate.
- Consequently, with the first division each of the two intermediate cells receives a single double-stranded chromosome from each homologous pair.
- The two daughter cells are not identical to each other or to the mother cell.

In meiosis II, there is no further DNA replication, and these 23 double-stranded chromosomes line up individually on the metaphase II plate.
- The double strands separate from each other.
- When meiosis is complete, four gametes (two pairs) have been produced from one somatic cell, each with only 23 chromosomes.

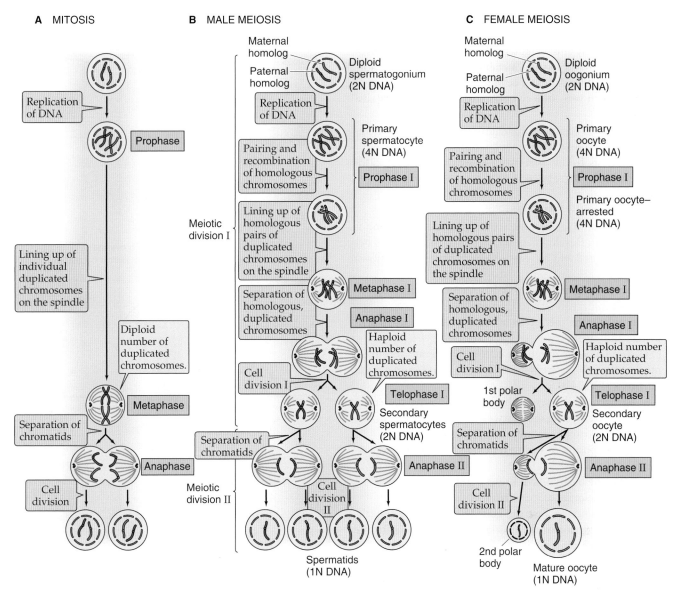

A MITOSIS   **B** MALE MEIOSIS   **C** FEMALE MEIOSIS

Fig. 34.7 Mitosis (A) and meiosis (B in males and C in females). Mitosis is the process of cell division. Meiosis produces gametes. In the development of the female gamete, meiosis is arrested in prophase I during fetal life, resumes at ovulation once menarche has occurred, is arrested in metaphase II, and resumes at fertilization. *DNA,* Deoxyribonucleic acid. (From: *Boron Medical Physiology,* 3rd Edition. Fig. 53.2.)

Meiosis and gametogenesis (the process by which gametes are formed and mature) differ significantly between the male and female reproductive systems.

- In the male, spermatogenesis occurs continuously throughout life, and a single germ cell normally produces four viable sperm.
- In the female, however, meiosis occurs in a limited time frame, and does not produce four fully functional gametes. Most oogonia begin the process of meiosis between the 12th and 20th week of fetal life. However, meiosis I is arrested at prophase I (DNA replicated and chromosomes condensed, but not attached to spindle).
- Consequently, at birth, the ovarian cortex houses primordial follicles, which consist of 4n *oocytes* that are suspended in

meiotic division, and a surrounding layer of ovarian granulosa cells.

- Granulosa cells are thought to mediate the arrest of meiosis I. Although approximately 7 million primordial germ cells migrate to the ovaries during embryogenesis, physiologic atrophy occurs during fetal development such that only about 2 million follicles remain at the time of birth.
- This atrophy continues in postnatal life, and by menarche (the onset of menstruation in adolescence), 400,000 follicles are distributed throughout the ovarian stroma.
- Of this number, only 300 to 400 will be released from the ovary (ovulated) before menopause; the rest will degenerate. Each month in the menstrual cycle, individual follicles are recruited for meiotic completion at the time of ovulation. However,

only a single ovum is generated because of unequal allocation of cytoplasm during cytokinesis I and II.

- In cytokinesis I, one daughter cell receives the majority of the cytoplasm and has the metabolic capacity to function, whereas the other daughter cell forms the first polar body, a small cell with very little cytoplasm which is ultimately discarded.
- Ovulation then occurs, with meiosis arrested again in metaphase II. It will only resume with fertilization.
- In cytokinesis II, the final ovum takes almost all the cytoplasm, while another polar body is formed.

Adolescence and Puberty

From infancy until adolescence, the reproductive system is largely quiescent. Development of the reproductive organs begins between ages 8 and 13 years in girls, a phase of life known as puberty.

- An unknown signal triggers GnRH secretion, which stimulates the pituitary to secrete LH and FSH.
- LH stimulates the theca cells of the ovarian follicles to synthesize androgens.
- FSH stimulates the granulosa cells to proliferate and make more of the enzyme aromatase, which converts androgens to estrogens (Fig. 34.8).

The estrogen level rises in the blood, exposing the entire body to its effects. Within the ovary, estrogen acts in a paracrine fashion to potentiate the influence of LH and FSH.

Increased exposure to estrogen heralds two primary developmental stages:

1. Thelarche, the beginning of breast development.
2. Menarche, the onset of menstruation.

Menarche occurs because the gonadotropins have reawakened the development of the ovarian follicles, leading to the onset of ovulation. Once follicular development has begun, the reproductive system enters into a self-sustaining monthly cycle of ovarian and uterine changes, including the vaginal bleeding of menses.

Around the time of menarche, growth hormone levels rise to promote the growth of the long bones. Shortly afterwards, adrenal androgens promote the growth of pubic and axillary hair, which is known as adrenarche.

Reproductive Maturity: Follicular Development and the Menstrual Cycle

It is customary to think of the neuroendocrine axes as controlled "from the top down."

- In other words, the hypothalamus stimulates target tissues and modulates their hormone production in accordance with feedback data, data on physiologic parameters, and circadian central nervous system rhythms.

The situation is different, however, in the HPG axis. Although hypothalamic GnRH does initiate puberty, afterwards the hypothalamic-pituitary-ovarian axis is largely controlled "from the bottom up." The ovarian follicles, on a predestined course much like that of embryologic development, set the pace of monthly ovulation, uterine buildup, and uterine shedding: the menstrual cycle.

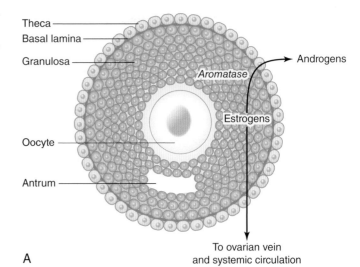

A

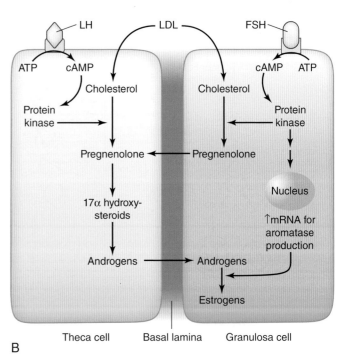

B

Fig. 34.8 Estrogen production by the ovarian follicle. A, A histologic view. B, A biochemical view. *ATP*, Adenosine triphosphate; *cAMP*, cyclic adenosine monophosphate; *FSH*, follicle-stimulating hormone; *LDL*, low-density lipoprotein; *LH*, luteinizing hormone; *mRNA*, messenger ribonucleic acid. (From Boron W, Boulpaep E. *Medical Physiology*, 3rd ed. Philadelphia: Saunders Elsevier; 2017. Fig. 53.2.)

The Follicular Phase

Each ovarian follicle contains an oocytes suspended in prophase I of meiosis. However, although the oocyte itself is arrested, the primordial follicles continue to develop throughout childhood (Fig. 34.9).

- Granulosa cells multiply and eventually secrete a fluid containing mucopolysaccharides, electrolytes, proteins, and numerous steroid and peptide hormones, creating a fluid known as antrum. All antral follicles generated before puberty undergo atresia (apoptosis).
- A thecal cell layer develops around the granulosa cell layer.
- The oocytes increase in size.

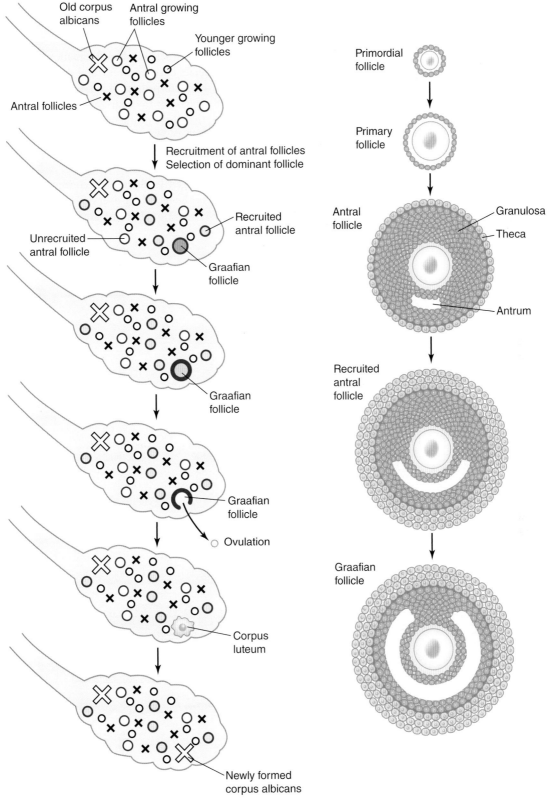

Fig. 34.9 Follicular development. Development is shown on the ovary on the left and shown apart from the ovary on the right. The *arrows* represent the passage of time. Although the drawings are not to scale, they correlate roughly with the actual size of the structures involved. The corpus luteum in particular takes up a substantial portion of the ovarian cortex before it regresses. Only the ovarian cortex is shown; the ovarian medulla, containing the ovarian blood vessels, is not depicted.

At puberty, pulsatile GnRH secretion increases in amplitude and frequency (one pulse every 60–200 minutes), which increases the size and frequency of LH and FSH pulses.

- With increased ovarian exposure to LH and FSH, recruitment begins among antral follicles.
- A group of around 10 follicles is recruited to develop further and swell in size, while nonrecruited follicles undergo atresia.
- The granulosa cells of the large, recruited follicles make estrogen, which stimulates the uterine endometrium to grow (Fig. 34.10).

Selection occurs when only one of the 10 follicles achieves a metabolic advantage and outgrows the others, leading to formation of the Graafian follicle.

- The Graafian follicle is especially sensitive to FSH from the pituitary, which enhances its advantage over the other follicles.

- As all the follicles pour estrogen and inhibin into the bloodstream, these ovarian hormones begin to inhibit FSH secretion from the pituitary gonadotrophs.
- Lacking the Graafian follicle's enhanced FSH sensitivity, the other follicles become atretic and die.
- This 2-week cultivation of a Graafian follicle is called the follicular phase of the ovarian cycle. This coincides with the proliferative phase of the uterine cycle, wherein endometrial growth is driven by increased follicular estrogen production.

Ovulation

Once the estrogen levels reach a concentration of more than 100 pg/mL in the blood for over 36 hours, it no longer inhibits LH and FSH secretion, but instead stimulates it.

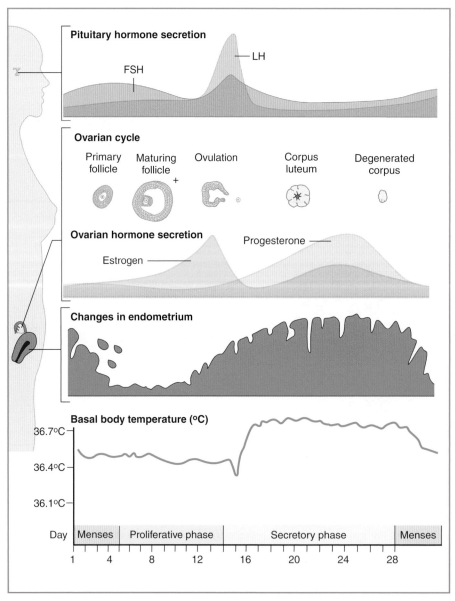

Fig. 34.10 Hormonal signaling in the menstrual cycle, under the control of follicular development. The ovarian, uterine, and body temperature cycles are also shown. *FSH*, Follicle-stimulating hormone; *LH*, luteinizing hormone. (From Carroll R. *Elsevier's Integrated Physiology.* Philadelphia: Mosby Elsevier; 2007. Fig. 14.9.)

The high estrogen level results in a shift from negative feedback to positive feedback.

- This results in the 48-hour midcycle surge of LH and FSH, wherein LH levels increase in excess of FSH levels.
- LH stimulates the follicle to resume meiosis.
- LH also promotes follicular inflammation, activates proteolytic enzymes, and initiates ovarian contractions. These, together with the pressure accumulated in the antrum by continued fluid secretion and the weakening of the follicular wall, lead to follicular rupture.
- The oocyte inside the follicle is ejected into the peritoneal cavity and clings to the ovarian capsule until it is swept into the fallopian tubes by the fallopian fimbria, which are a fingerlike fringe of tissue at the distal openings of the fallopian tubes.
- This is the process known as ovulation (see Clinical Correlation Box 34.2).

Clinical Correlation Box 34.2

Oral contraceptive pills (OCPs) capitalize on estrogen and progesterone's negative feedback effect on the hypothalamus and pituitary. By delivering daily doses of an estrogen and a progestin (which acts at the progesterone receptor), the pills inhibit the pituitary luteinizing hormone (LH) surge that is responsible for ovulation. The estrogen and progesterone combination also interferes with the normal changes of the uterine cycle so that the endometrium cannot mature to its full extent. An estrogen/progestin pill is typically taken daily for 3 weeks, when a sugar pill is substituted for 1 week. This withdrawal of steroidal support from the endometrium allows menstruation in mimicry of a normal menstrual cycle.

The Luteal Phase

By this point, the action of FSH during the follicular phase has now greatly increased the expression of LH receptors on the granulosa cells. This, in combination with the LH surge, now puts the follicle under the heavy influence of LH.

- Under this influence, the ruptured Graafian follicle transforms into a new tissue called the corpus luteum.
- This transformation is called luteinization and accounts for LH's name, luteinizing hormone.

The two major luteinizing effects of LH are a shift in enzyme expression and an alteration in the proliferative characteristics of the follicular cells.

- The shift in enzyme expression diverts the cells' steroidogenic pathway away from estrogen production and toward progesterone production.
- Meanwhile, the follicular cells begin proliferating rapidly and become heavily vascularized, allowing them to pour out progesterone.
- Over the next 2 weeks of the luteal phase renders the uterine lining secretory and supportive of a potential embryo. Thus, the luteal phase of the ovarian cycle corresponds with the secretory phase of the uterine cycle.

The corpus luteum is a transitory structure, fated for degeneration in 2 weeks' time unless rescued by the influence of a hormone called hCG.

- hCG is structurally similar to, but distinct from, LH and stimulates the LH receptors of the corpus luteum, thereby enabling the survival of the corpus luteum.

- The corpus luteum continues to produce progesterone, maintaining the endometrial lining of the uterus in a condition supportive of a developing embryo.
- hCG is produced by a part of the embryo itself called the trophoblast, the cells of which will later develop into the placenta (see Fast Fact Box 34.2).

Fast Fact Box 34.2

Home pregnancy tests measure the presence of human chorionic gonadotropin (hCG) in the urine with impressive accuracy and can be confirmed in the doctor's office with a blood test for the exact hCG level.

If pregnancy does not occur, however, no hCG is produced and the corpus luteum degenerates. The granulosa and theca cells become necrotic, and the corpus luteum is invaded by macrophages and leukocytes, a process called luteolysis.

- Luteolysis ends with the transformation of the corpus luteum into the corpus albicans, a scar-like structure in the ovary.
- As the corpus luteum degenerates, progesterone production falls and the endometrium degenerates, having lost its supporting hormone.
- The endometrium is then sloughed off in menstruation.

Concurrently, the decreased progesterone and estrogen production that follows luteolysis removes the inhibition from the hypothalamus and pituitary.

- During the luteal phase, estrogen and progesterone led to negative feedback on the brain, suppressing LH and FSH secretion.
- The removal of this negative feedback results in a bump in FSH secretion, which initiates recruitment of another 10 or so antral follicles for growth.
- This results in the beginning of a new follicular-proliferative phase.

This cycle will continue to repeat for all the reproductive years of a woman's life until the supply of antral follicles is exhausted.

The Uterine Cycle

The uterine cycle begins with the proliferative phase, in which endometrial growth occurs (Fig. 34.11). The proliferative phase coincides with the follicular phase of the ovarian cycle and takes place under the influence of estrogen from the growing follicles.

- The endometrium increases in thickness from 1 to 2 mm to 8 to 10 mm by day 14 (ovulation), when the proliferative phase ends.
- As basal endometrial cells proliferate, the stratum functionalis grows and its glands and arteries elongate.
- Estrogen also promotes the expression of progesterone receptors in the endometrium, preparing the endometrium for the transition into the progesterone-dominated luteal secretory phase.

After ovulation, progesterone from the corpus luteum initiates the secretory phase of the uterine cycle, lasting from day 15 to day 28 and coinciding with the luteal phase of the ovarian cycle.

- Estrogen levels fall, and progesterone downregulates the expression of estrogen receptors.

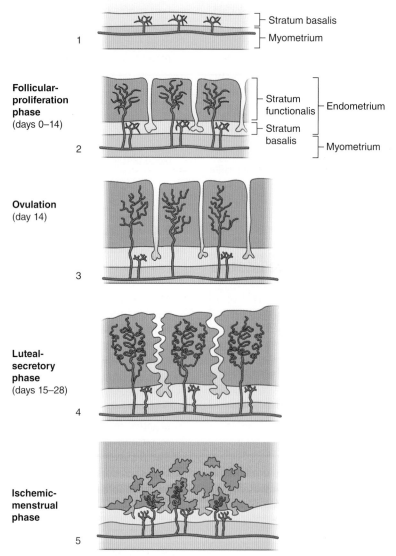

Fig. 34.11 The endometrium through the phases of the uterine cycle. The first three images show the progressive growth of the endometrium under the influence of follicular estrogen. The fourth image shows the increased tortuosity of the spiral arteries and endometrial glands under the influence of progesterone from the corpus luteum. The fifth image shows the breakdown of the endometrium and bleeding from ruptured spiral arteries under the influence of ischemia.

- Consequently, the high mitotic rate of the stratum basalis decreases, stopping endometrial growth.
- The endometrial mucus gland cells accumulate glycogen, glycoprotein, and glycolipid, and the glands and arteries become more coiled.
- Overall, the functionalis layer becomes a highly vascularized and nutrient-rich layer ready to support an embryo if one should arrive from a fallopian tube.

If conception does not occur, the uterine lining must be refreshed in anticipation of another ovarian cycle and possible conception.

- In the absence of pregnancy, the corpus luteum reaches the end of its allotted lifespan and degenerates into the corpus albicans.
- The functionalis, meanwhile, degenerates in parallel with the degeneration of the corpus luteum.

The two main mechanisms of endometrial remodeling are vasoconstriction and inflammation.

- Vasoconstriction of the spiral arteries may occur in response to increased levels of prostaglandins.
- The ischemia, or lack of blood flow, results in death of the spiral arteries' endothelium, with artery rupture, bleeding, and necrosis of the functionalis.
- Inflammation of the lining leads to enzymatic breakdown of the endometrium.

Fibrinolytic factors maintain bleeding to create a flow out of the uterus, and the entire functionalis is sloughed off over several days. The blood and shed endometrium exit the uterus by passing out of the cervix and then the vagina, resulting in menstruation (see Physiology Integration Box 34.1).

Physiology Integration Box 34.1

Many hormones promote changes in gene expression, leading to alteration of a tissue's receptivity to the signal of another hormone, such as with estrogen "priming" the endometrium for the secretory phase of the menstrual cycle by increasing progesterone receptors. This form of signaling is particularly common in the female reproductive system, as it relies on the genesis and degeneration of transient organs like the corpus luteum, the stratum functionalis, the placenta, and the lactating breast lobule.

Systemic Effects of Estrogen and Progesterone in Maturity

The breasts, vagina, cervix, hypothalamic thermoregulating center, and other parts of the body are also affected by the changing hormonal milieu during the menstrual cycle.

Estrogens have systemic effects, many of which share the function of tissue proliferation:

- During the estrogen surge in the follicular phase, there is growth not only of the follicles of the ovary and the functionalis of the uterus, but also in breast, cervical, and vaginal tissues.
- In addition, estrogen leads to the production of thin, clear, watery, and elastic mucus by the endocervical glands. This is most prominent during the follicular phase and immediately before the midcycle surge.
- The vaginal mucosa also responds to estrogen levels, subtly thickening and thinning over the menstrual cycle and noticeably undergoing atrophy at menopause.
- Finally, estrogen has also been shown to maintain bone density, which is one reason postmenopausal women suffer a decline in bone mass (osteoporosis).

Progesterone also has systemic effects, many of which share the function of tissue differentiation into secretory units.

- Stimulates the development of the secretory acinar glands in the breast.
- Converts the endocervical mucus from a thin, watery type to thick, opaque, viscous mucus.
- Leads to an increase of about 0.6°F in the basal body temperature. This increased temperature is apparent within 24 hours of ovulation and remains elevated for 11 or 12 days (or more, if a pregnancy occurs and maintains the corpus luteum).
- Finally, progesterone causes many symptoms commonly referred to as premenstrual syndrome, which occur just before menses, in concurrence with peak progesterone levels.
- Symptoms included breast tenderness, bloating, swelling of the extremities, and mood changes.

Menopause

Recall that the vast majority of antral follicles are not recruited for further growth and undergo atresia. Over many years, atresia of unrecruited follicles results in exhaustion of the oocyte store. As a woman approaches age 50 years, the groups of follicles recruited begin to dwindle in number.

- Fewer maturing follicles each month leads to decreased estrogen and inhibin production, as there is less follicular tissue available to synthesize these hormones.

- Declining estrogen and inhibin lessen the inhibition of FSH secretion from the pituitary.
- Increased FSH levels in turn may hasten the development of the follicle and shorten the cycle, leading to lighter or more irregular menstrual periods.
- Small follicle cohorts and abnormal patterns of follicular stimulation may also mean that some cycles do not even lead to ovulation.

This time of waning follicular recruitment and irregular periods is a transitional phase known as menopause. As the transition progresses toward total exhaustion of the stored oocyte pool and cessation of the menstrual cycle, women often experience a few characteristic symptoms in addition to irregular menses.

- The most common one is hot flashes—an intermittent and uncomfortable (but harmless) disturbance in temperature regulation related to decreasing estrogen levels.
- Hot flashes and other symptoms may be treated with short-term hormone replacement therapy (HRT)—exogenous estrogen— as is administered in oral contraceptives.

After the menopause transition is complete and the final menstrual period has occurred, estrogen levels decline in women.

- Low estrogen may lead to osteoporosis and fractures.
- However, long-term HRT may lead to increased risk of breast cancer, blood clotting, and coronary artery disease.

PATHOPHYSIOLOGY

Disorders of female reproduction fall into the following categories:

1. Disorders of sexual development
2. Disorders of fertility
3. Disorders of pregnancy
4. Disorders of parturition

Disordered of pregnancy and parturition will be discussed in the next chapter.

Disorders of Sexual Development

When the reproductive system does not develop in accordance with the XX or XY genotype, or when the sex chromosomes are abnormal or not intact, the result may be ambiguous genitalia at birth.

- Enzyme deficiencies in the fetus, the placenta, or the mother can create excess androgens and virilize a genotypically female fetus.
- Likewise, androgen insufficiencies or insensitivities can divert a genotypic male's reproductive development toward the default female phenotype.
- Mutations in the *SRY* gene that codes for TDF can also produce a female phenotype in a genetypically male fetus.
- Finally, abnormal sex genotypes can be caused by errors in chromosomal division during gametogenesis or during embryologic cell division.
  - Some result in phenotypically normal males or females with infertility.
  - Others lead to ambiguous phenotypes. Individuals who possess both male and female sex characteristics are described as hermaphroditic or hermaphrodites.

Disorders of Fertility

Once a couple has decided to have a child, the time to conception varies from one couple to another. The first ovulatory cycle may result in fertilization, or a number of cycles may pass before conception occurs.

- The diagnosis of infertility is made once a couple has tried to conceive without success for 1 year.
- Infertility can arise from either the male or female partner. Defects in female fertility can be classified by the location of the problem:
- Hypothalamic-pituitary factors
  - Hypothalamic dysfunction
    Malnutrition and strenuous exercise can suppress pituitary LH and FSH production, leading to a failure to ovulate; this is called hypogonadotropic hypogonadism.
  - Hyperprolactinemia
    Arises from prolactin-secreting pituitary tumor, which can suppress the pituitary gonadotrophs because of its inhibitory effect on GnRH secretion, leading to failed follicular development and anovulation.
- Ovarian factors
  - Polycystic ovary syndrome (single largest cause of ovulatory infertility)
    Excess ovarian androgens impair normal development of the Graafian follicle.
  - Disorders of sexual development
  - Endometriosis
  - Premature ovarian failure

Causes may be ischemic, toxic (including chemotherapeutics), traumatic, infectious, neoplastic, or autoimmune causes.
- Tubal factors (anything that obstructs the fallopian tube)
  - Pelvic inflammatory disease (usually because of chlamydia)
  - Pelvic adhesions
  - Endometriosis
  - Previous ectopic pregnancy
- Uterine factors
  - Uterine malformations
  - Uterine fibroids
- Cervical/vaginal factors
  - Cervical or vaginal obstruction

Endometriosis is a common condition in which endometrial cells grow in the peritoneum outside the uterus.
- Although this is a form of uncontrolled cell growth, endometriosis is not malignant.
- However, patients may suffer from pelvic pain and possible infertility. Endometriotic tissue can lead to development of peritoneal adhesions that distort the anatomy of the fallopian tubes and ovaries, which can mechanically interfere with the meeting of egg and sperm in the fallopian tube.
- Endometriomas on the ovary itself may also interfere with ovulation.

SUMMARY

- The female reproductive system is composed of the reproductive tract, the GnRH-producing center in the hypothalamus, and the pituitary gonadotrophs. The reproductive tract includes the vagina, cervix, uterus, fallopian tubes, and ovaries.
- The neuroendocrine system regulating reproductive function is called the HPG axis. Hypothalamic GnRH promotes the secretion of FSH and LH; FSH and LH stimulate ovarian responses, including the secretion of estrogen and progesterone.
- Estrogen and progesterone promote reversible (and at puberty irreversible) developments of the reproductive tract and feedback negatively on FSH and LH secretion.
- Ovarian follicles are the functional endocrine units of the ovary. A follicle is composed of one oocyte, theca, and granulosa cells.
- The default pathway of fetal gonadal and genital development is into the female.
- Primordial follicles undergoing meiosis is immediately arrested in prophase I.

- Meiosis remains arrested until puberty when it is resumed in one egg per month during ovulation. This oocyte arrests in metaphase II.
- Meiosis of the oocyte is completed only when the sperm penetrates the egg at fertilization.
- The ovarian follicles are the pelvic clock that controls the HPG axis from the bottom up.
- The phases of the menstrual cycle include:
  - Follicular phase
  - Mid-cycle LH surge
  - Ovulation
  - Luteal phase
  - Menstruation or pregnancy
- Over many years, atresia of unrecruited follicles results in exhaustion of the oocyte store. This leads to menopause—the cessation of monthly menstruation and fertility.
- Disorders of the female reproductive system can be divided into disorders of sexual development, fertility, pregnancy, and parturition.

REVIEW QUESTIONS

Directions: Each of the numbered items or incomplete statements in this section is followed by answers or by completions of the statement. Select the one lettered answer or completion that is best in each case.

1. A 26-year-old woman and her 28-year-old husband have been trying to conceive without success for more than a year. The man's sperm count and sperm quality are normal. Blood chemistries show a normal LH surge in the woman. If the woman has a history of pelvic inflammatory disease, the most likely cause of this couple's infertility is:
   A. Endometriosis
   B. An ovulatory defect
   C. Abnormal female reproductive tract anatomy
   D. Retrograde ejaculation
   E. Contraception

2. A 65-year-old postmenopausal woman who has been taking hormone replacement therapy (HRT) for 10 years is diagnosed with breast cancer. If the HRT contributed to the development of the carcinoma, it most likely did so through which mechanism?
   A. The mitogenic effect of estrogen
   B. The secretory effect of progesterone
   C. Progesterone's inhibition of prolactin
   D. Increased prolactin secretion
   E. Excess human chorionic somatomammotropin

3. A 29-year-old woman, 7 weeks pregnant, comes to the emergency room with a complaint of spotty vaginal bleeding and pelvic cramping. A transvaginal ultrasound shows no fetal heartbeat. A decrease in the plasma level of which of the following hormones may have caused her vaginal bleeding?
   A. Relaxin
   B. Human chorionic somatomammotropin (hCS)
   C. Estrogen
   D. Oxytocin
   E. Progesterone

ANSWERS TO REVIEW QUESTIONS

1. **The answer is C.** Scarring because of pelvic inflammatory disease can alter the anatomy of the female reproductive tract and prevent the egg from reaching the fallopian tube or prevent capacitated sperm from meeting the egg. The normal LH surge in the woman argues against an ovulatory defect, and the normal sperm count in the man argues against retrograde ejaculation as the cause of infertility.

2. **The answer is A.** Estrogen has a mitogenic (proliferative) effect on breast tissue, so estrogen-containing HRT can increase the risk of breast cancer in postmenopausal women. Progesterone, prolactin, and hCS all act on the breast, but they are not the principal ingredients of HRT and are not primarily mitogens.

3. **The answer is E.** The woman has likely had a spontaneous abortion. Fetal demise has led to trophoblast cell death and decreased hCG production. This in turn has led to luteolysis and decreased progesterone production. Decreased progesterone production has allowed the endometrium to begin to be sloughed off. Human chorionic somatomammotropin (hCS), different from hCG, affects maternal metabolism but does not support the corpus luteum.

35

Pregnancy and Parturition

THE ORGANS OF PREGNANCY

The placenta serves as the point of exchange between the circulatory systems of the mother and fetus; it is also a hormone-producing organ (Fig. 35.1A).

- The fully developed placenta is a round oval organ 15 to 20 cm in diameter and 2 to 3 cm thick, embedded in the uterine wall.
- It connects to the developing fetus via the umbilical cord and is expelled during birth.
- The placenta is composed of segments called cotyledons. Fingers of placental tissue (chorionic villi) extend into a pool of arterial maternal blood in the uterine wall, the intervillous space (Fig. 35.1B).
- The intervillous space is supplied by uterine spiral arteries, which have developed under the influence of progesterone.
- Bathed in the maternal blood of the intervillous space, the fetal capillaries of the villi passively absorb oxygen and nutrients and pass carbon dioxide and waste products into the maternal blood.
- The intervillous blood then drains back into the maternal circulation through the uterine veins in the decidua basalis.

The outer sheath of the villi is a layer called the chorion, which is composed of trophoblast cells. The chorionic barrier between the fetal villous blood and the maternal intervillous blood blocks the passage of most cells and large proteins.

- The barrier blocks peptide hormones but does allow the passage of steroid hormones.
- The chorion not only covers the villi but also extends beyond the placenta to envelop the entire amnion, the sac that contains the developing fetus in its amniotic fluid.

After a baby is born, the mother's body can continue to provide nourishment via the paired milk-producing mammary glands, or breasts (Fig. 35.2).

- The breasts are composed mainly of adipose and connective tissue.
- The mammary glandular tissue is divided into 15 to 20 lobules arranged in a radial pattern around the areola of the nipple.
  - Each lobule connects to the outside world through a network of lactiferous ducts.
  - The lactiferous ducts merge with each other as they approach the nipple, and there are about 5 to 10 duct openings on the nipple surface.
  - The lobules are composed of individual mammary alveoli. Each alveolus is lined with epithelial cells and a sublayer of myoepithelial cells.
- Lymphatic drainage from the breast is mainly to the axillary lymph nodes.

The Hormones of Pregnancy

Recall that human chorionic gonadotropin (hCG) maintains the corpus luteum and progesterone production. hCG is a heterodimeric glycoprotein synthesized and secreted by trophoblast cells of the placenta.

- Like luteinizing hormone (LH), follicle-stimulating hormone (FSH), and thyroid-stimulating hormone (TSH), hCG has an alpha and a beta subunit.
- The alpha subunit has the same amino acid sequence as that of LH, FSH, and TSH.
- The beta subunit is almost identical to that of LH but differs by having 31 extra amino acids at the carboxy terminus.
- hCG differs from the other three hormones in the number and type of carbohydrate side chains on the polypeptide subunits. Because hCG is more heavily glycosylated than LH, FSH, and TSH, it has a much longer half-life.

Relaxin, a polypeptide hormone secreted by the ovaries and other tissues, is active in many of the structures of pregnancy. It functions to relax the birth canal by proliferative effects on the surrounding tissues, which facilitates the delivery of a baby.

- Relaxin likely also acts through a nitric oxide-mediated mechanism to depress intestinal motility (which may be the reason for many of the gastrointestinal symptoms of pregnancy) and decreases blood vessel tone.

Prolactin is a polypeptide hormone synthesized and secreted by lactotroph cells in the anterior pituitary (see Clinical Correlation Box 35.1):

- It is structurally similar to growth hormone, as is its receptor.
- Breast tissue alveolar epithelial cells have prolactin receptors.

Oxytocin is a peptide product of hypothalamic magnocellular neurons and is released from the posterior pituitary.

- The cell bodies of the magnocellular neurons are located in the hypothalamic supraoptic and paraventricular nuclei.
- After production in these cell bodies, the oxytocin is packaged into secretory granules, transported down the axons within the infundibular stalk, and secreted at the axon terminals within the posterior pituitary.
- Oxytocin receptors are found on uterine myometrial cells and breast tissue myoepithelial cells. Oxytocin stimulates uterine contraction, and uterine contractions stimulate the release of additional oxytocin. This demonstrates a positive feedback loop that expedites parturition. But early in pregnancy, when parturition is not desirable because the fetus is not yet viable outside of the mother's body, a placental enzyme called oxytocinase, which also functions as a vasopressinase, inhibits the effects of oxytocin. However under circumstances such as a large placenta with multiple gestations the same enzyme can degrade arginine

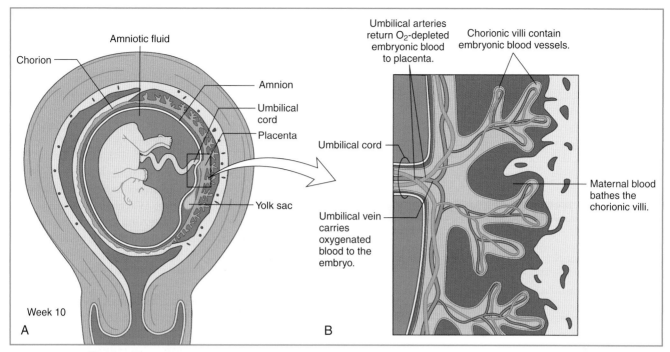

Fig. 35.1 The placenta, chorionic villi, and intervillous space. A, The position of the fetus and placenta within the uterus. B, A closer view of the villi and intervillous space. (From Carroll. *Elsevier's Integrated Physiology.* Fig. 16.3.)

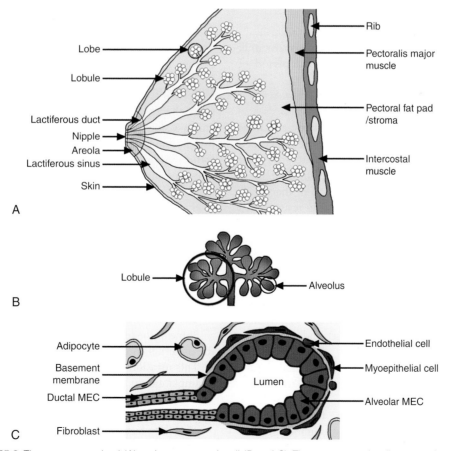

Fig. 35.2 The mammary gland (A) and mammary alveoli (B and C). The mammary alveoli are not drawn to scale; in reality, they are much smaller and more numerous. *MEC,* mammary epithelial cell. (From Truchet S, Honvo-Houéto E. Physiology of milk secretion. *Best Practice & Research: Clinical Endocrinology & Metabolism.* 2017;31(4);367–384; Fig. 2A–C.)

vasopressin, leading to large amounts of free water excretion in the urine of the mother, a condition known as diabetes insipidus of pregnancy.

Human chorionic somatomammotropin (hCS), also called human placental lactogen (hPL), is another protein hormone synthesized and secreted by the placenta. It strongly resembles prolactin and growth hormone and mimics their effects in the mother's body.

The prostaglandins are a family of related molecules derived from arachidonic acid. Among the many members of this family, prostaglandins E2 (PGE_2) and $F_2\alpha$ ($PGF_2\alpha$) are important in labor.

Clinical Correlation Box 35.1

Tumors which block the pituitary stalk and prevent the flow of dopamine from the hypothalamus to the anterior pituitary may result in hypooestrogenism with anovulatory infertility and a decrease in menstruation in women because of increased prolactin levels. Many women with hyperprolactemia also experience loss of libido, breast pain, and galactorrhea (breast milk production), and vaginal dryness.

SYSTEM FUNCTION: PREGNANCY

If pregnancy is achieved, the female reproductive system changes dramatically. The ovaries and uterus abandon their monthly cycles and instead promote:

- Growth of the fetus.
- Changes in the pelvis necessary to facilitate delivery.
- Development of the breasts necessary for lactation, or milk production, during the postpartum period, the period of time after birth.

Sexual Response in the Female

Fertilization may result from sexual intercourse between a male and female. In males and females, sexual intercourse is preceded by the condition of libido or desire, which leads to arousal or excitement in a sexual encounter. In the female, the excitement and plateau phases involve secretory lubrication of the vagina and elevation of the uterus in the pelvis. Orgasm is associated with spasm of the vaginal walls. Females can usually achieve arousal again shortly after orgasm, unlike males, who have a refractory period that increases with age.

Fertilization

Once ejaculated, sperm must undergo capacitation—cytologic changes that prepare the sperm for fusion with an egg—which occurs within the female reproductive tract and takes more than 1 hour.

- Capacitated sperm can last up to 2 days in the female reproductive tract, but for fertilization to occur, sperm must reach the oocyte within 24 hours of ovulation.

Pregnancy begins with a spermatozoon's fertilization of a secondary oocyte—an ovulated oocyte arrested in metaphase II of meiosis.

- The sperm swim from the vagina, through the cervix and uterus, and into the fallopian tube, where they encounter or wait for the oocyte in the ampulla.

- Estrogen-dependent proliferative-phase changes in the female reproductive tract encourage the sperm's progress:
  - Vaginal glycogen production acidifies the vagina and enhances sperm motility.
  - Watery cervical fluid promotes the sperm's passage, as does the enhanced contractility of the myometrium.
- Still, only one sperm in about a million reaches the ampulla. Shortly before or after the sperm's arrival, the oocyte is waved into the ampulla by the cilia lining the fallopian tube.

Each sperm cell in the ampulla penetrates the outer shell of the secondary oocyte, the corona radiata, by driving forward with flagellar movements. When one reaches the zona pellucida, a glycoprotein in the zona triggers the release of proteolytic enzymes from the acrosome, or head of the sperm (Fig. 35.3).

- The enzymes break down the zona and the sperm drives into the oocyte.
- Once a single sperm makes it through the zona pellucida, cortical granules in the oocyte release proteases in what is called the zona reaction and render the zona impenetrable to other sperm, thus ensuring that only one sperm fertilizes the egg.

Once inside the zona pellucida, the cell membranes of the sperm and egg fuse, making their cytoplasm continuous.

- This stimulates the nucleus of the secondary oocyte to exit its meiotic arrest and complete meiosis II, forming the mature haploid ovum and casting off a polar body.
- The nuclei of the mature ovum and the spermatozoon then fuse, forming a zygote with 46 chromosomes.

Development From Zygote to Embryo

Once the zygote begins to divide, it is called an embryo. The embryo slowly drifts down the fallopian tube, dividing as it travels, and enters the uterus approximately 3 days after fertilization. Although it increases in cell number along the way, it does not increase in size, which prevents it from becoming stuck in the fallopian tube.

- By the time it reaches the uterus, the embryo consists of about 12 cells clustered into a ball and is called a morula (Fig. 35.4).
- After another 3 days, the morula then develops into a blastocyst, an asymmetric ball of cells with a fluid-filled cavity inside, before it implants into the wall of the uterus.
- Thus the time from fertilization to implantation in the uterus is about 6 days.

Some of the cells of the blastocyst differentiate and grow into the maternal endometrial tissue.

- This invasion of fetal tissue into the endometrium is called implantation.
- The embryonic cells that invade the endometrium are known as trophoblasts. Importantly, it appears that the trophoblasts lack the major histocompatibility complexes by which a maternal immune response could be mounted against the foreign embryonic tissue.

Soon after implantation, the trophoblasts begin to produce hCG to maintain the corpus luteum.

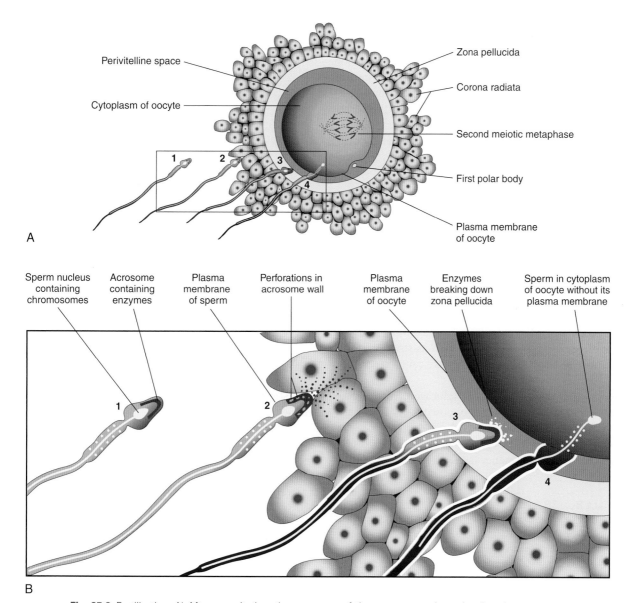

Fig. 35.3 Fertilization. A) After capacitation, the acrosome of the sperm can release its digestive enzymes. B) The enzymes digest part of the zona pellucida around the oocyte and ultimately merge the cytoplasm of the two gametes. The oocyte, arrested in metaphase II of meiosis, now resumes meiosis and generates a second polar body. (From Moore KL, Persaud TVN. *The Developing Human: Clinically Oriented Embryology.* 7th Edition. Philadelphia: WB Saunders; 2003.)

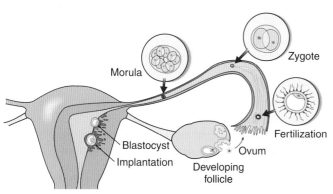

Fig. 35.4 Implantation. (From Spitz JL. *Textbook of Diagnostic Sonography.* Elsevier; 2018: p. 1177-1193; Fig. 49.1.)

The Placenta and the Hormones of Pregnancy

The placenta is a transient organ derived from embryonic tissue, which:

- Serves as the site of exchange between maternal and fetal circulations.
- Secretes hormones that maintain pregnancy.
  - Synthesized de novo: hCG and hCS.
  - Converted from maternal cholesterol: Progesterone.
  - Converted from fetal adrenal androgens: Estrogens.

Human Chorionic Gonadotropin and Human Chorionic Somatomammotropin

hCG from placental trophoblasts mimics the effects of LH and preserves the corpus luteum, and hence the endometrial functionalism, as described previously.

- hCG serum levels double approximately every 1.7 to 2 days during early pregnancy.
- It is easily detected and quantified in maternal peripheral blood.
- Trophoblastic production of hCG peaks at around the 10th week of gestation, then drops off and plateaus at a lower level.

hCG drives the secretion of progesterone from the corpus luteum, maintaining the endometrium but also by suppressing contraction of the myometrium. Progesterone secreted during pregnancy also thickens the cervical mucus and closes the cervical os to seal the uterus (see Fast Fact Box 35.1).

Fast Fact Box 35.1

If there is an early fetal demise and the production of human chorionic gonadotropin stops, the myometrium begins to contract and the endometrium begins to shed. This is known as spontaneous abortion, or miscarriage.

hCS is produced by the placenta beginning in the fourth or fifth week of gestation. In accordance with its structural similarity to growth hormone, hCS functions as a counterregulatory hormone, just as growth hormone does.

- The counterregulatory hormones (glucagon, cortisol, epinephrine, and growth hormone) oppose the effects of insulin and raise the blood glucose.
- While production of hCS begins early in pregnancy, it plays a larger role later in pregnancy (see Fast Fact Box 35.2).

Fast Fact Box 35.2

Human chorionic somatomammotropin (hCS) makes more circulating glucose available for fetal consumption. For this reason, it may contribute to gestational diabetes—high blood sugar levels associated with pregnancy.

Progesterone and Estrogen During Pregnancy

Around the 10th week of gestation, the developing placenta acquires the ability to convert maternal cholesterol into progesterone, thereby eliminating the dependence on the corpus luteum for progesterone to maintain the pregnancy.

Meanwhile, hCG stimulates the fetal adrenal glands to produce large amounts of androgens (mainly dehydroepiandrosterone), which circulate to the aromatase-rich placenta and are converted to estrogens. The placenta thus keeps the maternal circulation high in progesterone and estrogen.

- High levels of progesterone and estrogen feed back negatively on the hypothalamus and pituitary, suppressing LH and FSH secretion and thereby inhibiting follicular development and ovulation until the pregnancy ends.
- In addition, progesterone continues to maintain the quiescence of the myometrium and opposes the softening of the cervix seen during labor, preventing premature birth.
- Estrogen causes breast development in anticipation of lactation and stimulates prolactin production in the pituitary lactotrophs (see Clinical Correlation Box 35.2).

Clinical Correlation Box 35.2

Mifepristone, sometimes called "the abortion pill," serves as a competitive inhibitor of progesterone at its receptor. This leads to cervical softening and uterine contraction, which can lead to abortion within the first 9 weeks of pregnancy. It is sometimes used in combination with an orally or vaginally administered prostaglandin analog, misoprostol, which softens the cervical tissue just as endogenous prostaglandins do during labor. It can also prevent implantation of the embryo if administered within 72 hours of unprotected sex.

The Effects of Pregnancy Outside the Reproductive System

The organ systems must meet the added demand for energy, oxygen, and nutrients posed by the developing fetus. Thus a woman's body undergoes significant physiologic changes during pregnancy, which may be classified into two broad categories:
1. Altered organ function because of hormonal milieu
2. Physiologic adaption to mechanical and metabolic stresses

Changes in Metabolism

Early pregnancy is characterized by anabolism, while later pregnancy is characterized by catabolism. In a way, pregnancy constitutes a transfer of potential energy from mother to child.

- In early pregnancy, the synthesis of lipids, glycogen, and protein increases under the influence of insulin.
- In late pregnancy, high levels of placental hSC and corticotropin-releasing hormone (leading to increased cortisol, a counterregulatory hormone) promote the degradation of maternal lipids, glycogen, and proteins to supply fatty acids, glucose, and amino acids to the growing fetus.

For bone, transferring maternal stores to the fetus would compromise the integrity of the maternal skeleton. Consequently, the placenta recruits calcium needed for fetal ossification not from endogenous sources, but from dietary sources through ramping up vitamin D, which increases calcium absorption from the maternal intestines.

Finally, placental estrogen increases the hepatic synthesis of thyroid-binding globulin (TBG) and decreases the hepatic clearance of TBG.

- Increased TBG results in increased total maternal thyroxine levels, as more thyroid hormone is produced to fill the TBG reservoir.
- Maternal thyroxine demand increases independently of changes in TBG, which may reflect first-trimester losses of thyroxine to the fetus.

Cardiovascular, Hematologic, and Renal Changes

During pregnancy, several key cardiovascular changes occur:
- Decreased systemic vascular resistance (SVR)
  - Partially because of increased prostaglandins, which decrease blood vessel sensitivity to angiotensin II, a vasoconstrictor, and cause vasodilation.
  - Decidua basalis also adds parallel vasculature (the spiral arteries, intervillous space, and uterine veins), which increases the cross-sectional area of the circulatory system and thus reduces resistance.

- Increased cardiac output
- Increased activity of the renin-angiotensin-aldosterone system
  - Likely maintains blood pressure through extracellular fluid volume conservation rather than direct vasoconstriction during pregnancy.
  - Increases plasma volume by around 45% during third trimester, which can account for about 6 to 8 kg of weight gain during pregnancy.

These cardiovascular changes are accompanied by several hematologic changes:

- Increased erythrocyte volume
  - By 20% to 40%, depending on the availability of iron stores.
  - Occurs because of elevated erythropoietin levels.
- Decreased hematocrit
  - Occurs because the plasma volume generally increases in excess of the increase in blood cell mass.
  - Hematocrit is expected to drop by 4% to 7%.

For the renal system, increased systemic blood flow translates into:

- Increased renal blood flow
- Increased glomerular filtration rate (GFR)
  - GFR increases by nearly half again (then plateaus) by week 10.
- Decreased serum creatinine and urea nitrogen levels
  - Because of increased GFR results in lower serum creatinine and urea nitrogen levels.
- Increased urinary frequency and volume
  - Initially because of increased GFR.
  - Later in pregnancy, the uterus compresses the bladder, limiting bladder volume and increasing the frequency and urgency of urination.
- Decreased threshold for antidiuretic hormone secretion
  - Aids in increasing plasma volume, also supporting blood pressure in the face of decreased SVR (see Fast Fact Box 35.3).

Fast Fact Box 35.3

In late pregnancy, the gravid uterus can also compress the inferior vena cava (IVC), especially when the pregnant mother lies in the supine position (on her back) or on the right side (where the IVC is located). This compression results in impaired venous return to the heart and may lead to lightheadedness. For this reason, pregnant women are encouraged to lie on their left side.

Pulmonary Changes

Pulmonary function during pregnancy is influenced by two factors:

1. Decreased lung volumes owing to pressure from the enlarging uterus.
2. Increased tidal volumes because of progesterone's stimulatory effect.

As the uterus grows, it pushes up on the diaphragm, thus decreasing the space available in the thorax. Functional residual capacity (FRC)—the lung volume after a passive exhalation with breathing muscles at rest—decreases. However, the diaphragm can still contract normally, and airway function is normal.

Tidal volume, the size of each normal inhalation, increases during pregnancy because of progesterone's stimulation of increased central respiratory drive.

- Increased tidal volumes raise the partial pressure of oxygen (PO_2) and lead to respiratory alkalosis, which is compensated by increased renal excretion of bicarbonate.
- Increased PO_2 in maternal blood helps drive the diffusion of oxygen from the intervillous blood into the chorionic capillaries.
- The high oxygen affinity of fetal hemoglobin compared with adult hemoglobin further supports this oxygen transfer.

Table 35.1 summarizes the maternal changes during pregnancy.

Parturition

Parturition is the medical term for birth, which takes place after roughly 40 weeks of gestation in humans.

Uncoordinated uterine contractions (called Braxton-Hicks contractions) and cervical softening begin around 1 month before the end of gestation. However, parturition itself commences with the accelerated cervical dilation and coordinated uterine contractions known as labor.

- The contractions of labor, unlike Braxton-Hicks contractions, get increasingly stronger, longer, and closer together.
- Close to or during labor, the chorionic and amniotic membranes rupture under pressure (commonly referred to as "water breaking").
- The contractions ultimately drive the fetus out of the uterus and through the dilated cervix and vagina.

The preparation of the perineum for its role as birth canal is promoted by relaxin, which also acts to loosen the pelvic ligaments and soften the pubic symphysis.

The placenta is expelled soon after delivery of the baby, and intense uterine contractions, possibly driven by oxytocin, help staunch uterine bleeding via vasospasm and constriction of blood flow.

- When the placenta vacates the uterus, its hormonal influence goes with it.
- Placental hormones remain in the maternal blood for a duration dictated by their respective half-lives, then disappear.
- Placental progesterone and estrogen levels fall, releasing the hypothalamus and pituitary from their inhibition (see Physiology Integration Box 35.1).

Physiology Integration Box 35.1

The initiation of parturition in humans is not well understood.

- Oxytocin and locally acting prostaglandins promote uterine contractions, but they do not seem to be the initial or crucial elements in the signaling pathway.
- At labor, the myometrium may express increased numbers of oxytocin receptors.
- It has also been theorized that a change in the uterine ratio of progesterone and estrogen allows the myometrium to escape the inhibitory influence of progesterone.
- A critical fetal mass may also stretch the uterus to the point where reflex contractions begin.
- Another possibility is that fetal or maternal stress may trigger a rise in placental corticotropin-releasing hormone levels, which in turn may somehow trigger the cascade of events leading to birth.

- LH and FSH are once again secreted and follicular development resumes.

TABLE 35.1   Maternal Changes During Pregnancy

Maternal Organ or Parameter Affected During Pregnancy	Change During Pregnancy	Cause of Change
Myometrium	Contractions are suppressed	Progesterone At first produced in corpus luteum under influence of trophoblastic hCG, then produced directly by placenta
Cervix	Cervical os is closed, cervical connective tissue stabilized	Progesterone From corpus luteum and then placenta
Pituitary	LH and FSH secretion suppressed	Progesterone and estrogen From corpus luteum, then placenta
	Prolactin production increased	Estrogen From placenta
Ovary	Follicular development and ovulation suppressed	Low LH and FSH
Breast	Development of secretory apparatus, increase in size	Estrogen (from placenta) and prolactin (from pituitary)
Energy stores	Increase early in pregnancy	Insulin and other factors?
	Depleted to release fatty acids, glucose, and amino acids to fetus later in pregnancy	hCS, cortisol?
Serum calcium	Maternal ionized calcium remains stable, but gut absorption increases	Vitamin D (activated by placenta)
Thyroxine-binding globulin (TBG) and thyroxine level	Hepatic synthesis of TBG increased hepatic clearance of TBG decreased; total thyroxine level thus increased	Estrogen From placenta
Systemic vascular resistance (SVR)	Decreased	Prostaglandins (which decrease vessel sensitivity to angiotensin II) Addition of decidua basalis circuit
Cardiac output	Increased	?
ECF volume	Increased	RAA system
Red blood cell mass	Increased	Erythropoietin
Hematocrit	Decreased	ECF volume increased out of proportion in increases in RBC mass
Pedal edema	May appear in late pregnancy	Increased ECF volume
Venous return to the heart	May be decreased late in pregnancy in supine position	Uterine compression of inferior vena cava
GFR	Increased	Increased cardiac output Increased ECF volume
Bladder	Increased urinary frequency	Increased GFR Later in pregnancy, uterine compression of bladder
Osmoreceptor complex	ADH set point decreased; ADH more easily released	?
Functional residual volume	Decreased	Uterine compression of diaphragm at rest
Tidal volumes and P_aO_2	Increased	Progesterone From placenta

ECF, extracellular fluid; GFR, glomerular filtration rate; RAA, Renin-Angiotensin-Aldosterone; RBC, red blood cell; ADH, anti-diuretic hormone; LH, luteinizing hormone; FSH, follicle stimulating hormone; hCS, human chorionic somatomammotropin; hCG, human chorionic gonadotropin

Lactation and Mammary Physiology

The American Academy of Pediatrics advocates breastfeeding as "the ideal method of feeding and nurturing infants." Indeed, evolution has refined the breast's principal function—lactation—so that it serves the newborn child in every way possible.

- The reflex arc that governs milk production ensures that the supply of milk will always meet but not exceed the demands of the baby, thereby conserving maternal energy stores.
- In addition, a baby's suckling suppresses further menstrual cycles in its mother. This helps prevent another pregnancy too close to the first, so that maternal resources are conserved for the newborn exclusively.
- Breast milk is easily ingested by a naïve nervous and digestive system.
- Breast milk transmits physiologic gut flora to the infant (the symbiotic bacteria that inhabit the intestinal tract and protect

against harmful pathogens) and may pass on antibodies and factors that activate and modulate the naïve infantile immune system.

Breast Development

During pregnancy, the breasts undergo growth and development under the influence of estrogen, progesterone, prolactin, and hCS. In this state, the breasts differentiate into functional lactational units.

- The inactive terminal alveolar cells in the mammary gland lobules are converted into active milk-secreting units.
- After the birth of the baby, prolactin will be the main stimulus to the breast to produce milk.
- During pregnancy, however, the high levels of progesterone block this effect by inhibiting the action of prolactin at its receptors.

Postpartum Breast Function

Whereas progesterone helps the secretory apparatus to develop, it also inhibits its activation. During the high progesterone exposure of pregnancy, the breast cannot produce milk but instead produces colostrum.

- Colostrum is a thin fluid rich in nutrients and antibodies.
- It is secreted from the breast for the first 3 to 4 days of breastfeeding postpartum.

As maternal levels of estrogen and progesterone drop in the wake of placental expulsion, prolactin acts on the breasts unimpeded.

- Prolactin is cleared more slowly, taking at least 7 days to reach prepregnancy levels.
- This brief period of high prolactin levels without the inhibitory progesterone leads to the production of milk within the lobules of the mammary gland.

After this initial milk production, the newborn must suckle the nipples to maintain milk production and to elicit milk secretion. This is the reflex arc of lactation (Fig. 35.5).

- When the infant suckles at the breast, tactile sensors in the areola are activated, stimulating the hypothalamus and triggering the release of oxytocin from the posterior pituitary.
- Oxytocin travels through the bloodstream to the breast ductal systems, where it causes the myoepithelial cells that line the lactiferous ducts to contract, leading to the secretion of preformed milk from the ducts.

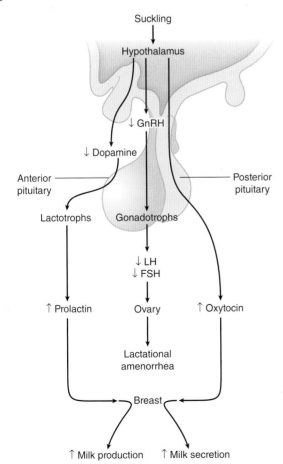

Fig. 35.5 The reflex arc of lactation. *FSH,* Follicle-stimulating hormone; *GnRH,* gonadotropin-releasing hormone; *LH,* luteinizing hormone.

The production of new milk is governed in a similar fashion but is activated by prolactin.

- Suckling at the breast not only promotes oxytocin secretion from the neurohypophysis, but also inhibits the hypothalamic production of the neurotransmitter dopamine.
- Because dopamine inhibits prolactin release from the anterior pituitary, decreased dopamine output leads to increased prolactin output.
- Prolactin then travels to the terminal ducts and causes milk production there.

The longer the infant suckles, the more prolactin is secreted and the more milk is produced. In this way, the infant regulates its own food supply.

- If the infant is not satisfied by the amount of milk in the breast at a given meal, it will suckle longer, the prolactin released during this feeding episode will be greater, and a larger supply of milk will be produced for the next meal.
- If a given meal is too large, the infant will stop suckling when full and the next meal will consequently be smaller.
- When suckling is discontinued for a prolonged period, milk production ceases and the breasts gradually return to their prepregnancy state.

Breastfeeding also suppresses ovarian function and fertility.

- This delay in return to normal menstrual cycles in a breastfeeding mother is called lactational amenorrhea.
- Suckling is thought to disrupt the pulsatile pattern of gonadotropin-releasing hormone release from the hypothalamus and LH and FSH release from the pituitary.
- Follicular development, ovulation, and endometrial development are thus suppressed (see Clinical Correlation Box 35.3).

Clinical Correlation Box 35.3

In vitro fertilization (IVF) is a form of assisted reproductive technology that involves the following phases:
- Superovulation: Pharmacologic stimulation of the ovary with recombinant follicle-stimulating hormone (FSH) to produce several Graafian follicles.
- Egg collection: Graafian follicles are aspirated from the ovary via a needle.
- Sperm preparation: Sperm are washed and selected for healthy appearance.
- In vitro insemination: Collected oocytes are placed in a test tube or Petri dish with thousands of sperm.
- Embryo transfer: Viable embryos are transferred into the uterus through a catheter, with supplemental progesterone given to ensure the uterus is hospitable for implantation. Unused embryos may be frozen.

Alternative methods include medical or surgical treatment of underlying causes of infertility, ovulation induction by recombinant FSH or estrogen antagonists, such as clomiphene citrate, intrauterine insemination (IUI), and intracytoplasmic sperm injection (ICSI).

Disorders of Pregnancy

An ectopic pregnancy, also known as a tubal pregnancy, is a pregnancy in which the embryo never passed from the fallopian tube to the uterus.

- The embryo grows, some of its cells differentiate into trophoblasts, and the trophoblasts ultimately begin to invade the fallopian tube as they would the endometrium.

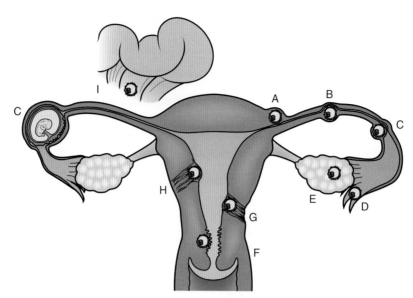

Fig. 35.6 Ectopic pregnancy. Ninety-five percent of ectopic pregnancies occur in the fallopian tube: in the interstitial (A), isthmic (B), ampullary (C, most common), and fimbrial (D) portions. Extratubal ectopic pregnancies may be found in ovarian (E), cervical (F), cesarean scar (G), myometrial scar (H), and abdominal (I) locations. (From Baltarowich OH, Scoutt LM. Ectopic pregnancy. In: *Callen's Ultrasonography in Obstetrics and Gynecology.* Elsevier; 2017: p. 966-1000. Fig. 33.1.)

- This can lead to severe hemorrhage.
- Although hCG is still produced by the ectopic trophoblasts, hCG levels are usually lower than in intrauterine pregnancies (Fig. 35.6).

A spontaneous abortion (miscarriage), mentioned earlier, is a fairly common complication of pregnancy.

- Although it usually represents a psychologic more than a physical threat to the mother, retained products of conception can lead to bleeding or infection.
- Miscarriages are most often managed surgically (by vacuum aspiration), but in pregnancies of less than 8 weeks' gestation, expectant management is possible and the body may expel the pregnancy on its own.

Even in a pregnancy that is successfully maintained, several diseases can arise as the direct result of pregnancy.

- In late pregnancy, the catabolic shift in maternal metabolism may result in low insulin reserve and high serum glucose, resulting in gestational diabetes mellitus.
- Preeclampsia is a very common and serious disorder of the endothelium, occurring after twenty weeks of pregnancy. It affects the liver, kidneys, and vascular system, leading to decreased placental perfusion and systemic vasoconstriction that can lead to multi-organ dysfunction. Its origin has been obscure because there has been no experimental animal model to elucidate it. However, recently preeclampsia has been shown to implicate a tyrosine kinase, sFLT-1, that originates in the placenta and increases maternal blood flow. While sFLT-1 increases the flow of nutrients to the fetus, the damage may be significant, including glomerular albuminuria and severe hypertension for the mother and placental ischemia for the fetus. If preeclampsia progresses to cause a new onset tonic clonic seizure in the mother, it is deemed ecclampsia. Magnesium sulfate is the treatment of choice to prevent such seizures.

The placenta is the source of 1,25 $(OH)_2$ vitamin D3. When the placenta is ischemic, this hormone production is reduced unless calcium is excreted in the maternal urine. Patients with preeclampsia have been found to have low urinary calcium excretion because of the association with placental health.

The placenta also produces an enzyme known as oxytocinase to prevent premature labor early in pregnancy. In multiple gestations, this enzyme level can be very high because of the large placental mass. Since oxytocin produced by the posterior pituitary gland is close in structure to vasopressin, an excess of oxytocinase/vasopressinase causes diabetes insipidus of pregnancy.

The placenta is also a source of renin, an enzyme that converts angiotensinogen to angiotensin I and II, which may be important for maternal vascular regulation.

Disorders of Parturition

A preterm birth is one that occurs before 37 weeks of gestation. It may occur spontaneously, or it may be induced by a doctor to protect the wellbeing of the mother or fetus.

- Preterm birth threatens the premature infant because its lungs and other organs are not fully developed and are not ready to negotiate extrauterine life.
- Inadequate surfactant production in the infant's lungs is a major complication of preterm birth because it compromises the infant's ability to breathe and oxygenate, leading to neonatal respiratory distress syndrome.

Causes of preterm labor are numerous and include:
- Infection of the reproductive tract or placental tissues
- Infection of the urinary tract
- Premature rupture of membranes (PROM)
- Preeclampsia or eclampsia
- Cervical incompetence

- Placental abruption (premature detachment of the placenta from the uterus)
- Multiple gestation
- Fetal distress (which may arise from many causes, including placental insufficiency, see Fast Fact Box 35.4)

Fast Fact Box 35.4

Fetal distress is assessed by monitoring the fetal heart rate (FHR), and fetal bradycardia (FHR <120 beats per minute) is suggestive of fetal distress.

If labor begins too soon, the underlying cause may sometimes be treated:
- Antibiotics may be administered for an infection of the membranes.
- Medications called tocolytics may also be used to forestall labor.
  - Terbutaline relaxes smooth muscle by sympathomimetic beta-2 agonism.
  - Magnesium sulfate's mechanism of tocolysis is still not understood.

Conditions, such as preeclampsia, PROM, or fetal distress, on the other hand, may necessitate induced labor with intravenous oxytocin and transvaginal prostaglandins to avert further risk to mother and fetus.

Other factors may necessitate a cesarean section, or abdominal surgery to deliver the fetus (Fig. 35.7).
- Causes include placenta previa (a placenta covering the cervix and positioned between the cervix and fetus—"placenta first"), unusual fetal positioning within the mother's pelvis, unsuccessful labor, hemorrhage, and fetal distress.
- A cesarean section may be performed in response to labor complications, or it may be planned.
- A complicated labor process may lead to hypoxic injury to the infant and consequent brain damage.

During parturition, fetal and maternal blood may mix in the uterus, which may lead to certain complications. For example, this may occur if the fetus has inherited from its father a different blood type than the mother's.
- This is because the mother's immune system may develop antibodies against that fetal red blood cell antigen.
- If the mother carries a second child with the same fetal blood antigens, the maternal antibodies may cross the placenta and attack the fetal red blood cells.

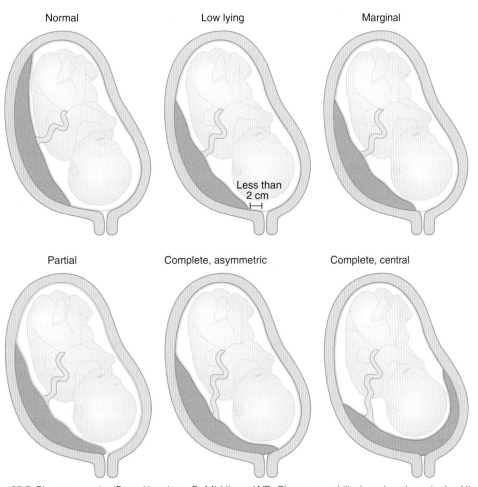

Fig. 35.7 Placenta previa. (From Hertzberg B, Middleton WD. Placenta, umbilical cord, and cervix. In: *Ultrasound: The Requisites*. Elsevier; 2016: p. 469-495; Fig. 20.11.)

This results in hemolytic anemia in the fetus, which may continue into infancy, when it is called hemolytic disease of the newborn (HDN).

- HDN can occur in response to foreign A or B blood types (ABO incompatibility), but it more commonly occurs in response to Rh factor on the fetal red blood cells.
- If the fetus is Rh positive and the mother is Rh negative, blood mixing will provoke a maternal immune reaction.
- For this reason, Rh-negative mothers are administered intravenous RhoGAM before parturition. RhoGAM is a preparation of antibody to Rh factor.
  - If any fetal red blood cells bearing the Rh factor mix with maternal blood, the RhoGAM antibodies bind to them.
  - Once bound to RhoGAM antibody, the Rh antigen does not elicit a maternal immune response.
- The maternal immune response to Rh factor is called Rh disease, or erythroblastosis fetalis (see Clinical Correlation Box 33.4).

Clinical Correlation Box 35.4

Prenatal diagnosis and prenatal screening are used to test for potential birth defects in a fetus before birth. Conditions or diseases commonly tested for include neural tube defects, Down syndrome, cystic fibrosis, or Tay-Sachs disease, among many others. Sex determination of the fetus is also a commonly requested test. Multiple methods are available, including chorionic villus sampling, amniocentesis, and ultrasound.

- In chorionic villus sampling, a sample of the chorionic villi is removed transcervically or transabdominally at around 10 to 12 weeks' gestation and is subsequently tested for genetic defects.
- Amniocentesis is performed later than chorionic villus sampling at around 16 to 22 weeks' gestation and involves removing a small amount of amniotic fluid from the amniotic sac, which is then tested for genetic defects.
- Finally, ultrasound is a noninvasive procedure which is commonly used to determine information, such as the progress of fetal growth and development or the sex of the fetus.

SUMMARY

- An egg must be fertilized within a day of ovulation. Fertility therefore lasts from around 2 days before ovulation to 1 day after.
- Fertilization stimulates the nucleus of the secondary oocyte to complete meiosis II and sperm and egg nuclei fuse, leading to the formation of a diploid zygote. Implantation takes place in the uterus 6 days later when embryonic trophoblasts invade the endometrium and start making hCG.
- The placenta serves as the point of exchange between the circulatory systems of the mother and fetus and is also a hormone-producing organ.

- Pregnancy leads to several key physiologic changes:
  - SVR drops.
  - Cardiac output and GFR increase.
  - FRC decreases, but tidal volume and P_aO_2 increase.
- Labor is the acceleration of uterine contractions and cervical softening and dilation that together lead to parturition (birth)

REVIEW QUESTIONS

Directions: Each of the numbered items or incomplete statements in this section is followed by answers or by completions of the statement. Select the one lettered answer or completion that is best in each case.

1. A 23-year-old woman is 34 weeks pregnant. She has no past medical history of any significant disease. Her body mass index prepregnancy was 28.5 kg/m² (normal range is 18.5–24.9 kg/m²). She notes increased urinary frequency and volume and feels profoundly fatigued. Her blood glucose is elevated, and a urinalysis shows significant glucosuria. Which of the following could contribute to her gestational diabetes?
   A. Increased concentrations of human growth hormone from the fetus acting on the mother through cortisol.
   B. Increased concentrations of human chorionic somatomammotropin ([hCS]; also known as human placental lactogen [hPL]) from the placenta.
   C. Increased concentrations of insulin from the mother's pancreatic beta islet cells in response to diffusion of glucose from the fetal circulation to the maternal circulation.
   D. Production of maternal antibodies that bind to glucagon and prevent it from agonizing its receptor.
2. A 28-year-old woman is pregnant, in her second trimester, when she presents with polyuria, constipation, fatigue,

nausea, and headaches. Her serum calcium concentration and parathyroid hormone (PTH) concentrations are elevated, and an ultrasound of her neck demonstrates a single enlarged parathyroid gland suggestive of a parathyroid adenoma. Which of the following might affect the baby within hours after birth?
   A. Rickets
   B. Hypomagnesemia
   C. Hyporeflexia
   D. Seizures
3. A 32-year-old woman with diabetes is pregnant. Knowing that plasma glucose can diffuse across the placenta from the maternal to the fetal circulation but that insulin (endogenous or exogenous) does not, which of the following do you expect in the case of this woman if she does not change her diabetes regimen and develops hyperglycemia during pregnancy? In utero, the fetus will have a(n) _____ serum concentration of _____ and after birth the fetus will have a(n) _____ serum concentration of _____.
   A. Increased…. Glucagon…. Increased…. Insulin
   B. Decreased…. Glucagon…. Increased…. Cortisol
   C. Increased…. Insulin…. Decreased…. Glucose
   D. Decreased…. Insulin…. Increased…. Glucose

ANSWERS TO REVIEW QUESTIONS

1. **The answer is B.** hCS, like many placental hormones, increases blood glucose and is believed to contribute to the pathophysiology of gestational diabetes. Growth hormone from the fetus is unlikely to reach significant levels in the mother (A). Whereas the increase in her own blood glucose levels (more likely than from the fetal circulation) may indeed increase her production and release of insulin, this would be expected to limit hyperglycemia (C). Glucagon increases the plasma glucose concentration, so in the unlikely event that maternal autoantibodies antagonized glucagon's effects, this would also tend to lower the plasma glucose, not increase it.

2. **The answer is D.** In utero, the baby will be exposed to an abnormally elevated calcium concentration because of the mother's hyperparathyroidism. Normally, the baby needs calcium from the mother in the development of well mineralized bone. Under the conditions in this case, the chronically elevated serum [Ca^{2+}] will suppress the baby's PTH production. With birth, the baby suffers an abrupt decrease in the supply of Ca^{2+} and since the baby's endogenous PTH production has been suppressed, hypocalcemia can result. This may lead to neonatal hyperreflexia and seizures. Hyporeflexia is more consistent with hypercalcemia. While low magnesium concentrations can stimulate PTH secretion, low PTS states are typically seen with a normal magnesium. Rickets is associated with low vitamin D levels and typically presents in children rather than in neonates.

3. **The answer is C.** Because glucose crosses the placenta, if the mother becomes hyperglycemic, the baby will also. This will increase fetal endogenous insulin production (and suppress fetal glucagon) in an attempt to limit the fetal hyperglycemia. After the baby is born, the supply of glucose from the maternal circulation via placental transfer will be stopped, the high concentration of insulin in the baby will drive down the plasma glucose. If the effects of chronically elevated insulin in the baby continue after parturition, the baby may become acutely hypoglycemic and suffer a neonatal seizure.

36

The Male Reproductive System

INTRODUCTION

The male reproductive system has three principal functions:

1. The differentiation and maintenance of the primary and secondary sex characteristics under the influence of the hormone testosterone, made in the testes.
2. Spermatogenesis: The creation of the male gametes inside the testes.
3. The penile delivery of sperm from the testes into the female's vagina in the act of procreation. This includes penile erection and ejaculation.

SYSTEM STRUCTURE

The male reproductive system is comprised not only the male genitals, but also the central nervous system (CNS) components—namely, the hypothalamus and pituitary regulate the performance of the male reproductive system.

- At the CNS level, male and female anatomy and histology are more or less the same
- For more details on the hypothalamic and pituitary structures involved in human reproduction, see the discussion in Chapter 29.

In the section that follows, we will focus on the anatomy and histology of the testes, the penis, and the ductal connections between the testes and penis.

The Testes

The male gonads, or testes, are each about 4 cm long and are suspended from the perineum in an external contractile sac called the scrotum (Fig. 36.1A).

- The testes are perfused by the spermatic arteries, which are closely apposed with the spermatic venous plexus.
- This permits countercurrent heat exchange between artery and vein, cooling the blood that flows to the testes.
- Countercurrent heat exchange helps keep the testicular temperature cool enough for optimal spermatogenesis (1° C–2° C cooler than body temperature).
- The external location of the testes in the scrotum serves as a second important cooling mechanism.

Because the testes develop within the abdomen, they descend into the scrotum during fetal life, reaching the deep inguinal rings around week 28 of gestation and inhabiting the scrotum by birth (see Clinical Correlation Box 36.1).

The testes are composed of coiled seminiferous tubules embedded in connective tissue (Fig. 36.1B).

- The connective tissue, which makes up about 20% of the testicular mass, contains Leydig cells, which make testosterone.
- The seminiferous tubules, constituting 80% of the testicular mass, generate the sperm.

The seminiferous tubules contain two main cell types:

- Spermatogonia are the germ cells that undergo meiosis to give rise to spermatids, the immediate precursors to spermatozoa.
  - Spermatogonia sit outside the blood-testis barrier near the basement membrane.
  - They continually conduct mitosis, the products of which are pushed toward the tubule lumen and undergo meiosis and differentiation into sperm cells.
- Sertoli cells, which completely envelop and protect the spermatids, sealing them off from any contact with the tubules' outer basement membrane or blood supply.
  - This Sertoli sheath hence forms a blood-testis barrier to protect the male gametes from any harmful bloodborne agents, as well as autoimmunity.
  - Sertoli cells also transport nutrients, oxygen, and hormones, such as testosterone, to the spermatids.
  - The Sertoli barrier is fluid and accommodates the passage of cells developing into spermatids.

The testes make around 120 million sperm a day. As they differentiate, the sperm migrate into the tubule lumen for transport distally to the rete testis, a plexus of ducts that collects sperm from each of roughly 900 seminiferous tubules.

- The rete testis empties into the epididymis, a single coiled tubule running from the top of the testis down its posterior aspect.
- In the epididymis, sperm are stored and undergo maturation before continuing their voyage outside the testis.

The Ducts and Penis

Each epididymis leads to a long, straight tube called the vas deferens (Fig. 36.1C).

- Each vas deferens enters the scrotum and then runs along the posterior pelvic wall.

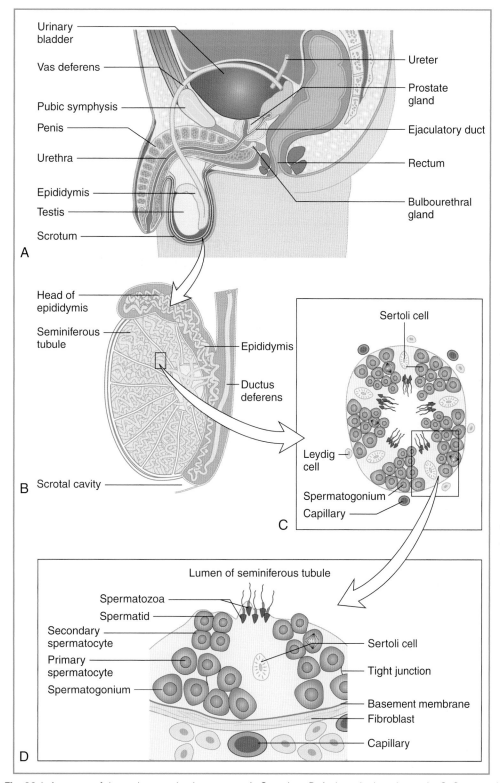

Fig. 36.1 Anatomy of the male reproductive system. A, Overview. B, A closer look at the testis. C, Gross and microscopic anatomy of the male reproductive system. The male reproductive system consists of the external penis, testis, and scrotum and the internal vas deferens, prostate gland, and bulbourethral gland. The histology of the testis is complex, revealing that maturation of the spermatozoa is supported by the Sertoli cells. (From Carroll. *Elsevier's Integrated Physiology.* Fig. 15.3.)

- Here the two vas deferens tubes widen into ampullae, which are attached to glands called the seminal vesicles, which secrete more than half the volume of the semen.
- The two ampullae each send an ejaculatory duct through the prostate gland, which subsequently joins the urethra (see Fast Fact Box 36.1).

Fast Fact Box 36.1

From this point onward, the male urethra serves as part of both the reproductive and urinary tracts, unlike female anatomy, in which the reproductive and urinary tracts are completely separate. Male physiology ensures that micturition and ejaculation do not occur simultaneously.

- The urethra next passes through the muscle tissue of the urogenital diaphragm, a consciously controllable sphincter. Sitting just under the urogenital diaphragm are the bulbourethral glands (also called Cowper's glands), which lubricate the urethra with mucus.

Finally, the urethra enters the penis. The cylindrical penis houses the urethra in erectile tissue, which helps effect the transition between the excretory and reproductive functions of the urethra (Fig. 36.2).

- The erectile tissue contains cavernous sinuses that fill with blood under circumstances of increased penile blood flow, leading to erection of the penis.
- When erect, the penis may be inserted into the vagina so that sperm may be delivered to the fallopian tubes.

The erectile tissue is present in three cylinders inside the penis, each called a corpus cavernosum and together called the corpora cavernosa.

- Two of the corpora lie dorsally and are sheathed by the ischiocavernosus muscles.

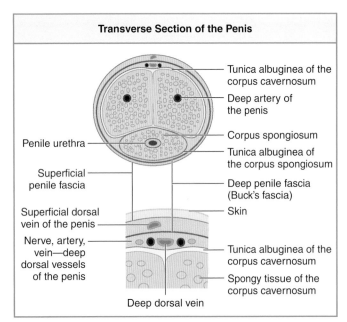

Transverse Section of the Penis

- Tunica albuginea of the corpus cavernosum
- Deep artery of the penis
- Corpus spongiosum
- Penile urethra
- Tunica albuginea of the corpus spongiosum
- Superficial penile fascia
- Deep penile fascia (Buck's fascia)
- Superficial dorsal vein of the penis
- Skin
- Nerve, artery, vein—deep dorsal vessels of the penis
- Tunica albuginea of the corpus cavernosum
- Spongy tissue of the corpus cavernosum
- Deep dorsal vein

Fig. 36.2 Cross section of the penis. (From Bogart. *Elsevier's Integrated Anatomy and Embryology.* Fig. 7.35.)

- One lies ventrally and is sheathed by the bulbospongiosus muscle. The ventral corpus cavernosum is also called the corpus spongiosum, and it is special in that it contains the urethra and forms the glans penis, the spongy head of the penis.
- The corpora are each supplied by a cavernous artery that gives out helicine arteries (see Fast Fact Box 36.2).

Fast Fact Box 36.2

The penis averages 8.8 cm (3.5 in) in length when flaccid and 12.9 cm (5.1 in) when erect, indicating no correlation between flaccid and erect size.

SYSTEM FUNCTION

Just as the female reproductive system, the activities of the male reproductive system are coordinated by the hypothalamic-pituitary-gonadal axis, in this case the hypothalamic-pituitary-testicular (HPT) axis (Fig. 36.3). (The gonadal HPT axis is not to be confused with the hypothalamic-pituitary-thyroid axis, also labeled HPT.)

- Gonadotropin-releasing hormone (GnRH) is the key hypothalamic hormone for both male and female reproductive systems.

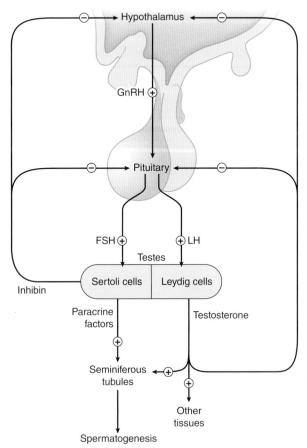

Fig. 36.3 Hypothalamic-pituitary-testicular axis. *Plus signs* represent stimulation; *minus signs* represent inhibition. *FSH,* Follicle-stimulating hormone; *GnRH,* gonadotropin-releasing hormone; *LH,* luteinizing hormone.

- Follicle-stimulating hormone (FSH) and luteinizing hormone (LH) are the key pituitary hormones for both systems, and are also known as gonadotropins (see Fast Fact Box 36.3).

Fast Fact Box 36.3

Gonadotropins are named for their female reproductive functions, but they act in the male patients nonetheless.

The same array of gonadal steroid hormones that is produced by the ovary is also synthesized by the male reproductive system, but in different proportions because of the differential expression of enzymes in the steroid synthesis pathway.

- The female gonad makes predominantly progesterone and estrogen, while the male gonad predominantly makes the androgen steroid hormone testosterone.
- Testosterone inhibits the secretion of GnRH, LH, and FSH in a classic negative-feedback loop.

The Hypothalamic-Pituitary-Testicular Axis

GnRH is the initial driver of testicular function. It is secreted in a pulsatile fashion (one pulse every 1–3 hours) and distributes to the pituitary gonadotrophs through the hypothalamic-pituitary portal circulation. There, the releasing hormone stimulates the LH- and FSH-secreting cells.

- Each GnRH pulse directly prompts an LH pulse from the gonadotrophs.
- More frequent or larger-amplitude GnRH pulses result in more frequent or larger-amplitude LH pulses.
- GnRH also increases FSH release, but the correlation between GnRH and FSH release is not as exact.

LH acts on the Leydig cells and promotes testosterone synthesis (Fig. 36.4):

- The LH signal is transduced by a seven-transmembrane receptor linked through a G protein to adenylyl cyclase, which produces cyclic adenosine monophosphate (cAMP).
- LH-dependent elevations in cAMP promote testosterone synthesis from cholesterol and promote the growth of Leydig cells.
  - Testosterone synthesis is increased by the activation and increased expression of key proteins involved in steroidogenesis, such as the steroidogenic acute regulatory (StAR) protein (see Fast Fact Box 36.4).

Fast Fact Box 36.4

The Leydig cells of the testis are unique in their ability to make testosterone in large amounts. Although the zona reticulata cells of the adrenal gland also make androgens, the adrenal pathway stops at androstenedione, the immediate precursor to testosterone. Certain peripheral tissues can make testosterone from androstenedione.

FSH, meanwhile, binds to receptors on the Sertoli cells and performs three main functions:

- Activates the production of proteins involved in spermatogenesis.
- Stimulates glucose metabolism, thereby providing energy to the sperm precursors (spermatogenesis will be discussed in more detail later).

- Upregulates the expression of the androgen receptor in Sertoli cells, thereby potentiating the influence of testosterone upon spermatogenesis.

Like all steroids, testosterone binds an intracellular receptor, which binds deoxyribonucleic acid (DNA) transcription factors and influences gene expression.

- The distribution of testosterone receptors in the body tissues determines the targets of testosterone action.
- Target tissues express 5α-reductase, an enzyme that converts testosterone to its more active form, dihydrotestosterone (DHT), which binds more avidly to the androgen receptor than does testosterone itself.

Testosterone from the Leydig cells passes through the Sertoli cells and into the seminiferous tubules, where, alongside FSH, it promotes spermatogenesis.

- The Sertoli cells make androgen-binding protein (ABP), which helps them to retain testosterone

Testosterone also acts systemically, promoting growth and sustaining gene expression in many peripheral tissues.

- Testosterone is transported in the blood by sex hormone-binding protein (SHBP), also called sex hormone-binding globulin, a liver-produced carrier protein that is structurally similar to ABP.
- It is thought that testosterone and SHBP itself may act at cell membrane receptors, in addition to testosterone's intracellular effects.

Finally, testosterone inhibits GnRH and gonadotropin secretion via negative feedback.

- Thus, testosterone limits its own production and action.
- Inhibin, a transforming growth factor-β glycoprotein hormone from the Sertoli cells, also inhibits the pituitary and hypothalamus.

Box 36.1 summarizes the actions of testosterone.

The Expression of Male Sex Characteristics

The male reproductive system begins to function during embryonic life. As soon as the testes are able to testosterone, the androgen begins to act on the body tissues.

- In the fetus, testosterone differentiates the fetus into a male with the appropriate primary sex characteristics; the male genitals.
- At puberty, testosterone causes sustained expression of the secondary sex characteristics, which are gender-based phenotypes other than the genitals, such as hair growth, muscle development, and a low voice.

BOX 36.1 Testosterone Actions

Causes and sustains expression of the male sex characteristics:
Embryologic development of male genitals and ducts
Growth of penis, testes, and prostate at puberty
Growth of hair, larynx
Promotion of positive nitrogen balance in muscles, bones, and skin (promotion of increased protein anabolism, requiring retention of more nitrogen-containing amino acids)
Increased libido and aggression
Causes spermatogenesis
Inhibits the hypothalamic-pituitary-testicular axis (negative feedback)

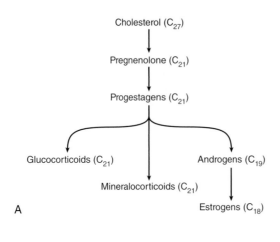

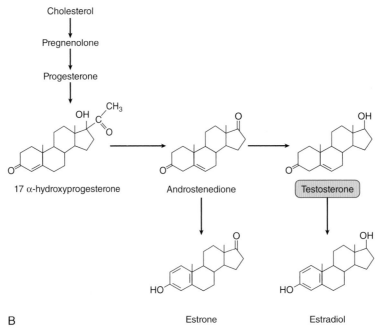

Fig. 36.4 Biosynthesis of androgens. A, The steroidal family tree. B, A closer look at testosterone and its androgen precursors.

Fetal Life and Infancy (Primary Sex Characteristics)

While the testes do act in utero, they cannot act before they have formed. Before 6 weeks of gestation, the gonads of genotypically male or female embryos have not begun to differentiate into either ovaries or testes.

- The undifferentiated gonad has an inner medullary (male) and an outer cortical (female) layer.
- In addition, the anatomic precursors of both males (the Wolffian ducts) and females (the Müllerian ducts) are present.

Only at 6 to 8 weeks of gestation is male sexual development initiated by the *SRY* gene, a gene on the short arm of the Y chromosome.

- *SRY* encodes a zinc finger DNA-binding protein called testis determining factor (TDF).
- Under the influence of TDF, the medullae of the indifferent gonads develop while the cortices regress.
- The previously indifferent gonads differentiate into testes:
  - Embryonic germ cells form spermatogonia.

- Coelomic epithelial cells form Sertoli cells.
- Mesenchymal stromal cells form Leydig cells.

Once formed, the Sertoli cells secrete a Müllerian-inhibiting factor, which causes regression of the Müllerian ducts. Meanwhile, human chorionic gonadotropin produced by the placenta—which is structurally related to LH—stimulates the Leydig cells to proliferate and secrete testosterone. Testosterone is reduced to DHT in target tissues by 5α-reductase, which leads to the formation of male genitalia (Fig. 36.5).

- The Wolffian ducts differentiate into the epididymis, vas deferens, and seminal vesicles.
- The genital tubercle transforms into the glans penis, the urethral folds grow into the penile shaft, and the urogenital sinus becomes the prostate gland.
- The genital swellings to fuse, forming the scrotum.

At its peak, the fetal testosterone level reaches 400 ng/dL, but by birth it falls below 50 ng/dL. The testosterone level remains low throughout childhood, until puberty.

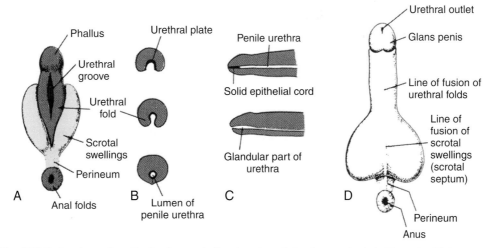

Fig. 36.5 Embryology of penile development. A) external genitalia at approximately 10 weeks, B) transverse sections through the phallus during penile urethra formation, C) development of the glandular urethra, D) normal newborn anatomy. (From Wan J, Rew K. Common penile problems. *Primary Care.* 2010;37(3):627-642, Fig. 1.)

Puberty and Beyond (Secondary Sex Characteristics)

Puberty is the process by which males and females achieve reproductive capacity, and it begins in both sexes with an increase in hypothalamic GnRH secretion. Gradual maturation of hypothalamic neurons probably plays a role in this pubertal change in GnRH secretion.

- As the child approaches adolescence, the hypothalamus gradually escapes feedback inhibition and GnRH secretion rises.
- LH and FSH secretion in turn rise.
- Testosterone secretion from the testes increases..

Increased testicular production of testosterone and other androgens at puberty has a host of effects.

- The penis, testes, and prostate gland all enlarge. From the beginning to the end of puberty, the testicular volume more than quadruples.
- Spermatogenesis commences.

Growth occurs in many tissues outside the reproductive system as well. This is because androgens are anabolic steroids; they promote the storage of energy in complex molecules. Increased protein synthesis is associated with increased:

- Skeletal muscle mass
- Bone density
- Skin thickness
- Hair (pubic, axillary, facial, chest, arms, and legs)
- Larynx (which lengthens the vocal folds, causing deepening of the voice and protrusion of the thyroid cartilage, or Adam's apple) (see Fast Fact Box 36.5)

Fast Fact Box 36.5

Muscle does not contain 5α-reductase, so it appears that testosterone, not dihydrotestosterone (DHT), promotes muscular protein anabolism. However, testosterone or DHT may promote muscular anabolism via extramuscular effects, such as the stimulation of growth hormone and insulin-like growth factor (IGF-1) production.

Collectively, the development of the secondary sex characteristics is called virilization (after the Latin vir for man). It appears that although testosterone promotes all of these effects—genital growth and spermatogenesis, hair growth, behavioral changes, and anabolism in peripheral tissues—certain androgen precursors, metabolic byproducts, and pharmaceutical androgen analogs preferentially effect peripheral anabolism. As a result, many of these metabolites and drugs are abused by bodybuilders and athletes (see Clinical Correlation Box 36.2 and Box 36.3).

Clinical Correlation Box 36.2

The Use and Abuse of Anabolic Steroids

Some athletes at amateur and professional levels use regimens of anabolic steroids as a strength and muscle-building strategy despite the fact that such a practice is illegal. The risks of anabolic steroid use include:

- Suppression of the hypothalamic-pituitary-testicular axis by negative feedback on the hypothalamus and pituitary, leading to decreased Follicle-stimulating hormone (FSH) and luteinizing hormone (LH) and testosterone levels. This leads to gonadal atrophy and impaired spermatogenesis.
- Increased peripheral metabolism of those androgens to estrogens, with feminizing effects such as gynecomastia (breast development in males).
- High cholesterol, high blood pressure, abnormal blood clotting, and other hematologic and cardiovascular risks.
- Irreversible virilization in women.

The effectiveness of anabolic steroids in building muscle has been controversial. However, recent literature has begun to support the notion that anabolic steroids do increase muscle mass in athletes. Older studies generally failed to reproduce the context, duration, and dosage used by competitive athletes. Anabolic steroids are obtained illegally via the black market. However, "dietary supplements" provide a legal way to obtain some varieties of anabolic steroids. The baseball player Mark McGwire is known to have used an androstenedione-containing dietary supplement during his record-breaking season. Although the effects of the supplement on athletic performance are a subject of controversy, data suggest that androstenedione does indeed have harmful cardiovascular effects.

Once testosterone levels rise during puberty, they reach a plateau and remain elevated until a man reaches his seventies, when they begin to decline. This event, called the male *climacteric*, may create some symptoms resembling those of female menopause. However, although testosterone does promote spermatogenesis, this testicular function is remarkably well preserved in men even after the climacteric.

The Haploid Life Cycle in the Male

As mentioned earlier, spermatogenesis begins with puberty and continues into the eighth decade of life. Spermatogenesis has three phases (Fig. 36.6):

- Spermatocytogenesis, during which the primordial spermatogonia divide by mitosis and differentiate into spermatocyt.
- Meiosis, resulting in four haploid gametes called spermatids, each with a quarter of the cytoplasm of the original spermatogonium.

- Spermiogenesis, during which the spermatids are nourished and physically reshaped by the surrounding Sertoli cells. The product of spermiogenesis is spermatozoa, or sperm.

The evolving group of cells spanning from spermatogonia to spermatozoa is sometimes called the spermatogenic series. After spermiogenesis, the epididymis and reproductive tract glands help prepare the sperm for fertilization.

Spermatocytogenesis and Meiosis

Not all spermatogonia enter into the spermatogenic series. If they did, they would be consumed—as happens to the oogonia in the ovary, eventually leading to menopause. Instead, the testis continually replenishes its own supply of spermatogonia. As they undergo mitosis, some of the new ones are committed to the spermatogenic series, while some remain undifferentiated.

- Undifferentiated stem cells are called type A spermatogonia.
  - These remain on the outside of the blood-testis barrier.
- Differentiated spermatogonia committed to becoming spermatocytes are called type B spermatogonia.
  - These cross the blood-testis barrier and become enveloped by the cytoplasmic processes of Sertoli cells.

Type B spermatogonia differentiate further and enlarge to become primary spermatocytes, which subsequently enter meiosis.

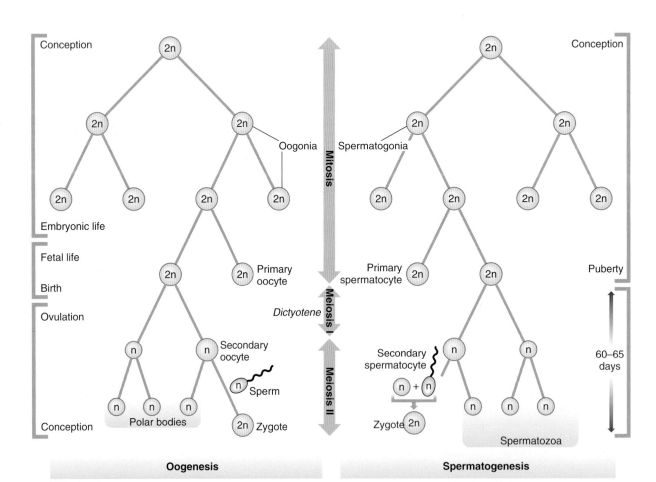

Fig. 36.6 Spermatogenesis and oogenesis compared. (From Chromosomes and cell division. In: *Turnpenny: Emery's Elements of Medical Genetics*. Elsevier; 2017: p. 24-41. Fig. 3.14.)

- This process takes around 3.5 weeks to complete, almost all of which is spent in prophase (when the newly replicated chromosomes condense).
- Each primary spermatocyte divides into two secondary spermatocytes.
- These in turn divide again into a total of four haploid spermatids.
    - Each spermatid contains either an X chromosome or a Y chromosome.
    - The male's gamete thus decides the sex of his offspring.

Spermiogenesis

Spermiogenesis begins once the spermatids are created and delivered into the embrace of the amoeboid Sertoli cells (Fig. 36.7). The spermatid then elongates and reorganizes its nuclear and cytoplasmic contents into a *spermatozoon* with a distinct head and tail. The structure of sperm cells enables them to swim up the female reproductive tract and fertilize oocytes.

- The head consists of a condensed nucleus surrounded by a thin layer of cytoplasm.
- The rest of the retained cytoplasm and cell membrane is shifted toward the opposite end of the sperm, the tail.
    - The tail also develops a flagellum for motility, which originates from one of the centrioles of the sperm cells. Consists of a central skeleton of microtubules called the axoneme.
    The axoneme is arranged in a 9 + 2 pattern (9 pairs of microtubules surrounding 2 central tubules) linked via a complex array of protein bridges.
    The sperm cell's mitochondria aggregate along the proximal end of the flagellum and supply energy for movement to the flagellum.

The anterior two-thirds of the head of the sperm cell is surrounded by a thick capsule known as the acrosome, formed from the Golgi apparatus.

- The Golgi apparatus contains numerous hydrolytic and proteolytic enzymes, similar to those found in lysosomes, and ultimately facilitates the sperm's penetration of the egg for fertilization as well as the mucus of the female cervix (see Oncology Box 36.1 and Pharmacology Box 36.1).

✳ ONCOLOGY BOX 36.1

Testicular germ cell tumors (GCTs) are the most common types of testicular cancers. Approximately 50% are pure seminoma while the other half are termed nonseminomatous germ cell tumors (NSGCTs). Patients often present with a testicular mass or testicular enlargement, but sometimes patients manifest symptoms attributed to metastatic disease, such as a cough from pulmonary involvement; nausea, vomiting, or bleeding from gastrointestinal involvement; or enlarged lymph nodes. In addition to symptoms, the diagnosis can be made with data from imaging studies, such as scrotal ultrasound and with the values of three biomarkers obtained from the blood: α fetoprotein, β human chorionic gonadotropin, and lactate dehydrogenase.

⬡ PHARMACOLOGY BOX 36.1

For many states of both seminoma and nonseminomatous germ cell tumors, orchiectomy is the primary treatment. Some patients benefit from radiotherapy. For those who require chemotherapy, cisplatin-based therapy. Cisplatin covalently binds to deoxyribonucleic acid (DNA), cross-linking it, denaturing the normal double helix structure, and thereby interfering with DNA function and replication.

Epididymal Sperm Maturation and Storage

After spermiogenesis is complete, the sperm pass out of the testis (through the rete testis) and into the epididymis, where growth and differentiation continue. The 120 million sperm produced each day in the seminiferous tubules are stored in the epididymis, as well as in the vas deferens and ampulla.

- After the first 24 hours in the epididymis, the sperm acquire the potential for motility.
- However, the epithelial cells of the epididymis secrete inhibitory proteins that suppress this potential.
- The sperm can thus remain in the excretory genital ducts in a deeply suppressed and inactive state for over a month without losing their potential for fertilization.

The epididymis also secretes a special nutrient fluid that is ultimately ejaculated with the sperm and is thought to mature the sperm.

- This fluid contains hormones, enzymes (such as glycosyltransferases and glycosidases), and nutrients that are essential to achieving fertilization and may aid in protecting the sperm against mutations.

Potentiation in the Ejaculate

The accessory genital glands—the seminal vesicles, prostate gland, and bulbourethral glands—also contribute to potentiation.

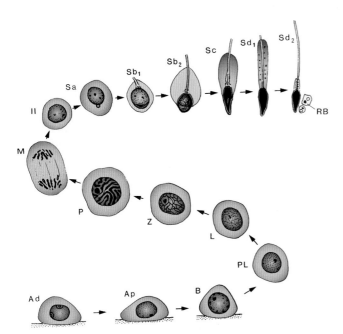

Fig. 36.7 Spermiogenesis (de Krester DM, Loveland K, O'Bryan M. Spermatogenesis. In: *Endocrinology: Adult and Pediatric.* Elsevier; 2016: p. 2325-2353.e9. Fig. 136.9.)

During ejaculation, their secretions dilute the epididymal inhibitory proteins, allowing the sperm's motile potential to be realized.

In addition, the glands make individual contributions to sperm preparation and support.

- The seminal vesicles secrete semen, a mucoid yellowish material containing nutrients and sperm-activating substances, such as fructose, citrate, inositol, prostaglandins, and fibrinogen.
  - Carbohydrates, such as fructose, provide a source of energy for the sperm mitochondria because they power the sperm's flagellar movements.
  - The prostaglandins are believed to aid the sperm by affecting the female genital tract—making the cervical mucus more receptive to the sperm, and dampening the peristaltic contractions of the uterus and fallopian tubes to prevent them from expelling the sperm.
- The prostate gland secretes a thin, milky, and alkaline fluid during ejaculation that mixes with the contents of the vas deferens.
  - This secretion contains calcium, zinc, and phosphate ions, citrate, acid phosphatase, and various clotting enzymes.
  - The clotting enzymes react with the fibrinogen of the seminal fluid, forming a weak coagulum that glues the semen inside the vagina and facilitates the passage of sperm through the cervix in larger numbers.
  - The alkalinity counteracts vaginal acidity, which is a natural defense against microbial pathogens that can also kill sperm or impair sperm motility.

Capacitation in the Female Reproductive Tract

Ejaculated sperm is not immediately capable of fertilizing the female oocyte. In the first few hours after ejaculation, the spermatozoa must undergo capacitation inside the female reproductive tract.

- First, the fluids of the female reproductive tract wash away more of the inhibitory factors of the male genital fluid.
  - This allows the flagella of the sperm to produce the whiplash motion that is needed for the sperm to swim to the oocyte in the fallopian tube.
- Second, the cell membrane of the head of the sperm is modified in preparation for the ultimate acrosomal reaction and penetration of the oocyte.

Fertilization

Once capacitated, the spermatozoa travel to the oocyte.

- There is an enormous rate of attrition among the hundreds of millions of ejaculated sperm; at most a few hundred reach the oocyte.

When the few hundred sperm reach the egg, they begin to try to penetrate the granulosa cells surrounding the secondary oocyte.

- The sperm's acrosome contains hyaluronidase and proteolytic enzymes, which open this path.

- As the anterior membrane of the acrosome reaches the zona pellucida (the glycoprotein coat surrounding the oocyte), it rapidly dissolves and releases the acrosomal enzymes.
- Within minutes, these enzymes open a pathway through the zona pellucida for the sperm cytoplasm to merge with the oocyte cytoplasm.
- From beginning to end, the process of fertilization takes about half an hour.

Penile Erection and Ejaculation

The penis allows the male to deliver semen directly to the internal female genital tract. There are two physiologic events crucial to this internal delivery of semen:

- Penile erection, which makes it possible for the penis to penetrate the vagina, bringing the urethral opening, or meatus, into close contact with the female cervix;.
- Penile ejaculation, in which the semen is secreted into the male reproductive ductal system, mixed with sperm, and then mechanically squirted out of the penis. Both of these events are initiated and controlled by the nervous system in connection with the subjective state of sexual arousal.

Sexual Response in the Male

William H. Masters and Virginia E. Johnson in 1966 described four phases of sexual response in males and females (Fig. 36.8):

- Excitement
- Plateau
- Orgasm
- Resolution

Desire or libido precedes excitement. Excitement that leads to erection derives from a combination of psychologic factors and genital stimulation.

- Erotic feelings can initiate an erection without physical stimulation, and physical stimulation can initiate erection in the absence of psychologic stimuli.
- The pudendal nerve transmits sensory information from the penis to the spinal cord and brain.

Erection

As excitement builds in the CNS, efferent parasympathetic fibers in the pelvic nerve discharge increasing numbers of impulses through the pelvic plexus to the smooth muscle of the penile cavernous artery, which runs down the center of each of the corpora cavernosa.

- This leads to the secretion of nitric oxide (NO, directly from the parasympathetic nerve terminals and also from the endothelial cells in the arterial vasculature).
- NO diffuses into the smooth muscle in the wall of the cavernous artery and relaxes it.
- NO-mediated arterial dilation leads to up to a 60-fold increase in penile blood flow, leading to swelling of the penis with blood.

When the spongy tissues are stretched to their full extent, intracavernous pressure then begins to rise.

- The penis becomes rigid and elevates.
- The increasing pressure eventually compresses the cavernous veins and reduces venous outflow, leading to a further increase in intracavernous pressure.

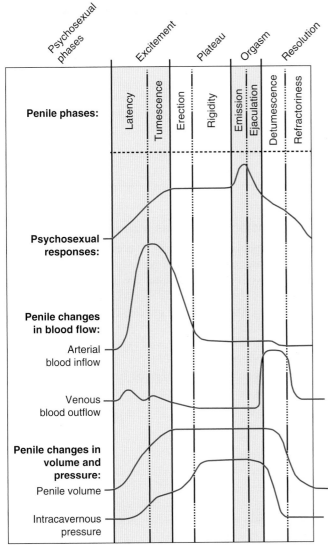

Fig. 36.8 Sexual response and changes in the penis.

Ejaculation

As sexual excitement continues to build, bulbourethral and urethral secretions lubricate the urethra. Of note, these secretions may contain small amounts of sperm that can lead to fertilization.

As genital stimulation excites the pudendal nerve more and more, a subjective sensation of orgasm ensues, followed immediately by the ejaculatory spinal cord reflex.

- At orgasm, the CNS likely releases the spinal reflex from its inhibition.
- Once the reflex is initiated, sympathetic nerves stimulate the closure of the bladder neck and contraction of the ampulla of the vas deferens, the seminal vesicles, and the prostate.
- The contractions cause the seminal vesicles and prostate to secrete their contents into the ejaculatory duct just as the sperm are propelled from the ampulla into the ejaculatory duct.
- This first stage of ejaculation is called emission.

Emission is directly followed by the rhythmic contraction of muscles surrounding the urethra: the bulbospongiosus muscle

that surrounds the corpus spongiosum, the urethral smooth muscle, and other pelvic floor muscles.

- These contractions expel the semen from the posterior urethra and out the penile meatus in spurts (see Fast Fact Box 36.6).

Fast Fact Box 36.6

The total ejaculate contains about 400 million sperm in about 3 to 4 mL of secretions. The normal sperm concentration ranges anywhere from 35 million to 200 million sperm per milliliter of fluid.

Resolution

If the sperm have been delivered into an ovulatory female reproductive tract, they now begin their journey toward the egg. Meanwhile, the resolution phase occurs a few minutes after ejaculation with detumescence (drainage of blood from the penis) and a refractory period of varying lengths, in which erection and ejaculation cannot be repeated.

- The cavernous arteries constrict, preventing arterial inflow, and venous outflow lowers the intracavernous pressure.
- As the pressure falls, the veins decompress and venous outflow increases further.
- This shift from net inflow to net outflow rapidly returns the penis to its flaccid state.

PATHOPHYSIOLOGY

Common problems associated with the male reproductive tract include:
- Erectile dysfunction (ED)
- Infertility
- Benign and malignant growth of the prostate
- Increased cardiovascular risk

Erectile Dysfunction

Some 10 to 20 million men suffer from ED, also known as impotence. Causes include:
- Vascular insufficiency
  - Atherosclerosis
  - Diabetes mellitus
  - Antihypertensive medication
- Psychologic factors (see Clinical Correlation Box 36.4).

Clinical Correlation Box 36.4

Treating Erectile Dysfunction

The popular drug Viagra (generic name, sildenafil citrate), introduced in 1998, is used to treat erectile dysfunction (ED). An internet search on the name at the time this chapter was written produced 17.4 million hits—an indication of the number of men seeking help for ED.

Viagra works by inhibiting the action of cyclic guanosine monophosphate (cGMP)-specific phosphodiesterase type 5 (PDE5). PDE5 is specific to the penis. When this enzyme is inhibited, the cGMP levels in smooth muscle rise, mimicking the effect of nitric oxide on the smooth muscle of the penile cavernous arteries. The smooth muscle relaxes, and penile blood flow increases. Cross-reactivity with other PDEs can cause vasodilation elsewhere in the body, however, leading to hypotension (low blood pressure).

Male Infertility

An estimated 10% to 15% of couples cannot conceive after 1 year of trying; they are considered to have infertility.

- In 20% of infertile couples, the cause is never discovered.
- In the remaining 80%, around half of the cases of infertility are because of a problem in the male reproductive system. Causes of male infertility include:
- Cryptorchidism results in sterility, as the spermatogonia cannot survive at the increased temperatures of the body cavity.
- Other abnormalities of the testes and genital tract may also impair fertility, including:
  - Environmental exposures (i.e., chemical, radiation)
  - Heat (because of tight underwear, fever, etc.)
  - Sexually transmitted infections
  - Mumps orchitis (can permanently destroy the seminiferous tubular epithelium)
  - Trauma
  - Varicoceles
  - Previous urogenital surgery (see Clinical Correlation Box 36.5)

Clinical Correlation Box 36.5

A varicocele is a dilation of the pampiniform plexus, the plexus of veins carrying deoxygenated blood from the testis along the spermatic cord. This plexus is vulnerable to valvular defects, leading to venous pooling and painful venous enlargement around the scrotum. This impairs cooling and can lead to male infertility.

The workup for male infertility includes a semen analysis, which assesses ejaculate volume, sperm count, sperm morphology and motility, semen pH, and white blood cell count.

- Sperm counts of less than 20 million sperm per milliliter render a male infertile.
- Abnormal morphology of the sperm, including multiple heads or tails and abnormally shaped heads or tails, will impair fertility.
- Abnormal functioning of the sperm heads (acrosomes) or tails (flagella), despite seemingly normal morphology, can also impair fertility.

A postcoital test may also be performed to evaluate the interaction between the sperm in the semen and the female cervical mucus.

- The inability of the sperm to penetrate the cervical mucosa may suggest an abnormality of the fluid contents of the semen or an abnormality of the acrosomal head of the sperm itself.

Analysis of serum FSH, testosterone, and TSH levels may also be helpful in diagnosing testicular disease.

- If the testes are damaged and fail to make sufficient testosterone, the serum testosterone level will be low and the FSH level will be high, resulting from hypothalamic disinhibition because of lack of negative feedback from testosterone.
- TSH levels aid in diagnosis because abnormal thyroid function interferes with spermatogenesis (see Clinical Correlation Box 36.6).

Clinical Correlation Box 36.6

As men age, testosterone levels gradually decrease. In certain cases, levels of testosterone drop to levels that manifest in very noticeable ways, including low libido or energy and depression. As a result, patients may elect to receive testosterone replacement therapy, in which exogenous testosterone is administered.

- Supplementation of testosterone has clinically significant effects, such as boosting mood, libido, and energy, and can in some cases be used to treat erectile dysfunction.
- Testosterone replacement therapy can be administered in a variety of ways, including via a gel that is absorbed through the skin, or via intramuscular injections.

Benign Prostatic Hyperplasia and Prostate Cancer

The development and growth of the prostate gland are stimulated by testosterone. This mitogenic (proliferative) effect on the prostate continues throughout life, often resulting in the development of benign prostatic hyperplasia (BPH).

- As many as 20% of men are affected by BPH before the age of 40 years.
- About 70% of men at age 60 years and 90% of men in their 70s show evidence of some BPH.

The main symptoms of BPH result from the enlarged prostate impinging on or obstructing the urethra, and include:
- Urinary frequency
- Urinary urgency
- Nocturia (waking at night to urinate)
- Urinary retention
- Urinary obstruction, which may predispose to urinary tract infections

Prostate cancer is by far the most common cancer in men and the second most frequent cause of male cancer deaths. Its incidence increases with age, and it often has an insidious onset. Therefore the cancer is frequently metastatic by the time of presentation.

- The medical community encourages screening by digital rectal exam (DRE) or the prostate-specific antigen (PSA) test for men above a certain age.
- Questionable results from a rectal examination are usually followed with transrectal ultrasound and/or an ultrasound-guided transrectal biopsy.

Testosterone is a growth stimulant for prostate cancer, just as it is for BPH. Certain therapies, especially those used in cases of known metastases, therefore aim at inhibiting testosterone production or preventing testosterone from stimulating the prostatic tissue, thereby slowing the growth and spread of the cancer. Men with both BPH and prostate cancer are candidates for transurethral prostate resection.

Heart Disease

Male gender is a risk factor for atherosclerosis. In 1999 in the United States, 49% more men than women died of heart disease. Many of the phenotypic differences between men and women may account for this statistic.

- Testosterone may increase the plasma level of low-density lipoproteins (LDL, or "bad" cholesterol) and decreases the level of high-density lipoproteins (HDL, or "good" cholesterol).

- High LDL levels and low HDL levels are both cardiac risk factors.

SUMMARY

- There are three principal functions of the male reproductive system:
  - The expression of male sex characteristics
  - Spermatogenesis (the creation of sperm)
  - The delivery of sperm into the female for procreation
- Male reproduction is coordinated by the hypothalamic-pituitary-testicular (HPT) axis, which is characterized by classic negative feedback. The hypothalamus secretes GnRH, which releases FSH and LH from the pituitary.
- FSH acts on the Sertoli cells in the seminiferous tubules of the testis and stimulates spermatogenesis.
- LH acts on the Leydig cells in the testicular parenchyma and stimulates secretion of the androgen steroid, testosterone. Testosterone inhibits GnRH and FSH/LH release.
- Testosterone is converted to its active form, dihydrotestosterone (DHT), at its sites of action.
- Testosterone causes development of the male genital system in utero and at puberty. It causes growth of the genitals; hair growth; the start of spermatogenesis; deepening of the voice; protein anabolism in muscle, bone, and skin; and increased libido and aggression.

- Spermatogenesis takes place in the seminiferous tubules of the testis and has three phases:
  - Spermatocytogenesis (mitosis and differentiation of some spermatogonia into spermatocytes)
  - Meiosis (resulting in four haploid spermatids)
  - Spermiogenesis (the production of spermatozoa from spermatids)
- Sperm was stored in the epididymis and vas deferens until ejaculation.
- The four phases of sexual arousal are excitement, plateau, orgasm, and resolution.
- If sperm are deposited into the vagina, they are capacitated, or rendered more motile and ready to fertilize, by the female reproductive tract. The acrosome, the head of the sperm cell, releases enzymes that digest a path into the oocyte, and fertilization occurs.
- Common problems associated with the male reproductive tract include erectile dysfunction, infertility, and benign and malignant growth of the prostate gland. Male gender is an independent cardiac risk factor.

REVIEW QUESTIONS

Directions: Each of the numbered items or incomplete statements in this section is followed by answers or by completions of the statement. Select the one lettered answer or completion that is best in each case.

1. The hypogastric nerve supplies sympathetic tone to the bladder and genitals. Its most important role in male reproductive function is probably that of stimulating:
   A. Spermatogenesis
   B. Testosterone production
   C. Urethral lubrication
   D. Erection
   E. Detumescence
   F. Capacitation of sperm
   G. Spermiogenesis
   H. Ejaculation

2. A 35-year-old man who is an avid bodybuilder complains of having developed what look like female breasts. A history reveals several years of drug abuse with a form of testoster-

one. Physical examination reveals acne, gynecomastia, and small testes. The mechanism behind his gynecomastia is:
   A. Negative feedback on the hypothalamus
   B. Suppression of gonadal function
   C. Positive nitrogen balance
   D. Increased testosterone metabolism
   E. Increased testosterone action

3. A 31-year-old man undergoes semen analysis after 1 year of trying unsuccessfully to impregnate his wife. If some of his sperm have abnormal flagella, this most likely reflects an error during which phase of sperm development?
   A. Spermatocytogenesis
   B. Epididymal maturation
   C. Mixing with seminal and prostatic fluid in the posterior urethra
   D. Spermiogenesis
   E. Meiosis

ANSWERS TO REVIEW QUESTIONS

1. **The answer is H.** Ejaculation is mediated by sympathetic impulses from the spinal cord. Remember "point and shoot": "p" for parasympathetic mediation of erection and "s" for sympathetic mediation of ejaculation. The pudendal nerve carries afferent information to the central nervous system, and the pelvic nerve carries efferent parasympathetic impulses.

2. **The answer is D.** The drug has increased the testosterone level, thereby increasing the peripheral metabolism of testosterone to estrogen, which has proliferative effects on the breast tissue of males and females. Although increased testosterone action at the androgen receptor, hypothalamic inhibition, and gonadal suppression all occur in this context, they do not cause gynecomastia.

3. **The answer is D.** Spermatids acquire their tails and become spermatozoa at the spermiogenesis phase of spermatogenesis. Thus it is here that abnormalities in tail morphology are likely to arise. Abnormalities at other stages of sperm development are more likely to lower the sperm count or reduce sperm motility or penetrative ability.

Endocrine Physiology

PRESENTATION: HISTORY AND PHYSICAL EXAMINATION

J.B is a 38 year old woman who presents to her primary care physician with a chief complaint of fatigue and weight gain. She was in her normal state of health until about 6 months ago. Since that time, she has been getting tired more easily and has lost over 12 pounds despite no significant change in her workout regime. In fact, she notes that her appetite has actually increased. Additionally, she reports diarrhea occurring 1 to 2 times per week. She has also found more hair than usual in her hairbrush. She diligently takes her medications as prescribed, exercises 3 times per week, and attempts to eat healthy. She does admit to occasional alcohol intake during the weekends.

On physical examination, J.B. appears anxious and has difficulty remaining still on the examination table. Her vital signs are notable for a blood pressure of 165/76 mm Hg, heart rate of 111 beats per minute, temperature 37.6° C, and a respiratory rate of 14 breaths per minute. When asked to extend her arms, she has a noticeable fine tremor of the extremities. On HEENT (head, eyes, ears nose, throat) examination, she has a slight bulging of her eyes, and her thyroid gland is enlarged and smooth. Her skin feels warm and moist. Her neurologic examination is notable for brisk reflexes. She is alert and oriented.

DISCUSSION

The review of systems and physical examination has revealed that J.B likely is suffering from hyperthyroidism.

The leading cause of hyperthyroidism is Graves disease, a condition that more commonly affects young woman. Graves disease is caused by a type of immunoglobulin (Ig)G known as thyroid-stimulating antibodies (TSAb). These antibodies bind to the thyroid stimulating hormone (TSH) receptor on the follicular cells of the thyroid. This stimulates the thyroid to generate significant amounts of thyroid hormone (T_3 and T_4) while the negative feedback loop of the hypothalamus-pituitary-thyroid axis is inhibited.

Hyperthyroidism can also be caused by a toxic adenoma or by multiple hyperfunctioning nodules. Thyrotoxicosis factitia is seen with ingestion of excessive thyroid hormone, and struma ovarii is seen when an ovarian teratoma has hyperactive thyroid tissue. However, these causes of hyperthyroidism are more rare.

A normally functioning thyroid gland has two hormone-producing cell types. As discussed in Chapter 30, the follicular cells are responsible for producing, storing and releasing triiodo-thyronine (T_3) and thyroxine (T_4), whereas the parafollicular cells secrete calcitonin. T_4 is the major circulating form within the body, however T_3 is the active form of thyroid hormone inside cells. When increased levels of T_3 and T_4 are secreted, multiple effects are seen throughout the body. Many of these can be identified with a thorough review of systems and physical exam, even in the absence of a laboratory evaluation (Box 36.1.1).

PRESENTATION: LABORATORY TESTS

Initial laboratory tests for hyperthyroidism should include a basic metabolic profile, a complete blood cell count, a thyroid-stimulating hormone level and T_3/T_4 Levels (Box 36.1.2 and Table 36.1.1).

J.B. is sent to the laboratory for a blood draw.

Basic metabolic panel: Na 141 mmol/L, K 4.2 mmol/L, Cl 101 mmol/L, CO2 24 mmol/L, blood urea nitrogen (BUN) 14 mg/dL, Cr 0.9 mg/dL, Glucose 88 mg/dL

Complete blood count: White blood cell 9.4 × 10³ cells/mcL, hemoglobin 13.7 g/dL, hematocrit 40%, platelets 250 × 10³/mcL

TSH: 0.4 µU/mL

Total triiodothyronine (T_3): 320 ng/dL

Total thyroxine (T_4): 20 mcg/dL

TSH-R antibodies: Positive

DISCUSSION

This laboratory evaluation helps us determine whether the hyperthyroidism is pituitary-dependent or not. TSH levels will be decreased if the thyroid is malfunctioning and secreting increased thyroid hormone, but TSH will be elevated if the pituitary is responsible for driving the thyroid to produce excess hormone. Additionally, it is helpful to review the levels of T_3 and T_4. If TSH levels are decreased while thyroid hormone levels are elevated, a thyroid-dependent etiology is suspected. The diagnosis of Graves disease can specifically be confirmed by looking for IgG antibodies (TSH-R antibodies).

In this case, the laboratory results confirm our suspicions. J.B. has reduced TSH with elevated thyroid hormone, suggesting a thyroid-dependent hyperthyroidism. The diagnosis is further confirmed with a positive antibody test.

TREATMENT

J.B. initially chose medical management to control her hyperthyroidism. She was prescribed propylthiouracil (PTU) to interfere with the synthesis of thyroid hormone by inhibiting *iodide* organification and iodotyrosine coupling. PTU also helps minimize peripheral conversion of T_4 to T_3. Unfortunately, she began having side effects from the medication, including headaches and dependent edema. She was seen in the office and a discussion was had about other potential options. Both radioiodine ablation of the active thyroid tissue and surgical resection were discussed. Ultimately, J.B opted for radioiodine ablation with the isotope ^{131}I, understanding that there is risk of treatment leading to hypothyroidism.

DISCUSSION

Management of Graves disease includes three possible treatment options.

Medical management revolves around slowing the production of thyroid hormone and decreasing the downstream effects of increased thyroid hormone. Propanolol or other beta-blockers can be used as needed to reduce symptoms of adrenergic excess, but does not constitute a definitive treatment as it does not treat the thyroid disease itself. Iodide can be given to temporarily inhibit the release of thyroid hormone, which occurs through a negative feedback mechanism known as the Wolff-Chaikoff effect. As we mentioned above, thionamides like PTU can be used to inhibit organification and coupling by interfering with thyroid peroxidase. For one-third of patients, this is sufficient for long-term control for their disease. Unfortunately, a significant number of patients will either have complications from the medication (as we saw with J.B.), the effects may not last long-term, or patients may have difficulty faithfully taking a daily medication.

Radioiodine ablation of active thyroid tissue is a more invasive option for management. J.B. underwent ablation with isotope ^{131}I, in which the overactive follicular cells selectively take up the radioactive isotope and are destroyed. Radioiodine ablation is highly effective, but may result in hypothyroidism requiring daily medication to replace thyroid hormone.

Surgical resection is generally regarded as a last resort, as ablation is effective and well tolerated. Complete resection of the thyroid gland is most effective, but carries an increased risk of damage to the recurrent laryngeal nerve leading to vocal cord paralysis. Partial resection of the thyroid gland has less risk of injury to the recurrent laryngeal nerve, but carries an increased risk of recurrence.

BOX 36.1.1 Signs and Symptoms of Hyperthyroidism

Fatigue	Amenorrhea	Weight loss
Tachycardia	Intolerance to heat	Muscle wasting
Fine tremor	Diarrhea	Proptosis
Restlessness	Irritability	Pretibial myxedema
Oligomenorrhea	Sweating	Leg swelling

TABLE 36.1.1 Thyroid Function Test Interpretation

		T4 Levels		
		Low	Normal	High
TSH	Low	Secondary Hypothyroidism (Pituitary Fail)		Primary Hyperthyroidism (Graves)
	Normal		Euthyroid	
	High	Primary Hypothyroidism (Hashimoto)		Secondary Hyperthyroidism

TSH, Thyroid stimulating hormone.

BOX 36.1.2 Common Thyroid Laboratory Tests

(Clinical Range)
Thyroid stimulating hormone <60 years old, <10 µU/mL
Female 2–16.8 µU/mL
>60 years old, Male 2–7.3 µU/mL, Female 2-16.8 µU/mL
Thyroxine (T4), total 5.0–12.0 mcg/dL
Thyroxine, free 0.8–2.3 ng/dL

Page numbers followed by *b* indicates boxes, *f* indicates figures and *t* indicates tables.